Target Organ Toxicology Series

Toxicology of the Liver

Second Edition

Editors

Gabriel L. Plaa, Ph.D.
Département de Pharmacologie
Faculté de Médecine
Université de Montréal
Montréal, Québec, Canada

William R. Hewitt, Ph.D.
Department of Project Management,
Research and Development
SmithKline Beecham Pharmaceuticals
Collegeville, Pennsylvania

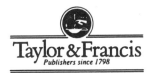

Taylor & Francis
Publishers since 1798

USA	Publishing Office	Taylor & Francis 1101 Vermont Avenue, NW, Suite 200 Washington, DC 20005-3521 Tel: (202) 289-2174 Fax: (202) 289-3665
	Distribution Center	Taylor & Francis 1900 Frost Road, Suite 101 Bristol, PA 19007-1598 Tel: (215) 785-5800 Fax: (215) 785-5515
UK		Taylor & Francis Ltd. 1 Gunpowder Square London EC4A 3DE Tel: 0171 583 0490 Fax: 0171 583 0581

TOXICOLOGY OF THE LIVER, 2/E

1 2 3 4 5 6 7 8 9 0   E B E B   9 0 9 8 7

This book was set in Times Roman. Composition and editorial services by TechBooks. Cover design by Michelle Fleitz.

A CIP catalog record for this book is available from the British Library.
∞ The paper in this publication meets the requirements of the ANSI Standard Z39.48-1984 (Permanence of Paper).

Library of Congress Cataloging-in-Publication Data

Toxicology of the liver / edited by Gabriel L. Plaa and William R.
    Hewitt – 2nd ed.
        p.   cm.
    Includes bibliographical references and index.
    ISBN 1-56032-719-7 (case : alk. paper)
    1. Hepatotoxicology.   I. Plaa, Gabriel L.   II. Hewitt, William R.
    [DNLM: 1. Liver – drug affects.   2. Poisoning.   WI 700 T766 1998]
    RC848.H48T89   1998
    616.3'8207 – dc21
    DNLM/DLC
    For Library of Congress   97-22577
                                                                      CIP

ISBN 1-56032-719-7 (case)

Toxicology of the Liver

Second Edition

Target Organ Toxicology Series

Series Editors
A. Wallace Hayes, John A. Thomas, and Donald E. Gardner

Contents

Part III: Cholestasis

Contributing Authors

Claude Barriault, Ph.D. *Département de Nutrition, Université de Montréal, Montréal, Québec, Canada H3C 3J7*

Guylaine Bouchard, M.Sc. *Département de Pharmacologie, Université de Montréal, Montréal, Québec, Canada H3C 3J7*

Kim L. R. Brouwer, Pharm.D., Ph.D. *School of Pharmacy, University of North Carolina, Chapel Hill, NC 27599-7360*

Steven D. Cohen, D.Sc. *Department of Pharmaceutical Sciences, School of Pharmacy, University of Connecticut, Storrs, CT 06269-2092*

Mario Comporti, Prof. *Istituto di Patologia Generale, Universita di Siena, 1-53100 Siena, Italy*

Andréa Monte Alto Costa, Ph.D. *CNRS-UPR 412, Institut de Biologie et Chimie des Protéines, Lyon, France, and Department de Histologia e Embriolgia, Universidade do Estado do Rio de Janeiro, Rio de Janeiro, Brazil*

Alexis Desmoulière, Ph.D. *CNRS-UPR 412, Institut de Biologie et Chimie des Protéines, Lyon, France*

Alexandra B. Duguay, Ph.D. *Département de Pharmacologie, Université de Montréal, Montréal, Québec, Canada H3C 3J7*

Patrick I. Eacho, Ph.D. *Lilly Research Laboratories, Eli Lilly and Company, Lilly Corporate Center, Indianapolis, IN 46285*

Sylvia M. Furst, Ph.D. *Boehringer Ingelheim Pharmaceuticals, Ridgefield, CN 06840*

A. Jay Gandolfi, Ph.D. *Department of Anesthesiology, College of Medicine, University of Arizona, Tuscon, AZ 85724*

Carol R. Gardner, Ph.D. *Toxicology Division, Environmental and Occupational Health Sciences Institute, Rutgers University and UMDNJ-Robert Wood Johnson Medical School, Piscataway, NJ 08855-1179*

William R. Hewitt, Ph.D. *Department of Project Management, Research and Development, SmithKline Beecham Pharmaceuticals, Collegeville, PA 19424-0989*

Debie J. Hoivik, Ph.D. *College of Veterinary Medicine, Texas A&M University, College Station, TX 77843*

Edward A. Khairallah, Ph.D.
(Deceased)

Lena M. King, *Parke Davis Research Institute, Mississauga, Ontario, Canada L5K 1B4*

James E. Klaunig, Ph.D. *Division of Toxicology, Department of Pharmacology and Toxicology, Indiana University School of Medicine, Indianapolis, IN 46202-5196*

Kyle L. Kolaja, Ph.D. *Division of Toxicology, Department of Pharmacology and Toxicology, Indiana University School of Medicine, Indianapolis, IN 46202-5196*

Debra L. Laskin, Ph.D. *Environmental and Occupational Health Sciences Institute, Rutgers University and UMDNJ-Robert Wood Johnson Medical School, Piscataway, NJ 08855-1179*

Jeffrey W. Lawrence, Ph.D. *Department of Biochemical Toxicology, Merck Research Laboratories, Merck and Company, Inc., West Point, PA 19486*

James W. Newberne, DVM, Ph.D. *University of Cincinnati College of Medicine, Cincinnati, OH 45267-0056*

Paul M. Newberne, DVM, Ph.D. *Division of Nutritional Pathology, Massachusetts Institute of Technology, Cambridge, MA 02139 and Department of Pathology, Boston University School of Medicine, Boston, MA 02118*

Gabriel L. Plaa, Ph.D. *Département de Pharmacologie, Université de Montréal, Montréal, Québec, Canada H3C 3J7*

Donald J. Reed, Ph.D. *Department of Biochemistry and Biophysics, Oregon State University, Corvallis, OR 97331*

Beatriz Tuchweber, Ph.D. *Département de Nutrition, Université de Montréal, Montréal, Québec, Canada H3C 3J7*

Mary Vore, Ph.D. *Graduate Center for Toxicology, University of Kentucky, Lexington, KY 40536-0305*

Ibrahim M. Yousef, Ph.D. *Département de Pharmacologie et Département de Nutrition, Faculté de Médecine, Université de Montréal, Montréal, Québec, Canada H3C 3J7*

Hyman J. Zimmerman, M.D. *George Washington University and Armed Forces Institute of Pathology, Washington, D.C. 20306-6000*

Preface

The growth in information and insight into the mechanisms, expressions, and consequences or outcomes of chemical-induced hepatotoxicity, since the publication of the first edition of this book, has been stimulating, daunting, and ultimately exhilarating. In the preface to the first edition, we indicated the intent to attempt to present the state of the art in chemical-induced liver injury, an understandable if somewhat naive goal. The intent of this second edition is to present state of the art reviews by recognized experts in selected areas of hepatotoxicity.

We freely admit to selection bias. Given the diversity of chemical classes involved, modes of exposure (e.g., occupational, medicinal, environmental, recreational), mechanisms of action, and manifestations of the liver to toxic insult, selectivity is required to keep the book to a single volume. The diversity of the approaches utilized to characterize how chemicals produce liver injury continues to expand. The physiologic, biochemical, and morphologic characteristics of hepatotoxicity all have been pursued, and new techniques in molecular biology and immunochemistry, among others, are contributing to the growth in understanding of the toxic events involved. In keeping with the multidisciplinary nature of the field, we have selected experts with differing approaches to discuss chemical-induced liver injury. The perspectives range from (a) clinical characterization of chemical hepatotoxicity to (b) microscopic characteristics of the different manifestations of liver responses to toxic insult to (c) examples of mechanisms by which chemicals can produce liver injury to (d) experimental models useful for the study of liver dysfunction.

As with the first edition, this book is written primarily for toxicologists who wish to enlarge their knowledge of hepatotoxicity induced by chemical agents. In addition, scientists and graduate students in related disciplines should find this a valuable source of basic information useful for a general comprehension of the problems associated with the liver as a critical target organ of chemical toxicity.

Gabriel L. Plaa
William R. Hewitt

PART I

Characterization of Chemical-Induced
Hepatotoxicity

Toxicology of the Liver, 2nd ed.,
Edited by Gabriel L. Plaa and William R. Hewitt
Copyright © 1998 Taylor & Francis

1

Drug-Induced Hepatic Disease

Hyman J. Zimmerman

*George Washington University and Armed Forces Institute of Pathology,
Washington, D.C. 20306-6000*

- **Types of Acute Hepatic Injury**
- **Subclinical Hepatic Injury**
- **Extrahepatic Manifestations of Drug-Induced Hepatic Injury**
- **Types of Chronic Hepatic Injury**
  - Chronic Cytotoxic Injury
  - Chronic Cholestatic Lesions
  - Vascular Lesions
  - Neoplastic Lesions
- **Mechanisms of Toxic Hepatic Injury**
  - Drugs as Intrinsic Hepatotoxicants
  - Idiosyncratic Hepatic Injury
  - Pathogenesis of Injury
  - Toxification and Detoxification of Drugs
- **Hepatic Injury Due to Large Doses of a Drug**
  - Acetaminophen (Paracetamol)
  - Aspirin
  - Iron Poisoning
  - Phenylbutazone
- **Hepatic Injury Caused by Specific Medicinal Agents**
  - Anesthetic Drugs
  - Neuroleptic Agents
  - Antidepressants
  - Anticonvulsants
  - Nonsteroidal Antiinflammatory Drugs (NSAIDs)
  - Other Drugs Used to Treat Arthritis
  - Antigout Drugs
  - Muscle Relaxants
  - Agents Used in the Treatment of Endocrine Disease and Related Conditions
  - Anabolic and Contraceptive Steroids
  - Antibacterial Agents
  - Antifungal Agents
  - Antiviral Agents

Adverse reactions to drugs appear to account for 2–5% of hospitalized cases of jaundice (1), for about 10% of cases of "hepatitis" among all adult patients, and for more than 40% of cases of "hepatitis" among patients over 50 (2). Drug-induced hepatic disease (DIHD) also has been estimated to account for 15–25% of cases of fulminant

TABLE 1. *Factors affecting susceptibility to drug-induced hepatic injury*

Age:	Adults more susceptible to injury from isoniazid, halothane, acetaminophen; children more susceptible to aspirin and valproate-associated injury.
Sex:	Females more susceptible than males to most forms of drug-induced hepatic injury, particularly chronic hepatitis.
Dose:	Dose dependence for drugs that are intrinsic hepatotoxins (e.g., acetaminophen, tetracycline) or produce injury because of metabolic idiosyncrasy (e.g., isoniazid, dantrolene). Little relevance of dose for hypersensitivity reactions.
Duration/Total dose:	Methotrexate-associated injury.
Route of administration:	Intravenous administration of tetracycline toxic; oral hardly toxic.
Drug interaction:	Valproate and chlorpromazine together lead to enhanced cholestasis. Oral contraceptive agents and troleandomycin together also lead to enhanced cholestasis. Rifampin and isoniazid are more hepatotoxic than either alone. Alcohol enhances hepatotoxic effects of chlorinated hydrocarbons, acetaminophen, methotrexate, isoniazid. Isoniazid enhances toxicity of acetaminophen.
Tissue oxygenation:	Tissue hypoxia enhances CCl_4 and halothane hepatotoxic effects. Hyperbaric oxygen inhibits CCl_4 toxicity.
Renal function:	Impairment enhances toxicity of tetracycline and probably that of allopurinol.
Effects of underlying disease:	AIDS enhances susceptibility to trimethoprim-sulfamethoxazole-oxacillin– and dapsone-associated hepatic injury. Active rheumatic fever enhances susceptibility to aspirin-associated hepatic injury.
Recognized genetic factors:	Slow metabolizers of debrisoquine are more susceptible to perhexiline maleate toxicity. Genetically defective epoxide hydrolase activity enhances susceptibility to phenytoin hepatic injury and to halothane-associated injury. HLA haplotypes affect susceptibility to nitrofurantoin and perhaps to halothane-associated injury. Acetylator phenotype may affect susceptibility to isoniazid toxicity.
Interval:	Daily doses of methotrexate are much more toxic than weekly ones.
Endocrine/Metabolic:	Hyperthyroidism enhances toxicity of CCl_4. Obesity enhances halothane toxicity, and obese diabetics are more susceptible to methotrexate injury.

Modified from reference (5).

hepatic failure (3, 4) and is a frequently incriminated cause of acute cholestatic jaundice (1). Also, a variety of chronic hepatic lesions of clinical importance are attributable to drugs.

Individual susceptibility to hepatic injury may be affected by genetic factors, age, sex, nutritional status, exposure to other drugs and chemicals, systemic disease, and other factors (Table 1). For the most part, the factors that affect vulnerability appear to result from their effects on conversion of the respective agents to a metabolite or on the detoxification or disposal of the metabolite (5).

Drug-induced hepatic disease may occur as an unexpected idiosyncratic reaction to a therapeutic dose of a drug or as an expected consequence of the intrinsic toxicity of an agent. The liver disease may be the only clinical manifestation of the adverse drug effect, or it may be accompanied by evident injury to other organs or by systemic manifestations. The injury may be acute or chronic. Acute injury may develop within several days of a toxic dose of a known hepatotoxicant; after 1–5 weeks of taking a drug that provokes hepatic injury by hypersensitivity; or after weeks to months of taking a drug that causes injury as the result of metabolic idiosyncrasy (1). Chronic hepatic injury follows long periods of taking a drug.

TYPES OF ACUTE HEPATIC INJURY

The types of acute hepatic injury are summarized in Table 2. Acute hepatic injury may be *cytotoxic* (cytolytic, hepatocellular), i.e., characterized by overt damage to hepatocytes; it may be *cholestatic*, i.e., manifested by arrested bile flow and jaundice; or it may be a mixture of the two. *Cytotoxic* injury includes necrosis, steatosis, or both. Hepatic necrosis leads to hepatocellular jaundice and a syndrome with biochemical

TABLE 2. *Clinical and biochemical reflections of drug-induced injury, acute syndrome*

Injury	Syndrome simulated	Biochemical response[1] AST-ALT[2]	ALP[3]	Example of cause[4]
Hepatocellular (cytotoxic)				
Necrosis	Hepatitis	8–500x	<3x	APAP, diclofenac INH
Steatosis	Reye's syndrome	8–20x	<3x	Tetra, VPA
Cholestasis				
Hepatocanalicular	Obstructive jaundice	<8x	>3x	Ajmaline CPZ, EE
Canalicular	Obstructive jaundice	<5x	<3x	Contraceptive, Anabolic steroids
Mixed	Obstructive jaundice or hepatitis	>8x	>3x	Sulindac

[1] Expressed as times (x) upper limit of normal.
[2] AST, ALT = Aspartate aminotransferase, alanine aminotransferase.
[3] ALP = alkaline phosphatase.
[4] APAP = acetaminophen, EE = erythromycin estolate, Tetra = tetracycline, VPA = valproic acid, INH = isoniazid, CPZ = chlorpromazine.

TABLE 3. *Estimated case fatality rates in drug-induced acute hepatocellular injury*

Halothane	~50%
Iproniazid	15%
Isoniazid	>10%
Dantrolene	~10%
Methyldopa	~30%
Phenytoin	~30%
Ticrynafen	~10%

values that resemble those of viral hepatitis. Severe cases may result in fulminant hepatic failure. Fatality rates of drug-induced hepatocellular jaundice have been 10% or more (5) (Table 3). Acute steatosis, such as that caused by parenteral tetracycline, leads to clinical and biochemical features resembling those of Reye's syndrome, which it also mimics histologically (1). In these conditions, the steatosis is microvesicular. Jaundice is usually relatively slight. Aminotransferase levels are usually not as high as those of hepatic necrosis. The illness, however, is serious and the prognosis grave. Known causes of microvesicular steatosis are listed in Table 4.

Cholestatic injury resembles extrahepatic obstructive jaundice in its clinical manifestations and biochemical parameters (1). Jaundice and pruritus are the main clinical manifestations. Aminotransferase levels are only modestly elevated—usually less than fivefold the upper limit of normal (ULN) and almost always less than eight times

TABLE 4. *Drug-induced steatosis*

Microvesicular	Macrovesicular
Acetylsalicylic acid[1]	Alcohol[2]
Aflatoxin	Asparaginase[4]
Alcohol ("alcohol foamy degeneration")[2]	Chromium toxicity
Amiodarone	Corticosteroids
Calcium hopantenate	Mercury poisoning
Camphor	Methotrexate
Cocaine	Minocycline
Desferrioxamine	Parenteral nutrition
Fluoroiodoarabinofuranosyl uracil (FIAU)	Perhexiline maleate
Hypoglycin A	Phosphorous poisoning[4]
Ibuprofen[3]	
Margosa oil	
Methylsalicylate[1]	
Piroxicam[3]	
Tetracyclines	
Tolmetin[3]	
Valproic acid	

[1] In overdose or as precipator of Reye's syndrome.
[2] Usual steatosis of alcohol excess is macrovesicular. Microvesicular is rare.
[3] Very rare cases.
[4] Mixture of microvesicular and macrovesicular.

TABLE 5. *Types of cholestatic jaundice caused by drugs*

Features	Canalicular jaundice	Hepatocanalicular jaundice
Examples of etiology	C-17 alkylated steroids (anabolic, contraceptives)	Chlorpromazine; erythromycin some oral antidiabetics; some antithyroid drugs
Character of syndrome	Resembles obstructive jaundice	Resembles obstructive jaundice
Clinical evidence of hypersensitivity	0	Frequent
Histological or biochemical evidence of parenchymal injury	Very rare	Occasional, minor
Biochemical features		
AST	<5x	<8x
ALT		
ALP	<3x	>3x
Histology		
Bile casts	+	+
Portal inflammation	0	+ (esp. early)
Parenchymal injury	0 or ±	± or +
Complications		
PBC-like syndrome	± or 0	+
Other terms	"Bland" cholestasis	"Cholangiolitic" cholestasis

± = Equivocally present, + = Definitely present, 0 or ± = absent or slight, ± or + = Equivocally or definitely present.
AST = aspartate aminotransferase; ALT = alanine aminotransferase; ALP = alkaline phosphatase; PBC = primary biliary cirrhosis.

the ULN. There are two main types of acute cholestatic injury (Table 5). One type is accompanied by portal inflammation and evident though slight hepatocyte injury. This type has been called *hepatocanalicular, cholangiolitic,* or *sensitivity cholestasis* or *cholestatic hepatitis*. The other, which is accompanied by little inflammation and even less hepatocyte injury, has been termed *canalicular, bland, pure,* or *steroid* cholestasis. The hepatocanalicular type is exemplified by chlorpromazine (CPZ) jaundice, and the canalicular type by anabolic or contraceptive steroid jaundice. Cholestatic injury, with a case fatality rate of less than 1%, has a far better prognosis than cytotoxic injury. An important exception was benoxaprofen jaundice. Despite its cholestatic nature, that entity appeared to have a high case-fatality rate, but the fatalities were not due to liver failure (6).

SUBCLINICAL HEPATIC INJURY

Injury reflected only by elevated serum enzyme levels is a common phenomenon. Some drugs lead to elevated aminotransferase levels and/or alkaline phosphatase levels in an incidence ranging from less than 5% to 50% of recipients (7). Most of the elevations are minor, i.e., less than three times the ULN, and they do not progress or may even subside despite continued administration of the respective drug. Nevertheless, the effort to prevent overt injury by drugs with a known toxic potential includes monitoring serum enzyme levels and withdrawal of the drug when a predetermined level (e.g., three or four times the ULN) is reached.

EXTRAHEPATIC MANIFESTATIONS OF DRUG-INDUCED HEPATIC INJURY

The clinical syndrome produced by acute hepatic injury may include systemic manifestations and evidence of injury to organs other than the liver. Traditional hallmarks of generalized hypersensitivity such as fever, rash, and eosinophilia are characteristic of reactions caused by some drugs (Table 6). In some instances, these features are accompanied by lymph node enlargement, lymphocytosis and "atypical" circulating lymphocytes, leading to a syndrome that resembles infectious mononucleosis and serum sickness.

Serologic markers of autoimmune response may be provoked by some drugs. Several forms of drug-induced injury lead to curious serologic markers. Iproniazid injury leads to an antimitochondral antibody (AMA-6) (8), ticrynafen injury (tienilic acid) leads to an antibody against an isoform of cytochrome P450 (P4502C 9/10) (9), dihydralazine hepatitis leads to another antiisoform (P4501A2) (10), clometacin injury leads to an antiactin antibody (11), and halothane hepatitis leads to an anticarboxylesterase antibody (12). The relationship to hepatic injury of such serologic phenomena, however, is far from consistent, as illustrated by procainamide, which leads to a very high (50–75%) incidence of antinuclear antibodies and "LE" factor in recipients and yet to extraordinarily rare instances of hepatic injury (1).

Some drugs produce liver disease only as part of the syndrome of generalized hypersensitivity, (e.g., phenytoin). Other drugs produce liver injury that may or may not be accompanied by the systemic manifestations of hypersensitivity (e.g., halothane, CPZ, erythromycin estolate). Drugs of a third group lead to hepatic injury that is accompanied relatively rarely by drug fever, rash, or eosinophilia (e.g., iproniazid, isoniazid) (Table 7). Organs other than the liver that may sustain injury as part of the syndrome of drug-induced jaundice include bone marrow, kidney, lung, skin, and vasculature.

TABLE 6. *Systemic manifestations that may be associated with drug hepatotoxicity*

Manifestations	Examples
Allergic	
Fever, rash, eosinophilia "Pseudomononucleosis"	Chlorpromazine, sulindac, phenytoin, dapone
Lymph node hyperplasia Lymphocytosis "Autoantibodies"	PAS, phenytoin, dapsone
Hemolytic anemia LE factor	Methyldopa, dapsone, oxyphenisatine
Bone marrow injury	Phenylbutazone, phenytoin
Renal injury	Anticonvulsants Methoxyflurane
Gastrointestinal (ulcer, pancreatitis)	Phenylbutazone Tetracycline, sulindac

From reference (1).
PAS = p-aminosalicyclic acid.

TABLE 7. *Association between hypersensitivity to drugs and hepatic injury induced by them*

	Hyper-sensitivity	Hepatic injury[1]	Accompanied by hypersensitivity[2]	Unaccompanied by hypersensitivity[3]	Incidence of trivial hepatic dysfunction[4]
Procainamide	5+	VR	−	−	?
Penicillin	4+	VR	−	−	?
Streptomycin	2+	VR	−	−	?
PAS	2+	+	+	0	?
DPH	2+	+	+	0	25%
CPZ	1+	+	+	+	20–50%
EE	1+	+	+	+	10–40%
TAO	1+	+	±	+	60%
Halothane	1+	+	+	+	20%

Symbol indicates relative incidence and prominence of clinical and serologic manifestation of hypersensitivity, e.g., rash, fever, eosinophil, antibodies to drug or components, "LE factor," antinuclear antibodies.

[1]VR = extremely rare, almost nonoccurring; + = accepted though uncommon phenomenon.
[2]+ = overt hepatic injury occurs in association with clinical evidence of hypersensitivity.
[3]+ = occurs without clinically evident hypersensitivity.
[4]? = no data. Actual figures refer to specific studies.
From reference (1).
PAS = p-aminosalicyclic acid; DPH = diphenylhydantoin; CPZ = chlorpromazine; EE = erythromycin estolate.

TYPES OF CHRONIC HEPATIC INJURY

The variety of chronic hepatic lesions that are drug-produced is listed in Table 8. The drugs that have been mainly incriminated in their production are shown in this table.

Chronic Cytotoxic Injury

Chronic Active Hepatitis

Drug-induced chronic active necroinflammatory disease behaves like "auto-immune" chronic active hepatitis (CAH) in many instances, with female predominance, "autoimmune" serologic markers (antinuclear antibody, smooth muscle antibody), hyperglobulinemia, and histologic features. Frequently incriminated drugs are listed in Table 9.

Steatosis

Chronic steatosis is mainly macrovesicular. It tends to have few clinical manifestations, in contrast to the acute, microvesicular type of drug-induced steatosis. The steatosis produced by ethanol, glucocorticoids, and methotrexate leads only to hepatomegaly as a clinical reflection. The lesion produced by asparaginase, although a form of chronic injury, may lead to micro- and macrovesicular steatosis and to clinical manifestations of hepatic insufficiency. The steatosis produced by asparaginase may be accompanied by necrosis. Another chronically evolving steatosis that is microvesicular is the one produced by valproate. This anticonvulsant can produce a form

TABLE 8. *Clinical and biochemical reflections of drug-induced injury, chronic syndrome*

Injury	Syndrome simulated[5]	Biochemical response[1] AST-ALT[2]	ALP[3]	Example of cause[4]
Hepatocellular				
Necroinflammatory	C.A.H. (Lupoid)	3–50x	1–3x	Nitrofurantoin Methyldopa
Steatosis	Alcoholic steatosis	1–3x	1–3x	MTX, GLC
Phospholipidosis				Amphophillic compounds
Pseudoalcoholic liver disease	Alcoholic liver disease	1–5x	Vx	Perhexiline, amiodarone
Cirrhosis				
Cholestatic injury				
Cholangiodestructive	P.B.C.	1–3x	3–20x	CPZ, ajmaline Haloperidol
Biliary sclerosis	Sclerosing cholangitis	1–5x	3–20x	FUDR
Granulomas		1–3x	3–20x	Many drugs
Vascular lesions				
Peliosis hepatis		1–3x	>3x	Anabolic steroids, OCs
Budd-Chiari	Congestive hepatopathy	2–20x	Vx	OCs
Venoocclusive disease				
Sinusoidal dilatation		1–3x	Vx	OCs
Pericellular and sinusoidal fibrosis		1–3x	Vx	Vitamin A
Portal hypertension				See text
Neoplasm				
Adenoma	Vx	Vx	Vx	OCs, As
Hepatocellular carcinoma	Vx	Vx	Vx	OCs, As
Cholicocellular carcinoma	Vx	Vx	Vx	?, As
Angiosarcoma				Vinyl chloride, estrogens, arsenic

[1] Expressed as times (x) upper limit of normal, Vx = Variable.
[2] AST, ALT = aspartate aminotransferase, alanine aminiotransferase.
[3] ALP = alkaline phosphatase.
[4] APAP = Acetaminophen, EE = erythromycin estolate; Tetra = tertracycline; MTX = methotrexate; VPA = valproic acid; FUDR = floxuridine; INH = isoniazid; CPZ = chlorpromazine; OC = oral contraceptives; GLC = glucocorticoids; AS = anabolic steroids.
[5] O.J = obstructive jaundice; C.A.H. = autoimmune type of chronic hepatitis; P.B.C. = primary biliary cirrhosis.

of chronic liver failure, somewhat resembling a slowly-evolving Reye's syndrome in that apparent hepatic encephalopathy is more severe than the apparent acute injury. A similar lesion in children has been caused by amiodarone.

Phospholipidosis

This lesion, which was first reported from Japan in recipients of a drug used to treat coronary disease (4,4'-diethylaminoethoxylhexestrol), has been seen in patients taking *perhexiline maleate, amiodarone*, and 4 *chloroquine*. A number of other amphophilic drugs can reproduce the lesion in experimental animals (1, 5).

TABLE 9. *Drugs incriminated as possible causes of chronic active hepatitis*

Drug
Acetaminophen[1]
Aspirin[1]
Clometacin
Dantrolene
Fenofibrate
Iproniazid[1]
Isoniazid[1]
Methyldopa
Nitrofurantoin
Oxyphenisatine
Papaverine
Propylthiouracil
Sulfonamide
Ticrynafen

[1] Chronic injury due to these drugs appears to reflect continued toxicity rather than immunological type of response.

The lesion, which consists of engorgement of lysosomes with phospholipids, is difficult to recognize by light microscopy. Presence of dramatically abnormal, lamellated lysosomes by electron microscopy permits ready recognition. The phospholipidosis may be accompanied by cirrhosis.

Clinical manifestations of phospholipidosis per se consist of hepatomegaly with or without other apparent hepatic injury. The neuropathy, pulmonary manifestations, and thyroid effects of phospholipidosis, however, are usually more prominent than the hepatic phospholipidosis. More important is the "pseudoalcoholic" liver disease (called *nonalcoholic steatohepatitis*) that also may accompany the phospholipidosis.

Pseudoalcoholic Liver Disease

This form of drug-induced injury resembles alcoholic liver disease morphologically and, to some degree, clinically. Morphologic changes consist of alcoholic hyalin (Mallory bodies), neutrophilic inflammation, variable steatosis, and cirrhosis. Hepatomegaly, ascites, spider angiomas, and a prominent abdominal venous pattern may make the presence of chronic liver disease with cirrhosis apparent, or hepatomegaly may be the only reflection of hepatic involvement.

Fibrosis and Cirrhosis

These changes, produced as a consequence of adverse drug effects, may result from chronic active hepatitis, methotrexate injury, the phospholipidosis-pseudoalcoholic lesion, chronic cholestatic injury, and lesions occluding the hepatic outflow tract.

Clinical manifestations of the fibrotic-cirrhotic lesion per se are those of portal hypertension coupled with those of the causative lesion.

Portal Hypertension

This entity may also be due to deposition of collagen in the periportal area and space of Disse and by reduction of portal vein caliber, a condition termed *noncirrhotic portal hypertension* and *hepatoportal sclerosis*. Hepatoportal sclerosis has been attributed to chronic exposure to inorganic arsenics, vinyl chloride, and copper sulfate. Other hepatic lesions that can lead to noncirrhotic portal hypertension are fibrosis in zone 3 due to vitamin A intoxication and nodular regenerative hyperplasia. Portal hypertension is particularly likely to result from preparation for bone marrow transplantation, which may lead to nodular regenerative hyperplasia or venoocclusive disease (5).

Chronic Cholestatic Lesions

Cirrhosis may also be a consequence of chronic drug-induced cholestasis (2). Two forms of chronic cholestasis may result from drug-induced injury. One is the *chronic intrahepatic cholestasis* that can evolve from some instances of acute cholestasis (1, 5). The other is the *biliary sclerosis* due to the ductal injury provoked by the chemotherapy of secondary hepatic carcinoma with infusion of floxuridine (FUDR) into the hepatic artery (1, 5) (Table 8).

Chronic Intrahepatic Cholestasis

A drug-induced syndrome resembling primary biliary cirrhosis has followed acute cholestasis due to organic arsenics, chlorpromazine, and a number of other drugs listed in Table 10 (1, 5).

Biliary Sclerosis

This term has been applied to the biliary tree injury produced by therapy of hepatic metastatic carcinoma with FUDR infused into the hepatic artery. In histology and in cholangiography, the lesion resembles sclerosing cholangitis. Obstructive biliary cirrhosis may be a consequence.

Vascular Lesions

A number of important vascular lesions can be produced by drug injury. Two involve interference with efferent blood flow and lead to congestive hepatopathy. They are thrombosis of the hepatic veins and occlusion of the hepatic venules. A third lesion is

TABLE 10. *Drugs incriminated in chronic cholestasis*

Aceprometazine (with meprobamate)
Ajmaline and related drugs
Amitriptyline
Ampicillin
Barbiturates
Carbamazepine
Carbutamide
Chlorpromazine
Cimetidine
Cyproheptadine
Haloperidol
Imipramine
Methyltestosterone
Norandrostenolone
Phenytoin
Prochlorperazine
Thiabendazole
Tiopronin
Tolbutamide
Troleandomycin
Xenalamine

peliosis hepatis. Additional lesions are sinusoidal dilatation, perisinusoidal fibrosis, and hepatoportal sclerosis (1, 5).

Hepatic Vein Thrombosis

Occlusion of the hepatic veins leads to the Budd-Chiari syndrome, characterized by tender hepatomegaly and abdominal pain, ascites, modestly elevated aminotransferase levels, and rarely, jaundice. At least 100 instances of hepatic vein occlusion have been reported in patients taking oral contraceptive steroids (5).

Venoocclusive Disease

Injury and occlusion of the central hepatic venules has long been known to be produced by pyrrolizidine alkaloids (1). It leads to hepatic congestion and can lead to fatal congestive cirrhosis. The clinical features and hepatic congestion are similar to the Budd-Chiari syndrome produced by hepatic vein thrombosis. Causes, in addition to the alkaloids, include urethane, thioguanine, azathioprine, indicine N-oxide, and a number of other oncotherapeutic agents, as well as irradiation (5).

Peliosis Hepatis

This lesion, which consists of blood-filled lakes, has been recorded as a rare consequence of taking contraceptive and anabolic steroids. Most instances have been seen in association with hepatic tumors or with cholestatic jaundice induced by the respective drug. The peliotic lesion may rupture and lead to the clinically dramatic syndrome of hemoperitoneum, or peliosis may be an incidental discovery at autopsy. Several drugs (hydroxyurea, azathioprine), other than the steroids, have been incriminated in the causation of the lesion (5).

Neoplastic Lesions

Only several drugs have been demonstrated or even suspected of producing tumors in humans. The etiologic role of contraceptive steroids in the development of liver cell adenoma, a benign tumor, is well established, and a role in hepatocarcinogensis is probable. A strong case for hepatocarcinogenesis also can be made for C-17 alkylated anabolic steroids (5).

MECHANISMS OF TOXIC HEPATIC INJURY

It has long been convenient to identify chemical agents that can damage the liver as *intrinsic* (true, predictable) hepatotoxicants or *idiosyncrasy*-dependent (unpredictable) hepatotoxicants (1) (Table 11). This dichotomy into toxicity and idiosyncrasy, however, is an overly simplified formulation. The potential for producing injury ranges from agents that damage the liver of all exposed members of a variety of species to some drugs that produce liver disease only in a particularly susceptible tiny proportion of exposed humans. Toxic effects in all depend on interplay between intrinsic toxicity and host vulnerability (Fig. 1). Nevertheless, it is helpful to distinguish agents that are mainly true toxicants from those that produce injury as idiosyncratic reactions and to recognize that even among drugs that produce idiosyncratic injury there are differences in apparent potential for injury (1).

Drugs as Intrinsic Hepatotoxicants

Potent intrinsic hepatotoxicants have been largely excluded from the clinical armamentarium. Carbon tetrachloride was once employed as a vermifuge; chloroform

TABLE 11. *Intrinsic and idiosyncratic hepatotoxicants*

Basis for hepatic injury	Experimental reproducibility	Dose dependence	Incidence in humans	Latent periods
Intrinsic hepatotoxicity (true, predictable hepatotoxic agents)	Yes[1]	Yes	High	Often short and relatively consistent
Idiosyncratic reaction (nonpredictable hepatotoxic agents)	No	No	Low	Often long and variable

[1]May apply only to some species. Depends on dose. When due to metabolic idiosyncrasy, may be reproducible experimentally in specially manipulated models.

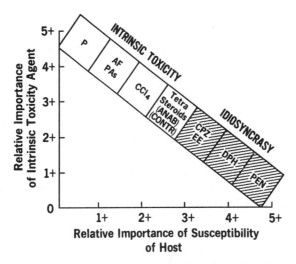

FIG. 1. Graphic formulation of relative importance of intrinsic toxicity of chemical agent and of susceptibility of exposed individual in the production of chemical hepatic injury. Note that interplay between susceptibility of host and toxicity of agent can be expressed as spectrum or as dichotomy. P = phosphorus; AF = aflatoxins; CCl_4 = carbon tetrachloride; tetra = tetracycline; ANAB = anabolic; CONTR = contraceptive; CPZ = chlorpromazine; EE = erythromycin estolate; DPH = phenytoin; PEN = penicillin K or G.

was used for anesthesia for over a century; and tannic acid was employed for the treatment of burns 4 decades ago and for bowel radiography 2 decades later. All are potent hepatotoxicants that were discarded when identified as the cause of hepatic necrosis (1).

A number of agents with some intrinsic hepatotoxic potential, however, are still employed in clinical medicine. Some, such as acetaminophen and ferrous salts, are hepatotoxic in large overdose (5) (acetaminophen can be hepatotoxic, even in modest doses, in unusually susceptible patients [e.g., alcoholics] [13]). Others, (e.g., tetracycline, asparaginase, anabolic steroids) show a dose-related toxicity that may become apparent even as therapeutic misadventures (1).

Idiosyncratic Hepatic Injury

By definition, the hepatic injury that occurs unpredictably in a small proportion of recipients of a drug is an expression of unusual individual susceptibility rather than of intrinsic toxicity of the offending agent (1). Idiosyncrasy may be immunologic (hypersensitivity) or metabolic (Table 12). The liver injury may be tentatively attributed to hypersensitivity when it is accompanied by clinical (fever, rash, eosinophilia) and histologic (eosinophilic or granulomatous inflammation in the liver) hallmarks of hypersensitivity. These characteristics, especially when supported by a prompt recurrence of the syndrome in response to readministration of the drug, permit the

TABLE 12. *Idiosyncratic reactions to drugs as cause of hepatic injury*

Type of idiosyncrasy dose	Duration of exposure	Clinical features, hypersensitivity (rash, fever, eosinophilia)	Response to challenge
Hypersensitivity	1–5 weeks	+	Prompt—one or two doses
Metabolic aberration	Variable—1 week, 12 months	−	Delayed—many days or weeks

inference that the hepatic injury is due to immunologic idiosyncrasy and that the drug or a metabolite has acted as a hapten (1). This form of injury usually develops after a "sensitization" period of 1–5 weeks. Examples of drugs in this category include sulfonanides, dapsone, and sulindac (5).

Lack of the clinical and histologic hallmarks of hypersensitivity and lack of prompt recurrence of the hepatic injury after one or two "challenge" doses of the suspected drug suggest an alternative mechanism for the liver damage, presumably the production of hepatotoxic metabolites or inability to detoxify them. This form of injury appears after widely variable latent periods ranging from weeks to months (1). Examples of drugs in this category are isoniazid, valproate, perhexiline maleate, and amiodarone (5).

That hypersensitivity-mediated reactions also can result from a metabolic defect is strongly suggested by the observations of Spielberg et al. (14). They found that patients (and their relatives) who had sustained hepatic injury in a hypersensitivity-type reaction to phenytoin had an apparent defect in converting the active metabolite (arene oxide) to the inactive dihydriodol. The active metabolite presumably could serve as a hapten or be cytotoxic.

Pathogenesis of Injury

Most toxic hepatic injury results from the action of the active metabolite of the drug or other chemical agent. The toxic metabolite may be a free radical or an electrophilic radical, or the metabolism may yield activated oxygen (15–17) (Table 13). Most intrinsic hepatotoxicants have the molecular property of being readily converted to active toxic metabolites in all individuals. Injury due to metabolic idiosyncrasy reflects the propensity of the injured individual to produce toxic metabolites from a drug to a greater degree than other individuals (1). Immunologic idiosyncrasy depends on the active metabolite's behaving as a hapten and/or because of a unique immune response of the individual (1).

Toxification and Detoxification of Drugs

Drug metabolism may be considered in two phases (Fig. 2), both microsomal. Phase I, which is cytochrome P450–mediated, is primarily oxidative and yields the active

---

TABLE 13. *Mechanisms by which hepatotoxic drugs lead to injury*

I. As a result of drug biotransformation
    A. Formation of free radical

Drug $\xrightarrow[\text{P450}]{\text{Cyt}}$ Free Radical $\longrightarrow$ Lipid Peroxidation $\longrightarrow$ Necrosis

e.g., Carbon Tetrachloride

    B. Formation of electrophilic intermediate

Drug $\xrightarrow[\text{P450}]{\text{Cyt}}$ Electrophile $\longrightarrow$ Covalent Binding $\longrightarrow$ Necrosis

    C. Production of "active oxygen" by drug oxidation

Drug $\xrightarrow[\text{P450}]{\text{Cyt}}$ Active Intermediate $\longrightarrow$ Conjugation $\longrightarrow$ Excretion

Active Oxygen $\longrightarrow$ Lipid Peroxidation $\longrightarrow$ Necrosis

e.g., Paraquat, ? Nitrofurantoin

II. As result of interference by untransformed drug with cell metabolism or integrity. For example, tetracycline interferes with exit of lipid from liver and with oxidation of fatty acid by the liver, causing steatosis.

---

intermediate metabolites that may be responsible for hepatic injury (18). Phase II, which is mainly conjugative, converts the active metabolite to nontoxic, more hydrophilic products by linking the metabolite to glutathione, glucuronate, or sulfate (1). Accordingly, Phase I reactions may be regarded as toxification and Phase II as detoxification (1, 15). Some injury reflects mainly toxification (e.g., CCl_4 toxicity), whereas other injury reflects both enhanced toxification (increased amount of active metabolite) and inadequate detoxification (decreased glutathione). The latter is exemplified by acetaminophen toxicity (17). Some injury reflects decreased detoxification of a reactive metabolite (e.g., phenytoin injury) (14).

Cytochrome P450, the key enzyme of phase I metabolism, is now known to be a family of isoforms. At least 30 have been identified in humans. Each isoform has specific substrates on which it can act, although there is some overlap. Indeed, the specificity of substrate relationship may have an important bearing on hepatotoxicity. For example, the isoform of P450 most involved in the conversion of acetaminophen

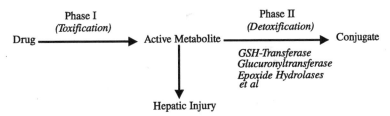

FIG. 2. Schematic representation of drug metabolism. Phase I is catalyzed by cytochrome P450, Phase II by one of the enzymes that converts the active intermediate to a nontoxic excretable product. The active metabolite can produce hepatic injury.

to a toxic intermediate, P4502E1, is the isoform induced by ethanol—explaining at least in part the enhancement by alcohol of acetaminophen toxicity (17–20). Another cardinal example of the relevance of P450 isoform multiplicity is the increased susceptibility of slow debrisoquine metabolizers to perhexiline maleate toxicity (21).

HEPATIC INJURY DUE TO LARGE DOSES OF A DRUG

Even lethal doses of some agents do not necessarily produce hepatic injury, and when a nonhepatotoxic agent is converted to an hepatotoxic one by increasing the dose, a degree of intrinsic hepatotoxicity has been exposed. Acetaminophen, aspirin, and ferrous sulfate are in this category (1, 5). They are not damaging to the liver in modest therapeutic doses but are distinctly hepatotoxic as an acute effect of a single large overdose or, in the case of aspirin and perhaps acetaminophen, as cumulative effect of large daily therapeutic doses. Phenylbutazone in therapeutic doses can lead to idiosyncratic hepatic injury but in poisonous, accidental overdose can lead to severe injury, seemingly as a manifestation of a degree of intrinsic toxicity (22).

Acetaminophen (Paracetamol)

Acetaminophen (APAP) is an intrinsic hepatotoxicant. It is a mild analgesic and antipyretic agent with very few side effects when taken in therapeutic doses of 1–4 g daily (5, 23) in most normal individuals. When taken in single large doses of 15 g or more (and in some instances lower doses) as a suicidal effort, it is a potent toxicant causing centrilobular (zone 3) necrosis and hepatic failure (23). The necrosis is in zone 3 because the peak concentration of the cytochrome P450 system and, consequently, of the active metabolite is in the hepatocytes of zone 3 (16). Intake of APAP with suicidal intent is the most common cause of liver failure in the United Kingdom (23).

The hepatic injury is produced by a toxic metabolite (Fig. 3). Normally, a small fraction of each dose is converted to an active metabolite that binds with glutathione (GSH) and is then excreted as mercapturic acid or a related molecule (16). Large doses lead to increased formation of the active metabolite. Metabolite, in excess of the available GSH, binds covalently to cytoplasmic proteins and, as an unexplained consequence, leads to necrosis. Only when the amount of toxic metabolite exceeds the available GSH, does necrosis occur (16). Accordingly, susceptibility to the hepatotoxic effects of a dose of APAP depends on *dose, rate of biotransformation of APAP,* and *tissue content of GSH*. Toxicity is enhanced by circumstances and agents that enhance activity of the P450 system or deplete stores of GSH. Recent studies have led to challenge the role of covalent binding in APAP injury and to the suggestion that oxidant stress leads to the injury (17). Administration of acetylcysteine during the first 16 hr (23) and perhaps 24 hr (24) after intake of APAP can prevent serious hepatic injury. Administration of cimetidine during the first few hours also appears to inhibit injury in experimental animals (25). Acetylcysteine benefit apparently derives from its repletion of GSH (25), and cimetidine benefit derives from its inhibition of the

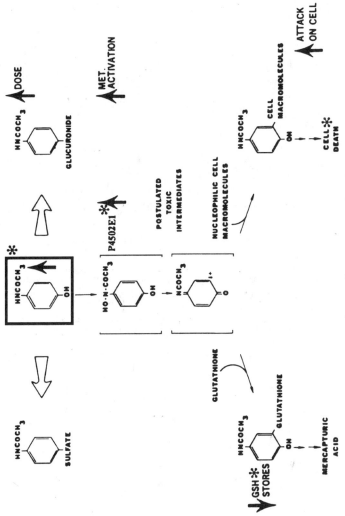

Pathways of acetaminophen disposition.

FIG. 3. Simplified presentation of metabolism of acetaminophen and of presumed mechanism of toxicity. Asterisk represents sites of pertinent to enhanced toxicity in the alcoholic person or other regular consumer of alcohol. Induction of P4502EI by alcohol intake and deficient conjugation with GSH is due to alcohol-inhibition of synthesis and impaired intake of protein as well as impaired conjugation with glucuronate due to fasting-associated impaired intake of carbohydrate.

19

cytochrome P450 system and prevention of production of the toxic metabolite (25). There is no evidence that cimetidine adds any benefit to the use of acetylcysteine in humans.

There are a number of instances of hepatic injury by APAP as a therapeutic misadventure (5, 13, 20). Several have involved multiple doses taken with therapeutic intent in a sufficiently short period to reach total doses large enough (e.g., 15 g) to produce hepatic injury. Other instances, however, have involved only moderately large total daily doses (4–10 g) or even approved doses (4 g or less) in alcoholics (13, 20) or other particularly susceptible individuals (e.g., those fasting) (26, 27). Alcoholics appear to have enhanced susceptibility to large single overdoses or to multiple therapeutic doses, as a presumed consequence of induction by ethanol of the isoform of P4502E1 involved in APAP metabolism and depletion of GSH associated with their disease and lifestyle (13, 19, 20). Both the inhibition of synthesis of GSH by alcohol (28) and the impaired nutrition secondary to alcohol use, presumably, contribute to deficient stores of GSH. In some instances even moderate intake of ethanol appears able to enhance the toxicity of APAP. Other circumstances associated with apparently enhanced susceptibility have involved wasting disease, malnutrition, and even fasting that might lead to depletion of GSH as well as of glucuronate, the latter leading to impaired glucuronidation and enhanced activity of the cytochrome P4502E1 pathway (13, 19, 20).

Aspirin

Aspirin and other salicylates can produce hepatic injury as a slowly evolving cumulative phenomenon, requiring days or weeks to develop or as the acute response to a poisonous overdose (29). The injury is dose-dependent, usually occurring at the doses of 4–6 g/day of aspirin, although instances of lower doses leading to hepatic injury have been reported. It is even more clearly related to blood levels, being much more likely to occur at levels above 25 mg or even 15 mg/dl than at lower ones. Susceptibility appears to be enhanced by active rheumatic fever, rheumatoid arthritis, or systemic lupus erythematosus and, perhaps, by preexisting liver disease but not recognizably by drugs or alcohol (29, 30).

The lesion in aspirin hepatic injury, which is nonzonal diffuse degeneration, stands in contrast to the zone 3 necrosis of APAP. Aspirin clearly has intrinsic hepatotoxic potential, but the mechanism for injury is not clear. The injury is usually nonthreatening. A lesion of special note and concern, however, is the microvesicular steatosis (Reye's syndrome) seen in children who had received aspirin after exposure to one of several viral illness (31). Large, single poisonous overdoses of aspirin also lead to microvesicular steatosis (32).

Iron Poisoning

Hepatic injury from *ferrous sulfate* poisoning is, like that due to APAP, the consequence of a single huge overdose, usually taken accidentally by children. The injury is distinctive, consisting mainly of necrosis in the lobular periphery (1, 5).

Phenylbutazone

The hepatic injury of very large doses of *phenylbutazone* is curious. A few cases of severe hepatic necrosis have been described in children and young adults taking large overdoses of the drug. The necrosis has been massive, with no clear-cut zonality reported. These instances of acute toxic effects of overdose suggest that intrinsic toxic potential may play a role even in the apparently idiosyncratic injury due to the drug (22).

HEPATIC INJURY CAUSED BY SPECIFIC MEDICINAL AGENTS

Over 1000 drugs have been implicated in instances of hepatic injury. There are differences among drugs. Some are far more likely than others to produce injury, and there are differences among individuals with regard to susceptibility to injury. There are also characteristic differences in the form of hepatic injury produced (Table 14).

Anesthetic Drugs

Volatile anesthetics that injure the liver produce hepatocellular injury. Known hepatotoxic ones of yesteryear include chloroform, trichloroethylene, divinyl ether, and tribromoethanol. None is still used as an anesthetic today. However, chloroform and trichloroethylene are still used in sniffing as a form of chemical abuse (1, 5).

Halothane

Little doubt remains that halothane can produce hepatic injury. Although decreasingly seen because of sharply decreased use of the drug and substitution of newer agents less threatening to the liver, halothane-associated liver disease continues to provide important lessons in drug-induced liver disease.

Incidence is greater after multiple exposures than after a single one (1). Figures as high as 1 in 10,000 on first exposure and 1 in 1000 on multiple exposure have been estimated (1). Even higher figures, in excess of 1%, have been recorded among women treated for carcinoma of the cervix with repeated radium implantation under halothane anesthesia (1, 5).

Importance and Clinical Setting

Despite the current low incidence, the formerly widespread use of halothane and the severity of halothane-induced injury established halothane as an important cause of acute hepatic failure recently (1, 5, 33). Furthermore, liver damage also has followed occupational exposure to halothane (1) and the sniffing of halothane as chemical abuse (34). Small amounts of halothane can produce injury in susceptible individuals even on exposure to halothane only as a contaminant of anesthesia machines (35, 36).

TABLE 14. *Types of acute hepatic injury caused by drugs in various therapeutic categories*

	Cytotoxic (hepatocellular) and mixed[2]	Cholestatic and mixed[2]	Some cytotoxic and some cholestatic[3]
Anesthetics[1]	Enflurane Fluroxene Halothane Isoflurane?[10] Methoxyflurane		
Neuro psychotropics	Amineptine Clozapine Cocaine Famoxitine Hydrazides (all) Maprotiline Metopimazine Methylphenidate Molindone Tranylcypromine Tricyclics (most) Zimelidine	Chlorpromazine (& other phenothiazines) Haloperidol Trimipramine Benzodiazepines	Chlordiazepoxide Diazepam Mianserin Trazodone Tricyclics (some)
Anticonvulsants	Phenytoin Progabide Valproate[5]		Carbamazepine Phenobarbital
Analgesic Antiinflammatory	Acetaminophen Chlorzoxazone Clomatacine	Benoxaprofen Diflunisal Penicillamine	Allopurinol[4] Gold compounds Naproxen
Anti–muscle spasm Antigout agents	Dantrolene Diclofenac Fenclozic acid Glafenine Ibuprofen Indomethacin Salicylates Pirprofen Tolmetin Zoxazolamine	Propoxyphene	Phenylbutazone[4] Piroxicam Sulindac
Hormonal derivatives and drugs used in endocrine disease	Acetohexamide Carbutamide Cyclofenil Glipizide Metahexamide Propylthiouracil[4] Tamoxifen Diethylstibestrol	Carbimazole Chlorpropamide[4] Tolazemide[4] Tolbutamide[4] Methimazole Methylthiouracil Anabolic and contraceptive steroids Danazol	Thiouracil
Antimicrobials	Amodiaquine Amphotericin B Antimonials Clindamycin Hycanthone	Amoxicillin-clavulante Erythromycin[7] Griseofulvin Thiabendazole Menelamine	Cephalosporins Chloramphenicol Clarithromycin Nitrofurandin[4] Penicillin[8]

Table continued on next page

TABLE 14. *Continued.*

	Cytotoxic (hepatocellular) and mixed[2]	Cholestatic and mixed[2]	Some cytotoxic and some cholestatic[3]
	Hydroxystilbamidine	Cloxacillin	Sulfamethoxazole
	Didanosine	Zidovudine	trimethoprim
	Ketoconazole	Dicloxacillin	Sulfadoxine
	Mebendazole	Floxacillin	pyrimethamine
	Mepacrine		Idoxyuridine
	Metronidazole		Zidovudine
	P-Aminosalicylate		Ampicillin
	Rifampin		Oxacillin
	Sulfonamides[4]		
	Sulfones		
	Tetracyclines[5]		
	Prothionamide		
Cardiovascular drugs	Amiodarone[5,11,12]	Ajmaline	Amrinone
	Aprindin	Captopril	Disopyramide
	Benziodarone	Chlorthalidone	Enalapril
	Diltiazem	Coumadin	
	Methyldopa	Phenindone	
	Mexiletine	Prajmaline	
	Hydralizines[4]	Propafenone	
	Nicotinic acid	Thiazides	
	Nifedipine[12]	Verapamil[4]	
	Papaverine		
	Perhexiline[5,11,12]		
	Procainamide		
	Pyridinol carbamate		
	Quinidine[4]		
	Suloctidil		
	Ticrynafen		
	Tocainamide		
	Labetolol		
	Lisinopril		
Antieoplastic[9]	Asparaginase[5,6]	Aminoglutethamide	Azathioprine
	Cis-platinum[5]	Busulfan	
	Cyclophosphamide	Floxuridine	
	Dacarbazine		
	DES[12]		
	Doxorubicin		
	Etoposide		
	Fluorouracil		
	Indicine-N-oxide		
	Methotrexate[6]		
	N-methyl-formamide[5]		
	Mithramycin		
	6-mercaptopurine		
	Nitrosoureas		
	Tamoxifen		
	Thioguanine[7]		
	Vincristine		
	Flutamide		

Table continued on next page

TABLE 14. *Continued.*

	Cytotoxic (hepatocellular) and mixed[2]	Cholestatic and mixed[2]	Some cytotoxic and some cholestatic[3]
Miscellaneous	Disulfiram Iodide ion Oxyphenisatin Phenazopyridine Tannic acid Vitamin A PABA	Propoxyphene Rapeseed oil- aniline[13] Methylene dianiline[14]	Cimetidine Ranitidine Etretinate Salizopyridine

[1] Hepatic injury produced by volatile anesthetic agents is always cytotoxic.

[2] Mixed forms of injury are categorized according to the predominant injury as cytotoxic or cholestatic.

[3] Refers to agents that are inconsistent in the form of injury produced, with some instances having been cholestatic and other cytotoxic.

[4] Can cause granulomas.

[5] Microvesicular steatosis. Valproate injury also includes necrosis in some cases.

[6] Macrovesicular steatosis.

[7] E-Estolate, E-Ethylsuccinate, E-Proprionate, E-Stearate.

[8] Semisynthetic penicillins and penicillin.

[9] Some of these agents alone or as combinations lead to venoocclusive disease.

[10] Two credible cases reported.

[11] Also leads to phospholipidosis.

[12] Can lead to changes resembling alcoholic liver disease (alcoholic hyaline).

[13] Responsible for "toxic oil" epidemic in Spain.

[14] Responsible for "Epping" jaundice.

Factors in Susceptibility

Susceptibility to hepatic injury from halothane appears to be greater in females, enhanced by advancing age and obesity, and probably by intake of alcohol, and it appears to be low in children (1, 5). Previous exposure to halothane is the single factor of most importance in predicting a subsequent, clinically apparent reaction. Many of the patients had had fever, with or without eosinophilia, after a prior exposure to halothane (1). There are hints of genetic factors in susceptibility (5).

Clinical Manifestations

The syndrome of halothane-induced hepatic injury includes features that appear to reflect hypersensitivity in more than half of the reported cases, followed or accompanied by manifestations of severe hepatic disease (1, 5). The onset is usually within 3–8 days but may be as late as 15 days after exposure. The interval between anesthesia and onset of illness is shorter in patients who have had prior exposure to halothane than in those who develop hepatic damage after the first exposure. Fatal cases are characterized by progressively deepening jaundice, prolonged prothrombin times with hemorrhagic phenomena, ascites, and coma. Serum bilirubin levels correlate somewhat with prognosis. Marked prolongation of the prothrombin time is the most important adverse prognostic sign.

Histologic Features

The hepatic injury caused by halothane is hepatocellular. Zone 3 (centrolobular) necrosis, resembling that of CCl_4 and of acetaminophen, is the most characteristic lesion (33).

Laboratory Manifestations

Levels of aminotransferases are very high (25–1000 times normal). Alkaline phosphatase levels are only moderately elevated (less than threefold) in most patients. Bilirubin levels may reach very high values, especially in patients with a fatal outcome in whom additional problems of renal failure and hemolysis may contribute. Hypoprothrombinemia is common and may be profound. Leukocytosis is usual, and eosinophilia occurs in about 50% of recognized cases (1).

Prognosis

The prognosis of patients with halothane-induced liver injury who develop jaundice has been grave, with the mortality rate ranging from 14% to 71% (1). Milder instances, however, probably go unreported or unrecognized.

Mechanism of Injury

Halothane-induced injury appears to involve, at least in part, immunologic reaction to a hepatocyte membrane component altered by a halothane metabolite. The altered component serves as a neoantigen (37, 38). The importance of multiple exposures, the incidence of fever and eosinophilia, the demonstration of sensitivity to planned or inadvertent reexposure, and reports of eosinophilic aggregates in the liver all support this view (1, 5). Particularly impressive is the report of an anesthesiologist in whom the role of halothane in the causation of cirrhosis was clearly established by deliberate reexposure that led to recurrence of clinical, biochemical, and histologic evidence of hepatitis (36).

There is also evidence for the role of a toxic metabolite (1). The zonal necrosis of halothane toxicity resembles the lesion of known toxicants, such as CCl_4, but is unlike the lesion of hypersensitivity-dependent hepatic injury (1). It supports the view that a toxic metabolite formed in zone 3 by the cytochrome P450 system contributes to or is responsible for the hepatic injury (1). Experimental studies support this possibility. There are two main pathways of halothane metabolism, one oxidative and the other reductive; and the pathway is critically dependent on oxygen concentration

(37). The reductive pathway leads to a necrogenic, free radical. The oxidative pathway yields a metabolite that produces no hepatic injury but reacts with hepatocyte microsomal proteins to produce a neoantigen. Accordingly, systemic or hepatic hypoxia would lead to reductive metabolism of halothane and formation of the free radical, whereas adequate oxygenation would trigger the immunologic response (37, 38). Neuberger and Williams (37) and Satoh et al. (38) believe that the immunologic response plays a major role in producing clinically severe injury. The frequency of zonal necrosis in halothane jaundice, however, suggests that the reductive pathway (and the free-radical that it yields) plays an important role, and it seems likely that periods of relative hepatic hypoxia, even if brief, may permit production of necrogenic metabolites (1, 5).

Methoxyflurane

Methoxyflurane is a halogenated ether closely resembling halothane in chemical structure and anesthetic properties. This agent also can produce hepatic necrosis similar to that of halothane (39). In addition, it leads to renal injury characterized by azotemia and a long-persisting defect in concentrating capacity as well as oxaluria and deposition of calcium oxalate crystals in the proximal tubules. The renal damage presumably results from the effects of fluoride metabolites on the kidney.

Enflurane

This halogenated anesthetic can lead to injury indistinguishable from that found with halothane and methoxyflurane (40). The incidence appears to be lower than that from halothane, presumably because a smaller percentage of the drug undergoes transformation. Prior exposure to enflurane or another haloalkane anesthetic can increase the risk of enflurane administration (40).

Isoflurane

This agent had appeared to provoke no instances of hepatic injury during its first few years of use, and even now very few cases have been reported. Nevertheless, there have now been several cases reported that appear to be reasonable examples of isoflurane-induced hepatic injury (41, 42). The oligotoxicity seems ascribable to the minimum biotransformation of the drug, which apparently is less than 1% (42).

Sevoflurane and Desflurane

Sevoflurane and desflurane are recently introduced fluorinated anesthetics that have thus far not been found to produce hepatic injury.

Neuroleptic Agents

Chlorpromazine

Chlorpromazine (CPZ) has a clear and well-studied profile of producing liver injury. In use for a half century, it is the most extensively studied neuroleptic, and the hepatic injury that it produces is the prototype of one type of cholestasis (1, 5, 43). Up to 1% of recipients develop jaundice, which usually appears within 1–5 weeks of the initiation of the CPZ (1).

Prodromal symptoms occur in 75% of patients. They may include fever, chills, and abdominal distress. Eosinophilia occurs in about 60% of cases. Severe itching is common. Readministration of small doses leads to prompt recurrence of hepatic dysfunction or jaundice in approximately half of the patients tested (1).

The CPZ-induced hepatic injury is primarily cholestatic (hepatocanalicular). Serum alkaline phosphatase values are greater than threefold the normal, while aminotransferase values are usually only slightly or moderately elevated. Liver biopsy in most patients reveals evidence of cholestasis with only slight hepatocyte degeneration and necrosis (1, 5, 43). Occasional acidophilic bodies are seen. The major inflammatory response is in the portal area, which contains many eosinophils, early in the course of illness (1). A small minority of patients with CPZ-induced injury develop a hepatocellular-type injury with hepatic necrosis and high aminotransferase levels (1, 5, 43).

The prognosis of CPZ jaundice is generally quite good. Two-thirds of patients recover fully within 8 weeks. Most of the remainder return to normal within 2–12 months (43). However, a small proportion of patients develop a prolonged cholestatic syndrome that may closely resemble primary biliary cirrhosis, characterized by marked hypercholesterolemia and even xanthomatosis. Histologic features may resemble those found in primary biliary cirrhosis with loss of interlobular bile ducts (vanishing bile duct syndrome). Most of these patients recover, although several have died (44).

Mechanism of Injury

Clinical features of CPZ-induced jaundice, along with the prompt recurrence of hepatic abnormality on reexposure to the drug, suggest that immunologic idiosyncrasy is responsible for the hepatic injury. However, there is evidence that there is also a toxic component to the injury. Chlorpromazine causes injury to hepatocytes in vitro and inhibits bile flow in intact monkeys and in perfused rat livers (1). Chlorpromazine, and particularly its hydroxylated metabolites, inhibit membrane Na^+K^+-ATPase and alter membrane fluidity (5). Its sulfoxide metabolite is inactive and nontoxic. Genetically determined ineffective sulfoxidation, accordingly, enhances susceptibility to CPZ toxicity (45). The manner in which immunologic factors and drug toxicity interact to produce jaundice is not clear.

Antidepressants

Iproniazid and Other Hydrazine Derivatives

Iproniazid, an amine oxidase inhibitor, was among the early drugs reported to damage the liver (46). The use of iproniazid led to liver injury sufficient to cause jaundice in approximately 1% of recipients. The onset of liver injury was insidious, with anorexia, malaise, fatigue, and jaundice usually appearing after 1–6 months of taking the drug. Biochemical, histologic, and clinical features indicated hepatocellular injury (1, 46). On liver biopsy there was evidence of extensive, diffuse parenchymal degeneration and necrosis. Instances of massive necrosis resembling the lesion of fatal viral hepatitis were observed.

The clinical deduction that the hepatic injury from iproniazid resulted from the production of hepatotoxic metabolites of the drug (46) found support in experimental studies conducted years later (47). Presumably, the responsible metabolites were formed in greater amounts in susceptible persons. The mortality rate for patients who developed clinically apparent jaundice was about 15% (46). Other hydrazides produce similar hepatic injury.

Other Antidepressants

Several amine oxidase inhibitors that are not hydrazine derivatives have been reported to produce hepatic injury, similar to that caused by hydrazine derivatives (1, 5). The hepatic injury in patients receiving the tricyclic antidepressants (amitriptyline, imipramine, and desipramine) may be either cholestatic or hepatocellular. A tetracyclic antidepressant, trazodone, has been incriminated in several instances of hepatic injury (48).

Anticonvulsants

Phenytoin (Diphenylhydantoin, DPH)

This drug has been a mainstay of anticonvulsant therapy for more than a half-century. Hepatocellular injury has been an infrequent but important adverse reaction to its use (1). Most cases of DPH-induced hepatic injury involve adults. The onset of liver disease is usually within 1–5 weeks of beginning the drug. The hepatic damage is mainly cytotoxic, with evidence of high aminotransferase values, often extensive hepatocellular necrosis, and poor prognosis. Rare reports have described cholestatic injury (1, 5). The clinical illness caused by DPH is often complex, with hepatic toxicity only part of a potentially devastating multisystemic problem. Almost all patients develop rash and fever, and some may develop the Stevens-Johnson syndrome. Ocular and other mucous membranes may be severely affected. Lymphadenopathy may be prominent and fever as high as 40°C has been described. Occasionally, extraordinarily high levels of leucocytes ($>30,000–50,000/mm^3$) may be found. Instances of curious lymph node changes resembling lymphoma have been described (1, 5). These clinical features support the view that DPH-induced injury is a manifestation of drug hypersensitivity. In support of this view is the occasional presence of the "pseudomononucleosis" syndrome of lymphadenopathy, lymphocytosis, and circulating atypical lymphocytes—a serum sickness–like illness suggesting the presence of circulating immune complexes (1). However, there is also evidence that DPH-induced liver injury results from the effects of a toxic intermediary molecule (14). The drug is metabolized by the cytochrome P450 system with the production of highly reactive arene oxide intermediates. Unless these intermediates are further converted to a nontoxic metabolite by the enzyme *epoxide hydrolase*, they bind covalently to tissue macromolecules, leading to hepatocyte injury or acting as hapten to form neoantigens. A genetically determined deficiency in epoxide hydrolase activity has been identified in patients with DPH-induced hepatic injury and in their family members (Fig. 4).

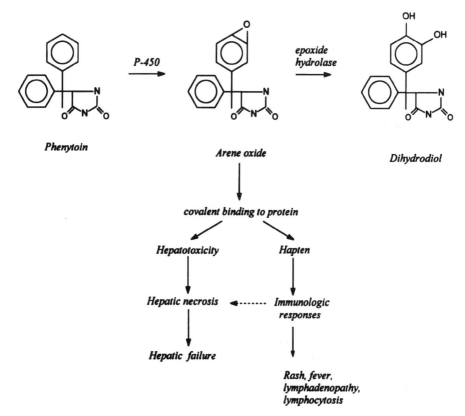

FIG. 4. Pathway of phenytoin metabolism and proposed role of the arene oxide metabolites in the pathogenesis of hepatotoxicity. From reference (14).

These observations suggest that susceptibility to hepatic liver injury is determined largely by genetic factors (14).

The prognosis for reported cases of DPH-induced hepatic injury has been poor, with a case-fatality rate of over 30% (1). Corticosteroid therapy is often used because the hepatic injury is accompanied by prominent features of hypersensitivity, but evidence of benefit is scant.

Sodium Valproate (VPA)

This anticonvulsant has been incriminated in a number of instances of fatal and nonfatal liver disease (49–51). In contrast to the case with most other drugs, children appear to be more susceptible than adults to the hepatic injury; those below the age of 2 years are particularly susceptible (49, 50). Clinically significant hepatic disease occurs in 0.01–0.5% of recipients. Incidence appears to be lower in patients on monotherapy than in those taking other anticonvulsants with the VPA. Increases in aminotransferase levels, often without associated symptoms, are frequent (6–44%) within the first 2 months of administration of VPA. There is no apparent relationship between these asymptomatic elevations of high incidence and the development of the very rare, severe hepatic injury (49).

The reactions have been characterized by gradual onset of signs suggesting liver disease, including changes in mental status and the development of progressive jaundice, elevated aminotransferase levels and coagulopathy (49–51). Histologic studies have revealed diffuse hepatocellular injury with microvesicular steatosis and in some cases necrosis (49–51).

The mechanism of valproate-induced liver injury is not known. Inhibition of mitochondrial oxidation of long-chain fatty acids leading to accumulation of these as the cause of the microvesicular fatty change is the prevailing hypothesis (52). Current views suggest that a metabolite of valproate is responsible for the inhibition of mitochondrial oxidative activity and that the responsible metabolite is 4 ENVPA, the *4-pentanoic derivative*. It has been suggested that infants with underlying familial defects of carnitine metabolism or of ornithine carbamoyltransferase function may be especially susceptible to hepatotoxicity from sodium valproate (53).

Carbamazepine

This iminostilbene derivative is useful in the treatment of trigeminal neuralgia, refractory seizures, and paresthesia from peripheral neuropathies. A number of instances of hepatic injury have been reported in recipients (54). Evaluation of the contribution of carbamazepine to hepatic toxicity is often made more difficult by the frequent concomitant administration of other drugs known to cause hepatic injury. The onset of carbamazepine liver injury is usually within 1 month of initiating therapy. The types of injury reported include granulomatous inflammation, cholestatic jaundice, and hepatocellular damage (5, 54). Development of a chronic cholestatic syndrome with disappearance of portal area bile ducts has been reported (55).

The mechanism for hepatic injury is unknown. Evidence of immunologic idiosyncrasy (hypersensitivity) as the cause of the injury include the onset of symptoms such as rash, fever, arthralgia, and elevated IgE levels within several weeks of beginning carbamazepine therapy.

Phenobarbital

This is a widely used drug rarely involved in significant hepatic injury. Only a few reports have appeared over a half-century of wide use (1, 5). In several of these instances the role of the drug in the hepatic injury has been proven by readministration. The mechanism appears to be immunologic idiosyncrasy.

Nonsteroidal Antiinflammatory Drugs (NSAIDs)

A number of NSAIDs can provoke hepatic injury in low incidence. For some of these drugs, the injury has been severe and even fatal (30, 56). One NSAID, benoxaprofen, was withdrawn shortly after its introduction when reports of fatal reactions involving liver and kidney injury appeared (57). There have been at least occasional instances of drug-induced liver injuries with most available NSAIDs. However, the hepatic injury induced by these drugs is not uniform with regard to frequency, character, or apparent mechanism of production (56). Most NSAIDs produce cyctoxic injury; a few lead to cholestatic injury (56). Although the mechanism in all appears to be idiosyncrasy, for some drugs it is immunologic (hypersensitivity) and for others, metabolic.

Phenylbutazone

Phenylbutazone has been incriminated in instances of hepatic injury for 4 decades. The injury appears to result from an immunologic idiosyncrasy in most instances, as deduced from the frequency of rash and fever and the usual onset of illness within 5 weeks of starting the drug (22). However, the hepatotoxic effect of poisonous overdose suggests that intrinsic toxicity may also play a role (22). Apparently, both sexes are affected equally. Several types of liver injury may occur. Hepatocellular injury is the most frequent form. Some patients develop cholestatic injury. A number of patients have had granulomatous liver injury. *Oxyphenbutazone* apparently produces a similar range of liver injuries.

Indomethacin

Several instances of hepatic injury including an instance of massive hepatic necrosis have been attributed to indomethacin (1, 5). Both hepatocellular and cholestatic types of injury have been reported. The incidence of indomethacin-induced hepatic toxicity appears to be low.

Sulindac

Sulindac is chemically related to indomethacin. However, sulindac has been incriminated in many more cases of hepatic injury. Both cholestatic and hepatocellular injury have been recorded. The cholestatic form is more frequent. The mechanism for the liver injury appears to be immunologic idiosyncrasy as judged by clinical features (58).

Ibuprofen

Ibuprofen appears to have a low incidence of hepatic injury. In the few reported cases the injury appears to have been hepatocellular (56), and at least one fatality has been attributed to liver injury. That patient had microvesicular steatosis (59). The mechanism for the putative hepatic injury from ibuprofen is unknown. The association with Stevens-Johnson syndrome and other hallmarks of hypersensitivity, in some instances, suggests that the drug may cause an immunologic-type reaction. There have been no reported instances of clinically apparent liver injury from low doses (200 mg three times a day) of ibuprofen. The closely related ibufenac was found to cause liver injury in a much higher incidence (5%) and was withdrawn from use (1).

Diclofenac

This widely used NSAID is a derivative of phenylacetic acid. At least 50 cases of hepatic injury from the drug have been reported, including some fatalities (60), and we have analyzed an additional 180 cases reported to the Food and Drug Administration (61). Women appear to be more susceptible to diclofenac injury than men (61). Also, curiously, patients with osteoarthritis appear to be more susceptible to the injury than do those with rheumatoid arthritis (61). The pattern of injury is regularly hepatocellular, usually with acute necrosis (60, 61). Chronic active hepatitis also has been attributed to the drug (61). The mechanism by which diclofenac leads to liver injury is unknown but is presumably metabolic idiosyncracy. However, anaphylactic shock also has been attributed to diclofenac (62).

Naproxen

Naproxen, a widely used NSAID, has been incriminated in hepatic injury. The jaundice may be hepatocellular, cholestatic, or mixed. The mechanism is unclear (30, 56, 63).

Piroxicam

There have been a few instances of hepatic injury attributed to piroxicam (30, 56, 63). Hepatocellular injury, fatal and nonfatal, as well as cholestasis have been described.

Benoxaprofen

This NSAID was briefly available in the United States, but was withdrawn when reports of fatal hepatic and renal insufficiency appeared (6, 30, 56, 63). The drug is of interest, even though now withdrawn, in part because of the high mortality rate that occurred in patients who developed jaundice while receiving the drug. Most patients with benoxaprofen-induced injury were elderly women. The strikingly slowed metabolism of the drug in elderly patients may have a bearing on the susceptibility to hepatic injury (56). The liver injury was predominantly cholestatic, with relatively little evidence of hepatic necrosis or inflammation. The mechanism of injury remains unknown. Presumably, the liver injury resulted from the effects of an undefined toxic metabolic product of benoxaprofen, perhaps a poorly soluble glucuronate. A remarkable and unexplained observation in patients with benoxaprofen-induced injuries was the high case-fatality rate, with 11 deaths among 14 reported patients (6, 56, 63). So high a fatality rate is strikingly paradoxic in such overtly cholestatic injury, since drug-induced cholestasis is rarely fatal (1, 56, 63). Prescott et al. (6) have suggested that death resulted from high blood levels of the drug due to severe cholestasis and renal failure, which together prevented its excretion.

Clometacin

This NSAID has been mainly used in France as an analgesic agent. It has led to hepatic injury that is predominantly hepatocellular, both acute and chronic (64–66). The chronic injury closely resembles the "autoimmune" type of chronic active hepatitis. Discontinuation of the drug appears to be followed by rapid recovery in patients with both acute and chronic injury. Readministration may lead to prompt reappearance of liver injury. Almost all affected patients have been elderly women. The drug is not in use in the United States.

Other Drugs Used to Treat Arthritis

Gold

Intrahepatic cholestasis is a rare complication of gold therapy for rheumatoid arthritis (1, 5, 67, 68). The liver injury apparently results from an idiosyncratic reaction presumably immunologic. Eosinophilia has been recorded, and elevated IgE antibodies have been found (69). Hepatocellular injury also has been described. Several cases have been fatal (70, 71). The liver injury from gold generally resolves within 3 months following cessation of therapy.

Propoxyphene

Rare instances of hepatotoxic effects of propoxyphene have been recorded (72). The injury has been cholestatic.

Antigout Drugs

Allopurinol

Allopurinol, a widely used xanthine oxidase inhibitor, has been incriminated as the cause of several types of hepatic injury. Minor biochemical abnormalities, hepatic granulomas, cholestasis, and severe hepatocellular injury all have been recorded. The liver injury generally disappears rapidly when the drug is withdrawn. In rare instances, fulminant hepatic failure associated with fever, exfoliative dermatitis, eosinophilia, and jaundice has been recorded (1, 5).

Probenecid

Probenecid, widely used in the treatment of gout, has rarely been incriminated in hepatic injury. There is one reported case of fatal hepatic necrosis from the drug (1).

Muscle Relaxants

Dantrolene

Dantrolene is a muscle relaxant that has been incriminated in instances of acute and subacute hepatic necrosis (73). In some patients, the subacute lesion resembles chronic active hepatitis. Evidence of liver damage usually does not appear until at least 6 weeks after starting the drug. Overt hepatic injury occurs in 0.5–1% of recipients. Dantrolene rarely affects children under the age of 10 years. Furthermore, dantrolene-induced injury has an apparent dose relationship, being rare at a dose below 200 mg/day.

Zoxazolamine

Zoxazolamine, a drug used to treat myospastic disease a quarter-century ago, was abandoned when a number of cases of severe injury were reported (1). *Chlorzox-azone*, a related drug in current use, also has been incriminated in rare instances of acute hepatocellular injury (74). Clinical features suggest metabolic rather than immunologic idiosyncrasy as the mechanism.

Agents Used in the Treatment of Endocrine Disease and Related Conditions

Thiourea Derivatives

There appear to be differences between the type of hepatic injury produced by the various derivatives of thiourea. The hepatic injury induced by thiourea, methimazole, carbimazole, and methylthiouracil is usually cholestatic, whereas that attributed to propylthiouracil has been mainly hepatocellular (1, 5). The mechanism for hepatic injury appears to be related to immunologic idiosyncrasy (hypersensitivity) as judged by the usual association of rash, fever, and eosinophilia; prompt recurrence in response to readministration; and the response of lymphocytes from affected patients to in vitro exposure to the drug (5).

Oral Hypoglycemic Drugs

Hepatic injury, predominantly cholestatic, has occurred in 0.5–1% of patients receiving chlorpropamide (1). Cholestasis also has been attributed to tolbutamide, tolazamide, and several other sulfonylurea derivatives (1, 5). Hepatocellular or mixed injury (1) as well as cholestatic injury (75) has been recorded in patients taking acetohexamide.

Sulfonylurea derivatives also can produce hepatic granulomas, which may develop in the absence of other evidence of hepatic injury (1). Only scattered (and incompletely documented) instances of hepatic injury have been ascribed to biguanides, and these injuries may have been coincidental (5).

Anabolic and Contraceptive Steroids

The hepatic effects of the C-17 alkylated anabolic steroids and of the oral contraceptive steroids have much in common (1, 5). Both groups of drugs are intrinsic, mild hepatotoxicants capable of producing acute, cholestatic jaundice (1, 5). Both groups, especially the anabolic steroids, have led to peliosis hepatis, and both have been implicated in hepatic tumor production (5, 76–85). Anabolic steroids appear more likely to produce peliosis (76), whereas contraceptive steroids lead to a dramatic form of sinusoidal dilatation not seen with anabolic steroids (5, 86). Both have been incriminated in the production of hepatocellular carcinoma (76–80). The contraceptive steroids have been more convincingly associated with the development of hepatic adenoma (1, 5, 80–87).

Only oral contraceptives have been incriminated in hepatic vein thrombosis and the Budd-Chiari syndrome (1, 5, 88). This lesion is presumably related to the thrombogenic effect of the estrogenic component of the contraceptive preparations (1, 5), especially in patients with an underlying tendency to develop thrombosis (88).

Evidence from a case control study suggests that the risk of hepatic vein thrombosis is more than doubled by the oral contraceptives (88).

Steroid-Induced Jaundice

The jaundice induced by the anabolic and contraceptive steroids is cholestatic, of the canalicular type (1, 5). Serum alkaline phosphatase levels remain normal or only slightly elevated. Aminotransferase levels are only slightly increased, although there are reports of an occasional patient who has high levels of aminotransferases (1). There is no portal inflammation or parenchymal injury found on liver biopsy. Steroid jaundice usually has its onset within the first 1–6 months of treatment. Onset is insidious, with pruritus and mild jaundice (serum bilirubin value usually <5 mg/dl). Rarely, jaundice is deep. The prognosis is excellent, with complete recovery usually occurring within a few weeks. Rarely, the jaundice may persist for months after the drugs are withdrawn. Contraceptive steroid jaundice resembles the cholestatic jaundice of pregnancy (1, 5).

The steroid-induced jaundice appears to result from the selective interference with bile excretion apparently related to an impaired uptake of bile acids from sinusoidal blood (5, 89). There is a loss of membrane fluidity and decrease in Na^+, K^+-ATPase in the plasma membrane (5, 87, 88a, 89). Impairment of canalicular contraction due to steroid-induced injury to the pericanalicular microfibrillar network probably also plays a role (88a).

The presence of an alkyl or ethinyl group on carbon 17 of the steroid appears to be essential for the production of cholestatic liver changes (1). Unsaturation of ring A, a characteristic of native estrogens, appears to enhance the adverse effect of steroids on hepatic function studies, as may be deduced in experimental animals, as well as from the greater adverse potency in humans of the estrogenic than of the progestational component of contraceptive preparations.

C-17 Alkylated Anabolic Steroids

The incidence of jaundice among patients who receive these agents is low, although some evidence of hepatic dysfunction occurs in almost all patients who have taken them in large doses (1). Genetic predisposition presumably plays a role.

Contraceptive Steroids

Women who have a personal or familial history of jaundice or pruritus from pregnancy are more likely to develop jaundice or pruritus from contraceptive steroids than are those without this background (1, 89). These observations and the clustering of cases of contraceptive steroid–induced jaundice in selected populations in Chile and Scandinavia, members of which have a high incidence of cholestatic jaundice of pregnancy, demonstrate the relevance of genetic susceptibility to this type of hepatic injury.

Steroid-Induced Liver Tumors

Hepatocellular carcinoma has been reported in recipients of the anabolic steroids (76, 77, 90) and of contraceptive steroids (78–80). Many of the patients with anabolic steroid-related tumors have received the agents for various types of anemia, although tumors have been reported in athletes ill-advisedly using the drugs for body building (77).

In view of the large number of women who have taken contraceptive steroids and the relatively smaller number of patients who have used anabolic steroids, hepatocarcinogenesis appears to be more readily attributable to the anabolic agents than to contraceptive steroids. The atypical character of the carcinomas described in recipients of these steroids has led to a questioning of the true carcinomatous nature of the tumors (90). Many of these tumors metastasize late if at all, and the incidence of elevated alpha-fetoprotein levels are low. Nevertheless, a potential carcinogenic role for both contraceptive and anabolic appears real.

Hepatic adenoma is clearly related to the taking of contraceptive steroids. Hepatic adenoma was first described as a complication of oral contraceptive therapy in 1973 (81). Since then a large number of cases of this tumor have been reported, over 90% of them in women taking contraceptive steroids. There is an apparent direct relationship between the duration of oral contraceptive use and the incidence of adenoma (1, 85). The adenoma may present as an asymptomatic or painful right upper abdominal mass or as a life-threatening hemoperitoneum secondary to rupture of the tumor (1, 5, 85). Anabolic steroids also have been incriminated in the development of adenoma but appear to be much less likely to lead to the tumor (76).

In many instances, hepatic adenomas regress when contraceptive steroid use is discontinued (89). However, some do not regress (91). Furthermore, a tumor that has apparently regressed may resume growth and rupture during pregnancy (5). There have also been reports of apparent transformation of the adenoma to hepatocellular carcinoma (83). These instances of recurrence during pregnancy and the potential carcinomatous transformation are sufficiently convincing that removal of the adenoma is preferable to depending on its regression.

Danazol

A number of reports have attributed liver injury to the use of danazol, a derivative of C-17 ethinyltestosterone (92–95). Cholestatic injury (92, 93), hepatic adenoma (94), and hepatocellular carcinoma (95) have each been described.

Antibacterial Agents

Tetracyclines

Tetracyclines lead to dose-related hepatic and pancreatic toxicity (1, 5). The multiple instances of severe hepatic toxicity in patients who were receiving tetracycline intravenously has led to a virtual abandonment of this route of administration of the drug. Nevertheless, the drug is of interest as the prototype of an important form of drug-induced injury. The characteristic lesion is microvesicular steatosis, resembling the fatty liver of pregnancy or Reye's syndrome (1, 5). The prognosis is poor. Indeed, most patients with recorded cases of clinically overt tetracycline-associated liver disease have died (1). A rare instance of macrovesicular steatosis to be provoked by a tetracycline derivative has been attributed to minocycline (96). Microvascular steatosis can be reproduced by administration of tetracycline to experimental animals (1). Recent reports described about 10 cases of acute and chronic hepatic injury resembling autoimmune hepatitis in patients taking minocycline by mouth (96a,b,c).

The biochemical features of tetracycline-induced liver disease also resemble those associated with Reye's syndrome. Bilirubin levels are usually below 10 mg/dl. Levels of aminotransferases are less elevated than those of hepatic necrosis, rarely more than 15-fold elevated, and in the majority of patients, less than fivefold the normal (1).

The mechanism for the hepatic injury is clearly hepatotoxicity of the drug and appears to be the result of inhibition of transport of lipid from the liver, coupled with inhibition of mitochondrial oxidation of fatty acids (1, 5).

Erythromycins

Early reports suggested that erythromycin estolate (EE) was the only derivative that produced liver injury (1). However, the ethylsuccinate, propionate, and stearate esters of erythromycin also have been incriminated in the production of cholestatic jaundice (5). Clinically apparent jaundice occurs in 1–2% of adult recipients of EE but very rarely in children (1). The pattern of injury is usually cholestatic (hepatocanalicular), with high values for serum alkaline phosphatase and modestly elevated serum aminotransferase values. Liver biopsy usually shows bile casts and a prominent portal inflammatory infiltration that is often rich in eosinophils. Uncommonly, an erythromycin can lead to hepatic necrosis (1). An instance of fulminant hepatic failure has been attributed to the use of intravenous erythromycin lactobionate (97).

Typically jaundice, pruritus, abdominal pain, and elevated aminotransferase levels appear 2–21 days after initiation of the erythromycin. The hepatic injury may develop after a much shorter interval on reexposure of susceptible individuals. The symptoms of liver disease usually subside promptly when the drug is withdrawn.

The clinical hallmarks of hypersensitivity that accompany the hepatic injury all suggest immunologic idiosyncrasy to be the mechanism of injury. However, the high incidence of hepatic dysfunction in recipients of EE (1) and the demonstration that the drug can damage isolated hepatocytes (98) and the in-vitro perfused liver (99) suggest that intrinsic hepatotoxicity contributes to the hepatic injury (1).

Triacetyloleandomycin (Troleandomycin)

This agent produced jaundice in 4% and hepatic dysfunction in over 50% of one group of patients who had been taking 2 g/day for 2 or more weeks (100). The histologic features and the pattern of hepatic dysfunction produced by this drug were those of mixed-cholestatic jaundice. There also are a number of reports describing young women who, while regularly taking oral contraceptives, developed intrahepatic cholestasis 2–20 days after beginning the triacetyloleandomycin (101). Triacetyloleandomycin apparently interferes with the metabolism of the oral contraceptive, thereby leading to the cholestasis (101).

Penicillin

Hypersensitivity reactions from penicillin, especially with fever and rash, are common, but reports of hepatic injury due to penicillin are exceedingly rare (1, 5). Among the huge number of recipients of penicillin, very few instances of liver damage have been recorded (1). The few reported instances of penicillin-induced liver injury have been cholestatic or hepatocellular with usually rapid reversal of injury upon withdrawal and generally associated with generalized hypersensitivity (1, 5).

Several semisynthetic penicillin derivatives, however, seem to produce jaundice or biochemical evidence of hepatic injury more commonly (1, 5) (Table 14). Cloxacillin (102) and flucloxacillin have been associated with severe cholestasis. The cholestatic reaction attributed to flucloxacillin may last for many months after withdrawal of the drug (103).

Amoxicillin/Clavulanic Acid

A number of patients receiving this preparation have developed predominately cholestatic liver injury (104–106). The onset of apparent liver injury was usually within 2 weeks of beginning the drug, although it may follow withdrawal of the drug by several weeks. The rarity of hepatic injury in recipients of amoxicillin suggests that the hepatotoxicity may result from the clavulanic acid component or from the combination. The mechanism of the injury is unknown. The prompt recurrence in response to readministration (105) suggests immunologic idiosyncrasy.

Organic Arsenics

The description by Hanger and Gutman over a half-century ago (107) of arsphenamine-induced cholestatic jaundice is a milestone in the history of drug-induced liver disease. Their account of drug-induced "intrahepatic obstructive" jaundice is a classic description of intrahepatic cholestasis, including the inference that the injury resulted from a hypersensitivity reaction. Fever and eosinophilia often appeared at the time liver injury was noted.

The biochemical abnormality found in patients with arsphenamine-induced liver injury closely simulated that of obstructive jaundice. Alkaline phosphatase levels were usually more than fourfold increased, and hypercholesterolemia was common. Prominent cholestasis and a variable portal inflammatory infiltration was seen on liver biopsy. Occasionally, the arsphenamine-induced injury persisted for many months and a syndrome resembling primary biliary cirrhosis developed (1, 5).

Sulfonamides

Acute hepatitis has been provoked by a variety of sulfonamide derivatives. Granulomatous liver injury also has been reported. Sulfonamides have also been implicated in the production of a chronic active hepatitis (1, 5, 108).

Most instances of acute hepatic injury attributed to sulfonamides are hepatocellular, although instances of cholestatic jaundice also have been described, and the hepatic damage is best characterized as mixed hepatocellular (1). The rash, fever, eosinophilia, and tissue eosinophils and granulomas seen in many of the patients and the relatively fixed latent period of 5–14 days that usually precedes the onset of injury suggest that hypersensitivity is the mechanism for the hepatic damage (1). One patient developed cholestatic jaundice from use of a sulfanilamide vaginal cream (109).

Sulfamethoxazole-Trimethoprim

There are multiple reports of liver injury caused by use of this combination drug (5, 108). Most affected patients have a predominantly cholestatic injury, and the cholestasis initiated by trimethoprim-sulfamethoxazole may be severe and last many months (108, 110, 111). It is probable that the trimethoprim contributes to the cholestatic injury (112). However, about 30% of patients have had hepatocellular injury, and fulminant hepatocellular failure has been recorded (5, 108, 113). Many features including fever, skin rash, arthralgias, and eosinophilia suggest at least an element of hypersensitivity in the mechanism. Patients with human immunodeficiency virus (HIV) infection are particularly susceptible to hepatic injury from this preparation (5).

Pyrimethamine-Sulfadoxine

This combination is widely used as prophylaxis against falciparum malaria in travelers and against *Pneumocystis carinii* pneumonia in patients with acquired immunodeficiency syndrome (AIDS) (5). Occasional instances of hepatic toxicity have been reported in recipients of the combination, and several patients have died of massive hepatic necrosis (114, 115). Some of the affected patients have had eosinophilia and granulocytopenia. Others have developed a Stevens-Johnson syndrome with exfoliative dermatitis (5). In addition, instances of granulomatous hepatitis following the use of pyrimethamine-sulfadoxine have been recorded (116). Whether the hepatic injury occurs from one of the two component drugs or from additive effects of the combination is unknown.

Sulfasalazine

Sulfasalazine is a sulfonamide derivative that is widely used in the treatment of inflammatory bowel disease. There have been a number of reports of sulfasalazine-induced liver injury (5) resembling that found in other sulfonamide-induced injuries. Fever, rash, arthralgias, and hepatitis usually develop within 1–4 weeks of starting the drug. Low serum complement and circulating immune complexes have been found in patients with sulfasalazine-induced injury (5).

Sulfones

These agents appear to produce hepatic injury more often than do sulfonamides (1, 5). The incidence of abnormalities has been reported to be about 5% in recipients of the prototypic compound, 4-4'-dapsone. The injury appears to be of the mixed hepatocellular type. The mechanism is not clear, but there are strong suggestions of immunologic idiosyncrasy.

Nitrofurantoin

This antimicrobial is widely used in the treatment of urinary tract infection. Acute and chronic liver injury has been attributed to the use of the drug (1, 5, 108, 117). Acute injury may be either cholestatic or hepatocellular (1). Hallmarks of hypersensitivity including fever and eosinophilia suggest that the mechanism is immunologic idiosyncrasy (1, 5).

Nitrofurantoin has been incrimanted in at least 50 published cases of chronic active hepatitis, almost all in females (1, 5, 108, 117–119). The chronic active hepatitis resembles to a remarkable degree the syndrome of idiopathic autoimmune chronic active hepatitis. The mechanism causing the liver injury is unknown, presumably immunologic idiosyncrasy. Several patients have been reported to have HLA-B8 antigen (119), which also is present in approximately 75% of patients with idiopathic, autoimmune chronic active hepatitis (5, 119).

Antituberculous Drugs

In most instances tuberculosis is treated by a combination of several drugs, making it difficult to assess the contribution of an individual agent to hepatic injury. Furthermore, drug–drug interactions may compound difficulties in assessment (1, 5). Nevertheless, observations from the use of p-aminosalicylic acid alone or with streptomycin, and the use of isoniazid alone for chemoprophylaxis of tuberculosis, have permitted deduction of the hepatotoxic potential of each (1, 5). Isoniazid is a well-established cause of drug-induced injury (1, 5, 120, 121). Streptomycin and dihydrostreptomycin appear to essentially not damage the liver; ethambutol rarely can be incriminated (5). Rifampin has been implicated in several cases of hepatic injury (1, 5). Rifampin also is an established inducer of cytochrome P450 (5, 122). As a result of the induction, the metabolism of isoniazid is enhanced, and its hepatotoxic threat may be enhanced (122).

p-Aminosalicylic Acid (PAS)

This drug was once widely used in the treatment of tuberculosis, and its use was accompanied by a generalized hypersensitivity reaction in 0.3–5% of recipients (1, 43). Hepatic injury occurred as part of the multisystemic syndrome. The PAS-induced reaction, which appeared after 1–5 weeks of taking the drug, occurs in a setting of fever, rash, eosinophilia, lymphadenopathy, and often atypical circulating lympho-cytes (pseudomononucleosis) and at times the Stevens-Johnson syndrome (1, 43). The PAS-induced liver injury is characterized by elevated serum aminotransferase levels in the range of hepatocellular injury and high serum alkaline phosphatase levels, yielding a pattern of mixed jaundice. Fatalities have been reported (1, 43).

Isoniazid (INH)

The recognition and appreciation of isoniazid-induced liver injury was a milestone in the understanding of drug-induced liver injury. Isoniazid had appeared to show extraordinarily slight potential for producing hepatic injury during the first 2 decades following introduction of the drug (1). Only a few instances of liver injury had been attributed to INH, most of them in patients who also had been receiving other agents. In the late 1960s the drug began to be used alone as chemoprophylaxis to prevent the emergence of tuberculosis. It soon became apparent that INH, used as a sole agent, could cause liver damage.

The incidence of clinically apparent jaundice developing among recipients of INH approaches 1% (120). Clinically evident hepatic injury is quite rare in patients under the age of 20 years and rises to greater than 2% in patients above 50 (1, 5, 120, 123). Females are apparently more likely to develop severe INH-induced injury than are males (123). Alcoholics appear to be at increased risk of developing injury (123). Minor elevations (< threefold) of serum aminotransferase levels occur in 10–20 % of patients during the first 2 months of treatment (1, 5).

Clinical features of isoniazid-induced liver injury resemble those found in acute viral hepatitis. Anorexia, fatigue, nausea, and vomiting are frequent prodromal fea-tures. The liver injury may be severe, with peak values for aminotransferase levels as high as 4000 IU. About 15% of cases of symptomatic INH-induced injury appear within the first month of therapy, and about 50% within the first 2 months. In the remaining 50% of cases, onset may be delayed from 3 to 12 months (120). Continued administration of isoniazid after prodromal symptoms have appeared may enhance the severity of injury and increase the risk of death (120). Isoniazid-induced hepatic necrosis is apparently the result of the production of toxic intermediates, which are highly reactive moieties that bind covalently to cell macromolecules and lead to cell necrosis (124).

Rifampin

The role of rifampin in producing hepatic injury is unclear. It has rarely been incriminated in hepatic injury while being taken alone, but more often in combination with isoniazid (1, 5). The injury attributed to rifampin when being taken with isoniazid usually appears during the first month of therapy (125). Rifampin-induced liver injury is mainly hepatocellular, or mixed (125). Hepatocellular necrosis is characteristic and tends to be most prominent in zone 3. There is considerable experimental and clinical evidence that rifampin and isoniazid together cause more hepatotoxicity than either drug alone (1, 5, 122). The apparently increased incidence is presumably due to induction by rifampin of the isoform of cytochrome P450 (P4502E1) involved in the conversion of isoniazid to its toxic metabolite (122). A similar relationship exists between isoniazid and acetaminophen. Isoniazid in its ability to induce P4502E1 can enhance the toxicity of acetaminophen (126).

Antifungal Agents

Griseofulvin

Griseofulvin is an antifungal agent that is a known experimental hepatotoxin producing in mice hepatic necrosis, hepatocellular carcinoma, and toxic porphyria as well as lesions similar to alcoholic hyaline (1, 5). Humans have developed porphyrinuria, and patients with acute intermittent porphyria in remission may relapse while taking the drug (1, 5). Only two unequivocal instances of liver injury from griseofulvin have been reported, both cholestatic. In one patient the cholestasis was prolonged. Other vague references to liver damage in humans have appeared (1, 5).

Ketoconazole (KCZ)

This drug is an imidazole derivative widely used as an antimycotic agent. Hepatocellular necrosis with jaundice has been recorded in about 0.1% of recipients, and abnormalities in biochemical tests without jaundice have been found in 8–12% of patients receiving the drug (127–129). Symptomatic hepatic reactions occur mainly within the first 1–6 months of treatment. Most reported instances of KCZ-induced liver injury have occurred in patients over 40 years old, especially women. Eosinophilia, rash, and fever have been uncommon, and the presumed mechanism of injury is metabolic idiosyncrasy. The most common histologic manifestation of KCZ-induced injury is diffuse hepatocellular necrosis with a predominance of zone 3 injury. Predominantly cholestatic injury also has been reported but is much less frequent than hepatocellular injury (127–129). A few instances of fulminant hepatocellular necrosis have been reported. Fatalities have ranged from 0% to 19% in published reports (127–128). Several ot her imidazole derivatives have been incriminated in instances of hepatocellular injury (5–130).

Flucytosine

Flucytosine is an antifungal agent that is converted to 5-fluorouracil. Transient elevations of aminotransferase levels occur in 10% of recipients, and occasional instances of frank hepatic necrosis have been reported (130, 131).

Antiviral Agents

Most antiviral agents do not pose serious hepatotoxic problems. *Idoxyuridine, xenelamine, vidarabine*, and *cytarabine* have all been reported to produce cholestatic jaundice as well as instances of hepatocellular injury (1, 5). *Zidovudine* has been reported to lead to cholestatic injury but rarely (132); also it has been incriminated in instances of severe steatosis (133). The related antiviral agent, *didanosine*, leads to a high incidence of abnormal aminotransferase levels (134) and has led to hepatic failure with microvesicular steatosis (135). Fialuridine, a nucleosidase that gave promise of being effective for treatment of chronic hepatitis B, proved to be a cause of severe liver disease during clinical trials. The injury was characterized by mitochondrial damage, lactic acid acidosis, and histologic changes that included microvesicular steatosis and necrosis (136).

Antiprotozoal Agents

Most agents used to treat malaria, amebiasis, and other protozoan disease have caused little overt injury. *Amodiaquine* has led to a number of instances of hepatocellular injury, several fatal (137). Quinine has been reported to lead to hepatic granulomas (138). Other antiprotozoan agents incriminated in hepatic injury are listed in Table 13.

Antihelminthic Agents

Chlorinated hydrocarbons and organic antimonials, long used as antihelmintics, are known to cause hepatic injury but have been abandoned largely (1). *Hycanthone*, which was used as treatment for schistosomiasis, was found to produce hepatocellular injury and, in some cases, fatal necrosis (1). *Piperazine* has been reported to cause acute liver injury, and *niclofolan* has been reported to lead to cholestatic jaundice in a patient with fascioliasis (1).

Thiabendazole has led to a few instances of prolonged intrahepatic cholestasis. Several have progressed to a chronic cholestatic syndrome that resembles primary biliary cirrhosis (1, 5, 130).

Drugs Used in Cardiovascular Disease

Calcium Channel Blocking Agents

Verapamil, nifedipine, and *diltiazem* have each been incriminated in cases of hepatocellular injury resembling alcoholic liver disease (Mallory bodies) (5, 130, 138a). These agents also have led to scattered instances of hepatocellular and cholestatic injury. Diltiazem has led to granulomas (5, 130). There are no useful data on the mechanisms involved.

Other Antihypertensive Agents

Methyldopa has been incriminated in many instances of acute hepatocellular injury and in a handful of cases of cholestatic injury (1, 5, 108, 130). In addition, this drug is one of the most prominent of the drugs involved in production of chronic active hepatitis (5, 108). The hepatic injury has been attributed to immunologic idiosyncrasy, although there is also evidence that the drug can be converted to a toxic metabolite (5).

The angiotensin-converting enzyme (ACE) inhibitors, *captopril, enalapril*, and *lisinopril*, have each been incriminated in hepatic injury. Most, though not all, of the captopril cases have had cholestatic jaundice (139). Enalapril has been considered responsible for instances of acute hepatocellular and cholestatic injury (140), and lisinopril has been incriminated in cases of hepatocellular injury (141). Immunologic idiosyncrasy has been inferred to be responsible for these cases.

Hydralazine and *dihydralazine* have led to a number of instances of hepatocellular disease as well as hepatic granulomas. The known ability to provoke a syndrome resembling systemic lupus erthyematosis supports the likelihood that immunologic mechanisms are responsible for the injury (5, 108).

Diuretics

Diuretic agents include a number of drugs that have been implicated in instances of jaundice. Almost all have been cholestatic (108, 130). An exception is the injury produced by *ticrynafen* (tienilic acid). A large number of cases of acute hepatocellular injury and a few with chronic hepatitis were reported shortly after the drug was introduced for clinical use in the United States, and the drug was abandoned (142). There is evidence supporting both immunologic (143) and metabolic idiosyncrasy (142) as the responsible mechanisms.

Adrenergic Blocking Agents

Debrisoquine is of great interest as a measure of activity of P4502D6 (18) but is not employed clinically and not implicated in hepatic injury. Several *beta-adrenergic blocking agents* have been incriminated in hepatic injury. *Labetelol* (144) and one of its four enantimorphs, *dilevalol*, (145) as well as *acebutolol* (146) and *metoprolol* (147) have been incriminated in hepatocellular injury. *Atenolol* has been implicated in an instance of cholestatic jaundice (148).

Antiarrhythmics

A variety of antiarrhythmic agents can produce hepatic injury. *Quinidine* has led to a number of cases of hepatocellular injury often accompanied by fever and granulomas, which are presumably due to immunologic idiosyncrasy (5). *Ajmaline* and its congeners, which are chemically similar to quinidine, produce hepatic injury, also accompanied by hallmarks of hypersensitivy (5). The injury, however, is cholestatic. Several other antiarrhythmics are listed in Table 14.

Antianginal Drugs

Amiodarone is a potent antiarrhythmic that at one time was used in the treatment of coronary disease. In common with two other drugs used to treat angina, it is a cause of an interesting and important form of drug-induced liver injury (5, 108, 149, 150).

Amiodarone, perhexiline maleate (PHM), and *4,4-diethylaminoethoxyhexestrol* (CORALGIL) are cationic, amphophilic compounds that produce *phospholipidosis* as a regular dose- and duration-dependent form of injury (149, 150). These three drugs also produce a lesion closely resembling alcoholic hepatitis as an uncommon idiosyncratic reaction. The phospholipidosis consists of engorgement of lysosomes with phospholipid (151). The alcoholic hepatitis–like disease (pseudoalcoholic liver disease [PSALD]) consists of Mallory body formation, usually accompanied by steatosis and, in some patients, cirrhosis (108, 150, 152). The phospholipidosis appears to be the result of binding within lysosomes of phospholipid drug complexes that are resistant to phospholipase activity as well as of inhibition of lysosomal phospholipase by the drug or metabolite (151). The PSALD develops in an estimated 1–3% of recipients of amiodarone who presumably have aberrant metabolism of the drug (149, 150). The PHM-induced PSALD occurs in patients whose ability to metabolize the drug is genetically impaired, an impairment marked by defective metabolism of debrosoquine (21). Although a similar genetic basis for CORALGIL or amiodarone-induced liver disease has not been demonstrated, the strikingly similar lesions produced by the three drugs suggests a similar pathogenesis.

The clinical manifestations include chronic liver disease as well as the effects of phospholipid deposits in the lung, thyroid, cornea, peripheral nerves, and skin (149–151). A variety of other amphophilic compounds can produce phospholipidosis *without* leading to the Mallory body lesion (108, 138a). There also are other agents (diethylstilbestrol, alcohol, griseofulvin in mice) that lead to the Mallory body lesion without phospholipidosis (Table 15). Apparently the two types of injury reflect a different pathogenesis.

Fibrates

Clofibrate, fenofibrate, and *gemfibrozil* are chemically related and have similar effects on blood lipids and the liver. All can produce elevated serum enzyme levels. Clofibrate-elevated aminotransferase levels have been attributed to muscle injury (153), but this drug also has led to instances of cholestatic (154) and granuloma hepatitis (155). *Fenofibrate* appears more prone to produce hepatic injury, having led to a number of instances of cholestasis (156–158) as well as of chronic hepatitis with autoimmune serologic markers (10). Gemfibrozil has led to little identified injury. However, all three drugs can lead to a striking degree of peroxisome proliferation in experimental animals, a phenomenon that has been linked to hepatocarcinogenesis (159). However, there is little induction of peroxisome proliferation in humans and no evidence of carcinogenesis by these agents.

Nicotinic Acid

This agent and its derivatives, also employed to treat hypercholesterolemia, have caused hepatic dysfunction in about one-third and jaundice in 3–5% of long-term recipients, especially of the delayed-absorption preparation (1, 5, 108). The demonstration of parenchymal degeneration and necrosis on biopsy and the high serum levels of aminotransferases indicate the hepatocellular nature of the damage. Indeed, massive necrosis has been reported (160, 161). Employment of large doses of nicotinic acid to treat psychiatric disease has led to jaundice with features of both hepatocellular injury and cholestasis (1, 5).

Hydroxymethylutaryl-Coenzyme A Reductase Inhibitors

Lovastin has been found to produce elevated aminotransferase levels to more than three times normal in 1–2% of recipients and to lesser elevations more frequently (162). Rarely, instances of overt hepatocellular injury have been reported (163). Simvastatin and provastatin appear to have similar effects (164).

Oncotherapeutic and Immunosuppressive Agents

The hepatic injury produced by oncotherapeutic agents is similar to that produced by other agents, for the most part. However, cirrhosis attributable to intrinsic drug toxicity, seen with methotrexate therapy, is not seen with most other drug-induced

TABLE 15. *Herbal products that can lead to hepatic injury*

Harbal product	Source	Active ingredient[2]	Ostensible effect	Hepatic injury[3]	Reference
Comfrey	Syphytum spp.	PAs	Nutritional supplement	VOD	192
Gordolobo yerba tea	Senecio spp.	PAs	Health aid	VOD	193
Mate tea	Ilex	PAs	Health aid	VOD	194
Chinese herb preparations					
Medicinal tea	Compositae spp.	?PAs[1]	Medicinal	VOD	195
"Chinese herbs"	"Fu-san-chi"	?Glycerrhyza	Medicinal	Hepatitis	196
Jin Bu Auan	Lycopodium serratum	?Levotetrahydro-palmitine	Anodyne hypnotic	"Hepatitis" Also microvesicular steatosis	197
Germander	Tencrium Chainaedrys	Furanoditerpinoids	Weight loss	Necrosis, zone 3	198
Chaparral leaf	Larria tridanta Larria divariatae ("Creosote bush," "Greasewood")	Nordihydroguaiaretic (NDGA) acid	Medicinal	Necrosis, zone 3	199–202
Mistletoe (plus other herbs)			Health aid	"Chronic" "Hepatitis"	203
Margosa oil	Azadirachta indica	Pulegone	Abortifacient	Microvesicular steatosis	130
Pennyroyal oil	Labiatae spp.	Isonpolegone	Also medicinal	Necrosis, microvesicular steatosis	130

[1] The content of this preparation are not clear. The entity is suggested in view of the character of the injury.
[2] PA = pyrrolizidine alkaloids.
[3] VOD = Veno occlusive disease.

hepatic injuries (165). Venoocclusive disease, the dramatic lesion characteristically produced by pyrrolizidine alkaloids, is produced by a number of cancer chemotherapy agents and protocols (108, 165, 166). Another unique drug-induced lesion is the ductal injury seen as a complication of pump infusion therapy of metastatic carcinoma to the liver, which leads to sclerosing cholangitis (108, 165–167).

Antimetabolites and Related Agents

Methotrexate has been found to produce hepatic steatosis, fibrosis, and even cirrhosis (165–171). Most prominent have been the reports of the development of liver disease in patients with psoriasis. While patients with rheumatoid arthritis seem less susceptible to the injury, they also can develop hepatic disease (168). The likelihood of liver damage in patients with psoriasis seems directly related to the duration of therapy and inversely related to the length of the interval between doses (168). Other important factors that have been especially emphasized are age, obesity, diabetes, and alcoholism (168). Indeed, it has become increasingly clear that in the absence of alcohol use and obesity or diabetes, methotrexate hepatotoxicity poses only a minor threat (172). Although there is clear progression of injury with increasing cumulative dose, the injury is usually minor.

Slight elevations of aminotransferase levels are often found for 1 or 2 days after a dose of methotrexate and may remain mildly abnormal; the mild elevations have little value in the recognition of hepatic injury (1, 5, 168). Liver biopsy is essential for identification of damage (170) and continues to be employed in the treatment of psoriasis with methotrexate. The lower doses of drug and lesser incidence of liver injury in patients with rheumatoid arthritis has led to a recommendation by Kremer et al. (170a) of a protocol not mandatory for defining the role of liver biopsy.

Antipyrimidines

Azauridine and azacitidine produce steatosis and hepatocellular necrosis in experimental animals (173). Cytarabine has been reported to produce both hepatocellular and cholestatic injury (1, 5, 108, 165, 166). 5-Fluorouracil can produce hepatic injury when given intravenously but not by the oral route (1).

Floxuridine is perhaps the most important of the antipyrimidines as a cause of hepatic injury. When administered by pump infusion into the hepatic artery for treatment of metastatic carcinoma of the liver, floxuridine can lead to sclerosing cholangitis (biliary sclerosis). The lesion has been ascribed to injury of the arterial supply of the ducts (167).

Antipurines

The important members of the antipurine groups are *6-mercaptopurine, azathioprine,* and *thioguanine.* 6-Mercaptopurine, an agent employed for the treatment of leukemia and to a lesser extent for immunosuppression, has been reported to produce hepatic injury in 6–40% of recipients (173). The injury is mixed. There is prominent cholestasis but predominant hepatocellular injury. Fatal hepatic necrosis has occurred. Possible potentiation of the hepatotoxicity of 6-mercaptopurine by doxorubin has been described (174).

6-Chloropurine has led to similar hepatic injury (173). Thioguanine has been reported to cause jaundice and venoocclusive disease (1, 166).

Azathioprine, a derivative of 6-mercaptopurine used mainly as an immunosuppressant, has been reported to cause cholestatic injury (1, 5, 165, 166). The drug has also been incriminated in a number of instances of hepatocellular injury and even of fatal hepatic necrosis (165, 166). An even more important observation is the recent suggestion that azathioprine can lead to vascular lesions, including venoocclusive disease, and peliosis hepatis (5, 165, 166). The mechanism of azathioprine-related hepatic injury is unknown. The suggestion that it may be related to the conversion of the drug to 6-mercaptopurine seems paradoxic, because some of the lesions are not seen with 6-mercaptopurine (1).

L-Asparaginase

This agent, although an enzyme, behaves like an antimetabolite (1, 5). By catalyzing the domination of asparagine, it apparently deprives the neoplastic cell of the amino acid, although some investigators have attributed hepatic injury to a contaminant of the enzyme rather than to asparagine deprivation. Large doses of L-asparaginase lead to hepatic necrosis (165).

Antineoplastic Antibiotics

Some antineoplastic antibiotics produce hepatic necrosis. Others cause steatosis, perhaps by a mechanism related to the antineoplastic effects (1). *Cyclosporine,* the antibiotic widely used as an immunosuppressive, appears to have dose-related cholestatic effects in experimental models (175) and in humans (176). In humans, the incidence of cholestatic injury has been estimated to be 50–60%. The cholestasis, however, is usually mild and poses little threat. *Interleukin-2,* the cytokine that has shown promise in oncotherapy, can lead to cholestasis (177). Etoposide can lead to hepatocellular injury (178).

Alkaloids

The vinca alkaloids, vincristine and vinblastine, lead to rare instances of hepatic injury in humans (165, 166). Coupled with irradiation, these agents can lead to hepatic necrosis.

Indicine-N-oxide can lead to venoocclusive disease and the associated zone 3 necrosis (130). This is to be expected because the drug is in the family of pyrrolizidine alkaloids, the classic cause of venoocclusive disease (1, 5, 130).

Alkylating Agents

The ethylenimine derivatives, mechlorethamine and melphalan, seem free of responsibility for hepatic injury (165). Chlorambucil and cyclophosphamide have been incriminated in instances of hepatocellular jaundice with necrosis (165, 166). Cholestatic jaundice has been attributed to an alkyl sulfonate (Busulfan) (165).

Nitrosoureas

Nitrosoureas have dose-related hepatotoxic effects in experimental animals. Of special note is the toxicity of dacarbazine. This cytostatic drug used as adjuvant therapy in patients with malignant melanoma has been associated with frequent transient aminotransferase elevations and has led to instances of acute venoocclusive disease (1, 5, 166).

Other Antitumor Agents

Urethane, formerly used to treat leukemia and multiple myeloma, is a known hepatotoxicant and hepatocarcinogen. It can produce venoocclusive disease with zone 3 necrosis and fibrosis (1, 5). The synthetic antiandrogenic drug *flutamide*, used in the treatment of prostatic cancer and other types of tumors, has been reported to cause instances of severe hepatocellular injury as well as cases of cholestasis (179).

Miscellaneous Drugs

A number of other agents are listed in Table 14. Several warrant special comment.

Oxphenisatin

Oxphenisatin, a component of many laxative preparations, is an established cause of acute and chronic liver injury. The acute injury resembles acute viral hepatitis, and the chronic injury resembles autoimmune chronic active hepatitis (CAH). Indeed, oxyphenisatin-induced injury is the prototype of drug-induced CAH. The drug has been banned in the United States but remains available in some parts of the world.

H_2 Blockers

The risk of hepatic injury with these drugs is very low. However, rare instances of liver injury, both cholestatic and hepatocellular, have been described in recipients of cimetidine and ranitidine (5).

Penicillamine

Rare instances of hepatic injury (predominantly cholestatic) have been attributed to this drug. In one patient the relationship of the penicillamine to the liver injury was established by return of the injury after rechallenge (1, 5, 180).

Disulfiram

Instances of hepatocellular injury have been reported in patients receiving disulfiram, usually during the first few weeks of use. Fatal cases have occurred. The mechanism appears to be immunologic idiosyncrasy (5, 130).

Vitamin A

Chronic vitamin A intoxication results from intake of excessive amounts of the agents. Daily doses five times the normal daily requirements have been reported to lead to liver injury. The injury consists of pericellular fibrosis, central vein sclerosis, or even cirrhosis. The clinical picture resembles that of cirrhosis (1, 5, 130).

Etretinate

A number of patients receiving this derivative of vitamin A for the treatment of psoriasis have developed hepatic abnormalities, including elevation of serum aminotransferase levels, periportal fibrosis, CAH, and even cirrhosis (180–184). There is some evidence to support a hypersensitivity reaction as the cause of etretinate injury, with the concomitant findings of eosinophilia and fever in some (182). Reappearance of etretinate-induced liver injury upon challenge has been demonstrated (182). Acitretin, a metabolite of etretinate, that is under investigation for treatment for psoriasis, has also been reported to cause severe hepatic injury that progressed to cirrhosis (185).

Cocaine

This agent of abuse, long known to produce serious systemic, cardiac, and neurologic injury, has been shown to produce hepatic injury in experimental animals and in humans (186, 187). In mice, cocaine leads to dose- and time-dependency toxicity manifested by elevated aminotransferase levels and by necrosis and steatosis (186). The necrosis has been described as zonal, but the zones involved have varied, according to the strain of mouse and the status of the cytochrome P450 system. In humans, the reported cases have shown coagulative necrosis involving zone 3, zone 2, or the entire acinus as well as microvesicular steatosis.

Herbal Remedies and Other Plant Toxins

A discussion of drug-induced hepatic injury would hardly be complete without reference to herbal drug employed as folk medicine, nontraditional and unconventional remedies, health aids, or nutritional supplements. The agents listed in Table 15 have received attention in the recent literature (188–203). These plant products tend to produce hepatocellular or mixed injury. Several of them lead to venoocclusive disease. Several are known toxicants with dose-related hepatotoxic effects (pyrrolizidine-alkaloids, pennyroyal, and margosia oil); others appear to reflect an idiosyncratic response of the involved individuals.

REFERENCES

1. Zimmerman HJ. *Hepatotoxicity: the adverse effects of drugs and other chemicals on the liver*. New York: Appleton-Century-Crofts, 1978.
2. Benhamou JP. Drug-induced hepatitis: clinical aspects. In Fillastre JP, ed. *Hepatotoxicity of drugs*. Rousen: University de Rousen, 1986:23–30.
3. Hoofnagle JH, Carithers RL, Shapiro C, Ascher N. Fulminant hepatic failure: summary of a workshop. *Hepatology* 1995;21:240–252.
4. Trey C, Davidson CS. The management of fulminant hepatic failure. *Prog Liver Dis* 1970;3:282–298.
5. Zimmerman HJ, Maddrey WC. Toxic and drug-induced hepatitis. In Schiff L, Schiff ER, eds. *Diseases of the liver*, 5th ed. Philadelphia: Lippincott, 1993:707–783.
6. Prescott LF, Leslie PJ, Padfield P. Side effects of benoxaprofen (letter). *Br Med J* 1982;284:1783–1784.
7. Lewis JH, Zimmerman HJ. Drug-induced liver disease. *Med Clin North Am* 1989;73:775–792.
8. Homberg JC, Stelly N, Andreis I, et al. A new antimitochondrial antibody (anti M6) in iproniazid-induced hepatitis. *Clin Exp Immunol* 1982;47:83–102.
9. Homberg JC, Andre C, Abulf N. A new anti-liver kidney microsome antibody (anti-LKM2) in tienilic acid induced hepatitis. *Clin Exp Immunol* 1984;55:561–570.
10. Bourdi M, Larrey D, Nataf J, et al. Anti-liver endoplasmic reticulum antibodies are directed against human cytochrome P4501A2. *J Clin Invest* 1990;85:1967–1973.
11. Homberg JC, Abuaf N, Helmg-Khali S, et al. Drug-induced hepatitis associated with anticytoplasmic organelle antibodies. *Hepatology* 1985;5:722–727.
12. Satoh H, Martin BM, Schulick AH, et al. Human anticytoplasmic antibodies in sera of patients with halothane-induced hepatitis are directed against a trifluoracetylated carboxylesterase. *Proc Nat Acad Sci USA* 1989;86:322–326.
13. Zimmerman HJ, Maddrey EC. Acetaminophen (Paracetamol) hepatotoxicity with regular intake of alcohol: analysis of instances of a therapeutic misadventure. *Hepatology* 1995;22:767–773.
14. Spielberg SP, Gordon GB, Blake DA, et al. Predisposition to phenytoin hepatotoxicity assessed in vitro. *N Engl J Med* 1981;305:722–727.
15. Kaplowitz N, Aw Ty, Simon FR, Stolz A. Drug-induced hepatotoxicity. *Ann Intern Med* 1986;104:826–839.
16. Mitchell JR, Thorgeirsson SS, Potter WZ, et al. Acetaminophen-induced hepatic injury: protective effect of glutathione in man and rationale for therapy. *Clin Pharmacol Ther* 1974;16:676–684.
17. Nelson SD. Molecular mechanism of the hepatotoxicity caused by acetaminophen. *Semin Liver Dis* 1990;10:267–278.
18. Watkins PB. Role of cytochromes P450 in drug metabolism and hepatotoxicity. *Semin Liver Dis* 1990;10:235–250.
19. Lieber CS. Interaction of alcohol with other drugs and nutrients: implication for the therapy of alcoholic liver disease. *Drugs (Suppl)* 1990;3:23–44.
20. Seeff LB, Cuccherini BA, Zimmerman HJ, et al. Acetaminophen hepatotoxicity in alcoholics: a therapeutic misadventure—a report of six cases and review of the literature. *Ann Intern Med* 1988; 104:399–404.

21. Morgan MY, Reshef R, Shah RR. Impaired oxidation of debrisoquine in patients with perhexiline liver injury. *Gut* 1984;25:1057–1064.
22. Benjamin SB, Ishak KG, Zimmerman HJ, et al. Phenylbutazone liver injury: a clinical-pathologic survey of 23 cases and review of the literature. *Hepatology* 1981;1:255–263.
23. Prescott LF. Paracetamol overdosage. *Drugs* 1983;25:290–314.
24. Keays R, Harrison PM, Wandon JA, et al. Intravenous acetylcysteine in paracetamol-induced fulminant hepatic failure: a prospective trial. *Br Med J* 1991;303:1026–1029.
25. Speeg KV Jr., Mitchell MC, Maldonado AL. Additive protection of cimetidine and N-acetylcysteine treatment against acetaminophen-induced hepatic necrosis in the rat. *J Pharmacol Exp Ther* 1985; 234:550–554.
26. Whitcomb DC, Block GD. Association of acetaminophen hepatotoxicity with fasting and ethanol use. *JAMA* 1994;72:1845–1850.
27. Price JF, Miller MG, Jollow DJ. Mechanism of fasting-induced potentiation of acetaminophen hepatotoxicity in the rat. *Biochem Pharmacol* 1987;36:427–453.
28. Lauterburg BH, Velez ME. Glutathione deficiency in alcoholics: risk factor for paracetamol. *Hepatology* 1988;29:1153–1157.
29. Zimmerman HJ. Effects of aspirin and acetaminophen on the liver. *Arch Intern Med* 1981;141:333–342.
30. Koff RS. Liver disease induced by nonsteroidal anti-inflammatory drugs. In Borda IT, Koff RS, eds. *NSAIDs: a profile of adverse effects*. St. Louis: Mosby Book, 1992:133–146.
31. Halpin TJ. Reye's syndrome and medication use. *JAMA* 1982;248:687–691.
32. Starko KM, Mullick FG. Hepatic and cerebral pathology findings in children with fatal salicylate intoxication: further evidence for a relation between salicylate and Reye's syndrome. *Lancet* 1983;1:326–328.
33. Benjamin SB, Goodman ZD, Ishak KG, et al. The morphologic spectrum of halothane-induced hepatic injury: analysis of 77 cases. *Hepatology* 1985;5:1163–1171.
34. Tucker SC, Patterson TE. Hepatitis and halothane sniffing. *Ann Intern Med* 1974;80:667–669.
35. Varma RR, Whitesell RC, Iskandarani MM. Halothane hepatitis without halothane: role of inapparent circuit contamination and its prevention. *Hepatology* 1985;5:1159–1163.
36. Klatskin G, Kimberg DV. Recurrent hepatitis attributable to halothane in an anesthetist. *N Engl J Med* 1969;280:515–522.
37. Neuberger J, Williams R. Halothane anaesthesia and liver damage. *Br Med J* 1984;89:1135–1139.
38. Satoh H, Fukuda Y, Anderson DK, et al. Immunological studies on the mechanism of halothane-induced hepatotoxicity: immunohistochemical evidence of trifluoroacetylated hepatocytes. *J Pharmacol Exp Ther* 1985;233:857–862.
39. Joshi PH, Conn HO. The syndrome of methoxyflurane-associated hepatitis. *Ann Intern Med* 1974;80:395–401.
40. Lewis JH, Zimmerman HJ, Ishak KG, Mullick FG. Enflurane hepatotoxicity: a clinico-pathologic study of 24 cases. *Ann Intern Med* 1983;98:984–992.
41. Brunt EM, White H, Marsh JW, et al. Fulminant hepatic failure after repeated exposure to isoflurane anesthesia: a case report. *Hepatology* 1991;13:1017–1021.
42. Zimmerman HJ. Even isoflurane. *Hepatology* 1991;13:1251–1253.
43. Zimmerman HJ. Clinical and laboratory manifestation of hepatotoxicity. *Ann NY Acad Sci* 1963;104:954–987.
44. Degott C, Feldman G, Larrey D, et al. Drug-induced prolonged cholestasis in adults: a histological semiquantative study demonstrating progressive ductopenia. *Hepatology* 1992;15:244–251.
45. Watson RG, Olomic A, Clements D, et al. A proposed mechanism for chlorpromazine jaundice-defective hepatic sulfoxidation combined with rapid hydroxylation. *J Hepatol* 1988;7:72–78.
46. Rosenblum LE, Korn RJ, Zimmerman HJ. Hepatocellular jaundice as a complication of iproniazid therapy. *Arch Intern Med* 1960;105:583–93.
47. Mitchell JR, Nelson SD, Thorgeirson SS, et al. Metabolic activation: biochemical basis for many drug-induced liver injuries. *Progr Liver Dis* 1976;5:259.
48. Sheikh KH, Nies AS. Trazodone and intrahepatic cholestasis (letter). *Ann Intern Med* 1983;99: 572.
49. Zimmerman HJ, Ishak KG. Valproate-induced hepatic injury: analyses of 23 fatal cases. *Hepatology* 1982;2:591–597.
50. Dreifuss FE, Langer DH, Moline KA, Maxwell JE. Valproic acid hepatic fatalities. II. US experience since 1984. *Neurology* 1989;39:201–207.

51. Powell-Jackson PR, Jackson JM, Williams R, et al. Hepatotoxicity to sodium valproate: a review. *GUT* 1984;25:673–681.
52. Eadie MJ, Hooper WD, Dickinson RG. Valproate-associated hepatotoxicity and its biochemical mechanisms. *Med Toxicol* 1988;3:85–106.
53. Appleton RE, Farrell K, Applegarth DA, et al. The high incidence of valproate hepatotoxicity in infants may relate to familial metabolic defects. *Can J Neurol Sci* 1990;17:145–148.
54. Williams SJ, Ruppin DC, Grierson JM, Farrell GC. Carbamazepine hepatitis: the clinicopathological spectrum. *J Gastroenterol Hepatol* 1986;1:159–168.
55. Forbes GM, Jeffrey GP, Shilkin KB, Reed WD. Carbamazepine hepatotoxicity: another case of the vanishing bile duct syndrome. *Gastroenterology* 1992;102:1385–1388.
56. Zimmerman HJ. Hepatic injury associated with nonsteroidal anti-inflammatory drugs. In: Lewis AJ, Furst DE, eds. *Nonsteroidal anti-inflammatory drugs: mechanism and clinical uses*, 2nd ed., New York: Marcel Dekker 1994:171–194.
57. Paulus HE. FDA arthritis advisory committee meeting. *Arthritis Rheum* 1982;25:1124.
58. Tarazi E, Harter JG, Zimmerman HJ, et al. Sulindac-associated hepatic injury: analysis of 91 cases reported to the FDA. *Gastroenterology* 1993;104:569–574.
59. Bravo JF, Jacobson MP, Mertens G. Fatty liver and pleural effusion with ibuprofen therapy. *Ann Intern Med* 1977;87:200–201.
60. Purcell P, Henry D, Melville G. Diclofenac hepatitis. *GUT* 1991;32:1381.
61. Banks T, Zimmerman HJ, Harter J, Ishak KG. Diclofenac-associated hepatic injury analysis of 181 cases. *Hepatology* 1995;22:820–827.
62. Dux S, Groslop I, Gartz M, Rosenfeld JB. Anaphylactic shock induced by diclofenac (letter). *Br Med J* 1983;286:1861.
63. Lewis JH. Hepatic toxicity of nonsteroidal anti-inflammatory drugs. *Clin Pharmacol* 1984;3:128–138.
64. Furet W, Breteau M. Accidents hépatique à la clometacine. *Therapie* 1984;39:523–529.
65. Goldfarb G, Pessayre D, Boisseau C, et al. Hépatite à la clometacine. *Gastroenterol Clin Biol* 1979;3:537.
66. Pessayre D, Degos F, Feldman G, et al. Chronic active hepatocellular and giant multinucleated hepatocytes in adults treated with clometacin. *Digestion* 1981;22:66–72.
67. Howrie DL, Gartner JC Jr. Gold-induced hepatotoxicity: case report and review of the literature. *J Rheumatol* 1982;9:727–730.
68. Schapira D, Nahir M, Scharf Y, Pollack S. Cholestatic jaundice induced by gold salts: treatment, clinical and immunological aspects. *J Rheumatol* 1984;11:843.
69. David P, Hughes GRV. A serial study of eosinophilia and raised IgE antibodies during gold therapy. *Ann Rheum Dis* 1975;34:203.
70. Fleischner GM, Morecki R, Hanaichi T, et al. Light and electron microscopical study of a case of gold salt-induced hepatotoxicity. *Hepatology* 1991;14:422–425.
71. Watkins PB, Schade R, Mills AD, et al. Fatal hepatic necrosis associated with parenteral gold therapy. *Dig Dis Sci* 1988;33:1025–1029.
72. Klein NC, Magida MG. Propoxyphene (Darvon) hepatotoxicity. *Dig Dis Sci* 1971;16:467–469.
73. Utili R, Boitnott JK, Zimmerman HJ. Dantrolene-associated hepatic injury: incidence and character. *Gastroenterology* 1977;72:610–616.
74. Powers BJ, Cattou EL, Zimmerman HJ. Chlorozoxazone hepatotoxicity: an analysis of 21 identified or presumed cases. *Arch Intern Med* 1986;146:1183–1186.
75. Rank JM, Olson RC. Reversible cholestatic hepatitis caused by acetohexamide. *Gastroenterology* 1989;96:1607–1608.
76. Ishak KG, Zimmerman HJ. Hepatotoxic effects of the anabolic androgenic steroids. *Semin Liver Dis* 1987;7:230–236.
77. Overly WL, Dankoff JA, Luang BK, Singh ND. Androgens and hepatocellular carcinoma in an athlete (letter). *Ann Intern Med* 1984;100:158–159.
78. Henderson BE, Preston-Martin S, Edmondson HA, et al. Hepatocellular carcinoma and oral contraceptives. *Br J Cancer* 1983;48:437–440.
79. Neuberger J, Forman D, Doll R, Williams JR, et al. Oral contraceptives and hepatocellular carcinoma. *Br Med J* 1986;292:1355–1357.
80. Mays ET, Christopher W. Hepatic tumors induced by sex steroids. *Semin Liver Dis* 1984;4:147–157.
81. Baum JK, Holtz F, Bobkstein JJ, Klein EW. Possible association between benign hepatomas and oral contraceptives. *Lancet* 1973;2:926–929.

82. Ishak KG, Rabin L. Benign tumors of the liver. *Med Clin North Am* 1975;59:995–1013.
83. Gordon SC, Reddy KR, Livingstone AS, et al. Resolution of a contraceptive-steroid induced adenoma with subsequent evolution into hepatocellular carcinoma. *Ann Intern Med* 1986;105:547–549.
84. Marks WH, Thompson N, Appleman H. Failure of hepatic adenomas (HCA) to regress after discontinuance of oral contraceptives. *Ann Surg* 1988;208:190–193.
85. Edmondson HA, Henderson B, Benton B. Liver-cell adenomas associated with use of oral contraceptives. *N Engl J Med* 1976;294:470–472.
86. Poulsen H, Winkler K. Liver disease with periportal sinusoidal dilation. *Digestion* 1973;8:441–446.
87. Zimmerman HJ, Lewis JH. Drug-induced cholestasis. *Med Toxicol.* 1987;2:112–160.
88. Valla D, Le MG, Poynard TM, et al. Risk of hepatic vein thrombosis in relation to recent use of oral contraceptives: a case control study. *Gastroenterology* 1986;90:807–811.
88a. Phillips MJ, Powell S, Oda M. Biology of disease mechanism of cholestasis. *Labor Invest* 1986;54:593–608.
89. Kreek MJ. Female sex steroids and cholestasis. *Semin Liver Dis* 1987;7:8–23.
90. Anthony PP. Liver tumours. *Bailliere's Clin Gastroenterol* 1988;2:501–522.
91. Edmondson HA, Reynolds TB, Henderson B, Benton B. Regression of liver cell adenomas associated with oral contraceptives. *Ann Intern Med* 1977;86:180–182.
92. Boue F, Caffin B, Delfraissy J-F. Danazol and cholestatic hepatitis. *Ann Intern Med* 1986;105:139–140.
93. Pearson K, Zimmerman HJ. Danazol and liver damage (letter). *Lancet* 1980;1:645.
94. Fermard JP, Lervy Y, Bouscary D, et al. Danazol-induced hepatocellular adenoma. *Am J Med* 1990;88:529.
95. Weill BJ, Menkes CSl, Cormier C, et al. Hepatocellular carcinoma after danazol therapy. *J Rheumatol* 1988;15:1447–1450.
96. Burette A, Finet C, Prigogine T, et al. Acute hepatic injury associated with minocycline. *Arch Intern Med* 1984;144:1491–1492.
96a. Herzog D, Hajoui O, Russi P, Alvarez F. Study of immune reactively of minocycline induced chronic active hepatitis. *Dig Sic Sci* 1997;42:1100–1103.
96b. Malcolm A, Heap TR, Eckstein RP, Lunzer MR. Minocycline induced liver injury. *Am J Gastroenterol* 1996;91:1641–1643.
96c. Gough A, Chapman S, Wagstaff K, et al. Minocycline induced autoimmune hepatitis and systemic lupus erythematosus-like syndrome. *BMJ* 1996;312:169–172.
97. Gholson CF, Warren GH. Fulminant hepatic failure associated with intravenous erythromycin lactobionate. *Arch Intern Med* 1990;150:215–216.
98. Zimmerman HJ, Kendler J, Libber S, Lukacs L. Hepatocyte suspensions as a model for demonstration of drug hepatotoxicity. *Biochem Pharmacol* 1974;23:2187–2189.
99. Kendler J, Anuras S, Laborda O, Zimmerman HJ. Perfusion of the isolated rat liver with erthromycin estolate and other derivatives. *Proc Soc Exp Biol Med* 1972;139:1272–1275.
100. Ticktin HE, Zimmerman HJ. Hepatic dysfunction and jaundice in patients receiving triacetyloleandomycin. *N Engl J Med* 1962;267:964–968.
101. Fevery J, Van Steenbergen W, Desmet V, et al. Severe intrahepatic cholestasis due to the combined intake of oral contraceptives and triacetyloleandomycin. *Acta Clin Belg* 1983;38:242–246.
102. Enat R, Pollack S, Ben-Arieh Y, et al. Cholestatic jaundice caused by cloxacillin: macrophage inhibition factor test in preventing rechallenge with hepatotoxic drugs. *Br Med J* 1980;2:982–983.
103. Turner IB, Eckstein RP, Riley JW, Lunzer MR. Prolonged hepatic cholestasis after flucloxacillin therapy. *Med J Aust* 1989;51:701–705.
104. Dawset JF, Gillow T, Heagerty, et al. Amoxicillin/clavulanic acid (Augmentin)-induced intrahepatic cholestasis. *Dig Dis Sci* 1989;34:1290–1293.
105. Reddy KR, Brillant P, Schiff ER, et al. Amoxicillin-clavulanate potassium-associated cholestasis. *Gastroenterology* 1989;96:1135–1141.
106. Stricker BH, Van den Broek JW, Keuning J, et al. Cholestasis hepatitis due to antibacterial combination of amoxicillin and clavulanic acid (Augmentin). *Dig Dis Sci* 1989;34:1576.
107. Hanger HM Jr, Gutman AB. Post-arsphenamine jaundice apparently due to obstruction of intrahepatic biliary tract. *JAMA* 1940;115:263.
108. Zimmerman HJ. Update of hepatotoxicity due to classes of drugs in common clinical use: nonsteroidal, anti-inflammatory drugs, antibiotics, antihypertensives and cardiac and psychotropic agents. *Semin Liver Dis* 1990;10:322–328

109. Magee G, Bokhari S, Layden TJ. Cholestatic hepatitis from use of sulfanilamide vaginal cream. *Dig Dis Sci* 1982;27:1044.
110. Oliver RM, Rickenbach MA, Thomas MR, Neville E. Intrahepatic cholestasis associated with co-trimoxazole. *Br J Clin Pract* 1987;41:975.
111. Munoz SJ, Martinez-Hernandez A, Maddrey WC. Intrahepatic cholestasis and phospholipidosis associated with the use of trimethoprim-sulfamethoxazole. *Hepatology* 1990;12:342–347.
112. Tanner AR. Hepatic cholestasis induced by trimethoprim. *Br Med J* 1987;293:1072–1073.
113. Alberti-Flor JJ, Hernandes ME, Ferrer JP. Fulminant liver failure and pancreatitis associated with the use of sulfamethoxazole-trimethoprim. *Gastroenterology* 1989;84:1577–1579.
114. Olsen VV, Loft S, Christensen KD. Serious reactions during malaria prophylaxis with pyrimethamine-sulfadoxine. *Lancet* 1982;2:994–995.
115. Zitelli BJ, Alexander J, Taylor S, et al. Fatal hepatic necrosis due to pyrimethamine-sulfadoxine (Fansidar). *Ann Intern Med* 1987;106:393–395.
116. Lazar HP, Murphy RL, Phair JP. Fansidar and hepatic granulomas. *Ann Intern Med* 1985;102:722.
117. Stricker BHC, Blotz APR, Class FHJ, et al. Hepatic injury associated with the use of nitrofurans: a clinicopathological study of 52 reported cases. *Hepatology* 1988;8:599–608.
118. Sharp JR, Ishak KG, Zimmerman HJ. Chronic active hepatitis and severe hepatic necrosis associated with nitrofurantoin. *Ann Intern Med* 1980;92:14–19.
119. Hatoff DE, Cohen M, Schweigert BF, Talbert WM. Nitrofurantoin: another cause of drug-induced chronic active hepatitis ? A report of a patient with HLA-B antigen. *Am J Med* 1979;67:117–121.
120. Black M, Mitchell JR, Zimmerman HJ, et al. Isoniazid-associated hepatitis in 114 patients. *Gastroenterology* 1975;69:289–302.
121. Maddrey WC. Isoniazid-induced liver disease. *Semin Liver Dis* 1981;1:129–133.
122. Pessayre D, Bentata M, Degott C, et al. Isoniazid-rifampin fulminant hepatitis: a possible consequence of the enhancement of isoniazid hepatotoxic by enzyme induction. *Gastroenterology* 1977;72:284–289.
123. Kopanoff DE, Snider DE Jr, Caras GJ. Isoniazid-related hepatitis: a US Public Health Service Cooperative Surveillance Study. *Am Rev Respir Dis* 1978;117:991–1001.
124. Mitchell JR, Thorgeirsson UP, Black M, et al. Increased incidence of isoniazid hepatitis in rapid acetylators: possible reaction to hydrazine metabolites. *Clin Pharmacol Ther* 1975;18:70–79.
125. Scheuer P, Summerfield JA, Lal S. Rifampicin hepatitis: a clinical and histological study. *Lancet* 1974;1:421–425.
126. Burk RF, Hill KE, Hunt RW Jr, Martin AE. Isoniazid potentiation of acetaminophen hepatotoxicity in the rat and 4-methylpyrazol inhibition of it. *Res Comm Chem Pathol Pharmacol* 1990;69:115–118.
127. Stricker BH, Blok AP, Bronkhorst FB, Van Parys GE. Ketoconazole-associated hepatic injury: a clinicopathological study of 55 cases. *J Hepatol* 1986;3:399–406.
128. Lake-Bakaar G, Scheuer PJ, Sherlock S. Hepatic reactions associated with ketoconazole in the United Kingdom. *Br Med J* 1987;294:419–422.
129. Lewis JH, Zimmerman HJ, Benson GD, Ishak KG. Hepatic injury associated with ketoconazole therapy. *Gastroenterology* 1984;86:503–513.
130. Stricker BH. *Drug-induced hepatic injury*. Amsterdam: Elsevier, 1992.
131. Record CO, Skinner JM, Sleight P, Speller DCE. Candida endocarditis treated with 5-fluorocytosine. *Br Med J* 1971;1:262–264.
132. Dubin G, Braffman MN. Zidovudine-induced hepatotoxicity. *Ann Intern Med* 1989;110:85–86.
133. Freiman JP, Helfet RE, Hamrell MR, Stein DS. Hepatomegaly with severe steatosis in HIV- seropositive patients. *AIDS* 1993;7:395.
134. Lambert JS, Seidlin M, Reichman RC, et al. 2′,3′-Dideoxyinosine (ddI) in patients with acquired immunodeficiency syndrome of AIDS-related complex. *N Engl J Med* 1990;322:1333–1340.
135. Lai KK, Gang DL, Zawacki JK, Cosley TP. Fulminant hepatic failure associated with 2,3′-dideoxyuridine (ddI). *Ann Intern Med* 1991;115:283–284.
136. Kleiner D. Personal communication, 1994.
137. Larrey D, Castot A, Pessayre D. Amodiaquine-induced hepatitis: a report of seven cases. *Ann Intern Med* 1986;104:801–803.
138. Katz B, Weeth M, Chopra S. Quinine-induced granulomatous hepatitis. *Br Med J* 1983;286:26–54.
138a. Zimmerman HJ, Ishak KG. Non-alcoholic steatohepatitis and other forms of pseudoalcoholic liver disease. In: Hall, P, ed. *Alcoholic liver disease pathology and pathogenesis*, 2nd ed. London: Edward Arnold, 1995:165–198.

139. Rahmat J, Gelfand RL, Gelfand M, et al. Captopril-associated cholestatic jaundice. *Ann Intern Med* 1985;102:56–58.
140. Rosellini SR, Costa PL, Gaudio M, et al. Hepatic injury related to enalapril (letter). *Gastroenterology* 1989;97:810.
141. Larrey D, Babany G, Bernau J, et al. Fulminant hepatitis after lisinopril administration. *Gastroenterology* 1990;99:1832–1834.
142. Zimmerman HJ, Lewis HJ, Ishak KG, Maddrey WC. Ticrynafen-associated hepatic injury:analysis of 340 cases. *Hepatology* 1984;4:315–323.
143. Neuberger J, Williams R. Immune reactions in tienilic acid associated hepatotoxicity. *Gut* 1989;30:515–518.
144. Clarke JA, Tanner LA, Zimmerman HJ. Labetotol and hepatocellular reaction. *Ann Intern Med.* 1990;113:210–213.
145. Vasca AJ, Victorino M, Vicotirino RMN. Hypersensitivity immune reaction as a mechanism for dilevol-associated hepatitis. *Ann Pharmacotherapy* 1992;26:924–926.
146. Tanner LA, Bosco LA, Zimmerman HJ. Hepatic toxicity after acebutolol therapy. *Ann Intern Med* 1989;111:533–534.
147. Larrey D, Henrion J, Heller F, et al. Metoprolol-induced hepatitis: rechallenge and drug-oxidation phenotyping. *Ann Intern Med* 1988;108:67–68.
148. Schwartz MS. Atenolol-associated cholestasis. *Am J Gastroenterol* 1989;184:108-1086.
149. Lewis JH, Ranard RC, Caruso A, et al. Amiodarone hepatotoxicity: prevalence and clinicopathologic correlation among 104 patients. *Gastroenterology* 1989;86:503–513.
150. Lewis JH, Mullick F, Ishak KG, et al. Histopathologic analysis of suspected amiodarone hepatotoxicity. *Hum Pathol* 1990;21:59–67.
151. Heath MF, Costa-Jussa FR, Jacobs JM, Jacobson W. The induction of pulmonary phospholipidosis and the inhibition of lysosomal phospholipases by amiodarone. *Br J Exp Pathol* 1985;66:391–397.
152. Pessayre D, Bichara M, Feldmann G, et al. Perhexiline maleate-induced cirrhosis. *Gastroenterology* 1979;76:170–177.
153. Smith AL, Macfie WG, Oliver MF. Clofibrate, serum enzymes and muscle pain. *Br Med J* 1970;2:86.
154. Valdes M, Jacobs WH. Intrahepatic cholestasis following the use of Atromid-S. *Am J Gastroenterol* 1976;66:69–71.
155. Pierce EH, Chesler DL. Possible association of granulomatous hepatitis with clofibrate therapy (letter). *N Engl J Med* 1978;299:314.
156. Vachon JM. Hépatite due au procetofene. *Nouv Presse Med* 1980;9:2740.
157. Aron E, Metman EH, Bougnoux P. Hepatite due au procetofene? Un case. *Nouv Presse Med* 1979;8:783.
158. Massen H, Furet Y. Hpatite au fenofibrate. *Cah Anesthesiol* 1986;34:249–250.
159. Popp JA, Marsman DS, Cattley RC, Conway JG. Hepatocarcinogenecity and peroxisome proliferation. *CIIT Activity* 1989;9:1–3.
160. Mullin GE, Greenson JK, Mitchell MC, et al. Fulminant hepatic failure after ingestion of sustained-released nicotinic acid. *Ann Intern Med* 1989;111:253–255.
161. Clementz GL, Holmes AW. Nicotinic acid induced fulminant hepatic failure. *J Clin Gastroenterol* 1987;5:582–584.
162. Tobert J, Shear CL, Chramos AN, Mantell GE. Clinical experience with lovastatin. *Am J Cardiol* 1990;65:23F–26F.
163. Raveh D, Arnon R, Israeli A, Eisenberg S. Lovastatin-induced hepatitis. *Isr J Med Sci* 1992;28:101–102.
164. Ballare M, Campanini M, Catania E, et al. Acute cholestatic during simvastatin administration. *Recent Prog Med* 1991;82:233–235.
165. Zimmerman HJ. Hepatotoxic effect of oncotherapeutic agents. *Prog Liver Dis* 1986;8:621–642.
166. Szol M, Oknuma T, Holland JF. Hepatic toxicity of drugs used for hematologic neoplasms. *Semin Liver Dis* 1987;7:237–256.
167. Ludwig J, Kim CH, Wiesner RH, Krom RA. Floxuridine-induced sclerosing cholangitis: an ischemic cholangiopathy? *Hepatology* 1989;9:215–218.
168. Lewis JH, Schiff ER. Methotrexate-induced chronic liver injuries: guidelines for detection and prevention. *Am J Gastroenterol* 1988;83:1337–1345.
169. Nyfors A, Poulsen H. Liver biopsies from psoriatics related to methotrexate therapy. I. Finding before and after nonmethotrexate therapy in 88 patients. *Acta Pathol Microbiol Scand Sec II* 1976;84:262–270.

170. Zaccharie H, Bjerring M. Methotrexate-induced liver cirrhosis: a follow-up. *Dermatologica* 1987;175:178–182.
170a. Kremer JM, Le RG, Tolman KG. Liver histology in rheumatoid arthritis patients receiving long-term methotrexate therapy: a prospective study with baseline and sequential biopsy samples. *Arthritis Rheum* 1989;32:121–127.
171. Gilbert SC, Klintman G, Menter A, Silverman A. Methotrexate induced cirrhosis requiring liver transplantation in three patients with psoriasis. *Arch Intern Med* 1990;150:889–891.
172. Kaplan MM. Methotrexate treatment of chronic cholestatic liver diseases: friend or foe. *Q J Med* 1989;72(NS):757–761.
173. Ellison RR, Silver RT, Ebgle RL Jr. Comparative study of 6-chloropurine and 6-mercaptopurine in acute leukemia in adults. *Ann Intern Med* 1989;51:322–328.
174. Rodriguez V, Bodey GP, McCredie, et al. Combination 6-mercaptopurine and adriamycin in refractory adult acute leukemia. *Clin Pharmacol Ther* 1975;18:462–466.
175. Stacey NH, Lotecka B. Inhibition of taurocholate and ouabain transport in isolated rat hepatocytes by cyclosporin A. *Gastroenterology* 1988;95:780–786.
176. Kassianides C, Nussenblatt R, Palestine AG, et al. Liver injury from cyclosporine A. *Dig Dis Sci* 1990;35:693–697.
177. Fisher B, Keenan AM, Garra BS, et al. Interleukin-2 induced profound, reversible cholestasis: a detailed analysis in treated patients. *J Clin Oncol* 1989;7:1852–1862.
178. Tran A, Housset C, Boboc B, et al. Etoposide (VP 16-213) induced hepatitis: report of three cases following standard dose treatment. *J Hepatol* 1991;12:36–39.
179. Moller S, Iverson P, Franzmann MD. Flutamide-induced liver failure. *J Hepatol* 1990;10:346–349.
180. Langan MN, Thomas P. Penicillamine-induced liver disease. *Am J Gastroenterol* 1987;82:1318–1319.
181. Camuto P, Schupack J, Orbuch P. Long-term effects of etretinate on the liver in psoriasis. *Am J Surg Pathol* 1987;11:30–37.
182. Khouri MR, Saul SH, Dlugosz AA, Soloway RD. Hepatocanalicular injury associated with vitamin A derivative etretinate: an idiosyncratic hypersensitivity reaction. *Dig Dis Sci* 1987;32:1207–1211.
183. Weiss V, West DP, Ackerman R, Robinson LA, et al. Hepatotoxic reactions in a patient treated with etretinate. *Arch Dermatol* 1984;120:104–106.
184. Weiss V, Layden T, Spinowitz A, et al. Chronic active hepatitis associated with etretinate therapy. *Br J Dermatol* 1985;112:591–597.
185. Van Ditzhuijsen TJM. Severe hepatotoxic reaction with progression to cirrhosis after use of a novel retinoid (acitretin). *Hepatology* 1990;11:185–188.
186. Mallat A, Dhumeaux D. Cocaine and the liver. *J Hepatol* 1991;12:272–278.
187. Silva MO, Roth D, Reddy KR, et al. Hepatic dysfunction accompanying acute cocaine intoxication. *J Hepatol* 1991;12:312–315.
188. Rosenburg DM, Kessler RC, Foster C, et al. Unconventional medicine in the United States. *N Engl J Med* 1993;28:246–252.
189. Larrey D. Liver involvement in the course of phototherapy. *Presse Med* 1994;23:691–692.
190. Koff RA. Herbal hepatotoxicity: revisiting a dangerous alternative. *JAMA* 1995;273:488.
191. Kane JA, Kane SP, Jain S. Hepatitis induced by traditional Chinese herb: possible toxic components. *Gut* 1995;35:146–147.
192. Ridker PM, Ohkuma S, McDermott WV, Trey C, Huxtable RJ. Hepatic veno-occlusive disease associated with the consumption of pyrrolizidine containing dietary supplement. *Gastroenterology* 1985;88:1050–1054.
193. Stillman AE, Huxtable R, Consroe P, et al. Hepatic veno-occlusive disease due to pyrrolizidone (Senecio) poisoning in Arizona. *Gastroenterology* 1977;73:349–352.
194. Mc Gee JO'D, Patrick RS, Wood CB, Blumgart LH. A case of veno-occlusive disease of the liver in Britain associated with herbal tea consumption. *J Clin Pathol* 1976;29:788–794.
195. Kumana CR, Ng M, Lin HJ, et al. Herbal tea induced hepatic veno-occlusive diseases: quantification of toxic alkaloid exposure in adults. *Gut* 1985;26:101–104.
196. Davies EG, Pollork J, Steal HM. Chronic herb for eczema (letter). *Lancet* 1990;336:177.
197. Woolf GM, Petrovic LM, Rojter SE, et al. Acute hepatitis associated with the Chinese herbal product Jin Bu Huan. *Ann Intern Med* 1994;121:729–735.
198. Larrey D, Vial T, Pauwels A, et al. Hepatitis after germander (*Teucrium chamaedrys*) administration: another instance of herbal medicine hepatotoxicity. *Ann Intern Med* 1992;117:129–132.
199. Katz M, Saibil F. Herbal hepatitis: subacute hepatic necrosis secondary to chaparral leaf. *J Clin Gastroenterol* 1990;2:203–206.

200. Clark F, Reed R. Chaparral-induced hepatitis: California and Texas, 1992. *Morbidity and Mortality Weekly Reports* 1992;41:812–814.
201. Alderman S, Kailas S, Goldfard S, et al. Cholestatic hepatitis after ingestion of chaparral leaf: confirmation by endoscopic retrograde cholangiopancreatography and liver biopsy. *J Clin Gastroenterol* 1994;19:242–247.
202. Gordon DW, Rosenthal G, Hart J, et al. Chaparral ingestion: the broadening spectrum of liver injury caused by herbal medications. *JAMA* 1990;273:489–490.
203. Harvey J, Colin-Jones DG. Mistletoe hepatitis. *Br Med J* 1981;282:186–187.

Toxicology of the Liver, 2nd ed.,
Edited by Gabriel L. Plaa and William R. Hewitt
Copyright © 1998 Taylor & Francis

2

Morphologic Characteristics of Chemical-Induced Hepatotoxicity in Laboratory Rodents

Paul M. Newberne

*Massachusetts Institute of Technology, Cambridge, MA 02139 and
Boston University School of Medicine, Boston, MA 02118*

James W. Newberne

University of Cincinnati College of Medicine, Cincinnati, OH 45267-0056

Numerous conferences, workshops, and reports dating back for more than a quarter of a century (1–8) have not resolved all of the questions regarding the most appropriate approach to evaluate the safety of drugs and chemicals in laboratory rodents. However, considerations described below, together with accurate diagnoses, can help to achieve this goal. In many cases the rodent liver is the primary target of injury from ingested drugs and other chemicals. The intent of this chapter is to introduce the reader to the complexity of the responses of the liver to injury and to aid in the recognition and interpretation of morphologic changes that can occur. Table 1 lists some components that impinge on the results and analyses of data from toxicity tests using rodents.

The selection of an appropriate species and strain of rodent for safety evaluation of chemicals will determine to a considerable degree the outcome of the study. Rats and mice have varying incidences of spontaneous lesions of the liver, which can complicate the interpretation of the results. It is important to know the historical background of these lesions as well as the incidence of such lesions in contemporary controls. In addition, the Syrian golden hamster has a very low incidence of spontaneous liver lesions, including tumors, and now that amyloidosis is under control, this species is also a useful test animal.

A large body of information is available on the liver disease profile of the Fischer 344 rat and the B6C3F1 hybrid mouse (9). Similar data are available on the second most widely used strain of rat, the Sprague-Dawley, favored by many pharmaceutical companies, as shown in Tables 2 and 3. Data in these tables illustrate the significance of spontaneous liver tumors (10, 11).

The diet and nutritional status of the test animal are two of the most important factors in toxicity studies; they are also often ignored (12–14). Natural food constituents in commercial diets (15) vary in quality and quantity; they sometimes contain toxic materials and estrogenic substances (16) indigenous to the plants used as protein sources. Oil seeds (soybean meal, peanut meal, cottonseed meal), major components of these diets, vary in protein quality and quantity; they may contain toxic principles such as aflatoxin and other mycotoxins and heavy metals. Many of these can have adverse effects on the results of safety tests, as can the effects of obesity, often seen with some strains of rats on long-term studies (12–14).

The dosing schedule of a compound depends on several factors, including the means by which the maximum tolerated dose (MTD), the highest dose to be used in

TABLE 1. *Factors influencing results of toxicity testing*

1. Selection of species and strain of animal
2. Housing and animal handling
3. Diet and nutrition
4. Dose and route of administration
5. Duration of tests
6. Spontaneous tumors of the liver
7. Diagnosis and interpretation of liver tumors

TABLE 2. *Spontaneous liver tumor in rats*[1]

Strain	Mean incidence (%)	
	Male	Female
Charles River CD	1.4 (2370)	2.7 (2070)
Osborne-Mendel	0.5 (380)	2.4 (290)
Alabama Strain	2.6 (1460)	1.3 (1170)
Sprague-Dawley #1	1.1 (870)	0.7 (760)
Sprague-Dawley #2	3.5 (585)	3.0 (568)
Sprague-Dawley #3	1.5 (159)	4.5 (171)
Wistar	1.8 (320)	1.1 (290)
Fischer 344	2.1 (2895)	3.7 (2600)

[1] Data derived from references 4, 12, 20, 24, 27, 34, 43, 46, and 51. Numbers in parentheses are numbers of animals examined.

long-term assays, is chosen for study; it is important that the MTD not compromise the animal by modifying metabolism or injuring vital organs so that valid interpretation of the results is impaired (17). The MTD is generally defined as the dose level of compound that permits the group of animals receiving it to attain an average body weight of about 90% of the body weight of a group of untreated controls. This observation, combined with absence of clinical signs or symptoms or of adverse metabolic analyses that might shorten survival significantly, is considered to be the appropriate MTD. Intermediate and lower doses are arbitrarily set so that one dose (the lowest dose) will likely result in no observed effect on the animals. The aim, in general, is to have a range of doses that will result in a dose–response relationship and allow for 50% or more of any treated group to survive until the end of the study, usually 18 months for mice and 24 months for rats. As a practical matter the MTD is usually established during a 90-day dose-ranging study using several doses (five or more), which also allows for the collection of important metabolic information.

There are other ways by which the MTD can be established. If a drug or chemical is an enzyme inducer, the level of enzyme induction and relative liver weight profiles in short-term studies can be used to set the highest dose for long-term chronic studies.

TABLE 3. *Spontaneous tumors in strains of mice[1]*

| | Mean incidence (%) | |
Strain	Male	Female
C3H	26.0 (320)	0 (0)
CBA	41.0 (285)	27.2 (229)
TF1	13.5 (107)	5.1 (91)
C3HE	78.0 (79)	0.0 (0)
CF1	20.1 (288)	13.0 (297)
CBA	41.1 (285)	27.0 (229)
CD1	7.1 (294)	0.0 (0)
CR White Swiss	2.0 (137)	1.5 (144)
B6C3F1	26.8 (5094)	6.3 (4086)

[1] Data compiled from references 4, 13–14, 26–27, 35–36, 41, 45, and 48–49. Numbers in parentheses are numbers of animals examined.

This method is illustrated by the graph shown in Fig. 1, which shows that on a multiple dose regimen the weight of the liver increases along with enzyme activity. At some point, however, there is a metabolic overload and the capacity of the liver and other organs to function normally is exceeded. The MTD is then set at a level that does not exceed the metabolic capacity and, in most instances, will allow for a normal lifespan and collection of essential data over about 2 years. The lower doses provide a range for dose–response relationship data.

If a chemical is not an enzyme inducer, data on its kinetics and metabolism may be used to set the highest dose (5, 18, 19). The promising alternative to the methods described above, "the relative systemic exposure ratio," is defined as the ratio of the plasma area under the concentration-time curve (AUC) of the drug or its major metabolites in rodents, at the conventional MTD, to the human plasma AUC at the projected maximum recommended daily dose (MRD). This systemic exposure ratio seems to be appropriate as a criterion, especially for high-dose selection for compounds with qualitatively similar metabolic profiles in rodents and humans, particularly those with low rodent toxicity. See references (5) and (19) for further details.

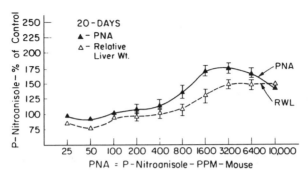

FIG. 1. Response of mouse liver to enzyme induction. Enzyme induction and relative liver weight increased with dose until metabolic capacity was exceeded. Highest dose for long-term studies (MTD) should be less than dose inducing peak enzyme level.

Once the dosing schedule has been decided, the dosing frequency must be established; in most situations the frequency is on a continuous basis, if administered in the diet, and 5–7 days each week, if given by intubation or by injection. If the route of administration of drug or chemical is to be oral in humans then it should be oral in the animal (diet or gavage); the same applies for topical or parenteral administration. Inhalation exposure should be used where humans are exposed by inhalation, assuming proper equipment and experienced personnel are available.

Traditionally, the time of initiation of tests has been soon after weaning (20, 21), although in utero exposure has been more widely accepted and extended in recent years (22). Generally accepted exposure periods for long-term studies in mice are 18 months and for rats, 24 months, a major portion of the lifespan of these species. A viable option is to hold the animals for an additional 6 months without further exposure.

Problems with diagnosis and interpretation of liver lesions in rodents (4, 9, 23–27) have been considerably reduced following the issuing of Guides for Toxicologic Pathology, by the Society of Toxicologic Pathology, in collaboration with the American Registry of Pathology (ARP) and the Armed Forces Institute of Pathology (AFIP). The most recent of these guides, issued in late 1994, addressed the rat liver (28).

The incidence of spontaneous liver tumors, which usually vary within and among strains and groups of the same strain, complicate the assessment of effects of chemical exposure. Generally, the spontaneous incidence of liver tumors in most rat strains is low, on the order of 1–3%. In mice, however, tumor incidence ranges from 5% to as high as 80% or 90% (Table 3). Histologic criteria for evaluating the biologic significance of many liver lesions, particularly proliferative changes that may lead to neoplasia, are now available (9, 29–35.) Attempts to agree on the significance of the various lesions, from early injury to undoubted neoplasia, and to develop markers to determine when parenchymal cells are irrevocably committed to neoplasia are ongoing (9, 36–40).

GENERAL MORPHOLOGY

The liver of mammalian species is not a homogeneous organ; rather, it is composed of a number of different types of cells, each with specific functions. There are two types of epithelial cells (hepatocytes and bile duct cells), a family of sinusoidal lining cells of several types, vascular (endothelial) lining cells, and other supporting stromal cells. All of these cell types are subject to injury from a variety of agents. The lesions found, grossly and microscopically, reflect the manner by which these cells respond to injury. Some lesions are acute, short-lived, and reversible; others are chronic and often irreversible. Some proliferative lesions are not included (i.e., hepatoblastoma, Kupffer, fat, or Ito cells) because they are not commonly seen as spontaneous or induced entities in rodents, as are those included in this chapter.

Categories used in describing liver lesions should be kept to a relatively few significant types, in keeping with reasonable completeness. This will tend to discourage statistical treatment of categories that are meaningless, in the biologic sense, but that may turn out to be of interest to statisticians when treated with one or another of the ever-growing number of statistical tests. The pathologist should make a judgment based on data that are biologically significant.

NONNEOPLASTIC LIVER LESIONS

Lipid Accumulation

One of the most common responses of the liver to a chemical insult is the accumulation of fat in parenchymal cells, most often in the periportal zone (Fig. 2). Chemicals interfere with the normal processing of lipids and other materials for secretion from the liver parenchyma; lipids thus accumulate. The condition is usually temporary and reversible in most cases, but with chronic poisoning fatty liver may be a more serious feature. Another type of nonxenobiotic fatty liver that progresses to cirrhosis and, ultimately, to hepatocellular carcinoma is the methyl group deficiency rat model (41–43), a unique type of fatty liver discussed briefly later in this chapter.

Focal fatty change occurs in the rodent liver without a specific lobular distribution. The cytoplasm of the cells in these foci contain clear spherical vacuoles ranging from small and multiple to large and solitary, filled with lipid (fat); the spherical nature of the vacuole is a result of the lipid/water surface tension interface. Nuclei may be centrally located or pushed to one side by the cytoplasmic vacuoles, and when a single large vacuole displaces the nucleus, a signet ring appearance to the cell may result; the significance of fat in parenchymal cells, with respect to chronic injury, is unclear.

Acute Necrosis

Acute death of liver cells exposed to a chemical may be as single cells, scattered through the lobule, or focal; in these cases cell death may be minor or massive and

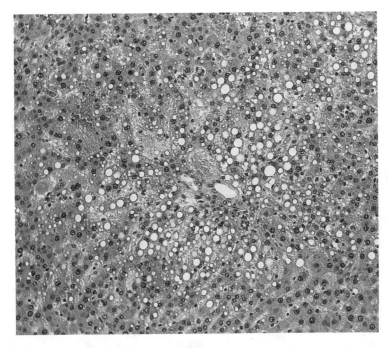

FIG. 2. Fatty infiltration in periportal area of the liver of a rat exposed to aflatoxin B1 48 hr earlier. H & E × 125.

with zonal preference (periportal, midzonal, centrilobular). An example of injury to parenchymal cells of the periportal zone is the acute lesion of aflatoxin B1 in the rat. Centrilobular necrosis is illustrated by the massive hemorrhagic necrosis produced by dimethylnitrosamine (DMN) (25). Midzonal injury with necrosis is rare but does occur in some chemical exposures such as phosphorus and in the eclampsia of pregnancy.

The role of necrosis and subsequent parenchymal proliferation, with a potential for progression to nongenotoxic hepatocellular carcinoma, are discussed later in this chapter.

Hypertrophy

Hypertrophy is typified by a simple enlargement of the parenchymal cells, a result of proliferation of smooth endoplasmic reticulum (SER) and, to a lesser extent, rough endoplasmic reticulum (RER), along with an increase in other normal cytoplasmic components. Hypertrophy may occur in any part of the lobule; it may be uniform as in centrilobular hypertrophy (Fig. 3), associated with enzyme induction, or as single-cell hypertrophy in the periportal zone (aflatoxin [AFB1], DEN, acetylaminofluorene

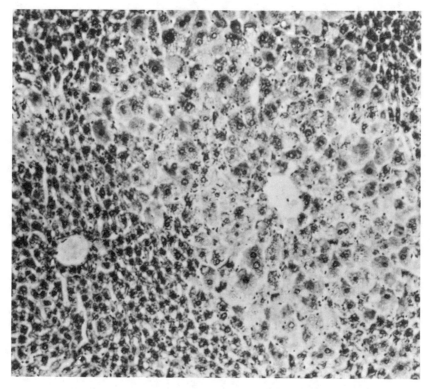

FIG. 3. Centrilobular hypertrophy, liver of rat fed phenobarbital, 1000 ppm, 20 weeks. H & E × 125.

[AAF]). The mouse liver is particularly striking when exposed for relatively long periods to inducers such as chlorinated hydrocarbon pesticides or to phenobarbital.

Foci of Cellular Alteration

These lesions consist of groups of hepatocytes that are modified in size, tinctorial characteristics, and lobe or lobular distribution. A consensus regarding these lesions has been reached (29a, 29b) and they are now classified collectively as *foci of cellular alteration* (9, 23, 26, 28–30, 33). Under this umbrella term are a number of subcategories; because of space limitations only the three most important ones are described in this chapter. Additional descriptions can be found in the guide (28).

Foci of cellular alteration are not usually observed grossly; occasionally, however, large foci may be seen as pinpoint lesions on the surface of the liver. Microscopically (Fig. 4), the cells may be smaller or larger than unaffected hepatocytes, however, and this and tinctorial properties of the cytoplasm are two of the key features that

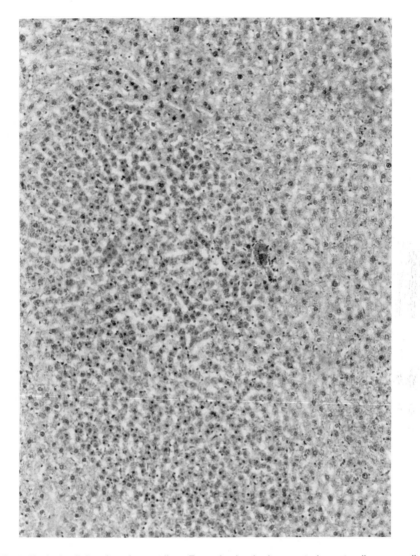

FIG. 4. Foci of cellular alteration, rat liver. Focus is clearly demarcated; most cells are smaller and stain more darkly than the surrounding liver cells, but atypia is absent. H & E × 100.

differentiate the various types of foci. Many of the foci contain more than one cell type; these should be diagnosed by the predominant cell type present. Nuclear characteristics can also serve as criteria in helping to differentiate types of foci; cellular atypia is generally absent, and the foci can vary in size from a few cells to lesions that occupy multiple hepatic lobules. The latter are generally sharply demarcated from the surrounding liver.

The hepatic lobular architecture within foci is generally unaltered. However, hepatic cords within foci may not be contiguous with the hepatic cords of adjacent normal liver. Large lesions and those with hypertrophied cells often distort or compress surrounding hepatic plates along a small portion of the periphery. This compression along the periphery of the focus is not as prominent a feature as is usually seen with neoplasms, an alteration which, along with preservation of hepatic lobular architecture, constitutes the main morphologic difference setting foci of cellular alteration apart from hepatocellular adenomas.

Enzyme alterations described in foci have led to the term *enzyme altered foci* as a synonym for altered foci (30, 38). Foci of cellular alteration in 2-year carcinogenicity studies, commonly observed as both spontaneous and induced lesions, include basophilic, eosinophilic, and clear-cell foci. These are described below.

Clear-Cell Foci (Hydropic Change)

These foci are composed of normal, slightly to markedly enlarged parenchymal cells with prominent membranes, sometimes frayed on the inner surface (Fig. 5).

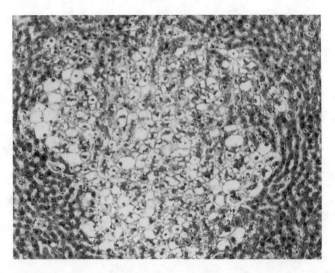

FIG. 5. Clear cell focus, composed of cells without staining, along with a few eosinophilic cells. H & E × 80.

The unstained cytoplasm contains abundant glycogen, which is dissolved during processing—thus, the "clear" appearance. These foci may exceed the size of a lobule and are assumed to be end-stage lesions, probably reversible. A few eosinophilic cells may be scattered throughout the lesion. The relevance of clear-cell foci to liver disease is not known.

Basophilic Foci

These foci are comprised of parenchymal cells, the cytoplasm of which stains more intensely basophilic than the surrounding parenchyma (Fig. 6). The nuclei may be irregular in size, but more often the cells are smaller than those of the surrounding parenchyma. Basophilic foci are sometimes seen in close association or intermingled with hydropic or, sometimes, fat-containing parenchymal cells. Such lesions are

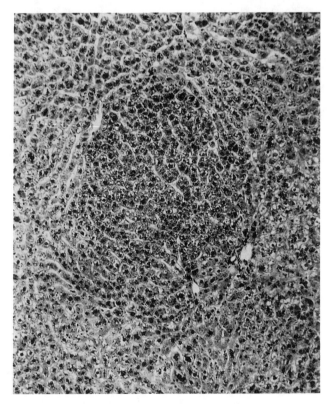

FIG. 6. Basophilic focus with parenchymal cells staining more deeply basophilic than surrounding parenchyma. Cords in the focus are contorted, and slight compression is noted along one aspect of the focal periphery. H & E × 100.

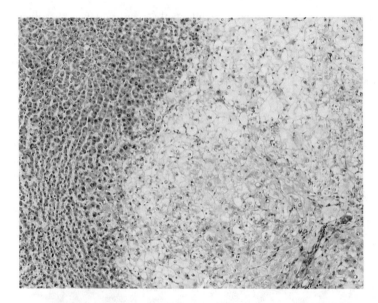

FIG. 7. Eosinophilic (ground-glass) focus. The cells of this focus stain intensely with eosin (acidophilic), the cytoplasm is increased, and nuclei are enlarged. Enlargement of cells causes some compression at the periphery of the focus. H & E × 80.

proliferative whether or not compression of surrounding cells is obvious. They label intensely with [³H]thymidine, and cell cords are tortuous because of the increased cellularity.

Eosinophilic Foci (Ground-Glass Changes)

Cellular alterations assigned to this category may be restricted to small areas or may encompass areas of a lobule or more (Fig. 7). The cells stain intensely with eosin (acidophilia), the cytoplasm is increased and with a ground-glass appearance, and the nuclei are enlarged; there are minimal irregularities of cords, and sinusoids are present. There is no obvious necrosis or parenchymal cell proliferation, nor do such areas appreciably compress the surrounding unaffected parenchyma.

Regenerative Hyperplasia

This term denotes a hepatocellular lesion associated with past or ongoing hepatocyte necrosis, along with other aspects of liver damage, including hepatocyte hyperplasia. It is a more extensive lesion than the hyperplastic nodule described previously (25), with some additional defining characteristics. Grossly, the liver may or may not be enlarged, but in severe cases, there is distortion of the shape of the lobes. The nodules

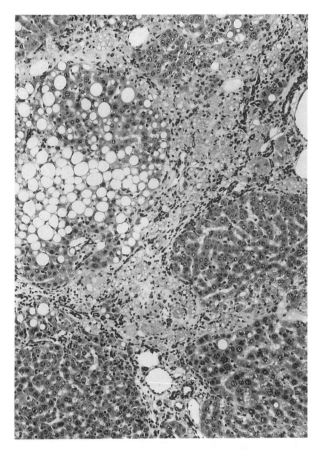

FIG. 8. Regenerative hyperplasia. Discrete nodular lesions of hepatocytes and hepatocyte damage including necrosis, fibrosis, inflammation, fat, and parenchymal hyperplasia. H & E × 100.

are clearly separated from adjacent parenchyma; color depends on lipid and glycogen content of the hepatocytes or the amount of blood present in the lesion.

There are two salient characteristics essential to diagnosis of regenerative hyperplasia (Fig. 8). One is the presence of one or more discrete nodular lesions of hepatocytes that lack the cytologic or histologic features of neoplasia; lobular architecture is distorted or missing in some areas of the section. The other essential feature is evidence of prior or ongoing hepatocyte damage (e.g., cytotoxicity, necrosis, degeneration, atrophy, fibrosis, inflammation, fat), which is often seen in the same histologic sections containing regenerative hyperplasia.

Other phenotypic and structural features may be observed in lesions of this category. Compression of adjacent hepatic parenchyma distorts the lobular architecture so that the central veins are partly collapsed, and portal areas may appear to be missing in a given section because they lie in a different plane. In some instances of extensive hyperplasia, chronic inflammation, hepatic degeneration, and oval cell proliferation (bile duct hyperplasia) may be present in portal areas and around the periphery of the nodules. Focal hyperplastic lesions are round in a two-dimensional view, within which there may be an increased number of mitoses, degenerating hepatocytes, and, occasionally, microgranulomas. In some cases, however, clear evidence of necrosis or cytotoxicity may not be present or is substantially reduced. This suggests that the regenerating hepatocytes in areas of regenerative hyperplasia are relatively resistant to the toxic effects of the chemical.

Related to regenerative hyperplasia or to the hyperplastic nodule (25) is the lesion formerly categorized as a neoplastic nodule (8); the diagnosis is still made by some pathologists, mainly Europeans, but currently the term is rarely used in North America. Although never clearly understood, the neoplastic nodule was not interpreted to be equivalent to the hyperplastic nodule but was close if not identical to the hepatocellular adenoma.

NEOPLASTIC LIVER LESIONS

Lesions to be described below are classified as either benign or malignant neoplasms and represent those liver lesions that are found routinely in the safety evaluation of drugs and other chemicals.

Hepatocellular Adenoma

Adenomas vary grossly in size and color, ranging in size from a few millimeters to several centimeters in diameter. They vary in color from normal to either lighter or darker than the surrounding tissue. These lesions may be round or spherical and often have an irregular border. More often than not they are solitary lesions, but they may be multiple.

Microscopically, adenomas are composed of nodules of parenchymal cells (Fig. 9) that are enlarged and eosinophilic (28); the lobular architecture is lost, and there is occasionally cellular atypia (karyomegaly, hyperchromasia, prominent nucleoli) but no clearly identifiable dysplasia. Adenomas may not be sharply demarcated from the more normal liver but are easily identified as proliferative lesions. The cells in an adenoma may form structures suggestive of trabeculae, but true trabeculae, as seen in carcinoma, are not a component of the adenoma. There is a lack of continuity of the nodule and the surrounding unaffected liver, with compression of at least a part of the surrounding parenchyma.

The cords of the adenoma often are perpendicular to or impinge obliquely on the cords of the adjacent liver, and within the tumor there is a loss of normal hepatic plate and lobular architecture. The cords may be arranged haphazardly, more than one cell layer thick, and with sinusoids compressed or, sometimes, dilated. Hepatocytes within

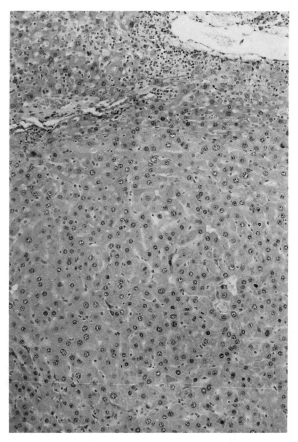

FIG. 9. Hepatocellular adenoma; large eosinophilic parenchymal cells and loss of lobular architecture and normal hepatic plate arrangement. Cords are arranged haphazardly, often more than one cell layer thick, and may impinge on the surrounding tissue in a perpendicular or oblique fashion. H & E × 120.

the adenoma vary in size and tinctorial characteristics; the latter may be eosinophilic, basophilic, or an admixture of both. Clear cells are variably present in the benign tumor, although adenomas composed primarily of clear cells are rarely observed. Except for occasional cellular atypia the cells in adenomas are comparable morphologically to those described for foci of cellular alteration. Fatty change and other degenerative changes may be present, but necrosis within an adenoma is uncommon. Oval cell proliferation (bile duct hyperplasia) and cystic degeneration (spongiosis hepatica) may also be observed. These lesions usually do not contain portal triads although triads are sometimes present because they have been enveloped as the adenoma grows by expansion.

Hepatocellular Carcinoma

Hepatocellular carcinomas may be found in any lobe of the liver; they vary in size, ranging from 1 cm to over 10 cm in diameter. The lesion protrudes above the liver surface and may be traversed by prominent blood vessels on the thickened capsule, an indication of angiogenesis. Hepatocellular carcinomas may vary in color but often resemble normal liver. The consistency of the tumor will vary depending on a number of factors, particularly the amount of necrosis and hemorrhage present. Three morphologic forms of hepatocellular carcinoma observed in rodents are described here: trabecular, glandular, and anaplastic.

Trabecular Carcinoma

The trabecular form (Fig. 10) is the most common as a response to tumorigenic chemicals. Hepatocytes may form a variety of patterns within the neoplasm. In the trabecular form the pattern is characterized by neoplastic cells forming multiple irregular trabeculae that are often several cells thick and contain a variably necrotic core that when lost, resembles a glandular pattern. The trabecular pattern generally constitutes a major portion of the lesion although it is often most obvious in that portion of the tumor where dilated vascular spaces separate the trabeculae. If such spaces are not present the tumor appears to be composed of packets or sheets of neoplastic cells. The individual cells approximate the appearance of normal hepatocytes; they are typically cuboidal with abundant cytoplasm and a centrally placed nucleus. The staining characteristics of the cytoplasm may be eosinophilic, basophilic, clear, or a mixture of types similar to those seen in foci of cellular alteration or in adenomas. Nuclei frequently vary in size, are large and hyperchromatic, and often have marginated chromatin.

Glandular (Acinar) Carcinoma

This type of carcinoma (Fig. 11), derived from liver cell parenchyma, is less common than the trabecular form. It is characterized by acinar formations with cells arranged around a central lumen, typical of some areas adjacent to or as a continuum with the trabecular patterns. More characteristic are cystic spaces, lined by flattened epithelium with varying amounts of stroma between the glandular elements. Some of the cystic spaces contain amorphous or necrotic material, presumably from the inflammatory infiltrate accompanying the development of some areas of the tumor. Viewed by electron microscopy, the cystic space is a dilated bile canaliculus, and there are wide variations in size and shape of cells lining the glandlike spaces; these range from flattened to cuboidal to low columnar epitheliallike cells. Some lining eosinophilic parenchymal cells have vesicular nuclei with prominent nucleoli arranged about a common dilated space. Other acini are formed by more basophilic, cuboidal cells.

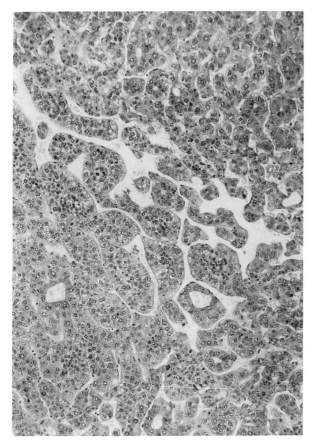

FIG. 10. Trabecular hepatocellular carcinoma, with neoplastic cells formed into trabeculae, irregular in size and staining characteristics. Necrotic cores have been lost in some of them, leaving an impression of glandular structures. H & E × 180.

In some poorly differentiated areas there are foci of hyperchromatic cells, distorted glandlike structures, abundant stroma, and reticulin with an appearance of cholangiocarcinoma. Such lesions are difficult to accurately diagnose by light microscopy but are clearly different from the more typical glandular or trabecular patterns.

Anaplastic Carcinoma

These tumors, rare in rodents, are composed of sheets of pleomorphic cells, many of which contain bizarre nuclei, and frequent mitotic figures. There are large, blood-filled spaces and areas of necrosis in the undifferentiated neoplasm, and the cells never

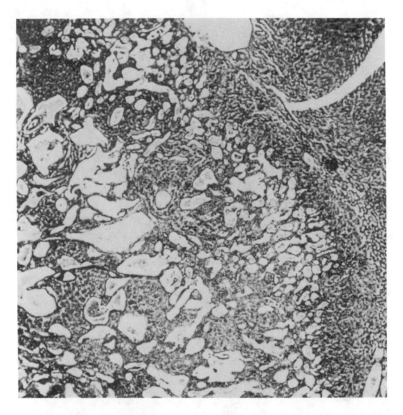

FIG. 11. Glandular (acinar) carcinoma, composed of acinar formations and cystic spaces lined by flattened epithelium. Eosinophilic or basophilic cells with vesicular nuclei arranged around a common dilated space are also observed. H & E × 80.

form a recognized pattern or organization. The blood-filled spaces may be lined by normal-appearing endothelium or, more often, by neoplastic cells. Cells abutting the blood-filled spaces may be more elongated but retain many of the features of cells of the trabecular lesions. Pleomorphic nuclei, necrosis, and variation in size and shape of cells typify this type of tumor (28).

INTRAHEPATIC BILIARY LESIONS

Bile Duct Hyperplasia

Bile duct hyperplasia (BDH) is a common lesion (Fig. 12) observed in the liver of rats exposed to a variety of chemicals and in the liver of untreated aging rats. It is generally considered to represent a physiologic response to toxic exposure. It is

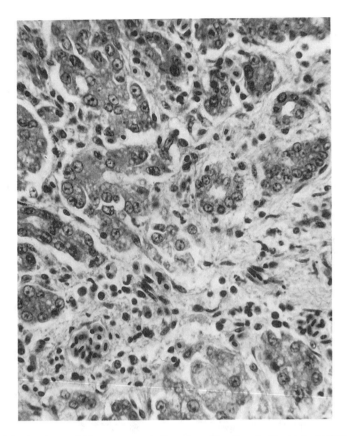

FIG. 12. Bile duct hyperplasia, composed of small, proliferating ducts, single or clusters of oval or cuboidal cells; epithelium is generally normal but may be somewhat distorted by proliferating epithelial cells. H & E × 200.

not clear whether these lesions may progress to benign or malignant tumors, but the prevailing weight of evidence is that they do not. Clearly, BDH associated with AFB1, AAF, DAB, and other selected true rodent hepatocarcinogens does not progress to cholangiocarcinoma.

The lesion consists of several small bile ducts occurring in a portal area accompanied by variable amounts of periductular fibrosis and inflammatory infiltrate. The epithelium is normal in morphology, but the ducts are sometimes dilated with or without mucoid debris in the lumen.

A number of investigators (44) have devoted intense efforts to demonstrate that "oval" cells, small epithelial cells with scanty, faintly basophilic cytoplasm and a prominent nucleolus, are different entities from the routine bile duct cells described above. The cells referred to as "oval" cells are indeed oval; they may be localized as single cells or appear as groups of cells between hepatocytes or as nearby areas of parenchymal cells that are reacting to severe toxicity and necrosis. Oval cells are bile duct–like cells that stream outward from the periportal zone along the sinusoids toward the centrilobular area. Some investigators believe that oval cells are stem cells for both bile duct epithelium and for hepatocytes, but others do not; the relation of oval cells to hepatocarcinogenesis is unclear.

SIMPLE BILIARY CYSTS

Simple biliary cysts (Fig. 13) are usually microscopic but may be observed grossly as a pale, translucent mass protruding from the liver. These lesions usually contain clear, viscous, or pale yellow fluid that escapes on incision. Microscopically, the simple cyst is a structure lined by flattened epithelium with occasional oval to cuboidal cells along some aspects of the limiting wall. The cysts may be single or multiple but do not reach

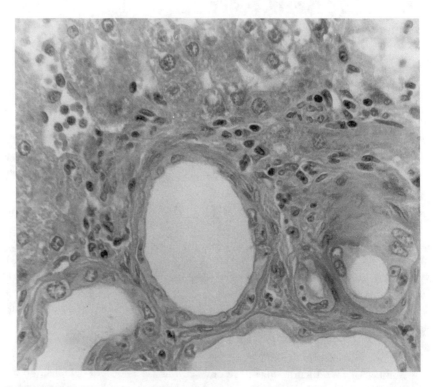

FIG. 13. Simple biliary cyst, a single or, sometimes, multiple compartmental structure lined by flattened epithelium with occasional oval or cuboidal cells along the limiting wall. H & E × 260.

the size of the multilocular type. The lumen is generally empty, but small amounts of intraluminal eosinophilic material may be present.

Multiloculated Cysts

Multiloculated biliary cysts are similar in appearance to simple biliary cysts but vary in size from microscopic to several centimeters in diameter. Larger lesions are divided into compartments by septa. Microscopically, these cysts are lined by flattened or low cuboidal cells separated by loose connective tissue. The cystic structures are divided into variable-sized compartments by fibrous connective tissue and lined by a single layer of flattened epithelium with occasional focal areas of cuboidal epithelium (28).

CHOLANGIOFIBROSIS (ADENOFIBROSIS, CHOLANGIOFIBROMA)

Cholangiofibrotic lesions (Fig. 14) vary in size from microscopic foci to grossly visible lesions up to 5 cm or more in diameter. Larger lesions are grossly visible as firm, pearly, white areas that may appear to be gritty when incised because of the dense connective tissue and variable calcified glandular structures and accompanying debris. An area of cholangiofibrosis is composed of atypical glandular structures lined by hyperbasophilic, sometimes dysplastic epithelium that may range from flattened to large cuboidal cells; goblet cells and occasional Paneth cells are sometimes seen within the same acinus. Some of the glands are typically crescent-shaped as a result of high columnar epithelium in one portion of the gland and attenuated epithelium on the other side. Mitotic figures are frequent in the epithelium, and the lumen is filled with mucin and necrotic debris derived from degenerated epithelium and white blood cells that mineralize in long-standing lesions. Connective tissue associated with these structures is densely sclerotic in the inner portions of the lesion; around the glandular structures the concentrically arranged connective tissue imparts a characteristic fibroadenomatous appearance to the area.

Cholangioma

Cholangiomas (28) vary from firm gray-white nodules to a spongy cystic structure, depending on the presence or absence of the latter. They can range in size from a few millimeters to very large masses up to several centimeters in diameter. In the solid forms margins are usually smooth; in the multilocular cystic forms the surface is irregular and similar in some respects to multilocular cysts. Cholangiomas are circumscribed but show evidence of expansion by compressing adjacent parenchyma. The neoplasms contain acini of generally uniform size, lined by a single layer of cuboidal cells. These cells contain round to oval nuclei located near the base of the cell, lending a histologic appearance similar to normal bile duct epithelium. In larger

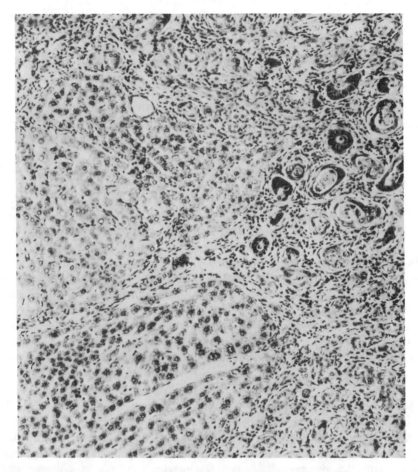

FIG. 14. Cholangiofibrosis lesion consisting of atypical glandular structures lined by hyperbasophilic, sometimes dysplastic epithelium, interspersed between sheets of relatively normal parenchymal cells. Mitotic figures are frequent, the lumen of glandlike structures contains mucin and other debris, and connective tissue may be prominent. H & E × 140.

lesions, which may be up to several centimeters in diameter, the lining epithelium is sometimes multilayered, but dysplasia is not observed. There is very little vascular stroma, and mitotic figures are rare.

CHOLANGIOCARCINOMA

Cholangiocarcinomas present as firm white to gray masses with an irregular border; when they protrude from the surface they may exhibit a spongy texture and exude clear or yellowish fluid when the surface is disturbed.

Microscopically, these tumors (28) have a glandular, solid, or papillary pattern, depending on the area examined. The major cellular component is cuboidal to columnar with basophilic cytoplasm and prominent hyperchromatic nuclei, commonly exhibiting cellular atypia and a high mitotic index. In some dilated glands the lining epithelium may be partially or completely absent, but when present, the cells are often piled up two or three cells thick. Mucin content varies, and the interstitium typically contains abundant scirrhous stroma. Microinvasion is present, and invasion of surrounding blood vessels and other tissues is not uncommon. Metastasis to other sites, however, is not common.

Hepatic Vascular Lesions

Angiectasis

Angiectasis usually is not observed grossly, although some larger lesions may appear as pinpoint dark red spots in the liver parenchyma. Further description and discussion of significance are in the open literature (28). Microscopically, hepatic angiectasis consists of dilated vascular spaces (sinusoids), filled with red blood cells. Disagreement on the nature and significance of such lesions is with respect to the presence or absence of lining cells and whether the hepatocytes are separated from direct exposure to blood flow by endothelial cells. In these tumors the spaces are lined by endothelial cells and the dilated spaces separate hepatic cords, most of which appear as convoluted plates. There is often compression of adjacent parenchyma because of dilated spaces, and often, this lesion is a component of other lesions such as foci of cellular alteration or hepatocellular neoplasms. Angiectasis can also be seen as a unique lesion and must be considered in the context of what other changes are present. In general, when angiectasis is a component of another lesion, such as foci of cellular alteration, it is not diagnosed separately.

ANGIOSARCOMA (HEMANGIOENDOTHELIALSARCOMA)

This tumor, derived from the vascular endothelium of the liver, is not uncommon in rodents as a spontaneous or induced neoplasm (45); it is seen more often in mice and hamsters than in rats. Some angiosarcomas are well differentiated, but others may be markedly anaplastic, displaying both vascular and solid patterns. Angiosarcomas must be distinguished from peliosis hepatis, the latter composed only of blood-filled spaces limited by hepatic cells and lacking an endothelial lining. This tumor must also be differentiated from telangiectasis, the latter a simple dilatation of the sinusoids, most often observed near the liver capsule.

The cells of an angiosarcoma may be composed of sheets that form syncytial structures or solid areas and an anastomosing network of irregular vascular spaces or channels filled with blood. The neoplastic endothelial cells vary considerably in size; they have pleomorphic nuclei, some of which are large and polygonal with vesicular nuclei and abundant cytoplasm, whereas others are small, elongated, and spindle-shaped. Mitotic figures are frequent and metastasis is common. Some areas may be difficult to distinguish from highly anaplastic fibrosarcomas. Isolated hepatocytes undergoing atrophy and necrosis, surrounded by tumor cells, are seen in most areas of infiltrating neoplasm.

CIRRHOSIS

Cirrhosis is a fibroproliferative disease that exhibits a number of competing entities; cells involved include hepatocytes, bile duct cells, endothelial cells, fibrocytes, and cells of the immune system (41–43). For the purposes of this chapter we will limit descriptions to two major types of cirrhosis: that which is induced by chronic exposure to chemicals (Fig. 15) such as AAF or carbon tetrachloride (CCl_4) and that which is due to methyl-group deficiency (Fig. 16), sometimes referred to as choline deficiency (13, 41, 42). Considerable progress in understanding the steatosis and ultimate cirrhosis of methyl-group deficiency has come from recent developments in digitizing liver sections and quantifying cellular molecules by computer assisted tissue analysis (CATA). This technology is described in part in a recent publication (13). In each

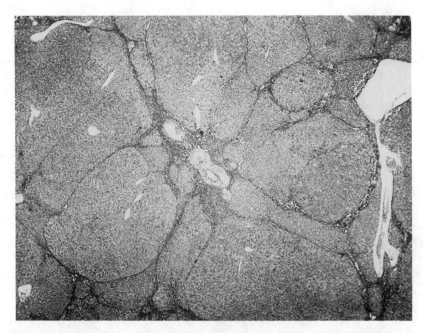

FIG. 15. Cirrhotic liver in rat exposed to AAF shows nodule formation, bile duct hyperplasia, and bridging fibrosis along with chronic injury, necrosis, and inflammation. H & E × 40.

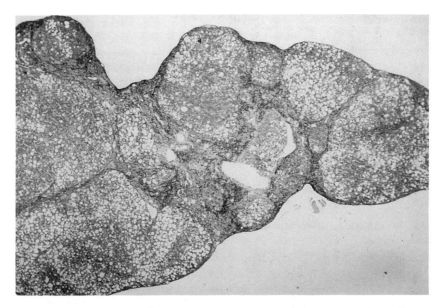

FIG. 16. Liver cirrhosis induced by chronic deficiency of methyl groups (choline deficiency). Nodule formation, similar to regenerative hyperplasia, is accompanied by necrosis, bile duct hyperplasia, inflammation, and bridging fibrosis. Some of these lesions progress to hepatocellular carcinoma. H & E × 40.

of these two types of cirrhosis there is hepatocyte necrosis and nodular hyperplasia, endothelial hyperplasia, bile duct hyperplasia, bridging fibrosis, and variable amounts of inflammatory infiltrate. The ratios of these various entities depends on a number of poorly understood factors. A detailed description and discussion of these two types of cirrhosis can be found in numerous literature references.

In the cirrhotic liver there is a mix of components that can vary considerably; in some parts of the liver more than one, and more often several, will be observed microscopically. The lesions induced by AAF or CCl₄ resemble the postnecrotic type of cirrhosis seen in humans, and this type is akin to the entity described under regenerative hyperplasia. The methyl-group (choline) deficiency type is similar to the micronodular type observed in humans associated with excessive alcohol consumption.

DISCUSSION

This chapter has drawn heavily on the literature accumulated over the past 3 decades relative to rodent liver pathology. Particularly useful has been the rich diversity of opinions of individuals and literature references now in abundance. The coming together of veterinary and human pathology, along with molecular biology, concerned primarily with diseases caused by chemical exposures has resulted in the emergence of a new subspecialty of pathology, that of toxicologic pathology. This discipline takes into account not only morphologic manifestations of toxic injury but some of the biochemical and metabolic alterations that account for them.

Molecular biology, with its genes and gels, would have been hard pressed to have achieved its notable successes over the past decade or so without taking into account some of the knowledge available on the spectrum of morphologic components of the liver. These cellular organelles can be altered in ways that modify cellular, organ, and whole-body functions, and a study of these constitutes toxicologic pathology.

The many lesions described above provide the basis for risk assessment of chemicals, even though most of them are not understood with regard to specific implications for human health. For example, foci of cellular alteration so elegantly described (29a, 29b) are present in the liver of aging rats, sometimes at an incidence approaching 100%, but the incidence of hepatic neoplasms is usually quite low (< 3–4%) in the same groups of animals. In addition, foci precede the development of hepatocellular neoplasms, even though the foci are reversible. Some pathologists believe them to be preneoplastic; others believe that foci may be end-stage lesions, only incidentally associated with tumor development. Current understanding (or lack of it) of the significance of the foci dictates that we should use caution when attempting to extrapolate the data on foci to human risk.

Distinguishing between benign and malignant tumors of hepatocellular origin raises questions and presents important challenges. The practice of combining hepatocellular adenomas and carcinomas in evaluating the results of a particular study, as is current NTP policy, reflects a level of ignorance but also admits that we have problems assigning risk based on the lesions.

Using the current system for evaluating rodent hepatic lesions, about half of the chemicals tested produce some form of cancer and about half of these induce liver tumors in mice (20, 46). By contrast, however, human liver cancer is uncommon in the United States and most other developed countries. Moreover, very few of the chemicals that induce tumors in rodents are associated with liver cancer in humans.

At the ultrastructural level, no significant differences exist between rodent liver tumors induced by any of several rodent hepatocarcinogens (aflatoxin, AAF, dimethylnitrosamine, dimethylaminoazobenzene). The ultrastructural organization of the rat liver cell carcinoma is remarkably similar to that of the human liver cell carcinoma. However, the organization of the two cell types (normal and neoplastic) at the ultrastructural level differs in important ways (24, 25, 34, 44, 46), although no single feature has been identified that clearly sets the two apart.

Bile duct hyperplasia, a common lesion of the untreated aged rat liver, is associated with exposure to many chemicals. Simple or multiloculated biliary cysts can destroy parenchymal cells, even though the cysts may be unrelated to chemical exposure. These lesions are considered by many pathologists to be degenerative, but some investigators believe them to be benign and refer to them as cholangiomas. This is an important point because in the mind of most regulatory scientists, the suffix—"oma" denotes tumorigenesis, if not carcinogenesis. Distinctions between biliary cysts and cholangiomas are not clear in the literature, and authors often give the diagnosis without a description of the criteria used to differentiate between the two.

Oval cells are seen in a number of situations, most often in association with lesions occasioned by severe toxicity and necrosis. One of the most remarkable examples is seen in the liver of a rat exposed to ethionine, an antimetabolite of the amino acid methionine. This is a true oval-cell hyperplasia, but even here the bile duct cells from which the hyperplasia derives do not go on to neoplasia. In the opinion of a majority of experienced pathologists, oval cells are simply proliferating bile duct cells. However, the hypothesis that these cells are a pluripotential cell from which either hepatocytes or bile duct epithelium may derive is attractive to some. Oval cells, unlike hepatocytes, are associated with a basement membrane, and this is an important distinguishing feature.

Cholangiofibrosis, a lesion sometimes observed in the liver of rodents, is an unusual morphologic entity, the significance of which is debatable; there is disagreement about its pathogenesis, its derivation, and as to whether it has neoplastic potential. A recent study (47) with furan reported that cholangiofibrosis progressed to cholangiocarcinoma with a low incidence of metastasis, suggesting a carcinogenic potential. Until further data are available, however, the nature of and implication for risk from this lesion remains unsettled.

The two types of tumors that derive from bile ducts, cholangiomas and cholangiocarcinomas, are rare in rodents but, as noted above, separation of benign and malignant lesions of bile duct origin remains a matter of some controversy; it depends primarily on the experience of the pathologist.

The manner in which the liver of rodents responds to toxic exposure can be influenced by many factors. Chemically induced cell necrosis and proliferation is an important consideration in attempting to understand mechanistic differences between genotoxic and nongenotoxic chemicals. Although it is not clear as yet how to best introduce it, information about induced necrosis and cell proliferation should be used in setting doses for bioassays, particularly where the traditional MTD determinations appear to be excessive (48). Opinions differ between regulatory scientists and others in the risk assessment field about the appropriateness of extrapolation of cancer risk from rodent models to humans, particularly the case where nongenotoxic agents exhibit liver-tumor activity only at very high dose levels.

The significance to public health of nongenotoxic chemicals may be equal to or more than that of genotoxic agents. The association of mutagenic and carcinogenic activity has been a useful concept enabling separation of chemicals into two broad classes: those that react with DNA in important ways (genotoxic), such as nonreversible covalent binding to DNA, and those that do not. This concept serves as the basis for most models of risk assessment and predictive assays.

The induction of cell death and proliferation by nongenotoxic chemicals raises the important question of how these events impinge on liver neoplasia. The stages of initiation, promotion, and progression in the pathogenesis of hepatocellular cancer are all accompanied by replication of hepatocytes; cell proliferation is required in the conversion of DNA adducts to mutations, as is the case for genotoxic substances. Mutations can also occur as spontaneous events after cells have been induced to undergo proliferation (19, 48). Thus, mutations and cytotoxicants may provide the environment during cell death and regeneration for a selective growth advantage and resistance to chemical toxicity of the newly forming hepatocytes, sufficient to escape growth control mechanisms. Clonal expansion, progression, and, ultimately, neoplasia may occur.

Increased tumor response in the liver is seen in a number of situations associated with rapid cell replication; for example, it is seen in the hepatectomized rodent liver, in the developing embryo, and in the young rodent liver. The early work (49, 50) used carbon tetrachloride and chloroform, both hepatotoxicants and both nongenotoxicants, to induce liver cancer. It was nearly a half-century before the significance of the work of Eschenbrenner and colleagues (49, 50) was fully recognized. These astute investigators pointed out two important observations: (1) tumors did not develop unless the dose of toxicant was sufficient to result in significant necrosis of hepatocytes; and (2) intermittent, as opposed to continuous, exposure to the toxicant was more efficient in producing tumors, indicating that the liver needed intermittent time to repair, even though repair was incomplete, allowing for increased genetic errors.

Another significant example of continuous cell death and hepatocyte regeneration that is linked to liver cell cancer is the choline-deficient rat model, first described by Copeland and Salmon (41). This methyl group–deficient rat liver undergoes a series of morphologic and metabolic changes manifested by fatty liver, fibrosis, cirrhosis, and, ultimately, hepatocellular carcinoma (41, 42, 51). Some of these important changes in hepatocytes are now amenable to quantitative analysis by computer-assisted technology (13). A salient feature of the deficient rat liver, in addition to steatosis, is continuous hepatocyte cell death and regeneration. However, in addition to the changes in the liver of the methyl-deficient rat, other changes are occurring as concommitants: a markedly depressed immunocompetence, diminished activity of some of the key drug-metabolizing enzymes (P450 family), increased sensitivity to known rat carcinogens, and a modified profile of some oncogenes.

In humans, a growing body of evidence suggests that liver damage and hepatocellular cancer are linked to cirrhosis and infection with hepatitis B and C, along with variable contributions from environmental contaminants. Based on these observations it seems that a promising approach to risk assessment in today's environment would be to find a way to link a physiologically based pharmacokinetic model with end points of cytotoxicity and induced cell proliferation, using the rodent model (5, 19, 36, 48). This should be particularly fruitful in those cases where the liver is the target of the chemical. Data derived from such a model should provide more accurate information regarding the relationships between dose and cancer risk, providing more confidence in advice offered by government, scientific, and media sources.

REFERENCES

1. Berenblum I. *Carcinogenicity testing*. Geneva: UICC Press, 1969.
2. Billups LH. Naturally-occurring neoplastic diseases in the rat. In: Melby EC, Altman NH, eds. *Handbook of laboratory animal science*, vol. 3. West Palm Beach: CRC Press, 1976:343–356.
3. Boyland EE. The biological examination of carcinogenic substances. *Br Med Bull* 1958;14:14–19.
4. Butler WH, Newberne PM, eds. *Mouse hepatic neoplasia*. Amsterdam: Elsevier Science Publishers, 1975.
5. Contrera JF. Emerging trends in nonclinical safety assessment for therapeutics. *Toxicol Pathol* 1994; 22:89–94.
6. Davidson CS, Leevy CM, Chamberlayne EC, eds. *Guidelines for detection of hepatotoxicity due to drugs and chemicals*. Washington, DC: US DHEW Publication 79-313, 1979.
7. Golberg L, ed. *Carcinogenesis testing of chemicals*. Cleveland: CRC Press, 1974.
8. Squire RA, Levitt MH. Report of a workshop on classification of specific heaptocellular lesions of rats. *Cancer Res* 1975;35:3214–3233.
9. Maronpot RR, Montgomery CA, Boorman GA, McConnell EE. National Toxicology Program nomenclature for hepato-proliferative lesions of rats. *Toxicol Pathol* 1986;14:263–273.
10. Coe JE, Ross MJ. Hamster female protein: a divergent acute phase protein in male and female Syrian hamsters. *J Exp Med* 1983;157:1421–1433.
11. Coe JE, Ross MJ. Amyloidosis and female protein in the Syrian hamster. *J Exp Med* 1990;171:1257–1267.
12. Keenan K, Smith PF, Soper KA. Effect of diet and dietary optimization (caloric restriction) on rat survival in carcinogenicity studies: an industrial viewpoint. In: McAuslane J, Lumley CF, Walker SR, eds. *The carcinogenicity debate*. Lancaster: Quay Publishing, 1992:77–102.
12a. Hart RW, Neumann DA, Robertson RT, eds. Dietary restriction: implications for the design and interpretation of toxicity and carcinogenicity studies. Washington, DC: ILSI Press, 1995.
13. Newberne PM, Sotnikov A. Diet: the neglected variable in chemical safety evaluation. *Toxicol Pathol* 1996;24:746–756.
14. National Academy of Sciences. *Control of laboratory animal diets*. Washington, DC: NAS Press, 1978:1–12.
15. Newberne PM, McConnell RG. Dietary nutrients and contaminants in laboratory animal experimentation. *J Environ Pathol Toxicol* 1981;4:105–122.
16. Coe JE, Ishak K, Ward JM, Ross MJ. Tamoxifen prevents induction of hepatic neoplasia by zeranol, an estrogenic food contaminant. *Proc Natl Acad Sci USA* 1992;89:1085–1089.
17. Ames BN, Gold LS. Chemical carcinogenesis: too many rodent carcinogens. *Proc Natl Acad Sci USA* 1990;87:7772–7776.
18. MacDonald JS, Lankas GR, Morrissey RE. Toxicokinetic and mechanistic considerations in the interpretation of the rodent bioassay. *Toxicol Pathol* 1994;l22:24–140.
19. Morgan DS, Kelvin AS, Kintner LB, Fish CF, Kerns WD, Rhodes G. The application of toxicokinetic data to dosage selection in toxicology studies. *Toxicol Pathol* 1994;22:112–123.
20. Selkirk JK, Soward SM, eds. *Compendium of abstracts from long-term cancer studies reported by the National Toxicology Program, National Institute of Environmental Health Sciences*, vol. 101, suppl. 1, Research Triangle Park: NIH NIEHS, April 1993.
21. FDA Advisory Committee. Protocols for safety evaluation: panel on carcinogenesis. *Toxicol Appl Pharmacol* 1971;20:419–438.
22. Toth B, Magee PN, Shubik P. Carcinogenesis study with dimethylnitrosamine administered orally to adult and subcutaneously to newborn BALB/c mice. *Cancer Res* 1964;24:1712–1721.
23. Hirota N, Williams GM. Persistence of growth of rat neoplastic nodules following cessation of carcinogen exposure. *J Natl Cancer Inst* 1979;63:1257–1275.
24. Newberne PM, Butler WH, eds. *Rat Hepatic Neoplasia*. Cambridge, MA: MIT Press, 1978.
25. Newberne PM. Assessment of the hepatocarcinogenic potential of chemicals: response of the liver. In: Plaa GL, Hewitt WR, eds. *Toxicology of the liver*. New York: Raven Press, 1982:243–290.
26. Ward JM. Morphology of foci of altered hepatocytes and naturally-occuring hepatocellular tumors in F344 rats. *Virchow Arch Pathol Anat* 1981;390:339–345.
27. Takayama S. Variation of histological diagnoses of mouse liver tumors by pathologists. In: Butler WH, Newberne PM, eds. *Mouse hepatic neoplasia*. Amsterdam: Elsevier, 1975:183–187.

28. Goodman DG, Maronpot RR, Newberne PM, Popp JA, Squire RA. Proliferative and selected other lesions in the liver of rats. *Guides for toxicologic pathology*. Washington, DC: AFIP 1994: 1–24.

29. Bannasch P. Sequential cellular alterations during hepatocarcinogenesis. In: Newberne P, Butler W, eds. *Rat hepatic neoplasia*. Cambridge, MA: MIT Press, 1978:58–99.

29a. Bannasch P, Zerban H, Hacker HJ. Foci of altered hepatocytes: rat. In: Jones TC, Popp JA, Mohr U, eds. *Digestive system: monographs on pathology of laboratory animals*, 2nd ed. Berlin: Springer, 1997:3–37.

29b. Ruebner BH, Bannasch P, Hinton DE, Cullen JM, Ward J. Foci of altered hepatocytes: mouse. In: Jones TC, Popp JA, Mohr U, eds. *Digestive system: monographs on pathology of laboratory animals*, 2nd ed. Berlin: Springer, 1997:38–49.

30. Bannasch P, Enzmann H, Klinek F, Weber E, Zerban H. Significance of sequential cellular changes inside and outside foci of altered hepatocytes during hepatocarcinogenesis. *Toxicol Pathol* 1989;17:617–629.

31. Newsholme SJ, Fish CJ. Morphology and incidence of hepatic foci of cellular alteration in Sprague-Dawley rats and mice. *Toxicol Pathol* 1994;10:95–109.

32. Popp JA. Hepatocellular carcinoma: liver, rat. In: Jones TC, Mohr U, Hunt RD, eds. *Digestive system: monographs on pathology of laboratory animals*. Berlin: Springer–Verlag, 1985:39–46.

33. Popp JA, Goldsworthy TL. Defining foci of cellular alteration in short-term and medium-term rat liver tumor liver models. *Toxicol Pathol* 1989;17:561–568.

34. Turusov VS. Tumors of the rat, Parts I and II. In: *Pathology of tumors in laboratory animals*, vol. 1. *Tumors of the rat*, 2nd ed. Lyon: IARC Press, 1990:1–748.

35. Williams GM. The significance of chemically-induced hepatocellular altered foci in rat liver and application to carcinogen detection. *Toxicol Pathol* 1989;167:663–674.

36. Butterworth BE, Popp JA, Connally RB, Goldsworthy TL. Chemically-induced cell proliferation in carcinogenesis. In: Vaino H, Magee P, McGregor DB, McMichael AJ, eds. *Mechanisms of carcinogenesis in risk identification*. Lyon: IARC Press, 1992:279–305.

37. Pitot HC, Campbell HA, Maronpot R. Critical parameters in the quantitation of the stages of initiation, promotion and progression in one model of hepatocarcinogenesis in the rat. *Toxicol Pathol* 1989;17:594–612.

38. Peraino C, Staffeldt EF, Carnea BA, Ludeman VA, Blomquist JA, Vesselinovitch SD. Characterization of histochemically detectable altered hepatic foci. *Cancer Res* 1984;44:3340–3347.

39. Tsude H, Sarma S, Rafalakshmi S, Subroff J, Farber E, Batzinger R, Youngman C, Bueding ME. Induction of hepatic lesions in mice with a single dose of hycanthone methanesulfonate after partial hepatectomy. *Cancer Res* 1979;39:4491–4496.

40. Williams GM, Watanabe K. Quantitative kinetics of the development of AAF-induced altered (hyperplastic) hepatocellular foci resistant to iron accumulation and of their reversion or persistence following removal of carcinogen. *J Natl Cancer Inst* 1978;61:113–121.

41. Copeland DH, Salmon WD. The occurrence of neoplasms in the liver, lungs, and other tissues of rats as a result of prolonged choline deficiency. *Am J Pathol* 1946;22:1059–1080.

42. Newberne PM. The methyl deficiency model: history, characteristics and research directions. *J Nutr Biochem* 1993;4:1–7.

42a. Newberne PM, Rogers AE. Nutritional fatty liver, cirrhosis and hepatocellular carcinoma: rat, mouse. In: Jones TC, Popp JA, Mohr V, eds. *Digestive system: monographs on pathology of laboratory animals*, 2nd ed. Berlin: Springer, 1997:143–151.

43. Rogers AE, Newberne PM. Aflatoxin B1 carcinogenesis in lipotrope-deficient rats. *Cancer Res* 1969;29:1965–1972.

44. Pack R, Heck R, Dienes HP, Oesch F, Steinberg P. Isolation, biochemical characterization, long-term culture, and phenotype modulation of oval cells from carcinogen-fed rats. *Exp Cell Res* 1993;204:198–209.

45. Eturk E, Cohen S, Price JM, Von Esch AJ, Crevetti AJ, Bryan, GC. The production of hemangioendothelialsarcoma in rats by feeding 5-acetamido-3-(5-nitro-2-furyl)-6H,2,4-oxadiazine. *Cancer Res* 1969;29:383–465.

46. Anonymous. *Proceedings: fifth mouse liver tumor workshop*. Washington, DC: International Life Sciences Institute, Nov/Dec 1994, 12/6:1–5.

47. National Toxicology Program (NTP). *Tech report series #402: USHHS publication* 1993:93-2857.

48. Conolly RB, Andersen ME. Biologically based pharmacodynamic models: tools for toxicological

research and risk assessment. In: Cho AK, ed. *Annual review of pharmacology and toxicology.* Palo Alto: Annual Reviews, 1991:503–523.

49. Eschenbrenner AB. Studies on hepatoma size and spacing of multiple doses in the induction of carbon tetrachloride hepatomas. *J Natl Cancer Inst* 1944;4:385–388.
50. Eschenbrenner AB. Induction of hepatomas in mice by repeated oral administration of chloroform, with observations on sex differences. *J Natl Cancer Inst* 1944;5:251–255.
51. Newberne PM, de Camargo JLV, Clark AJ. Choline deficiency, partial hepatectomy, and liver tumors in rats and mice. *Toxicol Pathol* 1982;10:95–109.

Toxicology of the Liver, 2nd ed.,
Edited by Gabriel L. Plaa and William R. Hewitt
Copyright © 1998 Taylor & Francis

3

Chemical-Induced Hepatocarcinogenesis

James E. Klaunig and Kyle L. Kolaja

Indiana University School of Medicine, Indianapolis, IN 46202-5196

- **The Multistage Model of Hepatocarcinogenesis**
- **Historic Perspective of Chemical-Induced Hepatic Carcinogenesis**
- **Mechanistic Classification of Hepatocarcinogens**
- **Alterations in Gene Expression during Hepatocarcinogenesis**
- **Quantification of Hepatic Focal Lesion Growth Induced by Hepatocarcinogens**
- **Mechanisms of Hepatic Tumor Promotion: Proliferation and Apoptosis**
- **Possible Cellular Mechanisms of Hepatic Lesion Growth**
  - Gap Junctional Intercellular Communication
  - Oxidative Stress
  - Mixed Function Oxidase System (MFOS)
  - Growth Factors, Oncogenes, Transcription Factors, and Tumor Suppressor Genes
- **Conclusions**
- **References**

The study of chemical-induced hepatocarcinogenesis has provided strong insight into the tumor formation process. A variety of chemicals and agents can increase the incidence, multiplicity, or time of onset of hepatic cancer. These compounds either damage DNA (genotoxic) or produce cancer through epigenetic (nongenotoxic) mechanisms. Compounds that produce hepatic cancer through these epigenetic mechanisms exert a variety of effects including changes in methylation, oxidative stress, gene expression, protein kinase C activity, gap junctional intercellular communication, mixed function oxidase activity, and growth factor expression. The most important effect nongenotoxic hepatocarcinogens have on hepatocytes is the induction of initiated cell growth through increased cell proliferation or decreased cell death (apoptosis). This chapter examines several aspects of chemical-induced hepatocarcinogenesis including the multistage model of hepatocarcinogenesis, quantification of lesion growth, the impact that carcinogens have on cell proliferation and apoptosis, and the possible mechanisms that are involved in carcinogen-induced imbalances in growth parameters that lead to hepatic cancer.

THE MULTISTAGE MODEL OF HEPATOCARCINOGENESIS

The induction of cancer in the liver by chemicals involves at least three definable stages: initiation, promotion, and progression (Fig. 1). Initiation is a two-step process that involves the nonlethal mutation of DNA followed by at least one round of DNA synthesis to fix the mutation. Depending on the location of the mutation in the genome, initiation can create a cell that either has all of the genetic damage necessary to produce a neoplasm without further modification or requires additional cellular modifications to produce a malignant hepatic tumor. Initiation can occur after a single genotoxic (DNA-damaging) event such as seen with x-rays, UV light, DNA-reactive compounds, or spontaneously through DNA repair infidelity. Once the genetic mutation is fixed, the initiated cell can remain dormant (quiescent) for a period of time (demonstrating the irreversible nature of this stage). For example, skin papillomas can emerge with TPA 43 weeks subsequent to initiation with DMBA (1). Similar memory by initiated cells has also been demonstrated in rodent liver (2, 3). The hepatic tumor-promoting agent phenobarbital (PB) was effective at enhancing lesion growth in rat liver after a 120-day interval between initiator and promoter treatment (4).

Tumor promotion is classically defined as the selective clonal expansion of initiated cells into islands of altered hepatocytes defined as focal lesions (3). Promotion results in the formation of putative hepatic focal lesions that have altered morphologic, enzymatic, and proliferative parameters when compared to normal hepatocytes (5). Enhancement of the promotion process by chemical compounds, unlike single-dose genotoxic carcinogens, requires continuous exposure over a prolonged period. Compounds that function as tumor promoters typically are nongenotoxic (non–DNA reactive), and their effect is directly related to treatment duration and exposure concentration (5). Tumor promotion, primarily a change in genetic expression, is considered a reversible process (3). Numerous studies have indicated that hepatic focal lesion number and volume decrease after removal of a promoting stimulus (2, 6, 7). In addition, the reversible nature of hepatic focal lesions is seen, as increased focal hepatocyte apoptosis is observed after withdraw of the promoter (8). Importantly, tumor promotion can be modulated by a diverse group of factors (e.g., diet, exercise, environmental exposure, prescription medicines, micronutrient status) that humans are subject to (6, 9), thus offering a possible stage of the cancer process to target for chemointervention.

Progression, the last stage in the hepatocarcinogenic process, is less defined than promotion and initiation. Progression is characterized by continued genetic change (aneuploidy or karyotypic instability), increased growth rate, metastasis, hormonal and growth factor responsiveness, and histopathologic uniqueness (10). Progression, like initiation, involves mutation of DNA that is fixed by DNA replication and is considered an irreversible process (3, 10). Unlike cells in the stage of initiation or promotion, those in progression may undergo continuous evolution toward autonomy from host defenses (10). The increasing loss of growth regulation observed in tumor progression coincides with phenotypic and genotypic changes. The hallmark of tumor progression is the onset of neoplasia.

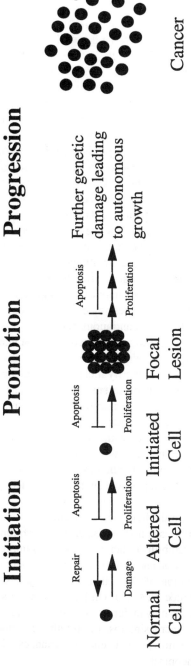

FIG. 1. The multistage model of hepatocarcinogenesis. Note that proliferation is required at all three stages of hepatic cancer development. Apoptosis can also be modulated to effect hepatocarcinogenesis. Chemical carcinogens can advance the cancer process by effecting any of the stages of cancer by either damaging DNA (e.g., initiation and progression) or by increasing cell proliferation or inhibiting apoptosis. Chemical-induced alterations in tissue growth mainly effect tumor promotion but can also enhance spontaneous genetic mutations in tumor initiation and progression.

HISTORIC PERSPECTIVE OF CHEMICAL-INDUCED
HEPATIC CARCINOGENESIS

The concept of hepatocarcinogenesis's being a multistage process finds its roots in numerous investigations involving chemical-induced skin carcinogenesis. Twort and Twort (11) applied oleic acid (5 days a week for 35 weeks) to mouse skin that was previously treated with the genotoxic carcinogen benzo(a)pyrene. Oleic acid was selected as the promoting compound because it had previously been shown to induce epidermal hyperplasia (12). In the 1940s, experiments showed that treatment with 3-methylcholanthrene or coal tar produced "latent tumor cells" in the epidermis of rabbits. Subsequent treatment with compounds or regimens that induced hyperplasia such as turpentine, chloroform, and cork wounding enhanced skin tumor formation (13, 14). Rous coined the term *initiation* to describe the presence of latent tumor cells that could be revealed by subsequent treatment of the same skin area with a hyperplasia-inducing factor, or promoter (13, 14).

Compounds can selectively exert their effects at different stages of the carcinogenesis process (1, 15, 16). Experiments by Berenblum and Harlan (16), showed that apportioned doses of either the initiating compound alone or the promoting compound alone were ineffective. Initiator treatment following promoter treatment (reverse-order) was also ineffective. This was in contrast to mice treated with initiator (DMBA) followed by promoter treatment (croton oil containing TPA), which resulted in neoplasia. These studies demonstrated that carcinogenic compounds can preferentially effect certain stages of cancer development.

Working from the studies on multistage cancer in the skin, a number of investigators probed for similar end points in the rodent liver (3, 17–21). Peraino et al. (18, 19) were among the first to show that hepatic cancer can be divided into at least two distinct stages, thus mimicking the results observed in skin tumorigenesis using 2-acetyl-aminofluorene (2-AAF) as an initiating carcinogen and PB as a tumor promoter. Similar to turpentine, TPA, or cork wounding in the skin model, PB treatment had been shown to cause hyperplasia and hypertrophy in the liver (18). Rats treated with 2-AAF and then PB (0.05% in diet) showed a 70% incidence of hepatic tumors. In contrast, the treatment with PB or 2-AAF alone induced a significantly lower incidence (5% and 25%, respectively). These studies support the premise that hepatic tumorigenesis in the rat occurs via at least two stages. Subsequent studies by others have further demonstrated that chemicals can preferentially act on a particular stage of hepatocarcinogenesis (3, 22–25). Thus, these results in the liver in concert with studies in other tissues helped to produce a new means of classification of carcinogens.

MECHANISTIC CLASSIFICATION OF HEPATOCARCINOGENS

Hepatocarcinogens appear to produce their carcinogenic effect through either genotoxic or nongenotoxic mechanisms. The ability of genotoxic carcinogens to react with DNA correlates directly with their mechanism of action. Initially, most if not

TABLE 1. *Ames assay positive compounds that are hepatocarcinogenic to rodents*

N-acetoxy-2-acetylaminofluorene	2-Acetylaminoflourene	2-Aminofluorene
N-hydroxy-2 acetylaminofluorene	2,7-Diaminofluorene	1,5-Napthalenediamine
N-hydroxy-2 aminofluorene	3-Nitro-p-acetophenitidine	4-Aminobiphenyl
5-Nitro-o-anisidine	Nithiazide	6-Nitro-benzimadole
3-Nitropropinoic acid	2,4-Diaminotoluene	P-nitrosodiphenylamine
5-Nitro-o-toluidine	4'4-Oxydianiline	Selenium sulfoxide
4'4-Thiodianiline	2,4-Toluene diisocyanate	2,6-Toluene diisocyanate
3,3-Dimethyloxybenzidine dihydrochlorine	2-Aminoanthraquinone	3-Amino-9-ethylcarbazole
1-Amino 2-methylanthraquinone	Bis(2-chloro-1-methylethyl) ether	1,3-Butadiene
4-Chloro-m-phenylenediamine	Chloramben	4-Chloro-o-phenylenediamine
5-Nitroacenapthalene	2-Nitronapthalene	Glycidol
H.C. Blue 1	H.C. Red 3	C.I. Acid red114
Dimethlnitrosamine	Diethylnitrosamine	Aflatoxin B1,B2,M2,G1
Di-n-propylnitrosamine	C.I. Basic 9 monohydrate	Nitrosoethylurea
C.I. Direct black 38	C.I. Direct brown 95	C.I. Disperse blue 1
C.I. Disperse yellow 14	C.I. Solvent yellow 14	Hydrazobenzene
4'4-methylene dianiline dihydrochloride	Lasocarpine	Azaserine
2-Methyl-1-nitroanthraquinone	Michler's ketone	P-cresidine
Cupferron	1,2-Dibromoethane	2,6-Dichloro-p-phenylenediamine
1,3-Dichloropropene	Di(p-ethylphenyl) dichloroether	Toxaphene

all carcinogens were considered to have genotoxic (DNA-damaging) activity (26). A genotoxic carcinogen is one in which a primary biological activity of the chemical or an ultimate metabolite reacts with DNA such that the information encoded within is permanently altered (27, 28). This alteration can be a point mutation, an insertion, a deletion, or changes in chromosomal structure or number. Typically, compounds that exert genotoxic activity can be identified (29). Numerous assays have been developed in bacterial or mammalian systems that when used with or without metabolic activation can detect the mutational activity of a chemical compound (27, 30). DNA reactivity does not itself mean that alteration of DNA is the only or absolute requirement for neoplastic transformation (31). There are mutagenic compounds that are noncarcinogenic after chronic administration (29, 31a, 32). Chronic exposure of the compound to a bioassay system indicates its carcinogenicity. Of the numerous chemical carcinogens that display genotoxic activity, a representative list of chemicals that are hepatocarcinogenic to rodents is shown in Table 1.

Single-dose exposure to a genotoxic hepatocarcinogen appears sufficient to produce neoplasia. Formation of presumptive initiated hepatocytes has been observed after as little as 4 days following a single application of diethylnitrosamine (33). Threshold doses of genotoxic carcinogens may be difficult to ascertain (9). Dose-responsive characteristics, however, have been observed in focal lesion formation in livers of carcinogen-treated rodents. A linear induction of ATPase-deficient focal lesions was observed in rats treated with diethylnitrosamine at doses of up to 30 mg/kg (34). Above 30 mg/kg, diethylnitrosamine produced carcinomas and no linearity of focal

TABLE 2. *Ames assay negative (nonmutagenic) compounds that are hepatocarcinogenic to rodents*

Carbon tetrachloride	Para-rosanaline	1,2-Dichloropropane
Ethyl carbamate	Safrole	1'Hydroxysafrole
Dieldrin	Cycasin	Dichlorophenyldichloroethylene
2,6-Dichloro-p-phenylenediamine	Amitrole	3'-Nitro-p-acetophenitide
Aldrin	6'-Nitrobenzimadazole	Toxaphene
11-Aminoundecanoic acid	Benzyl acetate	Chlorendic acid
Hexachloroethane	1,4-Dichlorobenzene	2,3,7,8-TCDD
Di(2-ethylhexyl) pthalate	Chlorodibromomethane	Bis-2 chloro-methylethylester
Furan	Di(2-ethylhexyl) adipate	Furfural
Dimethyl morpholinophoshoramidate	Wyeth-14,643	Pentachlorethane
PBB (Firemaster FF-1)	Hydrochlorothiazide	Monuron
1,1,2,2-Tetrachloroethane	Tetrachloroethylene	Trichloroethylene
Tris (2-ethylhexyl) phosphate	4-Vinylcyclohexene	Zearalenone
5-Nitro-o-toludine	Isophorone	Chlordane
Heptachlor	Dicofol	DDE
Tetrachlorvinphos	Chlorobenzilate	5-Chloro-o-toludine
Thioacetamide	Phenobarbital	2-Mercaptobenzothiazide
Chloroform	1,4 Dioxane	Nitrofen
2-Aminoanthraquinone	Trifluralin	Methyl carbamate
DDT	Ciprofibrate	Clofibrate
N-methylolacrylamide	Mirex	Pentochlorophenol
Phenylbutazone	Picloram	Piperonyl sulfoxide
Probenecid	2,4,6-Trichlorophenol	1,1,2-Trichloroethane
Benzofuran	Bromo dichloromethane	Chlorobenzene
C.I. Direct blue 6	C.I. Direct blue 6	Cinnamyl anthranilate
Diaminozide	Decabromobiphenyl oxide	2,7-Dichlorodibenzo-p-dioxin
2,4-Dithiobiurea	Ethylene thiourea (ETU)	Eugenol

lesion production was observed (34). A linear increase in the number and volume of altered hepatic foci in rats was observed with diethylnitrosamine and NNM at doses ranging from 10 to 250 mg/kg (35). In contrast, no detectable threshold or plateau was observed in the formation of GGT-positive foci following diethylnitrosamine treatment in rats (36, 37). The above studies suggest that genotoxic carcinogens have distinct effects, including single-dose efficacy, no observable lower threshold for focal lesion formation, and a linear relationship between number and volume of focal lesions at selected doses of the initiating carcinogen.

Besides genotoxic hepatic carcinogens, a number of drugs and chemicals induce hepatic cancer in rodents when administered at high doses for prolonged periods through non–DNA-damaging (nongenotoxic) mechanisms (Table 2). These compounds are considered to be nongenotoxic carcinogens because they lack genotoxicity as a primary biologic activity. The properties of these agents differ considerably from electrophilic DNA-reactive genotoxic carcinogens, which can produce carcinogenic results after a single low-dose exposure. Chronic exposure to nongenotoxic hepato-carcinogens leads to an increase in the incidence or multiplicity of hepatic lesions when compared to those of untreated rodents. Nongenotoxic compounds appear to act by cellular mechanisms other than the direct mutation of DNA. This is supported in part by experimental evidence: Nongenotoxic hepatocarcinogens have been shown to function at the stage of tumor promotion (3); many compounds that lack genotoxicity induce cancer (38); human cancer is mediated by several influences, many of which are considered nongenotoxic (6); and hormones (which are not mutagenic) have been shown to be hepatocarcinogenic (39). Nongenotoxic hepatocarcinogens produce hepatic cancer by functioning through lesser-defined epigenetic mechanisms.

Exposure to nongenotoxic hepatocarcinogens leads to changes in cell proliferation (in both normal and focal hepatocytes) or apoptosis in normal hepatocytes, among other effects, (40). An association has been made between induction of hepatic DNA synthesis in normal liver and hepatocarcinogenicity (29, 41). Based on this association, the target cell for induction of cancer by these compounds has been suggested to be the normal or naive liver (29). Cell proliferation and DNA synthesis are prerequisites for every stage of the cancer process (42). It has been proposed that the induction of DNA synthesis in a normally nondividing tissue such as the liver can lead to the spontaneous initiation of a replicating hepatocyte (29, 41). Controversy has developed over defining an exact mechanistic role in the onset of cancer to the increased DNA synthesis caused by carcinogen treatment (43). Although some investigators have purported that the increased level of DNA synthesis leads to an increased probability of causing a genetic mutation (29), others have proposed that there is no correlation between toxicity or increased cell proliferation and the onset of cancer (44, 45). Because hepatic cancer is a disease of loss of regulation of the cell cycle (uncontrolled growth), the relative significance of the induction of increased DNA synthesis or cell replication by hepatic carcinogens needs to be defined further.

The focal lesion in particular is a target for the growth stimulating effects of nongenotoxic carcinogens. Because the selective enhancement of cell growth is a characteristic of tumor promotion, many feel that hepatic nongenotoxic carcinogens exert their effect during the hepatic tumor promotion stage of cancer. Nongenotoxic agents as diverse as barbiturates, DDT, chlorinated hydrocarbon pesticides, polybrominated biphenyls, TCDD, polychlorinated biphenyls, lipid-lowering drugs, steroid hormones, bile acids, and dietary influences (fat, protein, carbohydrates, calories) all have been shown to modulate hepatic focal lesion growth (3, 5). Nongenotoxic hepatocarcinogens enhance the growth of hepatic focal lesions and appear to facilitate the conversion of a relatively small number of these foci into tumors. Thus, the initiated cell population appears to be the target for the enhancement of hepatic neoplastic production (3, 7, 27, 28, 46, 47).

Several proposals on the specific mechanism of action of nongenotoxic hepatocarcinogens have been put forward. Nongenotoxic carcinogens as noted above may function as tumor promoters and thus provide the signal that triggers expression of a specific gene in initiated cells that provides them with a selective growth advantage (48, 48a). This effect may be mediated through disturbance of hepatocyte membrane homeostasis (membrane damage, inhibition of gap junctional intercellular communication, modification of growth factor or hormone receptors, etc.) allowing initiated cells to escape normal growth regulation, which in turn results in their proliferation and the eventual growth of hepatic tumors. Changes in DNA fidelity in initiated cells may make initiated cells targets for subsequent interaction by nongenotoxic agents. For example, decreased DNA repair efficacy in hepatocytes in focal lesions has been reported (49). GSTP (glutathione-S-transferase; placental form)-positive hepatocytes (presumptive initiated cells) are able to continue to divide at a greater rate despite the presence of strand breaks and mispairing (50).

The classification of hepatic carcinogens into genotoxic and nongenotoxic groupings may be too simplistic. It is important to recognize that this classification system is in some cases arbitrary, and some genotoxic carcinogens may exhibit properties of nongenotoxic hepatocarcinogens and vice versa. In either case, the hepatic focal lesion represents an important stage in hepatic cancer development.

ALTERATIONS IN GENE EXPRESSION DURING HEPATOCARCINOGENESIS

Phenotypic and genotypic changes have been detected in both preneoplastic (foci) and neoplastic (adenomas and carcinomas) lesions during the cancer process (3, 39, 51, 52). Investigations into the biochemical, molecular, and morphologic alterations seen in preneoplastic and neoplastic hepatic lesions indicate that the process of neoplastic development in the liver involves complex changes in genetic expression that may be responsible for the selective enhancement of lesion growth and the acquisition of further genetic alterations, resulting in the subsequent progression to the malignant phenotype. Mellors and Seguira (51) detected an increase in alkaline phosphatase activity in hepatic lesions after treatment of rats with the carcinogen butter yellow. Carcinogen-induced preneoplastic and neoplastic hepatic lesions have been shown to be deficient in glucose-6-phosphatase activity compared to the surrounding normal liver in rats and mice (39, 52). Similarly, GGT (gamma-glutamyltransferase) activity has been shown to increase in focal and neoplastic lesions compared to normal liver carcinogen–treated rats (53). The accumulation of glycogen, or glycogenosis, in hepatic focal lesions of rats administered chemical carcinogens has also been reported (54).

Alteration in the expression of protein kinase C isozymes has also been observed in hepatic focal and neoplastic lesions in rats (55). The overexpression in hepatic foci of protein kinase C isoenzyme-a and protein kinase C isoenzyme-b has been reported to provide growth enhancement in rat liver, whereas overexpression of protein kinase C isoenzyme-d appears to inhibit focal growth (55). Overexpression of the oncogene ras-p21 has been demonstrated in focal and neoplastic lesions (56). Similarly, overexpression of c-myc and c-src oncogenes has been noted in focal and neoplastic liver (10, 57). Recent studies have also shown that c-jun is overexpressed in hepatic focal lesions in mice (58).

Despite the multitude of alterations in gene expression that have been observed, certain markers have been used preferentially as presumptive identifiers of hepatic focal lesions. GGTase overexpression has been used as a marker for hepatic lesions in rats and, occasionally, in mice (39, 53). In addition, the immunohistochemical detection of the expression of GSTP has also been used extensively to identify hepatic focal lesions in rats and is accepted as a marker of putative preneoplastic lesions (3, 56). However, neither GGT nor GSTP identify hepatic focal lesions produced by exposure to nongenotoxic hepatocarcinogens (e.g., peroxisome proliferators) (3, 39). In addition, both GGT and GSTP do not consistently identify spontaneous or chemical-induced lesions in male mice (3, 58, 59). In contrast to male mice, female mice have been shown to express GSTP in putative preneoplastic lesions (58). In addition, the expression of GSTP in rat hepatic focal lesions does not correlate with either c-jun or c-fos (60). These differences in the expression markers between mice and rats suggest that there are intrinsic differences in focal lesions between these two species, further indicating the need for a method of hepatic focal lesion detection that does not exhibit compound or species selectivity.

Morphologic investigations with light microscopy offer another way to examine hepatic focal lesions. In 1975, a committee (workshop) on the criteria to explain alterations in rat hepatic lesions was held (61). The criterion established at this meeting described the phenotypic diversity observed in focal and neoplastic lesions in rat liver. Focal lesions in rat liver were defined as basophilic, eosinophilic, clear, or mixed. In mouse liver, lesion classification has developed greatly from the original classifications of Walker, Thorpe, and Stevenson (62). In their paper, hepatic lesions were classified as A and B, with the latter being malignant carcinomas and the former being benign adenomas. Frith and Ward (63) later developed a lesion classification system that is similar to the rat model. The use of H & E to detect focal and neoplastic changes remains an essential method of altered hepatic focal lesion detection, especially when examining the growth of focal lesions in different species and chemical carcinogens.

QUANTIFICATION OF HEPATIC FOCAL LESION GROWTH INDUCED BY HEPATOCARCINOGENS

Defining and quantifying the appearance, disappearance, and growth of hepatic foci following carcinogen treatment requires a rigorous method of quantification (64). Initially, simple methods of gross observations of tumors followed by histochemical and histopathologic evaluation were used to describe the effects of hepatocarcinogens. This method was problematic because it included only neoplasms in the evaluation and offered little mechanistic information pertaining to lesion formation and growth. Because hepatic foci are considered to be presumptive precursors to hepatic neoplasia, an accurate method of quantification of focal lesion growth was needed (34). Models based on mathematic principles were used to define the number and volume of both focal and neoplastic lesions during chemical carcinogenesis. Stereology, the study of two-dimensional observations and conversion to three-dimensional results, offers a method of mathematic evaluation that can address treatment-induced effects on hepatic focal lesions.

Quantitative stereology was first used in early geologic research (65). In 1848, the French geologist Delesse first described how two-dimensional areas are proportional to three-dimensional volumes (65). In 1928, Wicksell was the first to apply stereology to biologic systems and determined the frequency and size of germinal centers inside the spleen (66). Scherer and Emmelot were among the first to adapt the mathematic principles used by Delesse to the enumeration of hepatic focal lesions (34). The validity of the mathematic models has been addressed by rigorously sectioning tissue, confirming the validity of the spherical nature of hepatic focal lesions, and introducing a lower limit of reproducible lesion detection (67). The use of stereology in hepatic cancer research enables the understanding of lesion growth and development.

The most reproducible method for determining the number of preneoplastic focal lesions per liver after treatment with an agent or those that occur naturally determines the number of focal lesions per cubic centimeter of liver (3). This method is considered to be more accurate than other methods that are based on two-dimensional parameters (3). In two-dimensional data, the mean diameter of all focal lesions must be identical for a correlation between the two-dimensional data and the actual response in three-dimensional liver (64). The stereologic methods described by Pugh, Campbell, and Bannasch have been used to determine the effects of nongenotoxic hepatocarcinogens on the growth of hepatic focal lesions (67–69).

Stereology can be used to determine the ability of a chemical to function as a complete carcinogen, tumor promoter, or initiating carcinogen (3, 5). The size of a hepatic focus will effect certain stereologic parameters. If a compound increases the number of lesions per liver as determined by stereology, the increase may be attributed to a variety of effects, including acting as a genotoxic agent and producing new initiated cell populations that grow into small detectable focal lesions (3), increasing the size of existing lesions such that their detectability in two-dimensional sections of a three-dimensional liver is increased (64), and enhancing the growth of focal lesions that were previously histologically unevident (70). Stereologic evaluation of hepatic focal lesion growth in properly designed studies can be an accurate estimator of a compound's ability to function at the stage of tumor promotion (3).

Another important stereologic parameter that indicates lesion growth is hepatic focal lesion volume. This parameter describes the volume of hepatic tissue that is focal compared to the normal surrounding liver. An increased volume of focal liver can be observed on the total population of altered hepatic foci or on a specific lesion phenotype. A rapid growth rate of focal lesions (increase in focal volume percentage) has been shown to correlate directly with increasing alterations from the normal genetic expression (3). Importantly, a small change in foci growth rate induced by a nongenotoxic hepatocarcinogen can contribute to a large increase in focal volume when extended over a period (21).

Phenotypic heterogeneity has been observed in spontaneous and chemical-induced hepatic focal lesions (69, 71). As previously noted, numerous genetic alterations exist during the stage of promotion, indicating a change toward a phenotype that is different from normal liver. Nongenotoxic hepatocarcinogens can selectively enhance the growth of certain focal phenotypic lesions. For example, phenobarbital promotes the growth of eosinophilic hepatic foci (7, 72–74). In contrast, peroxisome proliferators enhance the growth of basophilic lesions (6, 75, 76). Chronic treatment with phenobarbital or peroxisome proliferators produces hepatic adenomas that are eosinophilic and basophilic in phenotype, respectively (72, 73). This suggests that the preferential promoting activity nongenotoxic hepatocarcinogens may be exerted on certain focal phenotypically distinct lesions that are more likely to become neoplastic.

Alterations in stereologic parameters indicate an effect on lesion growth. Compounds that function at the stage of tumor promotion will increase the number and volume of hepatic focal lesions (Fig. 2). Stereologic data need to be coupled with cell

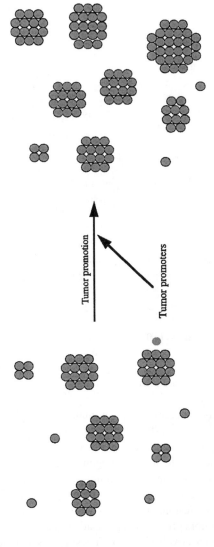

Hepatic focal lesion population

Hepatic focal lesion population

Tumor promotion

Tumor promoters

FIG. 2. The effect of tumor-promoting compounds on the growth of hepatic focal lesions and single, initiated cells. Note that not all initiated cells and focal lesions can be enhanced by tumor-promoting compounds, yet the overall effect of a tumor-promoting compound is to increase both the detectable size and the number of hepatic focal lesions.

kinetic data (cell proliferation and cell death [apoptosis]) in order to accurately study mechanisms of hepatic tumor promotion.

MECHANISMS OF HEPATIC TUMOR PROMOTION: PROLIFERATION AND APOPTOSIS

The ability of promoters to enhance neoplastic growth can also be explained by giving a growth stimulus to initiated hepatocytes that are neoplastic but would remain dormant otherwise. This hypothesis is supported by the promoter-dependent nature of hepatic focal lesions that regress after withdrawal of the promoting stimulus (3). In contrast, some focal lesions may be neoplastic and have sufficient ability to replicate. These lesions would appear in animals regardless of the promoter treatment. Nongenotoxic carcinogens may, however, enhance the acquisition of this phenotype (48a).

Chemical-induced focal lesion growth in rats appears to be a reversible event, as foci disappear upon removal of the promoting stimulus (77, 78). Three cycles of the compound 2-acetyl-aminofluorene (2-AAF; 3 weeks' feeding of 0.06% AAF, then 1 week on basal diet) resulted in the formation of macroscopic nodules that disappear a few months after the last cycle of treatment (77). DEN treatment of partial hepatectomized rats followed by continuous treatment by PB resulted in the formation of altered hepatic foci that disappeared upon PB removal (78). Also, DEN (200 mg/kg body weight) followed by partial hepatectomy and promoted with 2-AAF resulted in the formation of visible hyperplastic hepatic nodules (79). Subsequent removal of 2-AAF resulted in a decrease in the number and size of hyperplastic nodules. These studies suggest that some altered hepatic foci in rats may require the continuous presence of a nongenotoxic carcinogen or promoting agent to prevent their regression or disappearance and that nongenotoxic hepatocarcinogens enhance the growth of focal lesions in a reversible manner. These studies suggest that many focal lesions may still be under some control of the normal liver. Ultimately, the increased growth of hepatic focal lesions can be attributed to changes in cell proliferation or cell death.

Treatment of nongenotoxic hepatocarcinogens significantly elevates DNA synthesis in hepatic focal lesions when compared to untreated control preneoplastic lesions, possibly giving promoter-treated foci a selective growth advantage (7, 46–48, 48a). The exact cellular mechanism of this growth enhancement is relatively unclear. As shown in Fig. 3 chemical carcinogens have a multitude of effects on hepatocytes. Disturbances in oxidative stress, gene methylation, gene expression, protein kinase C activity, mixed function oxidase, and genetic integrity have been observed in carcinogen-treated liver.

Increased focal growth by nongenotoxic hepatocarcinogens has been considered to be the driving mechanism behind the carcinogenicity of these compounds (70). Growth of focal lesions can be through either increased focal cell replication or by decreasing the death rate of focal cells (42, 48a, 80, 81).

In focal hepatocytes, nongenotoxic hepatocarcinogens increase DNA synthesis and cell proliferation, leading to speculation that these compounds elicit their carcinogenic

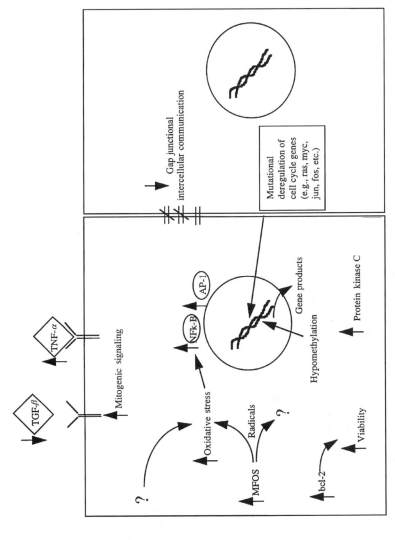

FIG. 3. The possible mechanisms of hepatocarcinogenesis and hepatic lesion growth. Chemical carcinogens can mutationally deregulate cell cycle genes, leading to uncontrolled cell proliferation or liberation from apoptosis. Some chemical carcinogens do not directly mutate DNA but modulate growth factors, suppressor genes, and protooncogenes; inhibit gap junctional intercellular communication; induce an oxidative stress, or alter the normal gene expression and regulation (e.g., hypomethylation) such that selective cell growth may occur.

105

effect through this growth mechanism (27, 70). Several nongenotoxic hepatocarcinogens, including TCDD, PB, a-hexachlorocyclohexane, cyproterone acetate, dieldrin, and Wyeth-14,643, induce hepatic DNA synthesis in focal lesions (47, 48, 48a, 70, 74, 82, 83). Because tumor promotion is defined as the selective clonal expansion of the initiated cell population into preneoplastic focal lesions, enhancement of focal lesion growth by increasing cell replication has led many investigators to ascribe the mechanism of action of nongenotoxic carcinogens at the tumor promotion stage (27).

Cell death in hepatic foci can occur by either necrosis or by apoptosis (programmed cell death) (84). Necrosis often occurs after severe cellular injury and leads to disruption of normal cellular homeostasis. In necrotic cells, mitochondrial dysfunction occurs and coincides with loss of cell membrane integrity, resulting in cell death. Necrosis frequently produces an inflammatory response in the tissue. Apoptosis, in contrast, occurs in single isolated cells and appears to be a controlled form of cell death, where mitochondrial function is maintained until very late in the process, occurs over the course of several hours, and, importantly, does not induce an immune response. The lack of an inflammatory response in apoptosis appears to be advantageous because it allows tissues to grow, develop, and remove unneeded cells without harming adjacent normal cells.

Apoptosis in hepatocytes occurs in morphologically evident stages. Apoptosis can be identified by morphologic criteria such as increased eosinophilia of the cytoplasm, separation from surrounding cells, condensation of the chromatin, and fragmentation of the cell into smaller vesicles that can be phagocytized by neighboring hepatocytes (8, 85). The first morphologically evident stage involves chromatin condensation, believed to be initiated by the activation of an endonuclease (86, 87). Fragmentation and the extracellular presence of small pieces of apoptotic bodies are subsequently observed. After fragmentation, the phagocytosis of the individual fragmented apoptotic bodies within viable hepatocytes was observed (85). The final stage of apoptosis is the fusion with lysosomes and degradation of the apoptotic bodies.

Inhibition of apoptosis has been suggested to be a possible mechanism of tumor promotion (80). Several nongenotoxic hepatocarcinogens including nafenopin, cyproterone acetate, TCDD, and PB have been shown to inhibit apoptosis in focal lesion hepatocytes in a manner that contributes to the hepatic tumor-promoting effect (6, 88). In contrast, treatment with Wyeth-14,643 has been shown to increase the incidence of apoptosis in rat liver (82). Similarly, methylpyrilene, a nongenotoxic hepatocarcinogen, has been shown to have no observable effect on normal and focal apoptosis in hepatocytes (82a). Because nongenotoxic hepatocarcinogens appear to effect apoptosis and cell proliferation, future studies should address the exact role of apoptosis in chemical carcinogen-induced hepatocarcinogenesis.

In the development of hepatocellular cancer, apoptosis does appear to be a pivotal cellular control mechanism. Dietary restriction (40% of control *ad libitum* intake) of otherwise untreated mice decreased cell proliferation and enhanced apoptosis (89, 90). Furthermore, the anticarcinogen perillyl alcohol has been shown to induce apoptosis in rat hepatic liver lesions, leading to a decrease in tumor volume (91). Apoptosis increases in the progression stage as a by-product of multiple karotypic changes

(92). Apoptosis in hepatic tumors may cause microcompensatory induction of cell proliferation and may be important in enhancing cell replication and conversion of hepatocytes to a malignant genotype (42). These studies suggest that apoptosis is an important regulatory factor and can be modulated in hepatocarcinogenicity.

Apoptosis has been clearly indicated as a mechanism for elimination of preneo-plastic and normal hepatocytes following removal of growth stimulus (78, 85, 88, 93). Cessation of treatment of dieldrin or PB, nongenotoxic hepatocarcinogens, in-creased the incidence of apoptosis in focal lesions, even 30 days after removal of the promoting agent (47). A similar pattern of enhanced focal apoptosis was observed after removal of PB in Wistar rats (85). In that study, a peak in apoptosis occurred 3–7 days after removal of PB, but the incidence of focal apoptosis was still significantly increased 42 days after cessation of PB treatment (85). These small but consistent increases in apoptosis can remove a large number of hepatocytes in a short period of time and result in a decreased number and volume of focal lesions (87). An alternative mechanism to explain the loss of focal lesions after promoter withdrawal proposes that focal hepatocytes revert to a phenotype histologically indiscernible from sur-rounding normal hepatocytes (94). It has been suggested that the actual number of focal lesions does not decrease after promoter cessation, but the rapid loss of vol-ume can be attributed to the loss of detectable phenotype (78). However, the rapid loss of foci volume, either through apoptosis or through reversion, would result in a decreased average volume of individual lesions and result in the observed decreased number of focal lesions (64). In studies in our laboratory, an increased incidence of apoptosis in focal lesions occurring after removal of either dieldrin or PB correlated with a decrease in the volume and number of focal lesions (47). The driving factors behind changes in proliferation and apoptosis are still unclear.

POSSIBLE CELLULAR MECHANISMS OF HEPATIC LESION GROWTH

Gap Junctional Intercellular Communication

Blockage of gap junctional intercellular communication (GJIC) may play an im-portant role in nongenotoxic hepatocarcinogenesis. Normal gap junctional intercel-lular communication allows the passage of small-molecular-weight water-soluble molecules (molecular weight < 1000) between adjacent hepatocytes. Through gap junctions, the passage of these small second messengers may function to maintain tissue homeostasis. This, in turn, may provide a system of checks and balances to prevent unneeded cell proliferation (95). In support of this hypothesis, the inhibition of GJIC appears to correlate with increasing hepatic DNA synthesis (96). In addition, most cancer cells exhibit a decreased or aberrant GJIC that appears to progressively decrease as the dysplasia of the cancer increases (95). Therefore, uncontrolled pro-liferation seen in hepatic cancer may be mediated by the down modulation of gap junctional intercellular communication.

Gap junctional intercellular communication can be controlled at several different levels including transcription (DNA), translation (RNA), protein stability, and post-translational modification of the gap junction pore. Rat hepatocellular carcinomas have decreased gene and protein expression (95). In addition, hepatic neoplasms displayed downregulated Cx 32 protein, possibly through alterations in the primary structure of the protein or by posttranslational modification (97). However, some hepatic tumors expressed abundant connexin mRNA without any observable immunoreactive protein, indicating that gap junctional protein expression can be regulated independently of gene translation (97). In any result, the modification of gap junctional intercellular communication appears to be a common factor in chemical-induced hepatocarcinogenesis.

Treatment with a nongenotoxic hepatocarcinogen alters gap junctional intercellular communication both in vivo and in vitro (97, 98). In hepatic focal lesions, greater cell proliferation is seen in foci with the lowest expression of gap junctional proteins (96). The nongenotoxic hepatocarcinogens PB and TCDD altered the immunohistochemistry of gap junctional proteins in hepatic focal lesions (97) and in cultured hepatocytes (99). Removal of the promoting stimulus (e.g., nongenotoxic hepatocarcinogen) lead to the reemergence of gap junctional expression in some focal lesions. This underscores both the reversible nature of the early stages of hepatocarcinogenesis and the significance of gap junctional intercellular communication in hepatic tumorogenesis.

The inhibition of cell-to-cell communication may enhance the cancer process in several ways but particularly at the tumor promotion stage (95). Initiated cells are held in check by cell-to-cell communication between normal cells and initiated cells. Blockage of gap junctional intercellular communication in initiated hepatocytes may remove the growth suppressive effects of the surrounding hepatocytes. Because second messengers (e.g., pH, Ca^{2+}, phosphorylation, and c-AMP) can modulate gap junctional intercellular communication, the prevention of the passage of these cellular molecules into the initiated cell from noninitiated hepatocytes may lead to a proliferative state (96).

Oxidative Stress

Oxidative stress, an imbalance in the prooxidant/antioxidant status of the cell in favor of the former that leads to potential damage (100), can participate at all stages of the hepatocarcinogenic process (101–103). The formation of oxidative stress has been proposed to be a mechanism by which some xenobiotics elicit their carcinogenic effects (102–105). Certain compounds can produce oxidative stress through biotransformation of the chemical into reactive intermediates (106), which, in turn, may lead to genotoxic damage (mutation, DNA strand breaks, or oxidative DNA damage). Chemical carcinogens can also produce oxidative stress by disrupting the normal prooxidant/antioxidant balance of a cell. Nongenotoxic hepatocarcinogens have been shown to increase oxidative radicals (107–109). Increased formation of reactive oxygen species can also modulate intracellular pH and intracellular Ca^{2+} concentrations, both of which can produce endonuclease activation and subsequent genotoxicity (110). In addition to reacting with important cellular macromolecules (lipids, DNA, and proteins), oxidative free radicals can induce the expression of immediate early genes such as c-myc, c-jun, and c-fos (106). The peroxisome proliferating hepatocarcinogens, Wyeth-14,643 and DEHP, increase the expression of c-jun and c-fos and induce oxidative stress in the liver (111). The transcription factors NFk-B and AP-1 (composed of c-jun and c-fos) are also stimulated by free oxygen radicals (112), which can lead to enhanced cell replication (113). NFk-B and AP-1 are also induced in B6C3F1 mice chronically exposed to dieldrin in a manner that correlates directly with hepatocyte proliferation and oxidative stress (unpublished observations). Oxidative stress, as well as several nongenotoxic compounds, has also been shown to inhibit gap junctional intercellular communication (114, 115).

The formation of reactive oxygen species can also stimulate protein kinase C (PKC) induction (107), which can lead to enhanced hepatocyte proliferation. The hepatocarcinogens carbon tetrachloride and cadmium, both of which appear to induce oxidative stress, have been shown to induce PKC activity (116). Similarly, peroxisome proliferators (Wyeth-14,642, perfluorooctanoate, clofibrate, ciprofibrate, DEHP, 2-ethylhexanol, and valproate) induce PKC activity in a manner that appears to correlate with carcinogenicity (117). Therefore, oxidative stress appears to be a plausible mechanism for the induction of hepatic cancer by nongenotoxic or genotoxic agents.

Dieldrin, a mouse-specific hepatocarcinogen, has been shown to selectively enhance the growth of mouse hepatic focal lesions (48). This effect was inhibited by vitamin E supplementation in the diet (48). Dieldrin has been demonstrated to induce oxidative damage selectively in mouse liver, increasing both hepatic 8-hydroxydeoxyguanosine (8-OHdGua), a marker of oxidant DNA damage, and malonyldialdehyde (MDA), a marker of lipid peroxidation in a dose-responsive manner (118). The oxidative stress by dieldrin may occur through several mechanisms. Dieldrin can activate macrophages, known producers of oxidative radicals (119). Also, Parke and Ioannides have suggested that compounds that induce cytochrome P450 like dieldrin generate oxidative radicals in a process called *futile cycling* (120). Dieldrin may also interact with hepatic enzymatic or nonenzymatic antioxidants. The latter suggestion is particularly intriguing because dieldrin and other nongenotoxic hepatic carcinogens can lower hepatic vitamin E levels substantially following treatment and the effects of dieldrin are prevented by vitamin E supplimentation.

Mixed Function Oxidase System (MFOS)

Hepatocarcinogens also induce cytologic changes such as hypertrophy and enzyme induction (22, 121). Hypertrophy, increases in cell size, is often attributed to induction of metabolic enzymes (24, 70). Parke and Ioannides suggested that compounds may induce P450 metabolic enzymes that react with the compound repeatedly, producing oxidative radicals in a process called *futile cycling* (120). Oxidative radicals and the oxidative stress has been implicated in all three stages of the carcinogenic process (122). Furthermore, Lubet et al. have shown that a linear correlation exists between a compound's ability to induce cytochrome P450 2B and the ability to function as a hepatic tumor promoter (123). This correlation exists for a variety of hepatocarcinogens including lindane, PB, DDT, valproic acid, barbital sodium, and diphenylhydantoin (123). Further studies with hamsters and monkeys expanded this correlation of cytochrome P450 induction and carcinogenicity (123). Cytochrome P450 2B generally detoxifies chemical compounds but can produce oxidative radicals through futile cycling (120). These studies indicate that the interaction between cytochrome P450 and certain chemical carcinogens may be a factor in determining the hepatocarcinogenicity of the compound.

Growth Factors, Oncogenes, Transcription Factors, and Tumor Suppressor Genes

Another common characteristic of hepatic chemical carcinogens is their ability to modulate the expression and responsiveness to proteins important in the regulation of tissue growth. Carcinogens can modulate the expression of the immediate early-response genes (e.g., c-myc, c-jun, and c-fos) (111). Growth factors such as TGF-b, TGF-a, EGF, and TNF-a have their normal physiologic functions altered by chemical carcinogens. In addition, the expression of bcl-2, an antiapoptosis gene, is altered in hepatic lesions (125). Other important regulators of the cell cycle (e.g., Rb, p53, ras, AP-1, and NFk-B) can also modulate hepatocarcinogenesis (124). Because the above factors are involved in tissue growth (e.g., cell proliferation and apoptosis), they may play a pivotal role in the hepatocarcinogenic process.

A number of cellular oncogenes (c-myc, bcl-2, Rb, p53, and TNF- a) and proteins regulate hepatocyte proliferation and apoptosis (125). The c-myc protooncogene (possibly a transcription factor) is a short-lived protein that is deregulated or elevated in virtually all tumors. The deregulation of c-myc leads to continuous cell proliferation as well as inability to differentiate (125). Surprisingly, c-myc also is a potent inducer of apoptosis, as its expression sensitizes many tissues to programmed cell death (126–128). In explanation of this phenomenon, it appears that c-myc over-expression is cytotoxic, especially when the appropriate exogenous growth factors are absent (129, 130). When cells that overexpress c-myc are in low serum media or treated with cytotoxic drugs (e.g., cyclohexamide), apoptosis is induced (130–132). The contrasting effects of c-myc overexpression may allow for a protective mechanism to prevent cell replication in unnecessary situations (125).

Overexpression of the protooncogene bcl-2 suppresses apoptosis (133–135). The protein bcl-2 is located on the endoplasmic reticulum, nucleus, and outer mitochondria membranes (136, 137). Bcl-2 was first identified as the site of reciprocal translocation in human follicular B cell lymphoma (136). However, bcl-2 overexpression has been observed in human hepatocellular carcinomas (138). The overexpression of bcl-2 protects a variety of cell types from apoptosis (133–135) as well as decreasing the sensitivity of the apoptotic inducing abilities of the overexpression of c-myc (139). The exact cellular mechanism of bcl-2 is unknown, but the end result is a protective inhibition of cell death. If the modulation of bcl-2 occurs in hepatic focal lesions, it may bestow a selective growth advantage by inhibiting the death process.

Tumor necrosis factor-α (TNF-α) has been shown to be an inducer of apoptosis as well as a stimulator of hepatocyte proliferation (140). The ability of TNF-α to induce apoptosis appears to depend on arrest at S-phase (141, 142). In contrast, TNF-α has been shown to be directly mitogenic to hepatocytes (143). TNF-α is secreted from activated Kupffer cells and has been suggested to be the mitogenic stimulus in peroxisome proliferator-treated liver (140). Because Kupffer cells secrete TNF-α, the modulation of TNF-α may be important in chemical-induced hepatic cancer for cytotoxic carcinogens in addition to peroxisome proliferators.

Loss or inactivation of retinoblastoma gene (Rb) and p53 tumor suppressor gene is involved in a number of human malignancies (144–150). Overexpression of p53 occurs shortly after genotoxic damage and leads to growth arrest at G1 (151). In addition, p53 sensitizes cells to apoptosis (152). Rb suppresses tumorigenicity and the neoplastic phenotype in certain tumor types but does not appear to lead to programmed cell death (153). However, little evidence for the role of these tumor suppressor genes in rodent chemical-induced hepatocarcinogenesis has been produced.

Altered expression of several genes involved in control of the cell cycle including the immediate early genes c-myc, c-jun and c-fos is involved in stimulating a cell from a resting phase into a proliferating phase (154). These genes can be mutation-activated by a genotoxic carcinogen, and nongenotoxic hepatocarcinogens can also increase the expression of these genes (111, 154). Because DNA is unwound and thus exposed during continued mRNA production, enhanced expression of these oncogenes can lead to the increased probability of chemical-induced or spontaneously induced genetic lesions (111). Treatment with the nongenotoxic hepatocarcinogens DEHP and Wyeth-14,643 led to the induction of c-jun (and jun-b and jun-d) and c-fos in a manner that correlated with both their carcinogenicity and their ability to induce DNA synthesis (111). In these studies, the induction of the immediate early genes could be blocked by a selective protein kinase C inhibitor. In furan-treated rats, a transient induction of c-myc and c-jun was seen in liver. However, the induction of c-fos and c-jun was not seen in mouse liver. Because furan increases hepatic DNA synthesis and is hepatocarcinogenic to both mice and rats, the changes in these immediate early genes appears to be independent of cell proliferation and carcinogenicity.

A positive regulator of hepatocyte growth is transforming growth factor alpha (TGF-α). TGF-α, not normally expressed in hepatocytes, binds to the EGF receptor. Overexpression of TGF-α due possibly to deregulation of the gene is seen in human hepatocellular carcinomas. TGF-α can enhance the growth of hepatic focal lesions and tumors and has been suggested to be a marker of progression in rodent hepatocarcinogenesis (155). In fact, TGF-α transgenic mice develop hepatocellular adenomas and carcinomas after 1 year (156). The stage of hepatocarcinogenesis on which TGF-α exerts its primary effect may be tumor promotion (157). Transgenic TGF-α mice do not develop hepatic cancer rapidly, suggesting that a mutational event must occur before neoplastic conversion by TGF-α alone can occur. Double transgenic (c-myc and TGF-α) develop hepatic cancer within 3–5 months, indicating that these two oncogenes may be sufficient to progress hepatocytes (157). In further support of TGF-α acting at the stage of tumor promotion, treatment of transgenic TGF-α overexpressing mice with either initiating carcinogen, diethylnitrosamine or dimethylnitrosamine, enhanced the formation of hepatic adenomas and carcinomas (158).

Chemical carcinogens may modulate the expression of TGF-α protein or the EGF receptor in a manner that bestows certain initiated cells with selective clonal growth. TGF-α overexpression is seen in hepatic focal lesions promoted by phenobarbital but not by the peroxisome proliferator Wyeth-14,643 or DEHP (159, unpublished observations). Morphologically, peroxisome proliferators promote the growth of weakly basophilic focal lesions and tumors, whereas phenobarbital enhances the growth of eosinophilic lesions (7, 72). This difference in morphology suggests that TGF-α may play a role in permitting eosinophilic lesions but not basophilic lesions to become neoplastic.

Another important regulator of hepatocyte growth is TGF-β (transforming growth factor beta). TGF-β is a negative growth regulator in hepatocytes (160, 161). TGF-β is secreted from nonhepatocytes in an inactive form and requires the physiologic activation by a proteolytic activity of mannose-6-phosphate/insulin growth factor II-receptor (M6P/IGFIIr). After activation, TGF-β is free to bind to TGF-β receptors and exert its physiologic activity. TGF-β inhibits hepatic proliferation both in vivo and in vitro (160), leading to the suggestion that TGF-β is the stimulus for apoptosis in hepatocytes. This induction of apoptosis exacts a cellular mechanism by which TGF-β functions as a negative-growth regulator.

Apoptosis and TGF-β have been suggested to be involved in hepatic tumor promotion (80, 160). TGF-β stimulates apoptosis in hepatocytes both in vitro and in vivo (160). TGF-β and the expression of its three receptors in hepatic focal tissue have been shown to be decreased by PB (160). TCDD downregulated the expression of TGF-β in human keratinocytes and may have a similar effect in hepatocytes (162). In addition, ethinyl estradiol inhibited hepatic focal lesion growth by increasing TGF-β in focal hepatocytes (163). Importantly, the loss of heterozygosity at the M6P/IGFII receptor and TGF-β receptors 1 and 2 was decreased in expression in human hepatocellular cancer (160). These studies indicate that TGF-β is an important regulatory growth factor in hepatic cancer in rodents and humans.

Although most of the discussion has focused on the changes in expression of cell cycle genes by nongenotoxic compounds, genotoxic carcinogens also enhance carcinogenicity by modulating these genes. Because of the DNA-reactive nature of genotoxic carcinogens, their primary effect is mutational activation or inactivation of oncogenes or suppressor genes, respectively. This mutational effect is considered to be a permanent change, while gene expression changes (those induced by nongenotoxic hepatocarcinogens) may be reversible. The mutation of a number of tumor suppressor genes and oncogenes can lead to conversion to a neoplastic phenotype. Loss of heterozygosity in mouse hepatic tumors was seen at loci known to harbor the following genes: Wilm's tumor, Rb, adenomatous polyposis coli (APC), deleted in colon cancer

(DCC), and mutated in colon cancer (MCC) (164). No role for p53 or neurofibromatous 1 or 2 in mouse hepatocarcinogenesis has been demonstrated (164). However, p53 mutations have been reported in human hepatocellular carcinomas, especially in regions of high aflatoxin B1 exposure (165–167).

The mutational activation of the ras protooncogene is frequently observed in both human and animal tumors (167–169). The mutations typically occur in three regions, corresponding to codons 12, 13, and 61 (167). Liver tumors from mice exhibit a variable degree of ras mutational activation depending on the carcinogen. For example, Ha-ras mutations were observed in all tumors produced by single-dose treatment of N-hydroxy-2-acetylaminofluorene, vinyl carbamate, 1'-hydroxy-2',3'-dehydroestragole in 12-day-old mice (170). In weanling mice given a single injection of diethylnitrosamine, 42% (14 of 33) of mouse liver tumors exhibited a detectable mutated Ha-ras gene (171). In spontaneous mouse liver tumors, 69% (33 of 48) of mouse liver tumors contained an activated oncogene, with 85% (28 of 33) having activated Ha-ras genes (171). In contrast, mutational Ha-ras activation is rarely seen in rat liver tumors. No activated protooncogenes were observed in 20 rat liver tumors produced by the Solt-Farber method (171). These studies suggest that unlike in the mouse, the mutational activation of Ha-ras protooncogene may not be important in the development of rat liver tumors.

DNA methylation plays an important role in normal development and carcinogenesis (172). In general, hypomethylation (e.g., decreased expression of DNA-5-methylcytosine) of DNA leads to increased gene expression. In carcinogenicity, the importance of mutagenesis cannot be refuted, but hypomethylation of certain gene products could facilitate neoplastic conversion (172). With the exception of tumor suppressor genes, hypomethylation leading to aberrant expression of cell cycle control genes could lead to unregulated cell division. The increased expression of mutated Ha-ras appears to be involved in transformation (173).

Tumor promotion, an operationally reversible stage in hepatocarcinogenesis, is often associated with changes in gene expression. As shown above, numerous genetic changes occur in hepatic focal lesions and neoplasms. Because DNA methylation status is one possible mechanism of regulation of gene activity, alterations in methylation induced by nongenotoxic hepatocarcinogens may contribute to the selective clonal expansion of initiated cells (172, 174). In chemical-induced hepatic tumors in mice, a decreased expression of 5-methylcytosine is seen compared to normal liver tissue. In addition, the regions of the DNA coding for Ha-ras and raf are hypomethylated in mouse liver tumors (175). Hypomethylation occurs reversibly during periods of cell replication (174). Thus, the promoting effect of hypomethylation is compatible with the current concept that tumor promotion is a reversible stage in hepatic tumorogenesis.

Hypermethylation also can contribute to the carcinogenic process. Tumor suppressor genes, which must be active to prevent progression through the cell cycle, may be hypermethylated and have their relative expression decreased. In addition, deamination of 5-methylcytosine bases to thymines can lead to G-C to A-T transitions, a mutation commonly seen in p53 tumor suppressor genes (174).

Feeding a diet deficient in methyl donors (e.g., a choline- and methionine-deficient diet) leads to the development of hepatic cancer in mice and rats. This deficiency in methyl donors leads to hypomethylation and increased expression of Ha-ras, c-myc, and c-fos as well as increased cell replication. It has been proposed that this persistent promoting effect is the driving factor behind the carcinogenicity of the feeding of a methyl-deficient diet.

CONCLUSIONS

The study of chemical-induced hepatocarcinogenesis offers strong insight into the multistage nature of tumor formation. Chemical carcinogens appear to elicit preferential activity at selected stages in hepatic cancer. While genotoxic carcinogens exert their primary effect on tumor initiation, nongenotoxic hepatocarcinogens appear to function mainly at tumor promotion. In either case, the enhancement of hepatic focal lesion growth and subsequent tumor formation is mediated through imbalances in the basic growth parameters, proliferation and death. The underlying mechanisms of the alterations that lead to hepatic cancer are complex but may involve inhibition of gap junctional intercellular communication, production of an oxidative stress, or modulation of the expression of important cell cycle genes.

REFERENCES

1. Berenblum I, Roe KL. An experimental analysis of the 'hair cycle effect' in mouse skin carcinogenesis. *Br J Cancer* 1958;12:402–413.
2. Glauert HP, Beaty MM, Clark TD, Greenwell WS, Tatum V, Chen L, Borges T, Clark TL, Srinivasan SR, Chow CK. Effect of dietary vitamin E on the development of altered hepatic foci and hepatic tumors induced by the peroxisome proliferator ciprofibrate *J Cancer Res Clin Oncol* 1990;116:351–356.
3. Pitot HC. Altered hepatic foci: their role in murine hepatocarcinogenesis. *Annu Rev Pharmacol Toxicol* 1990;30:465–500.
4. Peraino C, Richards WL, Stevens FJ. Multistage hepatocarcinogenesis. In: *Mechanisms of tumor promotion* New York: Wiley and Liss, 1981:2–53.
5. Diwan BA, Ward JM, Rice JM. Modification of liver tumor development in rodents. *Prog Exp Tumor Res* 1991;33:76–107.
6. Kraupp-Grasl B, Bursch W, Ruttkay-Nedecky B, Wagner A, Lauer B, Schulte-Hermann R. Food restriction eliminates preneoplastic cells through apoptosis and antagonizes carcinogenesis in rat liver. *Proc Natl Acad Sci USA* 1994;91:9995–9999.
7. Kolaja KL, Stevenson DE, Walborg EF Jr, Klaunig JE. Dose-dependence of phenobarbital promotion of preneoplastic hepatic lesions in F344 rats and B6C3F1 mice: effect of DNA synthesis and apoptosis. *Carcinogenesis* 1996;17:947–954.
8. Bursch W, Taper HS, Lauer B, Schulte-Hermann R. Quantitative histological and histochemical studies on the occurrence and stages of controlled cell death (apoptosis) during regression of rat liver hyperplasia. *Virchows Arch Cell Pathol* 1985;50:153–166.
9. Doll R, Peto R, eds. *The cause of cancer*, Oxford: Oxford Press, 1981.
10. Pitot HC. Progression: the terminal stage in carcinogenesis. *Jap J Cancer Res* 1989;80:599–607.
11. Twort JM, Twort CC. Comparative activity of some carcinogenic hydrocarbons. *Am J Cancer* 1939;35:80–85.
12. Twort CC, Ing HR. Untersuchungen uber krebserzeugende Agenzien. *Z Krebsforsch* 1928;27:309–351.
13. Rous P, Kidd JG. Conditional neoplasms and subthreshold neoplastic states: a study of tar tumors in rabbits. *J Exp Med* 1941;73:365–389.

14. Friedwald WF, Rous P. The initiating and promoting elements in tumor production. *J Exp Med* 1944;80:101–125.
15. Berenblum I. The cocarcinogenic action of croton resin. *Cancer Res* 1941;1:44–48.
16. Berenblum I, Harlan N. The significance of the sequencing of initiating and promoting actions in the process of skin carcinogenesis in the mouse. *Br J Cancer* 1955;9:268–271.
17. Farber E. Hepatic carcinogenesis. *Prog Liver Dis* 1972;2:173–182.
18. Peraino C, Fry R, Staffeldt E. Reduction and enhancement by phenobarbital of hepatocarcinogenesis induced by 2-acetyl amino fluorine. *Cancer Res* 1971;31:1506–1512.
19. Peraino C, Fry R, Staffeldt E. Enhancement of spontaneous hepatic tumorogenesis in C3H mice by dietary phenobarbital. *J Natl Cancer Inst* 1973;15:1349–1450.
20. Goldfarb S. A morphological and histochemical study of carcinogenesis of the liver in rat fed 3′-4-dimethylaminobenzene. *Cancer Res* 1973;33:119–128.
21. Goldfarb S, Pugh TD. Multistage rodent hepatocarcinogenesis. *Prog Liver Dis* 1986;8:597–620.
22. Schulte-Hermann R. Induction of liver growth by exogenous stimuli. *CRC Rev Toxicol* 1974;13:97–158.
23. Pitot HC, Barsness L, Goldsworthy T, Kitagawa T. Biochemical characterization of the stages of hepatocarcinogenesis after single dose of diethylnitrosamine. *Nature* 1978;271:456–458.
24. Schulte-Hermann R. Tumor promotion in the liver. *Archiv Toxicol* 1987;57:147–158.
25. Solt D, Farber E. New principles for the analysis of chemical carcinogenesis. *Nature* 1976;263:701–703.
26. Miller JA. A brief history of chemical carcinogenesis. *Cancer Lett* 1994;83:9–14.
27. Butterworth BE. Consideration of both genotoxic and nongenotoxic mechanism in predicting carcinogenesis potential. *Mutat Res* 1990;239:117–132.
28. Butterworth BE, Goldsworthy TL. The role of cell proliferation in multi-stage carcinogenesis. *Proc Soc Exp Biol Med* 1991;198:683–687.
29. Ames BN, Gold LS. Chemical carcinogenesis: too many rodent carcinogens. *Proc Natl Acad Sci USA* 1990;87:7772–7776.
30. Ashwood-Smith MJ. The genetic toxicology of aldrin and dieldrin. *Mutat Res* 1981;86:137–154.
31. Pitot HC, Sircia AE. The stages of initiation and promotion in hepatocarcinogenesis. *Biochim Biophys Acta.* 1980;605:191–215.
31a. Cunningham ML, Mathews HB. Relationship of hepatocarcinogenicity and hepatocellular proliferation induced by mutagenic noncarcinogens vs carcinogens. *Toxicol Appl Pharmacol* 1991;110:505–513.
32. Cunningham ML, Elwell MR, Mathews HB. Relationship of carcinogenicity and cellular proliferation induced by mutagenic noncarcinogens vs carcinogens. III. Organophosphates pesticides. *Toxicol Appl Pharmacol* 1994;124:363–369.
33. Cameron RG. Identification of the putative first cellular step of chemical hepatocarcinogenesis. *Cancer Lett* 1989;47:163–167.
34. Scherer E, Emmelot P. Kinetics of induction and growth of precancerous liver-cell foci, and liver tumor formation by diethylnitrosamine in the rat. *Eur J Cancer* 1975;11:689–696.
35. Moore M, Hacker HJ, Kunz HW, Bannasch P. Enhancement of NNM-induced carcinogenesis in the rat liver by phenobarbital: a combined morphological and enzyme histochemical approach. *Carcinogenesis* 1983;4:473–479.
36. Zerban H, Preussman R, Bannasch P. Dose-time relationship of the development of preneoplastic liver lesions induced in rats with low doses of N-nitrosodiethylamine. *Carcinogenesis* 1988;9:607–610.
37. Herren-Freund S, Pereira MA. Effect of phenobarbital on gammaglutamyl transpeptidase activity and the remodeling of nodules induced by the initiation-selection model. *Cancer Lett* 1985;27:153–161.
38. Tomatis L, Partensky C, Montesanto R. The predictive value of mouse liver tumor induction in carcinogenicity testing: a literature survey. *Int J Cancer* 1973;12:1–20.
39. Kemp CJ, Leary CN, Drinkwater NR. Promotion of murine hepatocarcinogenesis by testosterone is androgen receptor-dependent but not cell autonomous. *Proc Natl Acad Sci USA* 1989;86:7505–7509.
40. Yager JD, Shi YE. Synthetic estrogen and tamoxifen as promoters of hepatocarcinogenesis. *Preventive Med* 1991;20:27–37.
41. Cohen SM, Ellwein LB. Cell proliferation in carcinogenesis. *Science* 1990;249:1007–1011.
42. Columbano A, Ledda-Columbano GM, Lee G, Rajalakshmi S, Sarma DS. Inability of mitogen-induced liver hyperplasia to support the induction of enzyme-altered islands induced by liver carcinogens. *Cancer Res* 1987;47:5557–5559.

43. Melnick RL, Huff J. Liver carcinogenesis is not a predicted outcome of chemically induced hepatocyte proliferation. *Toxicol Ind Health* 1993;9:415–438.
44. Ward JM, Hagiwara A, Anderson L, Lindsey K, Diwan BA. The chronic hepatic or renal toxicity of DEHP, acetaminophen, sodium barbital, and phenobarbital in male B6C3F1 mice: autoradiographic, immunohistochemical, and biochemical evidence for levels of DNA synthesis not associated with carcinogenesis or tumor promotion. *Toxicol Appl Pharmacol* 1988;96:494–506.
45. Huff JE. Absence of morphologic correlation between chemical toxicity and chemical carcinogenesis. *Environ Health Perspec* 1993;101:45–53.
46. Klaunig JE. Selective induction of DNA synthesis in mouse preneoplastic and neoplastic hepatic lesions after exposure to phenobarbital. *Environ Health Perspec* 1993;101:235–249.
47. Kolaja KL, Stevenson DE, Walborg EF Jr, Klaunig JE. Reversibility of promoter-induced hepatic focal lesion growth in mice *Carcinogenesis* 1996;17:1403–1409.
48. Kolaja KL, Stevenson DE, Walborg EF Jr, Klaunig JE. Selective dieldrin promotion of hepatic focal lesions in mice. *Carcinogenesis* 1996;17:1243–1250.
48a. Williams GM. Epigenetic mechanisms of liver tumor promotion. In: *Mouse liver carcinogenesis: mechanisms and species comparisions*. New York: Alan R. Liss, Inc., 1996.
49. Mori H, Tanaka T, Nishikawa A, Willliams GM. Enhancing effects of phenobarbital on tumor formation. *J Natl Cancer Inst* 1982;69:1277–1282.
50. Stenius U, Hogberg J. GST-P positive hepatocytes isolated from rats bearing enzyme-altered foci show no signs of p53 induction and replicate even when their DNA contains strand breaks. *Carcinogenesis* 1995;16:1683–1686.
51. Mellors RC, Seguira K. Alkaline phosphatase activity and basophilia in hepatic cells following administration of butter yellow to rats. *Proc Soc Exp Biol Med* 1948;67:242–250.
52. Friedrich-Freska H, Gossner W, Borner P. Histochemische untersuchungen der cancerogenese in der rattenleber nach dauergaben von diethylnitrosamin. *Z Krebsforsch* 1969;72:226–235.
53. Fiala S, Fiala AE, Dixon B. Gammaglutamyl transpeptidases in transplantable chemically induced rat hepatomas and spontaneous mouse hepatomas. *J Natl Cancer Inst* 1972;48:1393–1401.
54. Bannasch P, Zerban H, Hacker HJ. Foci of altered hepatocytes in the rat. *Monogr Pathol Lab Anim* 1985;3:10–30.
55. LaPorta CAM, Comolli R. Membrane and nuclear protein kinase C activation in early stages of diethylnitrosamine-induced rat. *Carcinogenesis* 1994;15:1743–1747.
56. Sills RC, Goldsworthy TL, Sleight SD. Tumor-promoting effects of 2,3,7,8-tetrachlorodibenzo-p-dioxin and phenobarbital in initiated weanling Sprague-Dawley rats: a quantitative, phenotypic, and ras p21 protein study. *Toxicol Pathol* 1994;22:270–281.
57. Nagy P, Evart RP, Marsden E, Roach J, Thorgeirsson SS. Cellular distribution of c-myc transcripts during chemical carcinogenesis in rats. *Cancer Res* 1988;48:5522–5527.
58. Nakano H, Hatayama I, Satoh K, Suzuki S, Sato S, Tsuchida S. c-Jun expression in single cells and preneoplastic foci induced by diethylnitrosamine in B6C3F1 mice: comparision with the expression of pi-class glutathione S-transferase. *Carcinogenesis* 1994;15:1853–1857.
59. Hatayama I, Nishimura S, Narita T, Sato K. Sex-dependent expression of class pi glutathione S-transferase during chemical carcinogenesis in B6C3F1 mice. *Carcinogenesis* 1993;14:537–538.
60. Suzuki S, Satoh K, Nakano H, Hateyama I, Sato K, Tsuchida S. Lack of correlated expression between the glutathione-S-transferase P-form and the oncogene products c-Jun and c-Fos in rat tissues and preneoplastic foci. *Carcinogenesis* 1995;16:567–571.
61. Squire RA, Levitt MH. Report of a workshop on classification of specific hepatocellular lesions in rats. *Cancer Res* 1975;35:3214–3223.
62. Walker AIT, Thorpe E, Stevenson DE. The toxicology of dieldrin (HEOD). I. Long-term oral toxicity studies in mice. *Fd Cosmet Toxicol* 1973;11:415–432.
63. Frith CH, Ward JM. A morphologic classification of proliferative and neoplastic hepatic lesions in mice. *J Environ Pathol Toxicol* 1980;3:329–351.
64. Morris R. Testing statistical hypothesis about rat liver foci. *Toxicol Pathol* 1989;17:569–579.
65. Delasse M. Procede mecanique pour determiner la composition des roches. *Ann Mines* 1848; 13:379–388.
66. Wicksell SD. The corpuscle problem: a mathematical study of a biometric problem. *Biometrika* 1928;17:84–99.
67. Pugh TD, King JH, Koen H, Nychka D, Chover J, Wahba G, He Y, Goldfarb S. Reliable stereological method for estimating the number of microscopic hepatocellular foci from their transections. *Cancer Res* 1983;43:1261–1268.

68. Campbell HA, Pitot HC, Potter VR, Laishes BA. Application of quantitative stereology to the evaluation of enzyme-altered foci in rat liver. *Cancer Res* 1982;42:465–472.

69. Enzmann H, Bannasch P. Potential significance of hepatocellular heterogeneity of focal lesions at different stages in hepatocarcinogenesis. *Carcinogenesis* 1987;8:1606–1612.

70. Schulte-Hermann R, Timmermann-Trosnier I, Schupper J. Promotion of spontaneous preneoplastic cells in rat liver as a possible explanation of tumor production by nonmutagenic compounds. *Cancer Res* 1983;43:839–844.

71. Harada T, Maronpot RR, Morris R, Boorman GA. Morphological and stereological evaluation of spontaneous foci of cellular alteration in F344 rat liver. *Toxicol Pathol* 1989;17:489–499.

72. Ward JM, Ohshima M, Lynch P, Riggs C. Di(2-eythylhexyl) phthalate but not phenobarbital promotes diethylnitrosamine initiated hepatocellular proliferative lesions after short term exposure in male B6C3F1 mice. *Cancer Lett* 1984;24:49–55.

73. Ward JM, Lynch P, Riggs C. Rapid development of hepatocellular neoplasms in aging male C3H/HeNCr mice given phenobarbital. *Cancer Lett* 1988;39:9–18.

74. Schulte-Hermann R, Ohde G, Schupper J, Timmermann-Trosnier I. Enhanced proliferation of putative preneoplastic cells in rat liver following treatment with the tumor promoters phenobarbital, hexachlorocyclohexane, steroid compounds, and nafenopin. *Cancer Res* 1981;41:2556–2562.

75. Schulte-Hermann R, Krapp-Grasl B, Bursch W, Gerbracht U, Timmermann-Trosnier I. Effects of non-genotoxic hepatocarcinogens phenobarbital and nafenopin on phenotype and growth of different populations of altered foci in rat liver. *Toxicol Pathol* 1989;17:620–650.

76. Cattley RC, Popp JA. Differences between the promoting activities of the peroxisome proliferator Wyeth-14,643 and phenobarbital in rat liver. *Cancer Res* 1989;49:3246–3251.

77. Teebor GW, Becker FF. Regression and persistence of hyperplastic hepatic nodules induced by N-2-fluoroacetamide and their relationship to hepatocarcinogenesis. *Cancer Res* 1971;31:1–9.

78. Glauert HP, Schwarz M, Pitot HC. The phenotypic stability of altered hepatic foci: effect of the short-term withdrawl of phenobarbital and of the long-term feeding of purified diets after the withdrawal. *Carcinogenesis* 1986;7:117–121.

79. Enomoto K, Farber E. Kinetics of phenotypic maturation of remodeling hyperplastic nodules during liver carcinogenesis. *Cancer Res* 1982;42:2330–2338.

80. Schulte-Hermann R, Bursch W, Fesus L, Timmermann-Trosiener I, Krapp B, Liehr J. Role of cell death in hepatocarcinogenesis In: Bannasch P, Keppler D, Weber G, eds. *Liver cell cancer.* Dorderecht: Kluwer Academic Publishers, 1990:339–350.

81. Kraupp-Grasl B, Walduhor T, Huber W, Schulte-Hermann R. Glutathione-S-transferase isoenzyme patterns in different subtypes of enzyme-altered rat liver foci treated with the peroxisome proliferator nafenopin or with phenobarbital. *Carcinogenesis* 1993;14:2407–2412.

82. Marsman DS, Cattley RC, Conway JG, Popp JA. Relationship of hepatic peroxisome proliferation and replicative DNA synthesis to the hepatocarcinogenicity of the peroxisome proliferators DEHP and Wyeth 14,643 in rats. *Cancer Res* 1988;48:6739–6744.

82a. Richardson FC, Copple DM, Eacho PI. Effects of methapyrilene on DNA synthesis in mice and rats following continuous dietary exposure. *Carcinogenesis* 1992;13:2453–2457.

83. Lucier GW, Tritscher A, Goldsworthy T, Foley J, Clark G, Goldstein J, Maronpot R. Ovarian hormones enhance 2,3,7,8-tetrachlorodibenzo-p-dioxin-mediated increases in cell proliferation and preneoplastic foci in a two-stage model for rat hepatocarcinogenesis. *Cancer Res* 1991;51:1391–1397.

84. Ueda N, Shah SV. Apoptosis. *J Lab Clin Invest* 1996;124:169–177.

85. Bursch WB, Lauer B, Timmermann-Trosenier I, Barthel G, Schuppler J, Schulte-Hermann R. Controlled death (apoptosis) of normal and preneoplastic cells in rat liver following withdrawal of tumor promoters. *Carcinogenesis* 1984;5:453–458.

86. Kerr JFR, Wyllie AH, Currie AR. Apoptosis: a basic biological phenomenon with wide-ranging implications in tissue kinetics. *Br J Cancer* 1972;26:239–257.

87. Wyllie AH, Kerr JFR, Currie AR. Cell death: the significance of apoptosis. *Int Rev Cytol* 1980; 68:251–306.

88. Roberts RA, Soames AR, Gill JH, James NH, Wheldon EB. Nongenotoxic hepatocarcinogens stimulate DNA synthesis and their withdrawal induces apoptosis, but in different hepatocyte population. *Carcinogenesis* 1995;16:1693–1699.

89. James SJ, Muskhelishvilla L. Rates of apoptosis and proliferation vary with caloric intake and may influence incidence of spontaneous hepatoma in C57BL/6 x C3H F1 mice. *Cancer Res* 1994;54:5508–5510.

90. Kolaja KL, Bunting KA, Klaunig JE. Inhibition of tumor promotion and hepatocellular lesion growth by dietary restriction in mice. *Carcinogenesis* 1996;17:1657–1664.
91. Mills JJ, Chari RS, Boyer IJ, Gould MN, Jirtle R. Induction of apoptosis in liver tumors by the monoterpene perillyl alcohol. *Cancer Res* 1995;55:979–983.
92. Zerban H, Radig S, Kopp-Scneider A, Bannasch P. Cell proliferation and cell death (apoptosis) in hepatic preneoplastic and neoplasia are closely related to phenotypic cellular diversity and instability. *Carcinogenesis* 1994;15:2467–2473.
93. Bayly AC, Roberts RA, Dive C. Suppression of liver cell apoptosis in vitro by the non-genotoxic hepatocarcinogen and peroxisome proliferator nafenopin. *J Cell Biol* 1995;125:197–203.
94. Tatesumota M, Nagamine Y, Farber E. Redifferentation as a basis for remodeling of carcinogen-induced hepatocyte nodules to normal appearing liver. *Cancer Res* 1983;43:5049–5058.
95. Yamasaki H. Aberrant expression and function of gap junctions during carcinogenesis. *Environ Health Perspec* 1991;93:191–197.
96. Trosko JE, Goodman JI. Intercellular communication may facilate apoptosis: implications for tumor promotion. *Mol Carcinogenesis* 1994;11:8–12.
97. Neveu M, Hully J, Babcock K, Hertzberg E, Nicholson B, Paul D, Pitot HC. Multiple mechanisms are responsible for altered expression of gap junction genes during oncogenesis in rat liver. *J Cell Sci* 1994;107:83–95.
98. Klaunig JE, Baker TK. Morphologic evaluation of gap junctional intercellular communication. *Meth Toxicol* 1994;1:72–80.
99. Baker TK, Kwiatowski A, Klaunig JE. Inhibition of gap junctional intercellular communication by 2,3,7,8-tetrachlorodibenzo-p-dioxin (TCDD) in rat hepatocytes. *Carcinogenesis* 1995;16:2321–2326.
100. Sies H. Oxidative stress: from basic research to clinical application. *Am J Med* 1991;91:31s–38s.
101. Sun Y. Free radicals, antioxidant enzymes, and carcinogenesis. *Free Rad Biol Med* 1990;8:201–209.
102. Clayson DB, Mehta R, Iverson F. Oxidant damage: the effects of certain gentoxoic and operationally nongenotoxic carcinogens. *Mutat Res* 1994;317:25–42.
103. Klaunig JE, Bachowski S, Ketcham CA, Isenberg JS, Kolaja KL, Baker TK, Walborg EF Jr, Stevenson DE. Oxidative stress in nongenotoxic carcinogenesis. *Toxicol Lett* 1996;83:683–691.
104. Trush MA, Kensler TW. An overview of the relationship between oxidative stress and chemical carcinogenesis. *Free Rad Biol Med* 1991;10:201–209.
105. Cerrutti PA, Trump BF. Inflammation and oxidative stress in carcinogenesis. *Cancer Lett* 1991;3:1–7.
106. Crawford D. Oxidant stress induces the protooncogenes c-fos and c-myc in mouse epidermal cells. *Bull Cancer* 1990;77:501–502.
107. Gopalakrishna R, Anderson WB. Ca^{2+}- and phospholipid-independent activation of protein kinase C by selective oxidative modification of the regulatory domain *Proc Natl Acad Sci USA* 1989;86:6758–6762.
108. Buttke TM, Sandstrom PA. Oxidative stress as a mediator of apoptosis. *Immun Today* 1994;15:7–10.
109. Stevenson DE. The potential role of oxidative stress in nongenotoxic hepatocarcinogenesis in the mouse liver. *Prog Clin Biol Res* 1995;331:367–383.
110. Borek C. Free-radical processed in multistage carcinogenesis. *Free Rad Res Comm* 1991;12–13:745–750.
111. Ledwith BJ, Manam S, Troilo P, Josyln DJ, Gallaway SM, Nichols WM. Activation of immediate-early gene expression by peroxisome proliferators in vitro. *Mol Carcinogenesis* 1993;8:20–27.
112. Amsted P, Crawford D, Muehlematter D, Zbinden I, Larsson R, Cerutti P. Oxidant stress induces the proto-oncogenes, c-fos and c-jun in mouse epidermal cells. *Bull Cancer* 1990;77:501–502.
113. Bentley P, Bieri F, Muakkassah-Kelly S, Staeubli W, Waechter F. Mechanisms of tumor induction by peroxisome proliferators. *Arch Toxicol* 1988;12:240–247.
114. Trosko JE, Chang CC. Adaptive and nonadaptive consequences of chemical inhibition of intercellular communication. *Pharmacol Rev* 1984;36:137s–144s.
115. Ruch RJ, Klaunig JE. Antioxidant prevention of tumor promoter induced inhibition of mouse hepatocellular communication. *Cancer Lett* 1986;33:137–150.
116. Hirota N, Williams GM. The sensitivity and heterogeneity of histochemical markers for altered foci involved in liver carcinogenesis. *Am J Pathol* 1979;95:317–329.
117. Bojes HK, Keller BJ, Thurman RG. Wyeth-14,643 stimulates hepatic protein kinase C activity. *Toxicol Lett* 1992;62:317–322.

118. Bachowski S, Baker TK, Stevenson DE, Walborg EF Jr, Klaunig JE. The potential role of oxidative stress in nongenotoxic hepatocarcinogenesis in the mouse liver. *Prog Clin Biol Res* 1995;391: 385–396.

119. El Sisi AED, Earnst DL, Sipes IG. Vitamin A potentiation of carbon tetrachloride hepatotoxicity: role of liver macrophages and active oxygen species. *Toxicol Appl Pharmacol* 1992;119:295–301.

120. Parke DV, Ioannides C. Role of cytochrome p-450 in mouse liver tumor production. *Prog Clin Biol Res* 1990;331:215–230.

121. Stevenson DE, Walker AIT. Hepatic lesions produced in mice by dieldrin and other hepatic enzyme-inducing compounds. *J Eur Toxicol* 1969;2:83–84.

122. Trush MA, Kensler TW. An overview of the relationship between oxidative stress and chemical carcinogenesis. *Free Radical Biol Med* 1991;10:201–209.

123. Lubet RA, Nims RW, Ward JM, Rice JM, Diwan BA. Induction of cytochrome P-450 and its relationship to liver tumor promotion. *J Am Coll Toxicol* 1989;8:259–268.

124. Weinstein IB. Nonmutagenic mechanisms in carcinogenesis: role of protein kinase C in signal transduction and growth control. *Environ Health Perspec* 1991;93:175–179.

125. Harrington EA, Fanidi A, Evan GI. Oncogenes and cell death. *Curr Opin Gen Develop* 1994;4:120–129.

126. Langdon WY, Harris AW, Cory S. Growth of E mu-myc transgenic mice by Abelson murine leukemia virus and Harvey murine sarcoma virus. *Oncogene Res* 1988;2:403–409.

127. Dyall SD, Cory S, Adams JM. Bcl-2 gene promotes haemopoietic cell survival and co-operates with c-myc to immortalize pre-B cells. *Nature* 1988;335:440–442.

128. Nieman PE, Thomas SJ, Loring G. Induction of apoptosis during normal and neoplastic development B-cell development in the bursa of Fabricius. *Proc Natl Acad Sci USA* 1991;88:5857–5861.

129. Wurm F, Gwinn K, Kingston R. Inducible over-expression of the mouse c-myc protein in mammalian cells. *Proc Natl Acad Sci USA* 1986;83:5414–5418.

130. Evan G, Wyllie A, Gilbert C, Littlewoos T, Land H, Brooks M, Waters C, Penn L, Hancock D. Induction of apoptosis in fibroblasts by c-myc protein. *Cell* 1992;63:119–125.

131. Cohen J, Duke R, Fadok VA, Sellins KS. Apoptosis and programmed cell death in immunity. *Annu Rev Immunol* 1992;10:267–293.

132. Touchette N. Dying cells reveal new role for cancer genes. *J NIH Res* 1992;4:48–52.

133. Tsujimoto Y. Stress-resistance conferred by high level of Bcl-2 alpha protein in human B lymphoblastoid cell. *Oncogene* 1989;4:1331–1336.

134. Miyashita T, Reed JC. bcl-2 Gene transfer increases relative resistence of S49.1 and WEHI7.2 lymphoid cells to cell death and DNA fragmentation induced by glucocortoids and multiple chemotherapeutic drugs. *Cancer Res* 1992;52:5407–5411.

135. Walton MI, Whysong D, O'Connor PM, Hockenbery D, Korsmeyer SJ, Kohn KW. Constitutive expression of human bcl-2 modulates nitrogen mustard and camptothecin induced apoptosis. *Cancer Res* 1993;53:4251–4256.

136. Krajewski S, Tanaka S, Takayama S, Schibler M, Fenton W, Reed JC. Investigations of the subcellular-distribution of the bcl-2 oncoprotein-residence in the nuclear-envelope, endoplasmic reticulum, and outer mitochondria membranes. *Cancer Res* 1993;53:4701–4714.

137. Nakai M, Takeda A, Cleary ML, Endo T. The bcl-2 protein is inserted into the outer-membrane but not into the inner-membrane of the rat-liver mitochondria in vitro. *Biochem Biophys Res Comm* 1993;196:233–239.

138. Zhao M, Zhang NX, Economou M, Blaha I, Laissue JA, Zimmerman A. Immunohistochemical detection of bcl-2 protein in liver lesions:bcl-2 protein is expressed in hepatocellular carcinoma but not liver cell dysplasia. *Histopathol* 1994;25:237–245.

139. Fandidi A, Harrington E, Evan G. Co-operative interaction between c-myc and bcl-2 proto-oncogenes. *Nature* 1992;359:554–556.

140. Bojes H, Thurman R. Peroxisome proliferators activate Kupffer cells in vivo. *Cancer Res* 1996;56: 1–4.

141. Wallach D. Cytotoxins (tumour necrosis factor, lymphotoxin and others): molecular and functional characteristics and interactions with interferons. *Interferon* 1984;7:89–124.

142. Meikrantz W, Schlegel R. Apoptosis and the cell cycle. *J Cell Biochem* 1995;58:160–174.

143. Beyer HS, Theogides A. Tumor necrosis factor-a is a direct hepatocyte mitogen in the rat. *Biochem Mol Biol Int* 1993;4:176–187.

144. Hamel P, Gallie B, Phillips R. The retinoblastoma protein and cell cycle regulation. *Trends Genet* 1992;8:180–185.

145. Cobrinik D, Dowdy S, Hinds P. Mittnacht S, Weinberg R. The retinoblastoma protein and the regulation of cell cycling. *Trends Biochem Sci* 1992;17:312–315.
146. Weinburg RA. The retinoblastoma gene and cell growth control. *Trends Biochem Sci* 1990;15:199–202.
147. Goodrich D, Wang N, Qian YW, Lee EH, Lee WH. The retinoblastoma gene product regulates progression through the G1 phase of the cell cycle. *Cell* 1991;67:292–302.
148. Baker SJ, Markowitz S, Fearon ER, Willson JK, Vogelstein B. Suppression of human colorectal carcinoma cell growth by wild-type p53. *Science* 1990;249:921–915.
149. Diller L, Kassel J, Nelson CE, Gryka MA, Litwak G, Gebhardt M, Bressac B, Ozturk M, Baker SJ, Vogelstein B. p53 Functions as a cell cycle control protein in osteosarcomas. *Mol Cell Biol* 1990;10:5772–5782.
150. Martinez J, Georgoff I, Martinez J, Levine AJ. Cellular localization and cell cycle regulation by temperature-sensitive p53 protein. *Genes Dev* 1991;5:151–159.
151. Kastan MB, Onyekwere O, Sidransky D, Vogelstein B, Craig RW. Participation of p53 protein in the cellular response to DNA damage. *Cancer Res* 1991;51:6304–6311.
152. Lane DP. Cancer, p53, guardian of the genome. *Nature* 1992;358:15–16.
153. Bookstein R, Shew JY, Chen P, Scully P, Lee WY. Suppression of tumorigenicity of human prostate carcinoma cells by replacing mutated RB gene. *Science* 1990;247:712–715.
154. Butterworth BE, Sprankle CS, Goldsworthy SM, Wilson DM, Goldsworthy TL. Expression of myc, fos, and Ha-ras in the livers of furan-treated F344 rats and B6C3F1 mice. *Mol Carcinogenesis* 1994;9:24–32.
155. Dragan Y, Teeguarden J, Campbell H, Hsia S, Pitot HC. The quantification of altered hepatic foci during multi-stage hepatocarcinogenesis in the rat:transforming growth factor alpha expression as a marker for the stage of progression. *Cancer Letts* 1995;93:73–83.
156. Sandgren EP, Merlino G. Hepatocarcinogenesis in transgenic mice. *Prog Clin Biol Res* 1995;391:213–222.
157. Stromblad S, Erikkson LC, Andersson G. Increased expression of a sensivity to transforming growth factor-alpha: a promotive role during rat liver carcinogenesis. *Mol Carcinogenesis* 1994; 10:97–104.
158. Takagi H, Sharp R, Takayama H, Anver MR, Ward JM, Merlino G. Collaboration between growth factors and diverse chemical carcinogens in hepatocarcinogenesis of transforming growth factor alpha transgenic mice. *Cancer Res* 1993;53:4329–4336.
159. Miller RT, Cattley RC, Marsman DS, Lyght O, Popp JA. TGF alpha differentially expressed in liver foci induced by diethylnitrosamine initiation and peroxisome proliferator promotion. *Carcinogenesis* 1995;16:77–82.
160. Jirtle R, Hankins G, Reisenbichler H, Boyer I. Regulation of mannose-6-phosphate/insulin-like growth factor-II receptors and transforming growth factor beta during liver tumor promotion phenobarbital. *Carcinogenesis* 1994;15:1473–1478.
161. Oberhammer F, Pavelka M, Sharma S. Induction of apoptosis in cultured hepatocytes and in regressing liver by transforming growth factor b. *Proc Natl Acad Sci USA* 1991;89:5408–5412.
162. Fox TR, Best LL, Goldsworthy S, Mills JJ, Goldsworthy TL. Gene expression and cell proliferation in rat liver after 2,3,7,8-tetrachlorodibenzo-p-dioxin exposure. *Cancer Res* 1993;53:2265–2271.
163. Standeven AM, Goldsworthy TL. Promotion of preneoplastic lesions and induction of CYP2B by unleaded gasoline vapor in female B6C3F1 mouse liver. *Carcinogenesis* 1994;14:2137–2141.
164. Davis LM, Caspary WJ, Sakallah SA, Maronpot R, Wiseman R, Barett C, Elliot R, Hozier J. Loss of hetereozygosity in spontaneous and chemically induced tumors of the B6C3F1 mouse. *Carcinogenesis* 1994;15:1637–1645.
165. Hsu I, Metcalf R, Sun T, Welsh J, Wang N, Harris C. Mutational hot-spot in the p53 gene in human hepatocellular carcinomas. *Nature* 1991;350:427–428.
166. Bressac B, Kew M, Wands J, Ozturuk M. Selective G to T mutations of p53 in hepatocellular carcinoma from southern Africa. *Nature* 1991;350:429–430.
167. Cerrutti P, Hussain P, Pourzand C, Aguilar F. Mutagenesis of the H-ras protooncogene and the p53 tumor suppressor gene. *Cancer Res* 1994;54:1934–1938.
168. Balmain B, Brown K. Oncogene activation in chemical carcinogesis. *Adv Cancer Res* 1988;51:147–182.
169. Barbacid M. The ras oncogene in human cancer: a review. *Cancer Res* 1989;49:4682–4689.
170. Stowers SJ, Wiseman RW, Ward JM, Miller EC, Miller JA, Anderson MW. Detection of activated proto-oncogenes in n-nitrosodiethylamine-induced liver tumors: a comparison between B6C3F1 mice and Fischer 344 rats. *Carcinogenesis* 1988;9:271–276.

171. Reynolds SH, Stowers SJ, Patterson RM, Maronpot RR, Anderson MW. Oncogene activation in spontaneous and chemically induced rodent tumors: implications for risk analysis. *Environ Health Perspec* 1988;78:175–177.
172. Counts JL, Goodman JI. Hypomethylation of DNA: an epigenetic mechanism involved in tumor promotion. *Mol Carcinogenesis* 1994;11:185–188.
173. Finney RE, Bishop JM. Predisposition to neoplastic transformation caused by gene replacement of H-RAS 1. *Science* 1993;260:1524–1527.
174. Goodman JI, Counts JL. Hypomethylation of DNA: a possible nongenotoxic mechanism underlying the role of cell proliferation in carcinogenesis. *Environ Health Perspect* 1993;101:169–172.
175. Sawada N, Porier L, Moran S, Xu Y, Pitot HC. The effect of choline and methionine deficiencies on the number of and volume percentage of altered hepatic foci in the presence or absence of diethylnitrosamine initiation in rat liver. *Carcinogenesis* 1990;11:273–281.

PART II

Mechanisms of Hepatotoxicity

Toxicology of the Liver, 2nd ed.,
Edited by Gabriel L. Plaa and William R. Hewitt
Copyright © 1998 Taylor & Francis

4

An Overview of Peroxisome Proliferation

Jeffrey W. Lawrence and Patrick I. Eacho

*Lilly Research Laboratories, Eli Lilly and Company,
Lilly Corporate Center, Indianapolis, IN 46285*

- **The Phenomenom of Peroxisome Proliferation**
- **Extrahepatic Response of Rodents to Peroxisome Proliferators**
- **Agents That Cause Peroxisome Proliferation**
- **Mechanisms of Peroxisome Proliferation in Rodents**
- **Perturbations of Lipid Metabolism**
- **The Search for a Receptor**
- **The Peroxisome Proliferator Activated Receptor**
- **Interspecies Differences**
- **Human Responsiveness**
- **Hepatocarcinogenesis in Rodents**
- **Nongenotoxic Mechanisms of Carcinogenesis**
- **Human Relevance**
- **References**

THE PHENOMENOM OF PEROXISOME PROLIFERATION

Peroxisomes are cytoplasmic organelles that contain a homogeneous, granular, and electron-dense matrix surrounded by a single membrane (1). Nearly all eukaryotic cells contain peroxisomes, but the size and content vary from organ to organ (2, 3). Hepatic peroxisomes are round, measuring between 0.5 and 1 μm in diameter, and account for approximately 1–2% of the cytoplasmic volume in the rat liver (2, 4, 5). These organelles carry out a variety of enzymatic functions, many of which are involved in lipid metabolism, including H_2O_2 degradation, fatty acid activation and oxidation, plasmalogen (ether lipid) biosynthesis, and cholesterol biosynthesis (1–8).

The discovery of the remarkable phenomenon of xenobiotic-induced peroxisome proliferation has focused more attention on the study of peroxisomes. Clofibrate, a lipid-lowering drug used to treat hyperlipoproteinemias, was the first agent described to cause peroxisome proliferation in rodents (9, 10). Now, it is known that numerous agents, some chemically similar and others distinct from clofibrate, cause a marked increase in the number of hepatic peroxisomes in rodents (7, 11–13). Much of the interest in peroxisome proliferation over the years has centered around its association with the induction of liver cancer in rodents (14). It was proposed that the metabolic alterations associated with peroxisome proliferation have a causative role in the carcinogenic activity of these compounds (15). More recently, a great deal of research focus has been placed on the nuclear receptors that are activated by peroxisome proliferators (PPARs). An in-depth understanding of these receptors and the mechanisms involved in the induction of peroxisome proliferation will aid our ability to evaluate the human carcinogenic potential of these compounds. Numerous reviews and articles that detail various aspects of xenobiotic induced peroxisome proliferation are available (7, 11–13, 16–19). This chapter provides an overview of peroxisome proliferation, biochemical mechanisms of peroxisome proliferation, the relationship with carcinogenesis, and its relevance to humans.

The term *peroxisome proliferation* explicitly refers to an increase in the size and number of peroxisomes; when used in reference to the liver, however, it has become synonymous with the entire pleiotropic response, which includes induction of hepatomegaly and expression of numerous hepatic genes (9, 18, 20, 21). The development of hepatomegaly occurs rapidly during the first few days, and with continued treatment, a steady state is achieved within 2 weeks. This effect is sustained for the duration of treatment and reverses within 2 weeks after discontinuation of treatment (7, 22–24). The hepatomegaly is characterized by both hepatocellular hypertrophy and hyperplasia (7, 25, 26). Within the first few days of peroxisome proliferator treatment, a burst of replicative DNA synthesis occurs. The DNA synthetic rate generally returns to control levels within a few days to 2 weeks (23, 27). Some of the more potent peroxisome proliferators produce a sustained increase in replicative DNA synthesis during chronic treatment (23, 28). There is some evidence that cell proliferation induced by peroxisome proliferators plays a mechanistic role in hepatocarcinogenesis (23, 29). The expansion of the peroxisomal volume contributes to the hypertrophy of the liver cells. The peroxisome volume fraction increases from 2% in untreated rats to as much as 25% with administration of hypolipidemic agents (16, 30). The increase in peroxisome number begins within 24 hr and reaches steady levels within 2 weeks (9, 10, 31, 32). As with the hepatomegaly, the increase in the number of peroxisomes is sustained throughout treatment with the peroxisome proliferating agent (33). Peroxisomes display a zonal heterogeneity in rat liver. In normal rat liver, more peroxisomes are present in the centrilobular region than the periportal region (34). Peroxisome proliferation appears to concentrate in the centrilobular region (35–39). The more marked peroxisome proliferation in the centrilobular region corresponds with the predominantly centrilobular hepatocellular hypertrophy.

Many of the biochemical changes elicited by peroxisome proliferating agents involve fatty acid catabolism. The most extensively studied enzymatic system, the peroxisomal fatty acid β-oxidation system, can be induced up to 30-fold by the more active peroxisome proliferating agents (7, 30, 40). This system consists of three proteins that catalyze the oxidation of long-chain fatty acids to shorter products that can be further catabolized by the mitochondrial β-oxidation system. These proteins are acyl-CoA oxidase, enoyl-CoA hydratase/hydroxyacyl-CoA dehydrogenase (bifunctional protein), and thiolase (41–43). The induction of these proteins parallels the increase in peroxisome volume and is regulated at the transcriptional level (21, 44–48). The mRNA for acyl-CoA oxidase and the bifunctional protein increase within 1 hr after a single dose of ciprofibrate (21). By 16 hr, a 20-fold increase in mRNA is observed. Other peroxisomal enzymes induced by peroxisome proliferators include carnitine acetyl- and octanoyltransferases, dihydroxyacetone phosphate acyltransferase, and, to a lesser extent, catalase (41, 49–51). Urate oxidase, D-amino acid oxidase, and L-alpha-hydroxy acid oxidase activities are unaffected or lowered during peroxisome proliferator treatment (9, 26, 51, 52).

Peroxisome proliferators also produce changes in mitochondrial function and morphology. Clofibrate increases the number of mitochondria as a result of increased protein synthesis (53). Mitochondrial carnitine acetyltransferase activity increases 10-fold in response to clofibrate treatment (49). Mitochondrial β-oxidation also increases up to fourfold by clofibrate, fenofibrate, LY171883, and DEHP (54–57).

Proliferation of the smooth endoplasmic reticulum also contributes to the hepatocellular hypertrophy (9). Peroxisome proliferating agents induce a cytochrome P450 isozyme (P450 4A1) responsible for omega and omega-1 oxidation of fatty acids (58, 59). Lauric acid hydroxylase activity, which is catalyzed by P450 4A1, increases as much as 28-fold, whereas it is minimally induced by a classic P450 inducer such as phenobarbital (58, 60). Total cytochrome P450 levels are marginally affected by peroxisome proliferator treatment (25, 61–64).

EXTRAHEPATIC RESPONSE OF RODENTS
TO PEROXISOME PROLIFERATORS

Although peroxisome proliferation is generally regarded as a hepatic phenomenon, peroxisome proliferation and induction of peroxisomal enzymes are observed in several extrahepatic tissues in rodents. Peroxisomes in the kidney are localized primarily in the P3 segment of the proximal tubule (65). The hypolipidemic agent methylclofenapate causes marked proliferation of peroxisomes in mouse kidney; however, the degree of induction is less than in liver (66). In intestinal mucosa of rats, peroxisome number is increased and the corresponding peroxisomal enzymes are induced by clofibrate (67, 68). Peroxisomal β-oxidation and related mRNAs increase up to ninefold in the kidney and up to twofold in the heart and intestine, compared to 20- to 30-fold in the liver (20). Catalase in kidney, heart, and intestinal mucosa also increases, but to a lesser degree than in liver (20). Pulmonary type II cells and cerebral neurons also display a peroxisome proliferator response (69, 70). Interestingly, peroxisome proliferation was observed in skeletal muscle of transgenic mice that overexpress the lipoprotein lipase gene in muscle tissue (71). This may be related to the ability of fatty acids to activate PPAR and induce peroxisome proliferation (see below).

AGENTS THAT CAUSE PEROXISOME PROLIFERATION

Since the discovery of clofibrate as a peroxisome proliferator, many other chemicals have been identified as peroxisome proliferating agents. These include other hypolipidemic compounds (fibrates), phthalate ester plasticizers, leukotriene antagonists, and fatty acid–related compounds. The structures of some of these chemicals are illustrated in Fig. 1. Many of these compounds have important industrial applications and pharmacologic health benefits.

The hypolipidemic agents related to clofibrate compose the major group of agents that are classified as peroxisome proliferators (7, 17). These agents share the phenoxyisobutyric acid backbone but have various substitutions on the phenyl ring. Substitutions that increase lipophilicity of the compounds generally increase peroxisomal potency (12). Some of these agents are used clinically, including bezafibrate, ciprofibrate, clofibrate, fenofibrate, and beclobrate (33, 72, 73). Gemfibrozil, which is a modification of the fibrate backbone, is also used clinically and induces peroxisome proliferation (38, 74–76). Other hypolipidemic agents unrelated to clofibrate are aromatic or heteroaromatic analogs having a free carboxyl group or a function that serves as a precursor for the formation of an acidic function. Furthermore, metabolites of the hypolipidemic agents fenofibrate, beclobrate, and tiadenol are also active as peroxisome proliferators (77–79).

Phenoxy acid herbicides such as 2,4-dichlorophenoxyacetic acid (2,4-D), 2-methyl-4-chlorophenoxyacetic acid, and 2,4,5-trichlorophenoxyacetic acid (2,4,5-T) bear a close structural resemblance to clofibric acid (7, 80–87). It is interesting that these agents also have a hypotriglyceridemic effect (83–85). Structurally dissimilar herbicides including diphenyl ether lactofen, tridiphane, and fomesafen also induce peroxisome proliferation in rodents (18, 88, 89).

Phthalate ester plasticizers, major components used in the manufacturing of polyvinylchloride plastics, cause hepatic peroxisome proliferation in vivo. These agents include di(2-ethylhexyl)phthalate (DEHP), di(2-ethylhexyl)sebacate, and di(2-ethylhexyl)adipate (DEHA) (7, 82, 90). DEHP is hydrolyzed to the corresponding monoester (MEHP) and 2-ethylhexanol, which possess peroxisome proliferating activity in vivo (82, 90–92). The ultimate peroxisome proliferator derived from DEHP and MEHP is the mono 2-ethyl-5-oxo-hexyl phthalate (18, 93, 94). Mono(2-octyl) phthalate is more potent than the ethylhexyl analogs (94–97). Tri(2-ethylhexyl) trimellitate, di(2-ethylhexyl) terephthalate, and di(n-octyl) phthalate are weak inducers of peroxisome proliferation, possibly due to their rapid metabolism (98).

Leukotriene antagonists with the tetrazole-substituted acetophenone structure are a unique class of peroxisome proliferators (24, 99–101). These include LY171883 and structurally related leukotriene D4 antagonists (99). These agents lack the carboxylic acid function seen in most other peroxisome proliferators. Instead, they have an acidic tetrazole group, which is a bioisostere of the carboxylic acid (102).

Feeding rats diets rich in very long-chain fatty acids induces hepatic peroxisome proliferation (7, 103, 104). Likewise, metabolically stable fatty acid analogs also produce peroxisome proliferation in rodents. These include the perfluorinated n-decanoic,

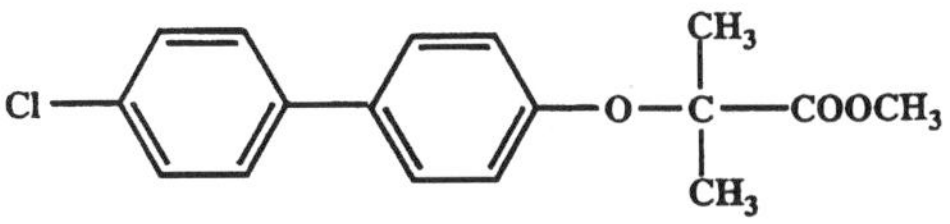

Methylclofenapate

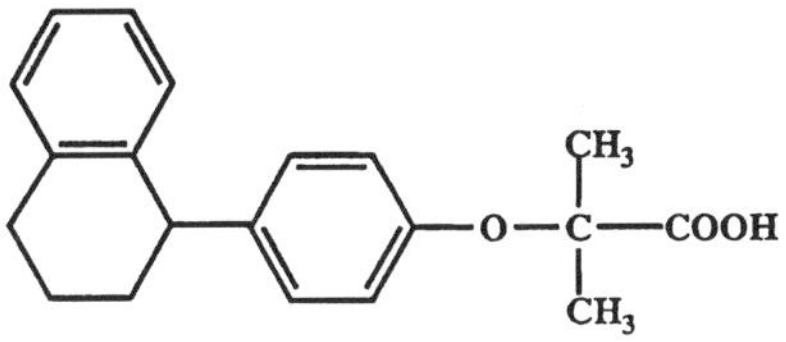

Nafenopin

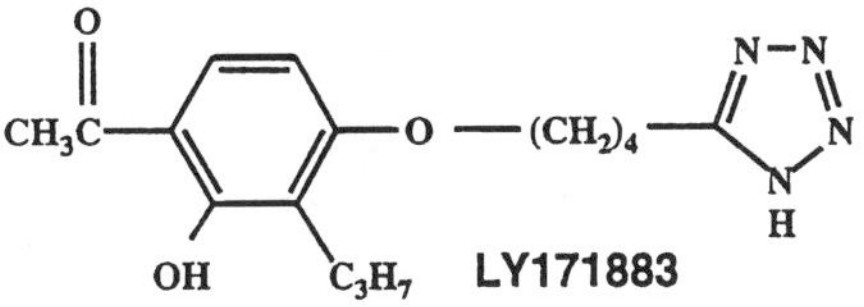

LY171883

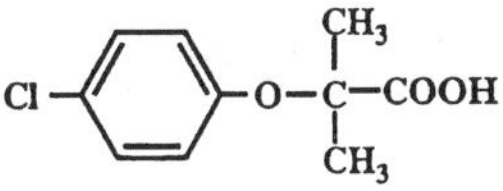

Clofibrate

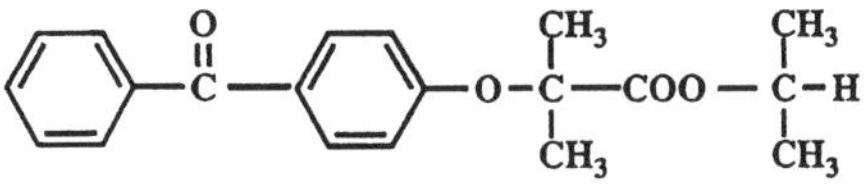

Fenofibrate

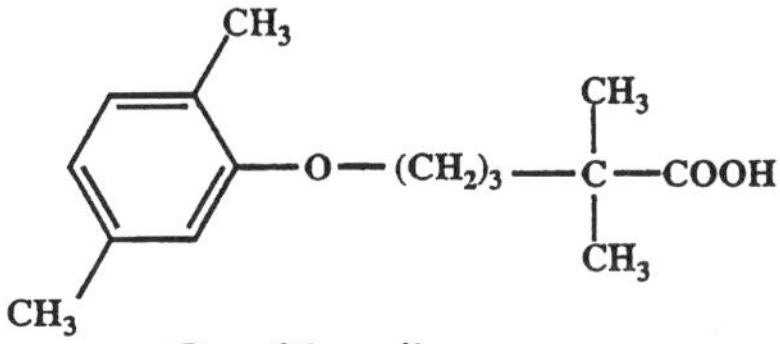

Gemfibrozil

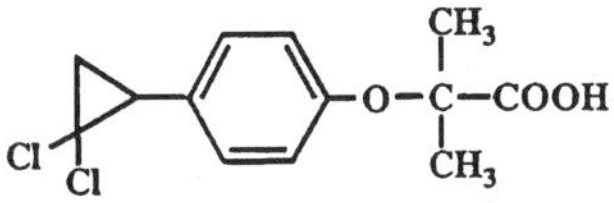

Ciprofibrate

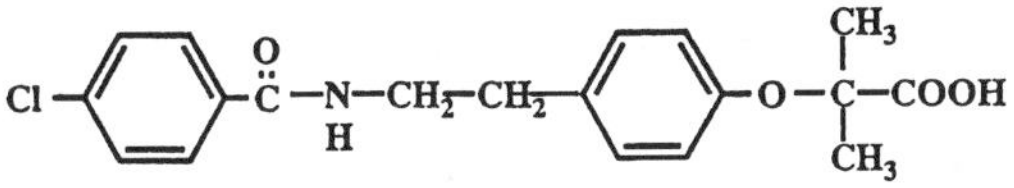

Bezafibrate

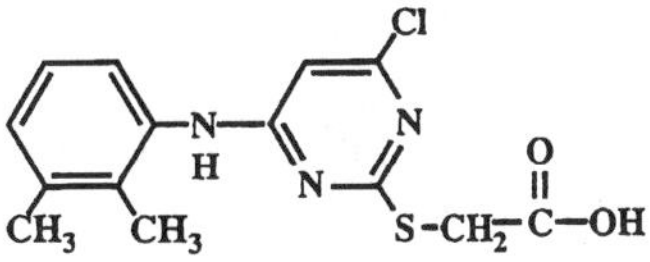

Wyeth-14,643

FIG. 1. Structures of some peroxisome proliferators.

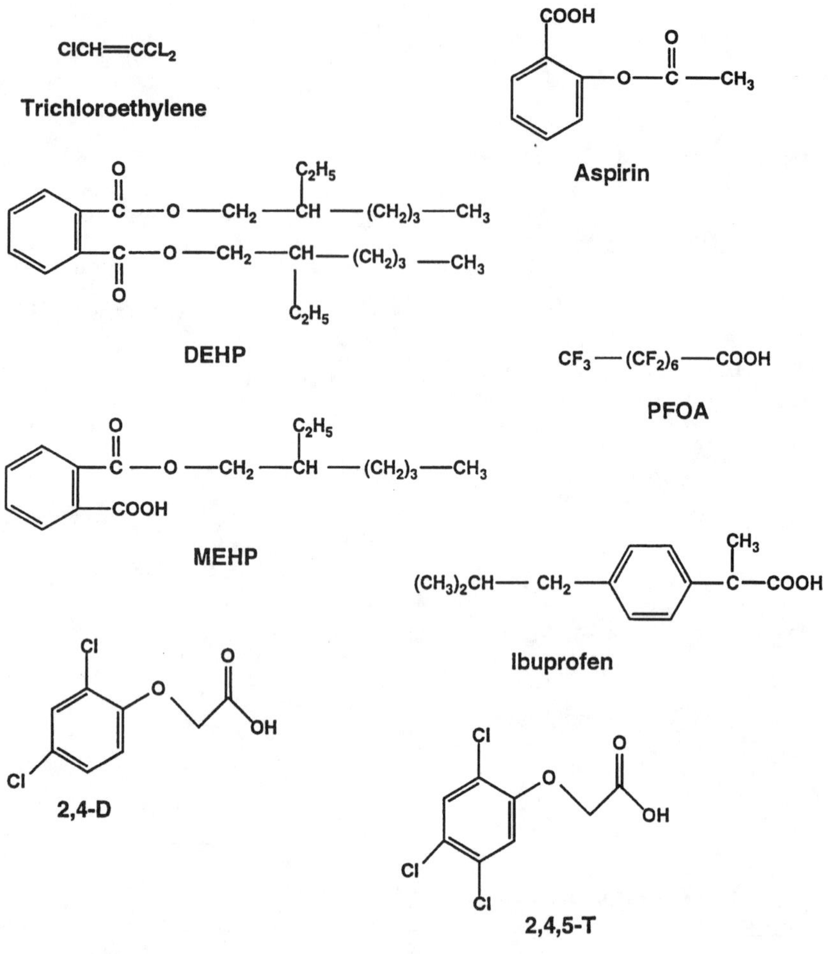

FIG. 1. *Continued.*

n-octanoic, and n-butanoic acids as well as the perfluorinated octane sulphonic acid and the non-β-oxidizable alkylthioacetic acids, 1,10-bis(carboxymethylthio)decane and 1-(carboxymethylthio)tetradecane (35, 105–111). Two related 2-methylpropen-oates, OKY-1581 and OKY-046, are as active as clofibrate in vivo (112). Long-chain dicarboxylic acids are also peroxisome proliferators (18). Trichloro- and dichloro-but not monochloroacetic acid are weak inducers of hepatic peroxisome proliferation (113–117).

Other compounds that produce hepatic peroxisome proliferation in rodents include aspirin and salicylic acid, ibuprofen, cetaben, valproic acid, 12-O-tetradecanoylphor-bol myristate-13-acetate, trichloroethylene, perchloroethylene, pentachloroethylene, 2,2,4-trimethylpentane, 2,2,4,4,6,8,8-heptamethylnonane, BM 15766, dehydroepian-dosterone, and phenothiazines including chlorpromazine (7, 17, 113, 115, 116,

118–129). The lipid-lowering agents nicotinic acid and cholestyramine produce small increases in peroxisome proliferation (130).

The peroxisome proliferators compose a group of agents with diverse chemical structures. However, most have some structural similarity to fatty acids. Two chemical features that seem to be important in peroxisome proliferators are an anionic group and a lipophilic backbone. Studies of the leukotriene antagonist series related to LY171883 indicate that the three-dimensional configuration of the molecule may be an important determinant of peroxisomal activity. Specifically, the ability of the compounds to form a compact conformation where the acidic group and the lipophilic backbone are in close proximity appears critical (131). The leukotriene antagonists share this property with the fatty acid oleate as well as other peroxisome proliferators such as clofibrate, Wyeth-14,643, and 5,8,11,14-eicosatetraynoic acid (131, 132). This suggests that the three-dimensional structures of peroxisome proliferators may be more similar than previously thought.

MECHANISMS OF PEROXISOME PROLIFERATION IN RODENTS

Considering that all peroxisome proliferators induce a similar pleiotropic response in rodent liver and that they share a common set of chemical–structural features, it is likely that they function by a common mechanism. This mechanism seems to involve PPAR-mediated modulation of gene expression (133, 134). The ability of these compounds to activate the PPAR in cotransfection assays suggests a direct action on PPAR in liver. An alternate hypothesis suggests that a fatty acid or other lipid metabolite activates the PPAR subsequent to peroxisome proliferation-induced perturbations of lipid metabolism (11, 18, 135, 136).

PERTURBATIONS OF LIPID METABOLISM

Many of the biochemical changes elicited by peroxisome proliferators are on enzymes involved in lipid metabolism. These include acyl-CoA oxidase, enoyl-CoA hydrotase, and carnitine transferases in peroxisomes, microsomal omega-oxidation of fatty acids, microsomal and mitochondrial carnitine acyltransferases, long-chain acyl-CoA hydrolase, and cytoplasmic fatty acid–binding protein (49, 58, 59, 80, 137–140). Thus, a major outcome of peroxisome proliferation is increased fatty acid catabolism. It has been proposed that the changes in gene expression in response to peroxisome proliferators may be an adaptive response to changes in lipid metabolism (18, 135, 136, 141). Support of this hypothesis is derived from observations that high-fat diets, starvation, and diabetes, all of which increase the influx of fatty acids to the liver, induce peroxisomal β-oxidation (142–144). Although the magnitude of the response in these cases is much smaller than those observed in xenobiotic-induced peroxisome proliferation, there may be common mechanisms. Peroxisome proliferators may exert their effects in the liver by virtue of their resemblance to fatty acids (131).

A metabolic perturbation caused by several peroxisome proliferators within the first 24 hr of treatment is transient lipid accumulation (31, 145, 146). Regression of the lipid coincides with the induction of the peroxisome proliferation and enzyme induction. The transient lipid accumulation caused by DEHP appears to result from inhibition of fatty acid oxidation (18, 135). A metabolite of DEHP, mono(2-ethyl-5-oxohexyl)phthalate, specifically inhibits medium-chain fatty acid oxidation in isolated mitochondria. In isolated hepatocytes, the metabolite inhibits fatty acid oxidation, causing an accumulation of medium-chain CoA esters and depletion of free CoA. It was proposed that the medium-chain acyl CoAs induce microsomal cytochrome P4504A1, leading to increased production of long-chain dicarboxylic acids, which, in turn, induce peroxisomal β-oxidation. According to this hypothesis, the induction of peroxisomal β-oxidation requires prior induction of microsomal omega-oxidation. In support of this hypothesis, it was shown that the induction of omega-oxidation by clofibrate precedes the induction of peroxisomal β-oxidation by several hours (147). Furthermore, the clofibrate-induced increases in peroxisomal acyl-CoA oxidase mRNA is blocked by inhibition of protein synthesis, whereas omega-oxidase mRNA is not affected. This supports the proposal that induction of the microsomal enzyme is required for the induction of peroxisomal enzymes. Thus, the metabolic perturbation hypothesis proposes that inhibition of fatty acid oxidation leads to peroxisome proliferation.

Other inhibitors of mitochondrial fatty acid oxidation, including valproic acid and POCA, induce peroxisome proliferation (120, 129, 148). The tetrazole-containing peroxisome proliferator LY171883 and a related analog inhibit hepatic fatty acid oxidation at the regulatory enzyme, carnitine palmitoyltransferase I (CPT-1) (320). Likewise, bezafibrate also inhibits CPT-1 (149). A generalized mechanism involving inhibition of fatty acid oxidation may not be applicable since two inhibitors of carnitine palmitoyltransferase I, POCA and 2-tetradecylglycidic acid (TDGA), attenuated the induction of peroxisomal β-oxidation by bezafibrate in cultured hepatocytes (150).

Bronfman et al. have proposed that the pharmacologically active forms of hypolipidemic agents are their CoA thioesters (151). CoA derivatives are formed in incubations of hepatic microsomes with ATP, CoA, and either clofibrate, nafenopin, or ciprofibrate. The reactivity of these agents correlates with their potency as peroxisome proliferators. The proposed role of fatty acyl-CoA esters in the regulation of peroxisomal enzymes is logical because CoA esters are known to exert regulatory control over other enzymes (152–154). However, some peroxisome proliferators such as LY171883 do not contain a carboxylic acid and should not be activated to CoA ester (24). Thus, the requirement for conversion to a CoA ester seems unlikely for some compounds. Nonetheless, the ultimate signal for the induction of peroxisome proliferation may be a lipid metabolite formed as a result of a perturbation in lipid metabolism. Such a metabolite may then bind and activate the PPAR, producing the cascade of effects that produce the pleiotropic response of peroxisome proliferation.

THE SEARCH FOR A RECEPTOR

It is now clear that a steroid hormone–like receptor is involved in the induction of the peroxisome proliferation response (134). The pursuit of this receptor was encouraged by several lines of evidence. These include tissue specificity of the peroxisomal response, the induction of similar changes in transplanted or cultured hepatocytes, the rapid onset of the transcriptional activation of inducible genes, the detection of specific binding proteins in liver cytosol, and, more recently, the cloning of a transcription factor that can be activated by peroxisome proliferators (21, 95, 117, 133, 155–162).

The first data supporting the receptor hypothesis were reported by Lalwani et al. (161, 162). A cytosolic protein was detected in liver and kidney that specifically binds ^{3}H-nafenopin. The binding was greater in liver than kidney, consistent with the stronger induction of peroxisome proliferation in liver. Several peroxisome proliferators displaced the ^{3}H-nafenopin, including clofibrate and ciprofibrate. More recently, a 70-kDa protein has been isolated using immobilized nafenopin, clofibrate, or ciprofibrate affinity chromatography (162). This protein has been identified as a member of the family of heat-shock proteins. These data did not, however, explain the activation of genes involved in the peroxisome proliferation response.

THE PEROXISOME PROLIFERATOR ACTIVATED RECEPTOR

In 1990, Issemann and Green reported cloning a member of the steroid hormone receptor superfamily that induced transcriptional activation in the presence of peroxisome proliferators (133). The discovery of this "receptor" has lead to an explosion of work in this field. These receptors bind to specific sequences in the promoter regions of responsive genes (peroxisome proliferator response elements or PPREs) which modulate transcriptional activity of the gene in either a positive or a negative fashion (133, 163, 164).

The first peroxisome proliferator–activated receptor to be cloned was the mouse PPARα (133). Additional homologs from rat, xenopus, and human have now been cloned (165–167). These have tentatively been classified into three groups based on similarities to the xenopus isoforms xPPARα, -β, and -γ (165). Mouse α and γ appear to be homologous to the xPPARα and -γ (133, 168). Mouse PPARδ and human NUC1 have been cloned and appear to be the homologs of xPPARβ (169–171). In the PPARγ class, two receptor subtypes have been identified, termed PPARγ1 and PPARγ2 (170, 172).

Steroid hormone receptors are single polypeptide molecules that have four characteristic domains, the N-terminal transactivation domain, the DNA binding domain, the hinge domain, and the ligand binding domain. The region of PPAR that is most homologous to other steroid receptors is the DNA binding domain, which contains two zinc-finger motifs (133, 173). This region gives the protein specificity for the DNA sequence (PPRE) to which it binds. A unique structural feature of PPARs is a D-box consisting of three amino acids (19). The D-box, located in the second zinc finger, is thought to be important for receptor dimerization (see below). Within the other zinc finger is the P-box, the portion responsible for determining the spacing between the half-site direct repeats in the PPRE (19).

Osumi et al. provided the pioneering work on the promoter structure of the acyl-CoA oxidase gene that allowed the identification of the PPRE (174–176). Within that promoter, the sequence of the peroxisome proliferator–sensitive positive enhancer was determined to be TGACCTTTGTCCT (−578 to −553). The consensus sequence for the PPRE was identified as direct repeat of TGACCT separated by one base-pair. This motif is known as a DR1, for direct repeat with one base-pair spacing. This element has now been found in the promoter of many peroxisome proliferator–responsive genes involved in lipid metabolism. These genes include enoyl-CoA hydratase/3-hydroxyacyl-CoA dehydrogenase, cytochrome P4504A6 and -4A1, fatty acid–binding protein, apo AI, apo AII, lipoprotein lipase, medium-chain acyl-CoA dehydrogenase, acyl-CoA synthase, acyl-CoA oxidase, HMG-CoA synthase, aP2 (adipocyte lipid-binding protein), phosphoenolpyruvate carboxykinase (PEPCK), and malic enzyme (19, 165, 172, 177–187). Other genes that probably contain a PPRE include 3-ketoacyl-CoA thiolase, apo CIII, carnitine palmitoyltransferase I, carnitine acyltransferase, carnitine octanoyltransferase, S14 (a putative lipogenic protein), and keritinocyte lipid-binding protein (164, 188–191). Recently, the human acyl-CoA oxidase promotor has been cloned (192). This promotor contains a functional PPRE that binds rat PPARα/RXRα heterodimers and is activated in co-transfection assays in the presence of peroxisome proliferators including ciprofibrate, Wyeth-14,643, and DEHP (193).

Initially, no binding of PPAR to its response elements was observed in band-shift assays in vitro (163, 194–197). Binding to the response element requires the addition of an accessory factor. This additional factor is now known to be the retinoid X receptor (RXR) and appears to be essential for transcriptional regulation. This is similar for other members of the nuclear hormone receptor superfamily (198). Thyroid hormone receptor (TR), vitamin D receptor (VDR), and retinoid receptor (RAR) all heterodimerize with RXR. PPAR has also been shown to heterodimerize with TR in vitro, but the in vivo significance of this dimerization is at present unclear (199). In cotransfection assays, induction of a reporter construct containing a PPRE was demonstrated to be strongest in the presence of both a peroxisome proliferator and 9-cis retinoic acid, the ligand for RXR (163). However, peroxisome proliferation still occurs in vitamin A–deficient rats (200). It is possible that the critical pool of retinol used for synthesis of the RXR ligand, 9-cis retinoic acid, may be resistant to depletion. Nevertheless, these experiments demonstrate that rats with severely depleted retinol pools respond to peroxisome proliferators.

The tissue-specific expression pattern of the different PPARs in rat has been recently detailed by Braissant et al. (201). The PPARα receptor is expressed in the rat at high levels in liver, kidney, intestinal mucosa, and heart (133, 169, 170, 201, 202). This correlates well with the tissue sensitivity to the induction of peroxisome proliferation (20). PPARs β and δ are more ubiquitously expressed, while PPARγ is located in adipocytes and the immune system (170, 172, 201, 203). Similar expression patterns for the PPARα are observed in human tissues (202). It is now clear that PPARγ2 is a fat-specific transcription factor that is important in adipocyte development, differentiation, and gene expression (172, 203). In mouse liver, PPARα levels display a zonal heterogeneity appearing most prominently in the centrilobular region, which is the zone in which the greatest peroxisome proliferation and hypertrophy are observed (204).

All peroxisome proliferators that have been tested have been shown to activate the PPARα in cotransfection assays. The rank order in potency of activation of PPARα correlates with the induction of peroxisome proliferation in vivo (133). The different PPARs, however, appear to be pharmacologically distinct (170, 205). The potent rodent hepatic peroxisome proliferator Wyeth-14,643 potently activates mPPARα but not mPPARδ or -γ. ETYA, the most potent activator for xPPARα, does not activate xPPARβ or γ. The mPPARγ is markedly activated by LY171883 and the antidiabetic thiazolidinediones (170, 205). Recently, it was demonstrated that fatty acids activate PPARα, suggesting that fatty acids may be the endogenous ligand for PPARα (169, 170, 196, 202, 206–209).

It is interesting to note that reporter gene constructs in yeast activation systems fail to demonstrate ligand responsiveness of PPAR (210). In these systems, constitutive expression is high, with virtually no increase in transcription in response to peroxisome proliferators. Whether a factor that bestows ligand responsivity is absent in yeast remains to be determined.

Binding studies with ^{3}H-nafenopin could not demonstrate specific binding to the PPAR protein (133). This suggested that PPARs are transcriptional activators in the peroxisome proliferation response but not receptors in the traditional sense. One possibility is that an accessory factor may be required to complete the receptor–effector complex. Alternatively, the inability to demonstrate nafenopin binding may be a technical problem. Based on the concentrations required to activate these receptors, the theoretic affinity constants for these receptors would probably be very low. Thus, ligands with higher specific activities may be required to demonstrate binding. Recently, specific binding of ^{3}H-BRL49653, an antidiabetic thiazolidinedione, has been demonstrated to PPARγ (205). Thus, it appears that PPARγ is the receptor for the antidiabetic thiazolidinediones. Although binding of ligand to PPARα has not been demonstrated, it is clear that PPARα is required for the induction of peroxisome proliferation in mice. In gene knockout experiments in homologous PPARα −/− mice, no peroxisome proliferation response after treatment with either clofibrate or Wyeth-14,643 was observed (211). The hepatomegaly response was also absent in these mice. These mice will be useful in determining the mechanism by which peroxisome proliferators produce their effects in rodents. These mice will also be vital in determining a role for PPARα activation in the induction of hepatocarcinogenesis (see below).

In addition to PPAR, there may be other proteins involved in the transcriptional response to peroxisome proliferators and fatty acids in the liver. Fatty acid–binding protein (FABP) is one that may have a role in peroxisome proliferator signaling. FABP is a 14-kDa protein that binds endogenous fatty acids and is believed to be involved in the uptake and intracellular transport of fatty acids (212–214). The peroxisome proliferator LY171883 was found to bind specifically to FABP, and the binding was competed by bezafibrate, ciprofibrate, clofibrate, and Wyeth-14,643 (215). The peroxisome proliferators also competed for oleic acid binding to FABP (215, 216). The rank order of potency was similar to that of their ability to induce peroxisome proliferation (215). This is not surprising in light of the structural features the peroxisome proliferators share with fatty acids (131).

Thus, the mechanism of peroxisome proliferation may include a direct action on the PPAR or activation by free fatty acids whose concentration increases as a result of a perturbation of lipid metabolism. FABP may have a role due to the peroxisome proliferator–induced displacement of endogenous fatty acids. FABP may also be involved in signal transduction to the nucleus. Preliminary data suggest that FABP facilitates the transport of fatty acids to the nucleus (217, 218). FABP may also transport peroxisome proliferators to the nucleus as fraudulent fatty acids. In this way, FABP may participate in fatty acid regulation of numerous genes including those associated with peroxisome proliferation as well as apo A-1, malic enzyme, glucose 6-phosphate dehydrogenase, and fatty acid synthase (219–224). Further work will be needed to clarify the role of FABP in the activation of PPAR.

INTERSPECIES DIFFERENCES

The peroxisome proliferation response that has been described above is most pronounced in rats and mice. Hamsters are responsive to peroxisome proliferators, but the magnitude of the response is smaller than in rats (24, 76, 225). Dogs and guinea pigs are relatively resistant to the effects of peroxisome proliferators (24, 76, 225–229). Marmosets and rhesus monkeys have been used in several studies involving peroxisome proliferators. Bezafibrate, clofibrate, and LY171883 have little or no effect on liver weight or peroxisomal β-oxidation in rhesus monkeys, and clobuzarit has no effect in the marmoset (24, 225, 228, 230). Nafenopin induced peroxisomal β-oxidation and laurate hydroxylase activity 2.5-fold in marmosets (227). In comparison, nafenopin produced a 10-fold induction of peroxisomal β-oxidation in the rat at a fivefold lower dose (227). Gemfibrozil increased the relative volume of peroxisomes 1.6-fold in rhesus monkey (76). A peroxisome proliferation response was elicited in monkey liver in dose-escalating studies involving ciprofibrate (up to 200 mg/kg) and DL-040 (up to 400 mg/kg) (231, 232). Peroxisome volume fraction and peroxisomal β-oxidation were increased approximately fivefold. By contrast, a dose of 25 mg/kg of ciprofibrate given to rats increases peroxisomal β-oxidation 25-fold (20). These results suggest that monkeys are not completely insensitive to peroxisome proliferators, but they are considerably less responsive than rats or mice.

The response to peroxisome proliferators occurs also in vitro in cultured rat hepatocytes. Increases in peroxisomal β-oxidation, omega-oxidation, were observed with MEHP in rat hepatocytes, but not guinea pig or marmoset hepatocytes (135, 233). Likewise, ciprofibrate, bezafibrate, and LY171883 induced marked increases in peroxisomal β-oxidation in rat hepatocytes, but no response was observed in dog or monkey hepatocytes (234). Hepatocytes from these nonresponsive species did respond to other enzyme inducers such as phenobarbital and were sensitive to the effects of epithelial growth factor (EGF) on replicative DNA synthesis, demonstrating that they were metabolically competent (135, 235, 236).

The in vivo and in vitro studies clearly demonstrate that larger species are unresponsive or considerably less responsive than rats or mice. This raises the question of whether the rodent carcinogenicity data are relevant to humans in light of the close relationship between the induction of peroxisome proliferation and hepatocarcinogenesis in rodents (see below).

HUMAN RESPONSIVENESS

The effect of clofibrate on human liver peroxisomes, first reported in 1980, involved biopsy samples from 67 hyperlipoproteinemic patients (237). Samples from treated patients exhibited hypertrophy of SER and an increased number of mitochondria and peroxisomes. These were subjective estimates without morphometric analysis. In a more thorough study of the livers of 16 patients treated with clofibrate for 3–4 months, the numeric density of peroxisomes increased 50% (238). Volume density was not significantly increased, suggesting that the peroxisomes were smaller. There was an increase in the number of mitochondria comparable to the increase in peroxisomes. However, untreated hyperlipoproteinemic patients have a significantly greater peroxisome volume density than normal individuals (239), and the authors concluded that the effect of clofibrate in human liver is unlike the hepatic peroxisome proliferation seen in rodents (238). Thus, the Hanefeld studies, although frequently cited as evidence for chemical-induced peroxisome proliferation in humans, do not support such an interpretation (237, 238).

There have been other clinical studies to evaluate peroxisome proliferation in humans. Biopsy samples from hyperlipoproteinemic patients treated with fenofibrate for up to 86 months show no evidence of hepatocellular hypertrophy (240). The number and volume of hepatic peroxisomes in this group are similar to those of untreated patients (240–243). Likewise, studies of the effects of gemfibrozil on peroxisomes in liver biopsy samples from eight patients treated for 17–27 months also show no increase in peroxisome number or volume compared to historical controls (74, 75).

Experiments performed with human hepatocytes in culture have provided data indicating an insensitivity to peroxisome proliferators. As discussed previously, cultured hepatocytes from several animal species display the pattern of interspecies differences in sensitivity to peroxisome proliferators that is seen in vivo. This is an important facet in the validation of the in vitro model. Human hepatocytes behave like dog, guinea pig, and marmoset hepatocytes in that they are unresponsive or far less sensitive than rodent hepatocytes to peroxisome proliferators. The functional viability of the human cells is maintained in culture, as demonstrated by the induction of cytochrome P450 by phenobarbital and stimulation of replicative DNA synthesis by EGF (135, 235, 236). Recently, human hepatocytes in culture were used to display the putative pharmacologic response to fenofibrate involved in the triglyceride-lowering effect (164). This effect, down-regulation of the apolipoprotein CIII gene, was observed in rat hepatocytes as well as the human cells. Whereas rat hepatocytes exhibited a marked increase in peroxisomal acyl-CoA oxidase mRNA in response to fenofibrate, no such effect was observed in the human hepatocytes. Thus, human hepatocytes display a pharmacologic response to fenofibrate but not the peroxisome proliferation-related response. Furthermore, the apo CIII gene response appears to be PPAR-mediated, which indicates that PPAR regulates gene expression in the human liver but does not activate a pleiotropic response like that observed in rodents. Even more puzzling is that the human acyl-CoA oxidase promotor contains a functional PPRE that is activated by peroxisome proliferators (193). These data suggest that other unknown factors influence the transcriptional regulation in humans and may account for the relative insensitivity displayed by larger mammals to peroxisome proliferators.

HEPATOCARCINOGENESIS IN RODENTS

The hepatocarcinogenicity of peroxisome proliferators in rodents was originally described in studies of nafenopin (244, 245). Subsequent studies of many peroxisome proliferators have indicated a strong correlation between the potency of inducing peroxisome proliferation and hepatocarcinogenicity (7, 246). For example, Wyeth-14,643, at a dose of 0.1%, causes a 100% incidence of liver tumors in rats after 1 year (23). DEHP, at a dose of 1.2%, causes only a 10% incidence of liver tumors after 2 years (247, 248). There is clearly an association between peroxisome proliferation and hepatocarcinogenesis in rodents, but the mechanistic link is not yet fully understood.

Induction of mutations into DNA is a well-established mechanism by which chemicals induce carcinogenesis (249). Numerous peroxisome proliferators have been evaluated in mutagenicity assays to determine if this mechanism could explain the hepatocarcinogenesis of peroxisome proliferators. A variety of tests have been performed, including the Ames Salmonella test, DNA repair, clastogenicity, and micronucleus assays (250–255). The bulk of the mutagenicity data has given negative results for genotoxic activity. There also are no DNA adducts detected by ^{32}P-postlabeling studies after treatment with clofibrate, fenofibrate, Wyeth-14,643, and DEHP (256). These studies indicate that peroxisome proliferators do not cause direct DNA damage.

Reddy and associates proposed that peroxisome proliferators could produce genetic damage through the production of free radicals and oxidative stress (7, 14, 15). This hypothesis was supported by the evidence that peroxisome proliferators produced a 20-fold increase in acyl-CoA oxidase in peroxisomes, which generates H_2O_2 (14, 137). The proliferation is associated with a twofold increase in catalase activity, which degrades H_2O_2. The net effect is proposed to be increased H_2O_2 leakage from peroxisomes, leading to generation of oxygen-free radicals and, ultimately, oxidative DNA damage. Increased H_2O_2 production was observed in liver homogenates from rats treated with peroxisome proliferators for short periods (257–260). However, long-term treatment with DEHP, clofibrate, or bezafibrate caused little or no increase in hepatic H_2O_2 production (261). Chu et al. have reported that CV-1 cells that overexpress the acyl-CoA oxidase gene generate greater amounts of H_2O_2 after exposure to linoleic acid (262). Subsequently, these cells became transformed as measured by their ability to grow in soft agar and to form adenocarcinomas when transplanted into nude mice. The data suggest that large amounts of H_2O_2 generated inside cells can lead to transformation. Oxidative defense mechanisms including vitamin E and glutathione peroxidase were found to be reduced by peroxisome proliferators (263–265). Accumulation of conjugated dienes and lipofuscin is also observed in rats treated chronically with peroxisome proliferators (251, 266). These products are thought to arise as a result of increased lipid peroxidation. The magnitude of the accumulation of lipofuscin and conjugated dienes was reported to correlate with hepatocarcinogenic potential (267).

Peroxisomes isolated from ciprofibrate-treated rats were found to nick circular SV40 viral DNA in the presence of palmitoyl-CoA (268). Peroxisomes from untreated rats did not affect the integrity of the DNA, suggesting that the peroxisome proliferator stimulated excess oxidative damage relative to control. However, the reactions in these studies were conducted under conditions where catalase was inhibited and the balance of H_2O_2 release was disturbed. Elliott and Elcombe failed to demonstrate DNA strand breaks in vivo after peroxisome proliferator treatment, suggesting that the oxidative defenses of the hepatocyte are not overwhelmed in response to increased H_2O_2 generation (264).

8-Hydroxydeoxyguanosine is a modified nucleotide that is usually formed by interaction of deoxyguanosine with free radicals (269, 270). It is used as a marker for oxidative damage to DNA. Kasai et al. (271) demonstrated increases in 8-hydroxy-deoxyguanosine in hepatic DNA from rats treated with ciprofibrate for 16–40 weeks (271). Other studies have demonstrated small increases in 8-hydroxydeoxyguanosine levels with DEHP and DEHA (272). However, Hegi et al. (273) failed to demonstrate increased 8-hydroxydeoxyguanosine levels following treatment with nafenopin for up to 8 weeks. Furthermore, there is considerably more 8-hydroxydeoxyguanosine in mitochondrial DNA than in nuclear DNA in rats, presumably arising from super-oxide leakage of the respiratory chain (274). Because Kasai et al. (271) measured 8-hydroxydeoxyguanosine in total liver DNA, much of the adducts may have originated from mitochondria.

If the oxidative stress hypothesis is the mechanism for liver carcinogenesis caused by peroxisome proliferators, there should be a correlation between the induction of peroxisomal β-oxidation and tumor formation. Marsman et al. (23) demonstrated that doses of DEHP and Wyeth-14,643 that produced similar induction of peroxisomal β-oxidation in rats induced a vastly different incidence of tumor responses (incidences of 10% and 100%, respectively). Ciprofibrate causes marked increases in peroxisomal β-oxidation in the kidney, but no tumors have been reported in this organ (16, 33). Thus, the data examining the peroxisome proliferator–induced DNA damage in rats has failed to provide conclusive evidence for the oxidative stress hypothesis.

NONGENOTOXIC MECHANISMS OF CARCINOGENESIS

Hepatocarcinogenesis induced by chemicals is described as a multistage process of initiation and promotion (275). An initiating agent causes genetic damage in a cell that creates the potential for malignant transformation. A promoting agent causes the selective growth of transformed cells. This selective growth fixes the lesion and clonally expands the population carrying the mutation, increasing the likelihood of the lesion's progressing to a carcinoma. As discussed above, peroxisome proliferators are negative in genotoxicity tests and do not appear to affect the integrity of DNA directly. Consistent with this, peroxisome proliferators do not appear to act as initiators in initiation-promotion protocols (276–278).

Tumor promotion by peroxisome proliferators has been clearly demonstrated in two-stage carcinogenicity models (279–282). These studies generally involve initiation with a genotoxin such as diethylnitrosamine, followed by treatment with the peroxisome-proliferating agent. The end points vary, but most of the studies measure enzyme-altered foci or tumor development. It is important to note that the selection of the focal marker is crucial because peroxisome proliferators produce foci that are phenotypically distinct from those produced by other promoters such as phenobarbital. Gamma-glutamyltransferase (GGT) and the placental form of glutathione S-transferase are commonly used markers that are expressed in phenobarbital–induced foci but not peroxisome proliferator–induced foci (283, 284). Several studies that failed to demonstrate promotional activity of peroxisome proliferators used the inappropriate marker, GGT (285–288). In fact, peroxisome proliferators have been shown to inhibit the formation of GGT-positive liver foci (289, 290). It is now evident that peroxisome proliferators induce basophilic foci when administered chronically in the absence of an initiating agent (281, 291). These basophilic foci have morphologic similarity to the tumors that appear subsequently, and the number of basophilic foci correlate with the number of tumors developed (292). The basophilic foci were proposed to develop as a result of the promotion of spontaneously initiated cells in rat liver. Cattley et al. (293) and Kraupp-Grasl et al. (294) demonstrated that older rats, which have more spontaneously initiated cells than younger rats, developed more tumors in response to peroxisome proliferators than rats exposed to the protocol at a younger age. The magnitude of peroxisome proliferation was similar in both young and old rats. Thus, promotion of spontaneously initiated cells in liver may account for the hepatocarcinogenesis of peroxisome proliferators.

The mitogenic effects of peroxisome proliferators probably play a key role in their hepatocarcinogenesis (23, 295). Increased cell replication in the normally quiescent liver may increase the probability of conversion of DNA lesions to mutations in the spontaneously initiated cells before they undergo repair. Increased proliferation rates may also increase the chance that a mutation will arise from the normal DNA replicative process (296). The mitogenic property of peroxisome proliferators upon hepatocytes can be reproduced in culture, suggesting direct mitogenic effects rather than a secondary response to stimuli produced in another organ (157, 295, 297).

The mitogenic effect of peroxisome proliferators in hepatocytes develops early in association with hepatomegaly (7, 23, 27, 298). Rates of DNA replication increase during the first day of treatment and generally return to normal after a few days. However, potent agents such as Wyeth-14,643 produce a sustained stimulation of replicative DNA synthesis (23, 299). The sustained response has been implicated in hepatocarcinogenesis. Wyeth-14,643 causes a chronic stimulation of cell proliferation and a 100% incidence of tumor formation in rats, whereas DEHP causes only a transient stimulation of cell proliferation and a 10% tumor incidence (23). Thus, sustained stimulation of proliferation of the general hepatocyte population may relate to tumorigenic potency but is not required for tumor formation. It seems more likely that induced replication of selected populations of hepatocytes is involved in hepatocarcinogenesis. The basophilic foci induced by peroxisome proliferators may be important in this regard. Using initiation–promotion protocols to compare phenobarbital and Wyeth-14,643, it was observed that phenobarbital induced the formation of many small foci whereas Wyeth-14,643 induced the formation of fewer but much larger foci (300). This observation has led to the belief that peroxisome proliferators selectively stimulate the growth of basophilic liver foci, which give rise to tumors. Indeed, direct measurement of DNA synthesis indicated that peroxisome proliferators increase the cell proliferation rate of these basophilic foci compared to normal hepatocytes (301, 302). Thus, the data suggest that cells in basophilic foci are uniquely sensitive to the mitogenic effects of peroxisome proliferators. An alternative hypothesis is that normal hepatocytes may become resistant to the proliferative effects of peroxisome proliferators whereas the basophilic cells retain responsiveness. This second possibility is consistent with the "selective growth" hypothesis of carcinogenesis (303).

There appear to be zonal differences in the mitogenic response to peroxisome proliferators in the rat liver. It is primarily hepatocytes in the periportal region of the rat liver lobule that undergo cellular division in the early response to peroxisome proliferators (23). The ploidy state of the cell may also determine its responsiveness to peroxisome proliferators. DEHP and methylclofenapate have been shown to stimulate DNA synthesis selectively in binucleated hepatocytes (304). Upon mitosis, this produces two tetraploid daughter cells. These data suggest that a specific population of cells may be susceptible to the proliferative effects of peroxisome proliferators. The relevance of these observations to hepatocarcinogenesis remains to be determined.

An additional factor that may influence the development of tumors in response to peroxisome proliferators is the difference in rate of cell division versus the rate of cell death. Apoptosis, the process of programmed cell death, is stimulated upon removal of promoting agents including phenobarbital and peroxisome proliferators (305, 306). If the promoter is returned to the system, the apoptopic process is inhibited. Likewise, if phenobarbital is used as a tumor promoter and then replaced by nafenopin, no apoptosis occurs (305). This suggests that peroxisome proliferators not only stimulate cell growth but also inhibit the process of apoptosis.

The mechanism by which peroxisome proliferators stimulate cell growth is at present unknown. Peroxisome proliferators have been found to activate protooncogenes that are also induced after partial hepatectomy (307, 308). Steady-state levels of mRNA for c-Ha-ras and c-myc increase after treatment with hypolipidemic agents (309). In cultured cells, c-fos and c-jun are induced by the peroxisome proliferator Wyeth-14,643 (310). Peroxisome proliferators decrease gap junctions on hepatocytes, which are critical to intercellular communication (311–315). This reduction of gap junctions is also observed during liver regeneration following partial hepatectomy. In the latter case, the number of gap junctions returns to normal when regeneration is complete. Likewise, during the process of tumorigenesis induced by phorbol esters, gap junctions become reduced progressively. Thus, the reduction of gap junctions in response to peroxisome proliferators may also have a role in carcinogenicity.

Other mechanisms have been proposed to play a role in peroxisome proliferator–induced hepatocarcinogenesis. For example, Ca^{2+} appears to play a key role in signaling cellular proliferation after partial hepatectomy or exposure to growth factors. Peroxisome proliferators have been shown to mobilize Ca^{2+} (316). Activation of protein kinase C also may play a role in peroxisome proliferator signal transduction (154). Interestingly, hepatic FABP was proposed to have a role in peroxisome proliferator–induced mitogenesis (317). At this time, it is unclear whether the mitogenic effects of peroxisome proliferators are mediated by PPAR. The PPAR is localized primarily in the centrilobular region of the rat liver, where the hepatocellular hypertrophy and proliferation of peroxisomes occur (204). In contrast, the hepatocellular DNA replication is localized primarily in the periportal region in response to peroxisome proliferators. These observations tend to argue against a role of PPAR in regulating the mitogenic response. However, PPAR −/− knockout mice show no hepatomegaly, suggesting that some of the mitogenic effects of peroxisome proliferators may be mediated by PPAR (211). Further studies will be required to determine if the regulatory regions of growth controlling protooncogenes or gap junction genes contain PPREs. It seems unlikely that a single mechanism will be responsible for the induction of hepatocarcinogenesis because of the numerous effects of peroxisome proliferators on hepatic gene expression.

HUMAN RELEVANCE

Peroxisome proliferators are clearly hepatocarcinogenic in rats and mice. It is thought that the tumor formation in response to these chemicals is related mechanistically to peroxisome proliferation or the associated cell proliferation. Thus, because humans are resistant to the hepatic effects of peroxisome proliferators, it is reasonable to conclude that this includes a resistance to the hepatocarcinogenic effects. However, the actual mechanisms of tumor production have not been defined, making the carcinogenic risk to humans difficult to assess.

Two studies have evaluated the incidence of cancer in humans treated with peroxisome proliferators. The World Health Organization sponsored a clinical trial with clofibrate that lasted approximately 5.8 years (318). In this study, a higher incidence of non–coronary heart disease deaths was reported. However, no significant differences in the incidence or distribution of neoplasia were observed. A Finnish study involving gemfibrozil included over 4000 patients (319). A borderline significant increase in basal cell carcinoma in the skin was measured, but no statistically significant increases in incidence or distribution of other specific types of cancers between the treatment and control groups occurred. This study is of limited value in determining the carcinogenic risk because of the short time periods involved in the treatments. Anecdotal information would also suggest that peroxisome proliferators do not present a carcinogenic risk to humans. The hypotriglyceridemic agents fenofibrate and bezafibrate, in addition to gemfibrozil, are widely used throughout the world, and there is no indication that they increase the cancer incidence. Likewise, ibuprofen induces peroxisome proliferation in rodents (118, 320) but is a safe and effective antiinflammatory agent in humans.

Other lines of evidence indicate that the risk to humans is very low. These agents are clearly nongenotoxic. Therefore, the human risk should be evaluated differently than for genotoxic compounds. The available data indicate that tumor formation is related to the development to the hepatic response, including liver enlargement, cell replication, and oxidative changes. In the absence of this response, it is reasonable to conclude that the compounds do not pose a carcinogenic risk to humans. Clinical epidemiologic and in vitro data indicate that the peroxisome proliferation response does not occur in humans. Therefore, if the association between peroxisome proliferation and hepatocarcinogenesis is consistent, then the strong implication is that humans are not at risk. Human risk will continue to be a subject of debate until the mechanism of peroxisome proliferation in rodents is clearly defined. Therefore, an understanding of the mechanisms involved in the induction of peroxisome proliferation will aid our ability to evaluate the human carcinogenic risk of these compounds.

REFERENCES

1. De Duve C. Microbodies in the living cell. *Sci Am* 1983;248:74–84.
2. Lazarow PB, Fujuki Y. Biogenesis of peroxisomes. *Annu Rev Cell Biol* 1985;1:489–530.
3. Reddy JK, Mannaerts GP. Peroxisomal lipid metabolism. *Annu Rev Nutr* 1994;14:343–370.
4. Kindl H, Lazarow PB. Peroxisomes and glyoxysomes. *Ann NY Acad Sci* 1982;386:1–550.
5. Tolbert NE. Metabolic pathways in peroxisomes and glyoxisomes. *Annu Rev Biochem* 1981;50:133–157.
6. Goldfischer S, Reddy JK. Peroxisomes (microbodies) in cell pathology. *Int Rev Exp Pathol* 1984;26:45–84.
7. Reddy JK, Lalwani ND. Carcinogenesis by hepatic peroxisome proliferators: evaluation of the risk of hypolipidemic drugs and industrial plasticizers to humans. *CRC Crit Rev Toxicol* 1983;12:1–58.
8. Mannaerts GP, Van Veldhoven PP. Metabolic role of mammalian peroxisomes. In: Gibson GG, Lake BG, eds. *Peroxisomes: biology and importance in toxicology and medicine.* London: Taylor & Francis, 1993:19–62.
9. Hess R, Staubli W, Reiss W. Nature of the hepatomegalic effect produced by ethylchlorophenoxyisobutyrate in the rat. *Nature* 1965;208:856–859.
10. Svoboda DJ, Azarnoff DL. Response of hepatic microbodies to a hypolipidemic agent, ethylchlorophenoxyisobutyrate (CPIB). *J Cell Biol* 1966;30:442–450.
11. Bentley P, Calder I, Elcombe C, Grasso P, Stringer D, Wiegand H-J. Hepatic peroxisome proliferation in rodents and its significance for humans. *Food Chem Toxicol* 1993;31:857–907.
12. Eacho PI, Feller DR. Hepatic peroxisome proliferation induced by hypolipidemic drugs and other chemicals. In: Witiak DK, Newman HAI, Feller DR, eds. *Antilipidemic drugs: medicinal, chemical and biochemical aspects.* Amsterdam: Elsevier, 1991:375–426.

13. Lake BG. Mechanisms of hepatocarcinogenicity of peroxisome-proliferating drugs and chemicals. *Annu Rev Pharmacol Toxicol* 1995;35:483–507.
14. Reddy JK, Azarnoff DL, Hignite CE. Hypolipidaemic hepatic peroxisome proliferators form a novel class of chemical carcinogens. *Nature* 1980;283:397–398.
15. Reddy JK, Rao MS. Oxidative DNA damage caused by persistent peroxisome proliferation. *Mutat Res* 1989;214:63–68.
16. Rao MS, Reddy JK. Peroxisome proliferation and hepatocarcinogenesis. *Carcinogenesis* 1987;8:631–636.
17. Hawkins JM, Jones WE, Bonner FW, Gibson GG. The effect of peroxisome proliferators on microsomal, peroxisomal and mitochondrial enzyme activities in the liver and kidney. *Drug Metab Rev* 1987;18:441–515.
18. Lock EA, Mitchell AM, Elcombe CR. Biochemical mechanisms of induction of hepatic peroxisome proliferation. *Annu Rev Pharmacol Toxicol* 1989;29:145–163.
19. Schoonjans K, Watanabe M, Suzuki H, et al. Induction of the acyl-coenzyme A synthase gene by fibrates and fatty acids is mediated by peroxisome proliferator response element in the C promotor. *J Biol Chem* 1995;270:19269–19276.
20. Nemali MR, Usuda N, Reddy MK, et al. Comparison of constitutive and inducible levels of expression of peroxisomal β-oxidation and catalase genes in liver and extrahepatic tissues of rat. *Cancer Res* 1988;48:5316–5324.
21. Reddy JK, Goel SK, Nemali MR, et al. Transcriptional regulation of peroxisomal fatty acyl-CoA oxidase and enoyl-CoA hydratase/3-hydroxyacyl-CoA dehydrogenase in rat liver peroxisome proliferators. *Proc Natl Acad Sci* 1986;83:1747–1751.
22. Fitzgerald JE, Sanyer JL, Schardein JL, Lake RS, McGuire EJ, de la Iglesia FA. Carcinogen bioassay and mutagenicity studies with the hypolipidemic agent gemfibrozil. *J Natl Cancer Inst* 1981;67:1105–1116.
23. Marsman DS, Cattley RC, Conway JG, Popp JA. Relationship of hepatic peroxisome proliferation and replicative DNA synthesis to the hepatocarcinogenicity of the peroxisome proliferators, di(2-ethylhexyl) phthalate and [4-chloro-6(2,3,-xylidino)-2-pyrimidiny[thio] acetic acid (Wyeth-14,643) in rats. *Cancer Res* 1988;48:6739–6744.
24. Eacho PI, Foxworthy PS, Johnson WD, Hoover DM, White SL. Hepatic peroxisomal changes induced by a tetrazole-substituted alkoxyacetophenone in rats and comparison with other species. *Toxicol Appl Pharmacol* 1986;83:430–437.
25. Beckett RB, Weiss R, Stitzel RE, Cenedella RJ. Studies on the hepatomegaly caused by the hypolipidaemic drugs nafenopin and clofibrate. *Toxicol Appl Pharmacol* 1972;23:42–53.
26. Moody DE, Reddy JK. The hepatic effects of hypolipidemic drugs on hepatic peroxisomes and peroxisome-associated enzymes. *Am J Pathol* 1978;90:435–446.
27. Styles JA, Kelly M, Pritchard NR, Elcombe CR. A species comparison of acute hyperplasia induced by the peroxisome proliferator methylclofenapate: involvement of the binucleated hepatocyte. *Carcinogenesis* 1988;9:1647–1655.
28. Moody DE, Rao MS, Reddy JK. Mitogenic effect in mouse liver induced by a hypolipidemic drug nafenopin. *Virchows Arch B Cell Pathol* 1977;23:291–296.
29. Smith-Oliver T, Butterworth BE. Correlation of the carcinogenic potential of DEHP with induced hyperplasia rather than genotoxic activity. *Mutat Res* 1987;188:21–28.
30. Lalwani ND, Reddy MK, Qureshi SA, Sirtori CR, Abiko Y, Reddy JK. Evaluation of selected hypolipidemic agents for the induction of peroxisomal enzymes and peroxisome proliferation in the rat liver. *Human Toxicol* 1983;2:27–48.
31. Price SC, Hinton RH, Mitchell FE, et al. Time and dose study on the response of rats to the hypolipidemic drug fenofibrate. *Toxicology* 1986;41:169–191.
32. Lake BGJ, Pels Rijcken WR, Gray TJB, Gangolli SD. Comparative studies of the hepatic effects of di- and mono-n-octylphthalates, di-(2-ethylhexyl) phthlate and clofibrate in the rat. *Acta Pharmacol Toxicol* 1984;54:167–176.
33. Witiak DT, Newman HAI, Feller DR. *Clofibrate and related analogs: a comprehensive review.* New York: Dekker, Inc., 1977.
34. Loud AV. A quantitative stereological description of the ultrastructure of normal rat liver parenchymal cells. *J Cell Biol* 1968;37:27–46.
35. Just WW, Gorgas K, Hartl FU, Heinemann P, Salzer M, Schimassek H. Biochemical effects and zonal heterogeneity of peroxisome proliferation induced by perfluorocarboxylic acids in rat liver. *Hepatology* 1989;9:570–581.

36. Lindauer M, Beier K, Volkl A, Fahimi H. Zonal heterogeneity of peroxisomal enzymes in rat liver: differential induction by three divergent hypolipidemic drugs. *Hepatology* 1994;20:475–486.
37. Moody DE, Reddy JK. Morphometric analysis of the ultrastructural changes in rat liver induced by the peroxisome proliferator SaH-42-348. *J Cell Biol* 1976;71:768–780.
38. Gorgas K, Krisans SK. Zonal heterogeneity of peroxisome proliferation and morphology in rat liver after gemfibrozil treatment. *J Lipid Res* 1989;30:1859–1875.
39. Baumgart E, Stegmeier K, Schmidt FH, Fahimi HD. Proliferation of peroxisomes in pericentral hepatocytes of rat liver after administration of a new hypocholesterolemic agent (BM 15766): sex-dependent ultrastructural differences. *Lab Invest* 1987;56:554–564.
40. Lalwani ND, Reddy MK, Qureshi SA, Moehle CM, Hayashi H, Reddy JK. Noninhibitory effect of antioxidants ethoxyquin, 2(3)-tert-butyl-4-hydroxyanisole and 3,5-di-tert-butyl-4-hydroxytoluene on hepatic peroxisome proliferation and peroxisomal fatty acid β-oxidation induced by a hypolipidemic agent in rats. *Cancer Res* 1983;43:1680–1687.
41. Lazarow PB, de Duve C. A fatty acyl-CoA oxidizing system in rat liver peroxisomes; enhancement by clofibrate, a hypolipidemic drug. *Proc Natl Acad Sci USA* 1976;73:2043–2046.
42. Lazarow PB. Rat liver peroxisomes catalyze the β-oxidation of fatty acids. *J Biol Chem* 1978;253: 1522–1528.
43. Hashimoto T. Comparison of the enzymes of lipid β-oxidation in peroxisomes and mitochondria. In: Fahimi HD, Sies H, eds. *Peroxisomes in biology and medicine.* Berlin: Springer-Verlag, 1987:97–104.
44. Watanabe T, Lalwani ND, Reddy JK. Specific changes in the protein composition of rat liver in response to the peroxisome proliferators, ciprofibrate, Wyeth-14,643, and di(2-ethylhexyl) phthalate. *Biochem J* 1985;227:767–775.
45. Chatterjee B, Demyan WF, Lalwani ND, Reddy JK, Roy AK. Reversible alteration of hepatic messenger RNA for peroxisomal and non-peroxisomal proteins induced by the hypolipidemic drug Wyeth-14,643. *Biochem J* 1983;214:879–883.
46. McQuaid S, Russell SEH, White SA, Pearson CM, Elcombe CR, Humphries P. Analysis of transcripts homologous to acyl-CoA oxidase and enoyl-CoA hydratase/3-hydroxyacyl-CoA dehydrogenase induced in rat liver by methylclofenapate. *Cancer Lett* 1987;37:115–124.
47. Hijikata M, Wen J-K, Osumi T, Hashimoto T. Rat peroxisomal 3-ketoacyl-CoA thiolase gene. *J Biol Chem* 1990;265:4600–4606.
48. Osumi T, Ozasa H, Hashimoto T. Molecular cloning of cDNA for rat acyl-CoA oxidase. *J Biol Chem* 1984;259:2031–2034.
49. Markwell MAK, Bieber LL, Tolbert NE. Differential increase of hepatic peroxisomal, mitochondrial and microsomal carnitine acyltransferases in clofibrate-fed rats. *Biochem Pharmacol* 1977;26:1697–1702.
50. Chatterjee B, Song CS, Kim JM, Roy AK. Cloning, sequencing and regulation of rat liver carnitine octanoyltransferase transcriptional stimulation of the enzyme during peroxisome proliferation. *Biochemistry* 1988;27:9000–9006.
51. Pollard AD, Brindley, DN. Effect of chronic clofibrate feeding on the activities of enzymes involved in glycerolipid synthesis and in peroxisomal metabolism in rat liver. *Biochem Pharmacol* 1982;31:1650–1652.
52. Leighton F, Coloma L, Koenig C. Structure, composition, physical properties, and turnover of proliferated peroxisomes: a study of the chronic effects of Su-13437 on rat liver. *J Cell Biol* 1975;67:281–309.
53. Lipsky, NG, Pedersen PL. Perturbation by clofibrate of mitochondrial levels in animal cells. *J Biol Chem* 1982;257:1473–1481.
54. Ganning AE, Olsson MJ, Peterson E, Dallner G. Fatty acid oxidation in hepatic peroxisomes and mitochondria after treatment of rats with di(2-ethylhexyl) phthalate. *Pharmacol Toxicol* 1989;65:265–268.
55. Mannaerts GP, Debeer LJ, Thomas J, De Schepper PJ. Mitochondrial and peroxisomal fatty acid oxidation in liver homogenates and isolated hepatocytes from control and clofibrate-treated rats. *J Biol Chem* 1979;254:4585–4595.
56. Van Veldhoven P, Declercq PE, Debeer LJ, Mannaerts GP. Effects of benofluorex and fenofibrate treatment on mitochondrial and peroxisomal marker enzymes in rat liver. *Biochem Pharmacol* 1984;33:1153–1155.
57. Foxworthy PS, Perry DN, Hoover DM, Eacho PI. Changes in hepatic lipid metabolism associated with lipid accumulation and its reversal in rats given the peroxisome proliferator LY171883. *Toxicol Appl Pharmacol* 1990;106:375–383.
58. Orton TC, Parker GL. The effect of hypolipidemic agents on the hepatic microsomal drug-metabolizing enzyme system of the rat: induction of the cytochrome(s) P450 with specificity toward terminal hydroxylation of lauric acid. *Drug Metab Dispos* 1982;10:110–115.

59. Gibson GG, Orton TC, Tamburini PP. Cytochrome P450 induction by clofibrate: purification and properties of a hepatic cytochrome P450 relatively specific for the 12- and 11-hydroxylation of dodecanoic acid (lauric acid). *Biochem J* 1982;203:161–168.

60. Okita RT, Masters BSS. Effect of phenobarbital treatment and cytochrome P450 inhibitors on the laurate omega- and (omega-1)-hydroxylase activities of rat liver microsomes. *Drug Metab Dispos* 1980;8:147–151.

61. Platt DS, Cockrill BL. Biochemical changes in rat liver in response to treatment with drugs and other agents. I. Effects of anticonvulsant, anti-inflammatory, hypocholesterolaemic and adrenergic β-blocking-agents. *Biochem Pharmacol* 1969;18:429–444.

62. Facino RM, Carini M. Effect of the hypolipidaemic drug bezafibrate on the hepatic MFO system of the rat: Heterogeneity in mono-oxygenase responses. *Pharmacol Res Commun* 1981;13:861–871.

63. Eacho PI, Foxworthy PS, Johnson WD, van Lier RBL. Characterization of liver enlargement induced by compound LY171883 in rats. *Fundam Appl Toxicol* 1985;5:794–803.

64. Lewis NJ, Witiak DT, Feller DR. Influence of clofibrate (ethyl-4-chlorophenoxyisobutyrate) on hepatic drug metabolism in male rats. *Proc Soc Exp Biol Med* 1974;145:281–285.

65. Beard ME, Novikoff AB. Distribution of peroxisomes (microbodies) in the nephron of the rat: a cytochemical study. *J Cell Biol* 1969;42:501–518.

66. Lalwani ND, Reddy MK, Mangkornkanok-Mark M, Reddy JK. Induction, immunochemical identity and immuno fluorescence localization of an 80,000 molecular-weight peroxisome-proliferation associated polypeptide (polypeptide PPA-80) and peroxisomal enoyl-CoA hydratase of mouse liver and renal cortex. *Biochem J* 1981;198:177–186.

67. Small GM, Burdett K, Connock MJ. Clofibrate-induced changes in enzyme activities in liver, kidneys and small intestine of male mice. *Ann NY Acad Sci* 1982;386:460–463.

68. Svoboda DJ. Response of micro peroxisomes in rat small intestinal mucosa to CPIB, a hypolipidemic drug. *Biochem Pharmacol* 1976;25:2750–2752.

69. Fringes B, Gorgas K, Reith A. Clofibrate increases the number of peroxisomes and lamellar bodies in alveolar cells type II of the rat lung. *Eur J Cell Biol* 1988;46:136–143.

70. Dabholkar AS. Peroxisomes in the rat brain and the effects of di-(2-ethylhexyl) phthalate during postnatal development. *Acta Anat* 1988;131:218–221.

71. Levak-Frank S, Radner H, Walsh A, et al. Muscle-specific overexpression of lipoprotein lipase causes a severe myopathy characterized by proliferation of mitochondria and peroxisomes in transgenic mice. *J Clin Invest* 1995;96:976–986.

72. Feller DR, Hagerman LM, Newman HAI, Witiak DT. Antilipidemic drugs. In: Foye WO, ed. *Principles of medicinal chemistry*. Philadelphia: Lea and Febiger, 1989:481–501.

73. Hagerman LM, Newman HAI, Feller DR, Witiak DT. Antilipidemic agents. In: Verderame M, ed. *CRC handbook of cardiovascular and antiinflammatory drugs*. Boca Raton: CRC Press Inc., 1986: 225–260.

74. de la Iglesia FA, Pinn SM, Lucas J, McGuire EJ. Quantitative sterology of peroxisomes in hepatocytes from hyperlipoproteinemic patients receiving gemfibrozil. *Micron* 1981;12:97–98.

75. de la Iglesia FA, Lewis JE, Buchanan RA, Marcus EL, McMahon G. Light and electron microscopy of liver in hyperlipoproteinemic patients under long-term gemfibrozil treatment. *Atherosclerosis* 1982;43:19–37.

76. Gray RH, de la Iglesia FA. Quantitative microscopy comparison of peroxisome proliferation by the lipid-regulating agent gemfibrozil in several species. *Hepatology* 1984;4:520–530.

77. Kocarek TA, Feller DR. Induction of peroxisomal fatty acyl-CoA oxidase and microsomal laurate hydroxylase activities by beclobric acid and two metabolites in primary cultures of rat hepatocytes. *Biochem Pharmacol* 1987;36:3027–3032.

78. Pourbaiz S, Heller F, Harvengt C. Effect of fenofibrate and LF 2151 on hepatic peroxisomes in hamsters. *Biochem Pharmacol* 1984;33:3661–3366.

79. Facino RM, Carini M, Tofanetti O. Carboxylic metabolites of tiadenol as proximate inducers of hepatic peroxisomal beta-oxidation activity. *Pharmacol Res Commun* 1988;20:265–276.

80. Katoh H, Nakajima S, Kawashima Y, Kozuka H, Uchiyama M. Induction of rat hepatic long-chain acyl-CoA hydrolases by various peroxisome proliferators. *Biochem Pharmacol* 1984;33:1081–1085.

81. Lundgren B, Meijer J, DePierre JW. Induction of cytosolic and microsomal hydrolases and proliferation of peroxisomes and mitochondria in mouse liver after dietary exposure to p-chlorophenoxyacetic acid, 2,4-dichlorophenoxyacetic acid, and 2,4,5-trichlorophenoxyacetic acid. *Biochem Pharmacol* 1987;36:815–821.

82. Lundgren B, Meijer J, DePierre JW. Examination of the structural requirements for proliferation of peroxisomes and mitochondria in mouse liver by hypolipidemic agents, with special emphasis on structural analogues of 2-ethylhexanoic acid. *Eur J Biochem* 1987;163:423–431.
83. Kawashima Y, Katoh S, Nakajima H, Kozuka H, Uchiyama M. Effects of 2,4-dichlorophenoxyacetic acid and 2,4,5-trichlorophenoxyacetic acid on peroxisomal enzymes in rat liver. *Biochem Pharmacol* 1984;33:241–245.
84. Hietanen E, Ahotupa M, Heinonen T, et al. Enhanced peroxisomal beta-oxidation of fatty acids and glutathione metabolism in rats exposed to phenoxyacetic acids. *Toxicology* 1985;32:103–111.
85. Vainio H, Linnainmaa K, Kahonen M, et al. Hypolipidemia and peroxisome proliferation induced by phenoxyacetic acid herbicides in rats. *Biochem Pharmacol* 1983;32:2775–2779.
86. Lewis DFV, Lake FG, Gray TJB, Gangolli SD. Structure activity requirements for induction of peroxisomal enzyme activities in primary hepatocyte cultures. *Arch Toxicol* 1987[suppl. 11]:39–41.
87. Lake BG, Lewis DFV, Gray TJB. Structure-activity relationships for hepatic peroxisome proliferation. *Arch Toxicol* 1988[suppl. 12]:217–224.
88. Butler EG, Tanaka T, Ichida T, Maruyama H, Leber AP, Williams GM. Induction of hepatic peroxisome proliferation in mice by lactofen, a diphenyl ether herbicide. *Toxicol Appl Pharmacol* 1988;93:72–80.
89. Moody DE, Hammock BD. The effect of tridiphane [2-(3,5-dichlorophenyl)oxirane] on hepatic epoxide-metabolizing enzymes: indications of peroxisome proliferation. *Toxicol Appl Pharmacol* 1987;89:37–48.
90. Moody DE, Reddy JK. Hepatic peroxisome (microbody) proliferation in rats fed platicizers and related compounds. *Toxicol Appl Pharmacol* 1979;45:497–504.
91. Lhuguenot J-C, Mitchell AM, Milner G, Locke EA, Elcombe CR. The metabolism of di(2-ethylhexyl) phthalate (DEHP) and mono(2-ethylhexyl) phthalate (MEHP) in rats: in vivo and in vitro dose and time dependency of metabolism. *Toxicol Appl Pharmacol* 1985;80:11–22.
92. Thomas JA, Northup SJ. Toxicity and metabolism of monoethylhexylphthalate and diethylhexylphthalate: a survey of recent literature. *J Toxicol Environ Health* 1982;9:141–152.
93. Mitchell A, Lhuguenot J-C, Bridges JW, Elcombe CR. Identification of the proximate peroxisome proliferator(s) derived from di(2-ethylhexyl) phthalate. *Toxicol Appl Pharmacol* 1985;80:23–32.
94. Gray TJB, Lake BG, Beamand JA, Foster JR, Gangolli SD. Peroxisome proliferation in primary cultures of rat hepatocytes. *Toxicol Appl Pharmacol* 1983;67:15–25.
95. Gray TJB, Beamand JA, Lake BG, Foster JR, Gangolli SD. Peroxisome proliferation in cultured rat hepatocytes produced by clofibrate and phthalate ester metabolites. *Toxicol Lett* 1982;10:273–279.
96. Lake BG, Lewis DFV, Gray TJB, et al. Structure activity studies on the induction of peroxisomal enzyme activities by a series of phthalate monoesters in primary rat hepatocyte cultures. *Arch Toxicol* 1986[suppl. 9]:386–389.
97. Lake BG, Gray TJB, Lewis DFV, et al. Structure-activity relationships for induction of peroxisomal enzyme activities by phthalate monoesters in primary rat hepatocyte cultures. *Toxicol Ind Health* 1987;3:165–183.
98. DeAngelo AB, Garrett CT, Manolukas LA, Yario T. Di-n-octyl phthalate, a relatively ineffective peroxisome inducing straight chain isomer of the environmental contaminant di(2-ethylhexyl) phthalate, enhances the development of putative preneoplastic lesions in rat liver. *Toxicology* 1986;41:279–288.
99. Eacho PI, Foxworthy PS, Dillard RD, Whitesitt CA, Herron DK, Marshall WS. Induction of peroxisomal β-oxidation in the rat liver in vivo and in vitro by tetrazole-substituted acetophenones: structure-activity relationships. *Toxicol Appl Pharmacol* 1989;100:177–184.
100. Grossman SJ, DeLuca JG, Zamboni RJ, et al. Enantioselective induction of peroxisomal proliferation in CD-1 mice by leukotriene antagonists. *Toxicol Appl Pharmacol* 1992;116:217–224.
101. Kelley M, Groth-Watson A, Knoble D, Kornbrust D. Induction of peroxisomal enzymes by a tetrazole-substituted 2-quinolinylmethoxy leukotriene D_4 antagonist. *Fundam Appl Toxicol* 1994;23:298–303.
102. Thornber CW. Isosterism and molecular modification in drug design. *Chem Soc Rev* 1979;8:563–580.
103. Nilsson A, Arey H, Pedersen JI, Christiansen EN. The effect of high-fat diet on microsomal lauric acid hydroxylation in rat liver. *Biochim Biophys Acta* 1986;879:209–214.
104. Nilsson A, Prydz K, Rortveit T, Christiansen EN. Studies on the interrelated stimulation of microsomal omega-oxidation and peroxisomal beta-oxidation in rat liver with partally hydrogenated fish oil diet. *Biochim Biophys Acta* 1987;920:114–119.
105. Ikeda T, Aiba K, Fukuda K, Tanaka M. The induction of peroxisome proliferation in rat liver by perfluorinated fatty acids, metabolically inert derivatives of fatty acids. *J Biochem* 1985;98:475–482.

106. Van Rafelghem MJ, Mattie DR, Bruner RH, Andersen ME. Pathological and hepatic ultrastructural effects of a single dose of perflouro-n-decanoic acid in the rat. *Fundam Appl Toxicol* 1987;9:522–540.
107. Harrison EH, Lane JS, Liking S, Van Rafelghem MJ, Andersen ME. Perflouro-n-decanoic acid: induction of peroxisomal beta-oxidation by fatty acid with dioxin-like toxicity. *Lipids* 1988;23:115–119.
108. Borges T, Glauert HP, Chen LC, Chow CK, Robertson LW. Effect of the peroxisome proliferator perfluorodecanoic acid on growth and lipid metabolism in Sprague Dawley rats fed three dietary levels of selenium. *Arch Toxicol* 1990;64:26–30.
109. Berge RK, Aarsland A, Kryvi H, Bremer J, Aarsaether N. Alkylthioacetic acid (3-thia fatty acids): a new group of non-β-oxidizable, peroxisome-inducing fatty acid analogs. II. Dose response studies on hepatic peroxisomal and mitochondrial changes and long chain fatty acid metabolizing enzymes in rats. *Biochem Pharmacol* 1989;38:3969–3979.
110. Berge RK, Aarsland A, Kryvi H, Bremer J, Aarsaether N. Alkylthioacetic acid (3-thia fatty acids): a new group of non-β-oxidizable, peroxisome-inducing fatty acid analogs. I. A study on the structural requirements for proliferation of peroxisomes and mitochondria in rat liver. *Biochim Biophys Acta* 1989;1004:345–356.
111. Aarsland A, Aaraether N, Bremer J, Berge RK. Alkylthioacetic acid (3-thia fatty acids): a new group of non-β-oxidizable, peroxisome-inducing fatty acid analogs. III. Dissociation of cholesterol- and triglyceride-lowering effects and the induction of peroxisomal beta-oxidation. *J Lipid Res* 1989;30:1711–1718.
112. Watanabe T, Utsugi M, Mitsukawa M, Suga T, Fujitani H. Hypolipidemic effect and enhancement of peroxisomal beta-oxidation in the liver of rats by sodium-(E)-3-(4-(3-pyridylmethyl)phenyl)-2-methylpropenoate (OKY-1581), a potent inhibitor of TxA2 synthase. *J Pharmacobiodyn* 1986;9:1023–1031.
113. Elcombe, CR. Species differences in carcinogenicity and peroxisome proliferation due to trichloroethylene: a biochemical human hazard assessment. *Arch Toxicol Suppl* 1985;8:6–17.
114. DeAngelo AB, Daniel FB, McMillan L, Wernsing P, Savage RE, Jr. Species and strain sensitivity to the induction of peroxisome proliferation by chloroacetic acids. *Toxicol Appl Pharmacol* 1989;101:285–298.
115. Goldsworthy TL, Popp JA. Chlorinated hydrocarbon-induced peroxisomal enzyme activity in relation to species and organ carcinogenicity. *Toxicol Appl Pharmacol* 1987;88:225–233.
116. Odum J, Green T, Foster JR, Hext PM. The role of trichloroacetic acid and peroxisome proliferation in the differences in carcinogenicity of perchloroethylene in the mouse and rat. *Toxicol Appl Pharmacol* 1988;92:103–112.
117. Mitchell AM, Bridges JW, Elcombe CR. Factors influencing peroxisome proliferation in cultured rat hepatocytes. *Arch Toxicol* 1984;55:239–246.
118. Watanabe T, Suga T. Effects of some anti-inflammatory drugs on biochemical values and on hepatic peroxisomal enzymes of rat. *J Pharmacobiodyn* 1985;8:1060–1067.
119. Fort FL, Stein HH, Langenberg K, Lewkowski JP, Heyman A, Kesterson JW. Cetaben versus clofibrate comparison of toxicity and peroxisome proliferation in rats. *Toxicology* 1983;28:305–311.
120. Horie S, Suga T. Enhancement of peroxisomal β-oxidation in the liver of rats and mice treated with valproic acid. *Biochem Pharmacol* 1985;34:1357–1362.
121. Aarsaether N, Fosse R, Aarsland A, Berge RK. Effects of the tumor promotor 12-O-tetradecanoyl-phorbol 13-acetate on peroxisomal activities and enzyme activities involved in lipid metabolism in rat liver. *Biochim Biophys Acta* 1990;1042:86–93.
122. Elcombe CR, Rose MS, Pratt IS. Biochemical, histological and ultrastructural changes in rat and mouse liver following the administration of trichloroethylene: Possible relevance to species differences in hepatocarcinogenicity. *Toxicol Appl Pharmacol* 1985;79:365–376.
123. Lock EA, Stonard MD, Elcombe CR. The induction of omega- and beta-oxidation of fatty acids and effects on alpha1a-globulin content in the liver and kidney of rats administered 2,2,4-trimethylpentane. *Xenobiotica* 1987;17:513–522.
124. Ikeda T, Ida-Enomoto M, Mori I, et al. Induction of peroxisome proliferation in rat liver by dietary treatment with 2,2,4,4,6,8,8-heptamethylnonane. *Xenobiotica* 1988;18:1271–1280.
125. Wu H-Q, Masset-Brown J, Tweedie DJ, et al. Induction of microsomal NADPH-cytochrome P450 reductase and cytochrome P4504A1 by dehydro-epiandrosterone in rats: a possible peroxisome proliferator. *Cancer Res* 1989;49:2337–2343.
126. Leighton B, Tagliaferro AR, Newsholme EA. The effect of dehydro-epiandrosterone acetate on liver peroxisomal enzyme activities of male and female rats. *J Nutr* 1987;117:1287–1290.

127. Frenkel RA, Slaughter CA, Orth K, et al. Peroxisome proliferation and induction of peroxisomal enzymes in mouse and rat liver by dehydroepiandrosterone feeding. *J Steroid Biochem* 1990;35:333–342.

128. Van den Branden C, Vamecq J, Dacremont G, Premereur N, Roels F. Short and long term influence of phenothiazines on liver peroxisomal fatty acid oxidation in rodents. *FEBS Lett* 1987;222:21–26.

129. Vamecq J, Roels F, Van den Branden C, Draye J-P. Peroxisomal proliferation in heart and liver of mice receiving chlorpromazine, ethyl 2-(5-(4-chlorophenyl)pentyl)oxiran-2-carboxylic acid or high fat diet: a biochemical and morphometric comparative study. *Pediatr Res* 1987;22:748–754.

130. Bakke OM, Berge RK. Induction of peroxisomal enzymes and palmitoyl-CoA hydrolase in rats treated with cholestyramine and nicotinic acid. *Biochem Pharmacol* 1984;33:3077–3080.

131. Eacho PI, Foxworthy PS, Herron DK. Tetrazole substituted acetophenone peroxisome proliferators: structure-activity relationships and effects on hepatic lipid metabolism. In: Gibson GG, Lake BG, eds. *Peroxisomes: biology and importance in toxicology and medicine.* London: Taylor & Francis, 1993:343–372.

132. Eacho PI, Foxworthy PS, Lawrence JW, Herron DK, Noonan DJ. Common structural requirements for peroxisome proliferation by tetrazole and carboxylic acid containing compounds. *Ann NY Acad Sci* 1996;804:387–402.

133. Issemann I, Green S. Activation of a member of the steroid hormone receptor superfamily by peroxisome proliferators. *Nature* 1990;347:645–650.

134. Green S, Issemann I, Tugwood JD. The molecular mechanism of peroxisome proliferator action. In: Gibson G, Lake B, eds. *Peroxisomes: biology and importance in toxicology and molecular medicine.* London: Taylor & Francis, 1993:99–118.

135. Elcombe CR, Mitchell AM. Peroxisome proliferation due to di-(2-ethylhexyl) phthalate: species differences and possible mechanisms. *Environ Health Perspec* 1986;70:211–219.

136. Sharma R, Lake BG, Foster J, Gibson GG. Microsomal cytochrome P-450 induction and peroxisomal proliferation by hypolipidaemic agents in rat liver. *Biochem Pharmacol* 1988;37:1193–1201.

137. Nemali MR, Reddy MK, Usuda N, et al. Differential induction and regulation of peroxisomal enzymes: predictive value of peroxisome proliferation in identifying certain nonmutagenic carcinogens. *Toxicol Appl Pharmacol* 1989;97:72–87.

138. Brady PS, Marine KA, Brady LJ, Ramsey RR. Co-ordinate induction of hepatic mitochondrial and peroxisomal carnitine acyltransferase synthesis by diet and drugs. *Biochem J* 1989;260:93–100.

139. Solberg HE, Aas M, Daae LNW. The activity of the different carnitine acyltransferases in the liver of clofibrate fed rats. *Biochim Biophys Acta* 1972;280:434–439.

140. Kawashima Y, Nakagawa S, Tachibana Y, Kozuka H. Effects of peroxisome proliferators on fatty acid-binding protein in rat liver. *Biochem Biophys Res Commun* 1983;754:21–27.

141. Bremer J, Norum KR. Metabolism of very long-chain monounsaturated fatty acids (22:1) and the adaptation to their presence in the diet. *J Lipid Res* 1982;23:243–256.

142. Ishii H, Horie S, Suga T. Physiological role of peroxisomal β-oxidation in liver of fasted rats. *J Biochem (Tokyo)* 1980;87:1855–1858.

143. Horie S, Ishii H, Suga T. Changes in peroxisomal fatty acid oxidation in the diabetic rat liver. *J Biochem (Tokyo)* 1981;90:1691–1696.

144. Neat CE, Thomassen MS, Osmundsen H. Induction of peroxisomal β-oxidation in rat liver by high fat diets. *Biochem J* 1980;186:369–371.

145. Mann AH, Price SC, Mitchell FE, Grasso P, Hinton RH, Bridges JW. Comparison of the short term effects of di(2-ethylhexyl) phthalate, di(n-hexyl) phthalate and di(n-octyl) phthalate in rats. *Toxicol Appl Pharmacol* 1985;77:116–132.

146. Mitchell FE, Price SC, Hinton RH, Grasso P, Bridges JW. Time and dose-response study of the effects on rats of the plasticizer di-(2-ethylhexyl) phthalate. *Toxicol Appl Pharmacol* 1985;81:371–392.

147. Gibson GG, Milton MN, Elcombe CR. Induction of cytochrome P4504A1-mediated fatty acid hydroxylation: relevance to peroxisome proliferation. *Biochem Soc Trans* 1990;18:97–99.

148. Bone AJ, Sheratt HSA, Turnbull DM, Osmundsen H. Increased activity of peroxisomal β-oxidation in rat liver caused by ethyl 2-[5-(4-chlorophenyl)pentyl] oxiran-2-carboxylate: an inhibitor of mitochondrial β-oxidation. *Biochem Biophys Res Commun* 1982;104:708–712.

149. Eacho PI, Foxworthy PS. Inhibition of hepatic fatty acid oxidation by bezafibrate and bezafibroyl-CoA. *Biochem Biophys Res Commun* 1988;157:1148–1153.

150. Hertz R, Bar-Tana J. Prevention of peroxisomal proliferation by carnitine palmitoyltransferase inhibitors in cultured rat hepatocytes and in vivo. *Biochem J* 1987;245:387–392.
151. Bronfman M, Amigo L, Morales MN. Activation of hypolipidaemic drugs to acyl-coenzyme A thioesters. *Biochem J* 1986;239:781–784.
152. Powell GL, Tippett PS, Kiorpes TC, et al. Fatty acyl-CoA as an effector molecule in metabolism. *Fed Proc* 1985;44:81–84.
153. Kakar SS, Huang WH, Askari A. Control of cardiac sodium pump by long-chain acyl-coenzymes A. *J Biol Chem* 1987;262:42–45.
154. Bronfman M, Morales MN, Orellana A. Diacylglycerol activation of protein kinase C is modulated by long-chain acyl-CoA. *Biochem Biophys Res Commun* 1988;152:987–992.
155. Rao MS, Thorgeirsson S, Reddy MK, et al. Induction of peroxisome proliferation in hepatocytes transplanted into the anterior chamber of the eye: a model system for the evaluation of xenobiotic-induced effects. *Am J Pathol* 1986;124:519–527.
156. Reddy JK, Jirtle RL, Watanabe TK, Reddy NK, Michalopoulos G, Qureshi SA. Response of hepatocytes transplanted into synergistic hosts and heterotransplanted into athymic nude to peroxisome proliferators. *Cancer Res* 1984;44:2582–2589.
157. Bieri F, Bentley P, Waechter F, Staubli W. Use of primary cultures of adult rat hepatocytes to investigate mechanisms of action of nafenopin, a hepatocarcinogenic peroxisome proliferator. *Carcinogenesis* 1984;5:1033–1039.
158. Foxworthy PS, Eacho PI. Conditions influencing the induction of peroxisomal β-oxidation in cultured rat hepatocytes. *Toxicol Lett* 1986;30:189–196.
159. Furukawa K, Mochizuki Y, Sawada N. Properties of peroxisomes and their induction by clofibrate in normal adult rat hepatocytes in primary culture. *In Vitro* 1984;20:573–584.
160. Hardwick JP, Song BJ, Huberman E, Gonzalez FJ. Isolation, complementary DNA sequence and regulation of rat hepatic lauric acid omega-oxidation (cytochrome P450). *J Biol Chem* 1987;262:801–810.
161. Lalwani ND, Fahl WE, Reddy JK. Detection of a nafenopin-binding protein in rat liver cytosol associated with the induction of peroxisome proliferation by hypolipidemic compounds. *Biochem Biophys Res Commun* 1983;116:388–393.
162. Lalwani ND, Alvares K, Reddy MK, Reddy MN, Parikh I, Reddy JK. Peroxisome proliferator-binding protein: Identification and partial characterization of nafenopin-, clofibric acid-, and ciprofibrate-binding proteins from rat liver. *Proc Natl Acad Sci USA* 1987;84:5242–5246.
163. Kliewer SA, Umesono K, Noonan DJ, Heyman RA, Evans RM. Convergence of 9-cis retinoic acid and peroxisome proliferator signalling pathways through heterodimer formation of their receptors. *Nature* 1992;358:771–774.
164. Staels B, Vu-Dac N, Kosykh VA, et al. C-III expression independent of induction of peroxisomal acyl-coenzyme A oxidase: a potential mechanism for the hypolipidemic action of fibrates. *J Clin Invest* 1995;95:705–712.
165. Dreyer C, Krey G, Keller H, Givel F, Helftenbein G, Wahli W. Control of the peroxisomal β-oxidation pathway by a novel family of nuclear hormone receptors. *Cell* 1992;68:879–887.
166. Gottlicher M, Widmark E, Li Q, Gustafsson JA. Fatty acids activate a chimera of the clofibric acid-activated receptor and the glucocorticoid receptor. *Proc Natl Acad Sci USA* 1992;89:4653–4657.
167. Sher T, Yi H-F, McBride OW, Gonzalez FR. cDNA cloning, chromosomal mapping, and functional characterization of the human peroxisome proliferator activated receptor. *Biochemistry* 1993;32:5598–5604.
168. Zhu Y, Alveres K, Huang Q, Rao MS, Reddy JK. Cloning of a new member of the peroxisome proliferator-activated receptor gene family from mouse liver. *J Biol Chem* 1993;268:26817–26820.
169. Schmidt A, Endo N, Rutledge SJ, Vogel R, Shinar D, Rodan GA. Identification of a new member of the steroid hormone receptor superfamily that is activated by peroxisome proliferator and fatty acids. *Mol Endocrinol* 1992;6:1634–1641.
170. Kliewer SA, Forman BM, Blumberg B, et al. Differential expression and activation of a family of murine peroxisome proliferator-activated receptors. *Proc Natl Acad Sci USA* 1994;91:7355–7359.
171. Chen F, Law SW, O'Malley BW. Identification of two mPPAR related receptors and evidence of five subfamily members. *Biochem Biophys Res Commun* 1993;196:671–677.
172. Tontonoz P, Hu E, Graves RA, Budavari AI, Spiegelman BM. mPPARγ2: tissue-specific regulator of an adipocyte enhancer. *Genes & Dev* 1994;8:1224–1234.
173. Ribeiro RCJ, Kushner PJ, Baxter JD. The nuclear hormone receptor gene superfamily. *Annu Rev Med* 1995;46:443–453.

174. Osumi T, Ishii N, Miyazawa S, Hashimoto T. Isolation and structural characterization of the rat acyl-CoA oxidase gene. *J Biol Chem* 1987;262:8138–8143.
175. Osumi T, Wen J, Hashimoto T. Two *cis*-acting regulatory sequences in the peroxisome proliferator-responsive enhancer region of rat acyl-CoA oxidase gene. *Biochem Biophys Res Commun* 1991;175: 866–871.
176. Osumi T, Wen J-K, Taketani S, Hashimoto T. Molecular mechanisms involved in induction of peroxisomal β-oxidation enzymes by hypolipidaemic agents. In: Gibson GG, Lake BG, eds. *Peroxisomes: biology and importance in toxicology and medicine.* London: Taylor & Francis, 1993:149–172.
177. Zhang B, Marcus SL, Sajjadi FG, et al. Identification of a peroxisome proliferator-responsive element upstream of the gene encoding rat peroxisomal enoyl-CoA hydratase/3-hydroxyacyl-CoA dehydrogenase. *Proc Natl Acad Sci USA* 1992;89:7541–7545.
178. Muerhoff AS, Griffin KJ, Johnson EF. The peroxisome proliferator-activated receptor mediates the induction of CYP4A6, a cytochrome P450 fatty acid hydroxylase, by clofibric acid. *J Biol Chem* 1992;267:19051–19053.
179. Aldridge TC, Tugwood JD, Green S. Identification and characterization of DNA elements implicated in the regulation of CYP4A1 transcription. *Biochem J* 1995;306:473–479.
180. Issemann I, Prince R, Tugwood J, Green S. A role for fatty acids and liver fatty acid binding protein in peroxisome proliferation? *Biochem Soc Trans* 1992;20:824–827.
181. Vu-Dac N, Schoonjans K, Laine B, Fruchart J-C, Auwerx J, Staels B. Negative regulation of the human apolipoprotein A-I promotor by fibrates can be attenuated by the interaction of the peroxisome proliferator-activated receptor with its response element. *J Biol Chem* 1994;269:31012–31018.
182. Vu-Dac N, Schoonjans K, Kosykh V, et al. Fibrates increase human apolipoprotein A-II expression through activation of the peroxisome proliferator-activated receptor. *J Clin Invest* 1995;96:741–750.
183. Staels B, Auwerx J. Perturbation of the developmental gene expression in rat liver by fibric acid derivatives: lipoprotein lipase and alpha-fetoprotein as models. *Development* 1992;95:1035–1043.
184. Gulick Y, Cresci S, Caira T, Moore DD, Kelly DP. The peroxisome proliferator-activated receptor regulates mitochondrial fatty acid oxidative enzyme gene expression. *Proc Natl Acad Sci USA* 1994;91:11012–11016.
185. Rodriguez JC, Gil-Gomez G, Hegardt FG, Haro D. The peroxisome proliferator-activated receptor mediates the induction of the mitochondrial 3-hydroxy-3-methylglutaryl-CoA synthase gene by fatty acids. *J Biol Chem* 1994;267:18767–18772.
186. Tontonoz P, Hu E, Devine J, Beale EG, Spiegelman BM. PPARγ2 regulates adipose expression of the phosphoenolpyruvate carboxykinase gene. *Mol Cell Biol* 1995;15:351–357.
187. Castelein H, Gulick T, Declercq PE, Mannaerts GP, Moore DD, Baes MI. The peroxisome proliferator-activated receptor regulates malic enzyme gene expression. *J Biol Chem* 1994;269:26754–26758.
188. Osmundsen H, Bremer J, Pedersen JI. Metabolic aspects of peroxisomal beta-oxidation. *Biochem Biophys Acta* 1991;1085:141–158.
189. Thumelin S, Esser V, Charvy D, et al. Expression of liver carnitine palmitoyltransferase I and II genes during development in the rat. *Biochem J* 1994;300:583–587.
190. Jump DB, Ren B, Clarke S, Thelen A. Effects of fatty acids on hepatic gene expression. *Prostaglandins Leukot Essent Fatty Acids* 1995;52:107–111.
191. Ibrahimi A, Tebouli L, Gaillard D, et al. Evidence for a common mechanism of action for fatty acids and thiazolidinedione antidiabetic agents on gene expression in preadipose cells. *Mol Pharmacol* 1994;46:1070–1076.
192. Varansi U, Chu R, Chu S, Espinosa R, LeBeau MM, Reddy JK. Isolation of the human peroxisomal acyl-CoA oxidase gene: organization, promotor analysis, and chromosomal localization. *Proc Natl Acad Sci USA* 1994;91:3107–3111.
193. Varanasi U, Chu R, Huang Q, Castellon R, Yeldandi AV, Reddy JK. Identification of a peroxisome proliferator-responsive element upstream of the human peroxisomal fatty acyl-coenzyme A oxidase gene. *J Biol Chem* 1996;271:2147–2155.
194. Gearing KL, Gottlicher M, Teboul M, Widmark E, Gustafsson J-A. Interaction of the peroxisome-proliferator-activated receptor and retinoid X receptor. *Proc Natl Acad Sci USA* 1993;90:1440–1444.
195. Marcus SL, Miyata KS, Zhang B, Subramani S, Rachubinski RA, Capone JP. Diverse peroxisome proliferator-activated receptors bind to the peroxisome proliferator-responsive elements of the rat hydratase/dehydrogenase and fatty acyl-CoA oxidase genes but differentially induce expression. *Proc Natl Acad Sci USA* 1993;90:5723–5727.

196. Issemann I, Prince RA, Tugwood JD, Green S. The peroxisome proliferator-activated receptor: retinoid X receptor heterodimer is activated by fatty acids and fibrate hypolipidaemic drugs. *J Mol Endocrinol* 1993;11:37–47.
197. Bardot O, Aldridge TC, Latruffe N, Green S. PPAR-RXR heterodimer activates a peroxisome proliferator response element upstream of the bifunctional enzyme gene. *Biochem Biophys Res Commun* 1993;192:37–45.
198. Yu VC, Delsert C, Anderson B, et al. A coregulator that enhances binding of retinoic acid, thyroid hormone, and vitamin D receptors to their cognate elements. *Cell* 1991;67:1251–1266.
199. Bogazzi F, Hudson LD, Nikodem VM. A novel heterodimerization partner for thyroid hormone receptor. Peroxisome proliferator-activated receptor. *J Biol Chem* 1994;269:11683–11686.
200. Lawrence JW, Foxworthy PS, Perry DN, et al. Nafenopin induced peroxisome proliferation in vitamin A deficient rats. *Biochem Pharmacol* 1995;49:915–919.
201. Braissant Q, Foufelle F, Scotto C, Dauca M, Wahli W. Differential expression of peroxisome proliferator-activated receptors (PPARs): tissue distribution of PPAR-α, -β, and -γ in the adult rat. *Endocrinology* 1996;137:354–366.
202. Mukherjee R, Jow L, Noonan D, McDonnell DP. Human and rat peroxisome proliferator activated receptors (PPARs) demonstrate similar tissue distribution but different resposiveness to PPAR activators. *J Steroid Biochem Molec Biol* 1994;51:157–166.
203. Tontonoz P, Hu E, Spiegelman BM. Stimulation of adipogenesis in fibroblasts by PPARγ2, a lipid-activated transcription factor. *Cell* 1994;79:1147–1156.
204. Huang Q, Yeldandi AV, Alveres K, Ide H, Reddy JK, Rao MS. Localization of peroxisome proliferator-activated receptor in mouse and rat tissues and demonstration of its nuclear translocation in transfected CV-1 cells. *Int J Oncol* 1995;6:307–312.
205. Lehmann JM, Moore LB, Smith-Oliver TA, Kliewer SA. An antidiabetic thiazolidinedione is a high affinity ligand for peroxisome proliferator-activated receptor γ (PPARγ). *J Biol Chem* 1995;270:12953–12956.
206. Gottlicher M, Demoz A, Svensson D, Tollet P, Berge RK, Gustafsson JA. Structural and metabolic requirements for activators of the peroxisome proliferator-activated receptor. *Biochem Pharmacol* 1993;46:2177–2184.
207. Krey G, Keller H, Mahfoudi A, et al. Xenopus peroxisome prolifertor activated receptors: genomic organization, response element recognition, heterodimer formation with retinoid x receptor and activation by fatty acids. *J Steroid Biochem Molec Biol* 1993;47:65–73.
208. Dreyer C, Keller H, Mahfoudi A, Laudet V, Krey G, Wahli W. Positive regulation of the peroxisomal β-oxidation pathway by fatty acids through activation of the peroxisome proliferator-activated receptor (PPAR). *Biol Cell* 1993;77:67–76.
209. Bocos C, Gottlicher M, Gearing K, et al. Fatty acid activation of peroxisome proliferator-activated receptor (PPAR). *J Steroid Molec Biol* 1995;53:467–473.
210. Henry K, O'Brien ML, Clevenger W, Jow L, Noonan DJ. Peroxisome proliferator-activated receptor response specificities as defined in yeast and mammalian cell transcription assays. *Toxicol Appl Pharmacol* 1995;132:317–324.
211. Lee SS-T, Pineau T, Drago J, et al. Targeted disruption of the α isoform of the peroxisome proliferator-activated receptor gene in mice results in abolishment of the pleiotropic effects of peroxisome proliferators. *Mol Cell Biol* 1995;15:3012–3022.
212. Appelkvist EL, Dallner G. Possible involvement of fatty acid binding protein in peroxisomal β-oxidation of fatty acids. *Biochim Biophys Acta* 1980;617:156–160.
213. Peeters RA, Veerkamp JH, and Demel RA. Are fatty acid binding proteins involved in fatty acid transfer? *Biochim Biophys Acta* 1989;1002:8–13.
214. Glatz JFC, van der Vusse GJ. Cellular fatty acid binding proteins: current concepts and future directions. *Mol Cell Biochem* 1990;98:237–251.
215. Cannon JR, Eacho PI. Interaction of LY171883 and other peroxisome proliferators with fatty acid-binding protein isolated from rat liver. *Biochem J* 1991;280:387–391.
216. Brandes R, Kaikaus RM, Bass NM. Induction of fatty acid-binding protein by peroxisome proliferators in primary hepatocyte cultures and its relationship to the induction of peroxisomal β-oxidation. *Biochim Biophys Acta* 1990;1034:53–61.
217. Lawrence JW, Eacho PI. Hepatic fatty acid binding protein facilitated nuclear transport of fatty acids. *Toxicologist* 1995;14:315.
218. Eacho PI, Lawrence JW. Binding of hepatic fatty acid binding protein to a 33 kDa nuclear protein. *Toxicologist* 1995;14:315.

219. Williams SC, Grant SG, Reue K, Carrasquillo B, Lusis AJ, Kinniburgh AJ. Cis-acting determinants of basal and lipid regulated apolipoprotein A-IV expression in mice. *J Biol Chem* 1989;264:19009–19016.

220. Jump DB, Clarke SD, Thelen A, Liimatta M. Coordinate regulation of glycolytic and lipogenic gene expression by polyunsaturated fatty acids. *J Lipid Res* 1994;35:1076–1084.

221. Tomlinson JE, Nakayama R, Holten D. Repression of pentose phosphate pathway dehydrogenase synthesis and mRNA by dietary fat in rats. *J Nutr* 1988;118:408–415.

222. Clarke SD, Armstrong MK, Jump DB. Dietary polyunsaturated fats uniquely suppress rat liver fatty acid synthase and S14 mRNA content. *J Nutr* 1990;120:225–231.

223. Clarke SD, Armstrong MK, Jump DB. Nutritional control of rat liver fatty acid synthase and S14 mRNA abundance. *J Nutr* 1990;120:218–224.

224. Blake WL, Clarke SD. Suppression of rat hepatic fatty acid synthase and S14 gene transcription by dietary polyunsaturated fat. *J Nutr* 1991;120:1727–1729.

225. Watanabe T, Horie S, Yamada J, et al. Species differences in the effects of bezafibrate, a hypolipidemic agent, on hepatic peroxisome-associated enzymes. *Biochem Pharmacol* 1989;38:367–371.

226. Oesch F, Hartmann R, Timms C, et al. Time-dependence and differential induction of rat and guinea pig peroxisomal β-oxidation, palmitoyl-CoA hydrolase, cytosolic and microsomal epoxide hydrolase after treatment with hypolipidemic drugs. *J Cancer Res Clin Oncol* 1988;114:341–346.

227. Lake BG, Evans JG, Gray TJB, Korosi SA, North C. Comparative studies on nafenopin-induced hepatic peroxisome proliferation in the rat, syrian hamster, guinea pig, and marmoset. *Toxicol Appl Pharmacol* 1989;99:148–160.

228. Orton TC, Adam HK, Bentley M, Holloway B, Tucker MJ. Clobuzarit: species differences in the morphological and biochemical response of the liver following chronic administration. *Toxicol Appl Pharmacol* 1984;73:138–151.

229. Platt DS, Thorp JM. Changes in the weight and composition of the liver in the rat, dog and monkey treated with ethyl chlorophenoxyisobutyrate. *Biochem Pharmacol* 1966;15:915–925.

230. Hoover DM, Bendele AM, Foxworthy PS, Eacho PI. Effects of chronic treatment with the leukotriene D4 antagonist compound LY171883 on Fischer 344 rats and rhesus monkeys. *Fundam Appl Toxicol* 1990;14:123–130.

231. Reddy JK, Lalwani ND, Qureshi SA, Reddy MK, Moehle CM. Induction of hepatic peroxisome proliferation in non-rodent species, including primates. *Am J Pathol* 1984;114:171–183.

232. Lalwani ND, Reddy MK, Ghosh S, Barnard SD, Molello JA, Reddy JK. Induction of fatty acid β-oxidation and peroxisome proliferation in the liver of rhesus monkeys by DL-040, a new hypolipidemic agent. *Biochem Pharmacol* 1985;34:3473–3482.

233. Lake BGJ, Gray TJB, Gangolli SD. Hepatic effects of phthalate esters and related compounds: in vivo and in vitro correlations. *Environ Health Persp* 1986;67:283–290.

234. Foxworthy PS, White SL, Hoover DM, Eacho PI. Effect of ciprofibrate, bezafibrate, and LY171883 on peroxisomal β-oxidation in cultured rat, dog, and Rhesus monkey hepatocytes. *Toxicol Appl Pharmacol* 1990;104:386–394.

235. Blaauboer BJ, Van Holsteijn CWM, Bleumink R, et al. The effect of beclobric acid and clofibric acid on peroxisomal β-oxidation and peroxisome proliferation in primary cultures of rat, monkey and human hepatocytes. *Biochem Pharmacol* 1990;40:521–528.

236. James NH, Roberts RA. Species differences in the clonal expansion of hepatocytes in response to the coaction of epidermal growth factor and nafenopin, a rodent hepatocarcinogenic peroxisome proliferator. *Fundam Appl Toxicol* 1995;26:143–149.

237. Hanefeld M, Kemmer C, Leonhardt W, Kunze KD, Jaross W, Haller H. Effects of p-chlorophenoxyisobutyric acid (CPIB) on the human liver. *Atherosclerosis* 1980;36:159–172.

238. Hanefeld M, Kemmer C, Kadner E. Relationship between morphological changes and lipid-lowering action of p-chlorophenoxyisobutyric acid (CPIB) on hepatic mitochondria and peroxisomes in man. *Atherosclerosis* 1983;46:239–246.

239. Gariot P, Foliguet B, Drouin PB, Barrat E, Genton P, Debry G. Hypertrophy of liver peroxisomes in type II and type IV hyperlipoproteinemia. *Atherosclerosis* 1986;59:257–262.

240. Gariot P, Barrat E, Drouin P, et al. Morphometric study of human hepatic cell modifications induced by fenofibrate. *Metabolism* 1987;36:203–210.

241. Gariot P, Barrat E, Mejean L, Pointel JP, Drouin P, Debry G. Fenofibrate and human liver: Lack of proliferation of peroxisomes. *Arch Toxicol* 1983;53:151–163.

242. Blumcke S, Schwartzkopff W, Lobeck H, Edmondson NA, Prentice DE, Blane GF. Influence of fenofibrate on cellular and subcellular liver structure in hyperlipidemic patients. *Atherosclerosis* 1983;46:105–116.
243. Gariot P, Pointel JP, Barrat E, Drouin D, Debry G. Etude morphometrique des peroxysomes hepatiques chez des malades hyperlipoproteineniques traites par fenofibrate. *Biomed Pharmacother* 1984;38:101–106.
244. Reddy JK, Rao MS, Moody DE. Hepatocellular carcinomas in acatalase mice treated with nafenopin, a hypolipidemic peroxisome proliferator. *Cancer Res* 1976;36:1211–1217.
245. Reddy JK, Rao MS. Malignant tumors in rats fed nafenopin, a hepatic peroxisome proliferator. *J Natl Cancer Inst* 1977;59:1645–1650.
246. Stott WT. Chemically induced proliferation of peroxisomes: Implications for risk assessment. *Regul Toxicol Pharmacol* 1988;8:125–159.
247. Reddy JK, Moody DE, Azarnoff DL, Rao MS. Di(2-ethylhexyl) phthalate: an industrial plasticizer induces hypolipidemia and enhances hepatic catalase and carnitine acetyltransferase activities in rats and mice. *Life Sci* 1976;18:94–96.
248. Kluwe WM, Haseman JK, Douglas JF, Huff JE. The carcinogenicity of dietary di-(2-ethylhexyl) phthalate (DEHP) in Fischer 344 rats and B6C3F1 mice. *J Toxicol Environ Health* 1982;10:797–815.
249. Williams GM, Weisburger JH. Chemical carcinogens. In: Amdur MO, Doull J, Klaassen CD, eds. *Casarett and Doull's toxicology.* New York: Pergamon Press, 1991:127–200.
250. Warren JR, Simmon VF, Reddy JK. Properties of hypolipidemic peroxisome proliferators in the lymphocyte [^{3}H]thymidine and Salmonella mutagenesis assays. *Cancer Res* 1980;40:36–41.
251. Reddy JK, Lalwani ND, Reddy MK, Qureshi SA. Excessive accumulation of autofluorescent lipofuscin in the liver during hepatocarcinogenesis by methyl clofenapate and other hypolipidemic peroxisome proliferators. *Cancer Res* 1982;42:259–266.
252. Glauert HP, Reddy JK, Kennan WS, Sattler GL, Rao VS, Pitot HC. Effect of hypolipidemic peroxisome proliferators on unscheduled DNA synthesis in cultured hepatocytes and on mutagenesis in Salmonella. *Cancer Lett* 1984;24:147–156.
253. Bentley P, Bieri F, Mitchell F, Warchter F, Staubli W. Investigations on the mechanism of liver tumour induction by peroxisome proliferators. *Arch Toxicol* 1987;10:157–161.
254. Ashby J, Lefevre PA, Elcombe CR. Cell replication and unscheduled DNA synthesis (UDS) activity of low molecular weight chlorinated paraffins in rat liver in vivo. *Mutagenesis* 1990;5:515–518.
255. Butterworth BE, Bermudez E, Smith-Oliver T, et al. Lack of genotoxic activity of di(2-ethylhexyl) phthalate (DEHP) in rat and human hepatocytes. *Carcinogenesis* 1984;5:1329–1335.
256. Gupta RC, Goel SK, Earley K, Singh B, Reddy JK. ^{32}P-postlabeling analysis of peroxisome proliferator-DNA adduct formation in rat liver in vivo and hepatocytes in vitro. *Carcinogenesis* 1985;6:933–936.
257. Elliott BM, Dodd NJF, Elcombe CR. Increased hydroxyl radical production in liver peroxisomal fractions from rats treated with peroxisome proliferators. *Carcinogenesis* 1986;7:795–799.
258. Goel SK, Lalwani ND, Reddy JK. Peroxisome proliferation and lipid peroxidation in rat liver. *Cancer Res* 1986;46:1324–1330.
259. Tomaszewski KE, Agarwal DK, Melnick RL. In vitro steady-state levels of hydrogen peroxide after exposure of male F344 rats and female B6C3F1 mice to hepatic peroxisome proliferators. *Carcinogenesis* 1986;7:1871–1876.
260. Conway JG, Neptun DA, Garvey LK, Popp JA. Role of fatty acid acyl-coenzyme A oxidase in the efflux of oxidized glutathione from perfused livers of rats treated with the peroxisome proliferator nafenopin. *Cancer Res* 1987;47:4795–4800.
261. Tamura H, Iida T, Watanabe T, Suga T. Long-term effects of hypolipidemic peroxisome proliferator administration on hepatic hydrogen peroxide metabolism in rats. *Carcinogenesis* 1990;11:445–450.
262. Chu S, Huang Q, Alvares K, Yeldandi AV, Rao MS, Reddy JK. Transformation of mammalian cells by overexpressing H$_2$O$_2$-gene generating peroxisomal fatty acyl-CoA oxidase. *Proc Natl Acad Sci USA* 1995;92:7080–7084.
263. Lake BG, Evans JG, Walters DG, Price RJ. Comparison of the hepatic effects of nafenopin, a peroxisome proliferator, in rats fed adequate or vitamin E and selenium deficient diets. *Hum Exp Toxicol* 1991;10:87–88.
264. Elliott BM, Elcombe CR. Lack of DNA damage or lipid peroxidation measured in vivo in the rat liver following treatment with peroxisome proliferators. *Carcinogenesis* 1987;8:1213–1218.

265. Furukawa K, Numoto S, Furuya K, Furukawa NT, Williams GM. Effects of the hepatocarcinogen Nafenopin, a peroxisome proliferator, on the activities of rat liver glutathione-requiring enzymes and catalase in comparison to the action of phenobarbital. *Cancer Res* 1985;45:5011–5019.
266. Cattley RC, Conway JG, Popp JA. Association of persistent peroxisome proliferation and oxidative injury with hepatocarcinogenicity in female F-344 rats fed di(2-ethylhexyl) phthalate for 2 years. *Cancer Lett* 1987;38:15–22.
267. Conway JG, Tomaszewski KE, Olson MJ, Cattley RC, Marsman DS, Popp JA. Relationship of oxidative damage to the hepatocarcinogenicity of the peroxisome proliferators di(2-ethylhexyl) phthalate and Wyeth-14,643. *Carcinogenesis* 1989;10:513–519.
268. Fahl WE, Lalwani ND, Watanabe T, Goel SK, Reddy JK. DNA damage related to increased hydrogen peroxide generation by hypolipidemic drug-induced liver peroxisomes. *Proc Natl Acad Sci USA* 1984;81:7827–7830.
269. Kasai H, Nishimura S. Hydroxylation of guanosine in nucleosides and DNA at the C-8 position by heated glucose and oxygen radical-forming agents. *Environ Health Perspect* 1986;67:111–116.
270. Kasai H, Crain PF, Kuchino Y, Nishimura S, Ootsuyama A, Tanooka H. Formation of 8-hydroxyguanine moiety in cellular DNA by agents producing oxygen radicals and evidence for its repair. *Carcinogenesis* 1986;7:1849–1851.
271. Kasai H, Okada Y, Rao MS, Reddy JK. Formation of 8-hydroxydeoxy-guanosine in liver DNA of rats following long-term exposure to a peroxisome proliferator. *Cancer Res* 1989;49:2601–2605.
272. Takagi A, Sai K, Umemra T, Hasegawa R, Kurokawa Y. Significant increase of 8-hydroxy-deoxyguanosine in liver DNA of rats following short-term exposure to the peroxisome proliferators di(2-ethylhexyl) phthalate and di(2-ethylhexyl) adipate. *Jap J Cancer Res* 1990;81:213–215.
273. Hegi M, Ulrich D, Sagelsdorff P, Richter C, Lutz WK. No measurable increase in thymidine glycol or 8-hydroxydeoxyguanosine in liver DNA of rats treated with nafenopin or choline-devoid low methionine diet. *Mutat Res* 1990;238:325–329.
274. Richter C, Park JW, Ames BN. Normal oxidative damage to mitochondrial and nuclear DNA is extensive. *Proc Natl Acad Sci USA* 1988;85:6465–6467.
275. Schulte-Hermann R. Tumor promotion in the liver. *Arch Toxicol* 1985;57:147–158.
276. Garvey LK, Swenberg JA, Hamm TE, Popp JA. Di(2-ethylhexyl) phthalate: Lack of initiating activity in the liver of female F-344 rats. *Carcinogenesis* 1987;8:285–290.
277. Glauert HP, Clark TD. Lack of initiating activity of the peroxisome proliferator ciprofibrate in two-stage hepatocarcinogenesis. *Cancer Lett* 1989;43:95–100.
278. Williams GM, Maruyama H, Tanaka T. Lack of rapid initiating, promoting or sequential syncarcinogenic effects of di(2-ethylhexyl) phthalate in rat liver carcinogenesis. *Carcinogenesis* 1987;8:875–880.
279. Glauert HP, Beer D, Rao MS, et al. Induction of altered hepatic foci in rats by the administration of hypolipidemic peroxisome proliferators alone or following a single dose of diethylnitrosamine. *Cancer Res* 1986;46:4601–4606.
280. Lillehaug JR, Aarsaether N, Berge RK, Male R. Peroxisome proliferators show tumor-promoting but no direct transforming activity in vitro. *Int J Cancer* 1986;37:97–100.
281. Kraupp B, Huber W, Schulte-Hermann R. Liver growth and early cellular changes in response to peroxisome proliferation. *Biochem Soc Trans* 1990;18:89–92.
282. Reddy JK, Rao MS. Enhancement of Wyeth-14,643, a hepatic peroxisome proliferator, of diethyl-nitrosamine-initiated hepatic tumorigenesis in the rat. *Br J Cancer* 1978;38:537–543.
283. Rao MS, Tatematsu M, Sunnarao V, Ito N, Reddy JK. Analysis of peroxisome proliferator-induced preneoplastic lesions of rat liver for placental form of glutathione S-transferase and gamma-glutamyltranspeptidase. *Cancer Res* 1986;46:5287–5290.
284. Rao MS, Nemali MR, Usuda N, et al. Lack of expression of glutathione S-transferase P, gamma-glutamyltranspeptidase, and alpha-fetoprotein mRNAs in liver tumors induced by peroxisome proliferators. *Cancer Res* 1988;48:4919–4925.
285. Ward JM, Rice JM, Creasia D, Lynch P, Riggs C. Dissimilar patterns of promotion by di(2-ethylhexyl) phthalate and phenobarbital of hepatocellular neoplasia initiated by diethylnitrosamine in B6C3F1. *Carcinogenesis* 1983;4:1021–1029.
286. Numoto S, Mori H, Furuya K, Levine WG, Williams GM. Absence of a promoting or sequential syncarcinogenic effect in rat liver by the carcinogenic hypolipidemic drug nafenopin given after N-2-fluorenylacetamide. *Toxicol Appl Pharmacol* 1985;77:76–85.
287. DeAngelo AB, Garrett CT, Queral AE. Inhibition of phenobarbital and dietary choline deficiency promoted preneoplastic lesions in rat liver by environmental contaminant di(2-ethylhexyl) phthalate. *Cancer Lett* 1984;23:323–330.

288. Popp JA, Garvey LK, Hamm TE, Swenberg JA. Lack of hepatic promotional activity by the peroxi-somal proliferating hepatocarcinogen di(2-ethylhexyl) phthalate. *Carcinogenesis* 1985;6:141–144.
289. DeAngelo AB, Garrett CT. Inhibition of development of preneoplastic lesions in the livers of rats fed weakly carcinogenic environmental contaminant. *Cancer Lett* 1983;20:199–205.
290. Staubli W, Bentley P, Bieri F, Fryhlich E, Waechter F. Inhibitory effect of nafenopin upon the develop-ment of diethylnitrosamine induced enzyme-foci within the rat liver. *Carcinogenesis* 1984;5:41–46.
291. Marsman DS, Popp JA. Importance of basophilic hepatocellular foci in the development of hepato-cellular tumors induced by the peroxisome proliferator, Wyeth-14,643. *Proc Am Assoc Cancer Res* 1989;30:193.
292. Popp JA, Cattley RC. Peroxisome proliferators as initiators and promotors of rodent hepatocarcino-genesis. In: Gibson GG, Lake BG, eds. *Peroxisomes: biology and importance in toxicology and medicine.* London: Taylor & Francis, 1993:653–665.
293. Cattley RC, Marsman DS, Popp JA. Age-related susceptibility to the carcinogenic effect of the peroxisome proliferator Wyeth-14,643 in rat liver. *Carcinogenesis* 1991;12:469–473.
294. Kraupp-Grasl B, Huber W, Taper H, Schulte-Hermann R. Increased susceptibility of aged rats to hepatocarcinogenesis by the peroxisome proliferator nafenopin and the possible involvement of altered liver foci occurring spontaneously. *Cancer Res* 1991;51:666–671.
295. Butterworth BE, Loury DJ, Smith-Oliver T, Cattley RC. The potential role of chemically induced hyperplasia in the carcinogenic activity of the hypolipidemic carcinogens. *Toxicol Indust Health* 1987;3:129–149.
296. Loury DJ, Goldsworthy TL, Butterworth BE. The value of measuring cell replication as a predictive index of tissue specific tumorogenic potential. In: Butterworth BE, Slaga TJ, eds. *Nongenotoxic mechanisms in carcinogenesis.* New York: Cold Spring Harbor Laboratory, 1987:119–136.
297. Bieri F, Muakkassah-Kelly S, Waechter F, Sageldorff P, Staubli W, Bentley P. The significance of in vitro studies on peroxisomal proliferation. *Toxicol in Vitro* 1990;4:428–431.
298. Lanier TL, Berger EK, Eacho PI. Comparison of 5-bromo-2-deoxyuridine and [^{3}H]thymidine for studies of hepatocellular proliferation in rodents. *Carcinogenesis* 1989;10:1341–1343.
299. Eacho PI, Lanier TL, Brodhecker CA. Hepatocellular DNA synthesis in rats given peroxisome proliferating agents: comparison of Wyeth-14,643 to clofibric acid, nafenopin and LY171883. *Car-cinogenesis* 1991;12:1557–1561.
300. Cattley RC, Popp JA. Differences between the promoting activities of the peroxisome proliferator Wyeth-14,643 and phenobarbital in rat liver. *Cancer Res* 1989;49:3246–3251.
301. Schulte-Hermann R, Ohde G, Schuppler J, Timmermann-Trosiener I. Enhanced proliferation of pu-tative preneoplastic cells in the rat liver following treatment with the tumor promoters phenobarbital, hexachlorocyclohexane, steroid compounds, and nafenopin. *Cancer Res* 1981;41:2556–2562.
302. Schulte-Hermann R, Timmermann-Trosiener I, Schuppler J. Promotion of spontaneous preneoplastic cells in rat liver as a possible explanation of tumour production by nonmutagenic compounds. *Cancer Res* 1983;43:839–844.
303. Solt D, Farber E. Principle for the analysis of chemical carcinogenesis. *Nature* 1976;263:701–763.
304. Styles JA, Kelly M, Elcombe CR. A cytological comparison between regeneration, hyperplasia and early neoplasia in the rat liver. *Carcinogenesis* 1987;8:391–399.
305. Bursch W, Lauer B, Timmermann-Trosiener I, Barthel G, Schuppler J, Schulte-Hermann R. Con-trolled death (apoptosis) of normal and putative preneoplastic cells in rat liver following withdrawal of tumour promotors. *Carcinogenesis* 1984;5:457–458.
306. Bayly AC, Roberts RA, Dive C. Suppression of liver cell apoptosis in vitro by the non-genotoxic hepatocarcinogen and peroxisome proliferator nafenopin. *J Cell Biol* 1994;125:197–203.
307. Thompson NL, Mead JE, Braun L, Goyette M, Shank RR, Fausto N. Sequential protooncogene expression during rat liver regeneration. *Cancer Res* 1986;46:3111–3117.
308. Bieri F, Nemali MR, Muakkassah-Kelly S, et al. Increased peroxisomal enzyme mRNA levels in adult rat hepatocytes cultured in a chemically defined medium and treated with nafenopin. *Toxicol in Vitro* 1988;2:235–240.
309. Cherkaoui Malki M, Lone YC, Corral-Debrinski M, Latruffe N. Differential proto-oncogene mRNA induction from rats treated with peroxisome proliferators. *Biochem Biophys Res Comm* 1990;173:855–861.
310. Ledwith BJ, Manam S, Troilo P, Joslyn DJ, Galloway SM, Nichols WW. Activation of immediate-early gene expression by peroxisome proliferators in vitro. *Mol Carcinog* 1993;8:20–27.
311. Ruch RJ, Klaunig JE. Effects of tumor promotors, genotoxic carcinogens and hepatocytotoxins on mouse hepatocyte intercellular communication. *Cell Biol Toxicol* 1986;2:469–483.

312. Trosko JE, Chang CE, Madhukar BV, Klaunig JE. Chemical, oncogene and growth factor inhibition of gap junctional intercellular communication: an integrative hypothesis of carcinogenesis. *Pathobiology* 1990;58:265–268.
313. Klaunig JE, Ruch RJ. Role of inhibition of intercellular communication in carcinogenesis. *Lab Invest* 1990;62:135–146.
314. Klaunig JE, Ruch RJ, DeAngelo AB, Kaylor WH. Inhibition of mouse intercellular communication by phthalate monoesters. *Cancer Lett* 1988;43:65–71.
315. Klaunig JE, Ruch RJ, Lin EL. Effects of trichloroethylene and its metabolites on rodent hepatocyte intercellular communication. *Toxicol Appl Pharmacol* 1989;99:454–465.
316. Berridge MT. Inositol lipids and cell proliferation. *Biochim Biophys Acta* 1987;907:33–45.
317. Sorof S. Modulation of mitogenesis by liver fatty acid binding protein. *Cancer Metast Rev* 1994;13:317–336.
318. Oliver MF, Heady JA, Morris JN, Cooper J. A co-operative trial in the primary prevention of ischemic heart disease using clofibrate (report from the committee of principle investigators). *Br Heart J* 1978;40:1069–1118.
319. Frick H, Elo Haapa K, Heinonen OP. Helsinki heart study: primary-prevention trial with gemfibrozil in middle-aged men with dyslipidemia. *N Engl J Med* 1987;317:1235–1247.
320. Foxworthy PS, Perry DN, Eacho PI. Induction of peroxisomal β-oxidation by nonsteroidal anti-inflammatory drugs. *Toxicol Appl Pharmacol* 1993;118:271–274.
321. Foxworthy PS, Eacho PI. Inhibition of hepatic fatty acid oxidation at carnitine palmitoyl transferase I by the peroxisome proliferator 2-hydroxy-3-propyl-4-[6-(tetrazol-5-yl)hexyloxy] acetophenone. Biochem J. 1988;252:409.

Toxicology of the Liver, 2nd ed.,
Edited by Gabriel L. Plaa and William R. Hewitt
Copyright © 1998 Taylor & Francis

5

Acetaminophen-Induced Hepatotoxicity

Steven D. Cohen, Debie J. Hoivik, and Edward A. Khairallah*

University of Connecticut, Storrs, CT 06269

- · **Toxicology and Pathology**
- · **Biotransformation**
- · **Covalent Binding**
- · **Mitochondrial Injury**
- · **Oxidative Damage**
- · **Calcium Homeostasis**
- · **DNA Damage**
- · **Kupffer Cells**
- · **Summary**
- · **Acknowledgments**
- · **References**

Acetaminophen (N-acetyl-p-aminophenol, 4-acetamidophenol, 4 hydroxyacetanilide, paracetamol, APAP) is an analgesic and antipyretic that is used alone or in combination with other therapeutic agents. It is widely available in both prescription and nonprescription medications. APAP, first introduced with other coal tar analgesics in the late 19th century, did not come into wide use until 60 or more years later (1). It is considered equipotent to aspirin for relief of pain and fever but lacks antiinflammatory action (2). It is now among the most popular analgesics in most countries and is generally considered safe at therapeutic doses and relatively free from interactions with other drugs. However, in acute overdose it can produce fatal liver and kidney damage (3, 4).

TOXICOLOGY AND PATHOLOGY

Laboratory models have been developed for the study of APAP-induced hepatotoxicity in many species including dogs and cats (5); swine (6); and mouse, rat, hamsters, and guinea pigs (7, 8). Comparison of the dosages required for toxicity suggests that

---

*Deceased.

mice and hamsters, which respond to 400–600 mg APAP/kg, more closely approximate humans than do rats, which generally require doses of 1–2 g APAP/kg (4, 9, 10). In mice, glycogen loss and vacuolization of centrilobular hepatocytes is evident within the first few hours after both hepatotoxic (7, 11, 12) and nonhepatotoxic doses (11). After a nontoxic dose these effects disappear, but with a toxic dose, these early changes progress over the next several hours to result in coagulative centrilobular necrosis generally by 12–24 hr in rats, mice, and hamsters (7, 11–14). Single-cell necrosis has been detected by 3 hr (12). Early ultrastructural changes in mitochondria and plasma membrane have been suggested as being important for the development of APAP toxicity (11, 12). Biochemically, APAP hepatotoxicity is generally assessed by monitoring plasma for the appearance of hepatic enzymes, e.g., transaminases and sorbitol dehydrogenase (11, 15, 16), and there is generally good correlation with histopathology (11, 17, 18).

The majority of the mechanistic research studies have been conducted with mice, rats, and hamsters. Even among mice, toxicity varies with strain, age, and sex. Thus, DBA/2 mice are less susceptible than C57BL/6 (19), young mice are less sensitive than mature mice (17, 20, 21), and female mice are more sensitive than male mice (22). By contrast, in Sprague-Dawley rats males are more sensitive than females (23), neonates are more resistant than young rats, and sensitivity to APAP is diminished in 2-year-old rats (24, 25). Rats also exhibit strain differences in susceptibility to APAP (26). Other experimental variables can affect APAP toxicity. These include the vehicle employed for APAP delivery (27, 28), both lighting and feeding schedules (29), and dietary factors and nutritional status (30–37). Thus, it is important to be aware of these factors when designing and evaluating mechanistic studies and when comparing disparate results from apparently similar studies. It is also important to consider this when attempting to extrapolate mechanistic hypothesis from in vitro studies to toxicity in vivo.

Interestingly, the time course for development of toxicity can be influenced by many of the factors mentioned above. For example, 2-month-old B6C3F1 mice respond to 400 mg APAP/kg, administered in a saline vehicle, with maximal elevation of serum transaminases by 4 hr (15) and, similarly, early histopathologic evidence of severe necrosis (18). By contrast, in 3-month-old male CD-1 mice given 600 mg APAP/kg, administered in 50% propylene glycol, plasma enzymes and histopathologic evidence of similar injury are not significantly elevated until 8–12 or more hours after APAP (11, 17, 38). The slower manifestation of the toxicity in the latter model system better reflects the protracted time course in humans (4, 39). It likely results from a slowing of cytochrome P450–mediated APAP activation by the propylene glycol (27, 28) and may permit better temporal discrimination of the sequence of events causing cellular disruptions that eventually lead to cell death (40).

For purposes of this discussion we propose that APAP-induced hepatotoxicity fits the general multievent model (41) that invokes both initiation and progression events in toxicity. More than 20 years of APAP-related research has resulted in an accumulation of evidence for or against one proposed mechanism of toxicity or another. Analysis of this research leads one to the conclusion that there is no single mechanism responsible for APAP-induced hepatotoxicity. Rather, toxicity may be envisioned as resulting from a combination of multiple initiating and progression events. Each by itself is inadequate to mediate hepatotoxicity, but working in concert they are capable of destroying the cells and the organ. The evidence is overwhelming that the initiating events involve *activation* of APAP to a toxic electrophile and *covalent binding* of the electrophile to critical target macromolecules, e.g., protein arylation, with or without *oxidation* by the electrophile of critical target macromolecules. Subsequent to these initiating events a multitude of progression events comes into play; e.g., disruption of calcium homeostasis, disruption of redox balance, diminished mitochondrial function, diminished membrane integrity with lipid peroxidation, and altered nuclear function, along with activation of macrophages. The ultimate determinant of outcome will be how the cell handles these perturbations through repair of injured cells or through removal and replacement of injured and dead cells. It is within this framework that the discussion of mechanisms of toxicity is built in this chapter.

BIOTRANSFORMATION

Metabolism of APAP is crucial for the development of target organ toxicity, and the balance among APAP biotransformation pathways generally determines outcome. The early studies by Mitchell and coworkers (7, 9, 42–46) played a pivotal role in clarifying these relationships. They demonstrated the importance of mixed function oxidase activation of APAP, depletion of glutathione (GSH), and metabolite covalent binding to proteins in explaining the dosage threshold associated with APAP hepatotoxicity. In the 1980s, studies by Nelson and coworkers (47–50) documented the mechanism of formation from APAP of the toxic, reactive intermediate, N-acetyl-*p*-benzoquinoneimine (NAPQI) and clarified the nature of NAPQI binding to protein thiols, e.g., cysteine residues (51, 52).

After nontoxic doses APAP is primarily detoxified through conjugation with glucuronide and sulfate. In mice, hamsters, and rats these conjugates account for 75–80% of the APAP dose. The ratio of these two conjugates varies among species, with hamsters excreting approximately equal amounts of each, rats excreting more sulfate than glucuronide, and mice excreting more glucuronide than sulfate (9). Studies in isolated hepatocytes indicate that sulfate has a higher affinity for APAP but becomes rapidly saturated, whereas glucuronide has a higher capacity for APAP. By contrast, cytochrome P450 has a lower affinity for APAP, and NAPQI formation is greatest at high APAP concentrations (53). Cytochrome P450 also contributes to the production of catechol metabolites, which are unlikely produced in sufficient amounts to contribute to the toxicity (54), and identification of *p*-benzoquinone metabolites in mouse urine after APAP suggests that N-deacetylation also occurs (55). A very small percentage of a nontoxic dose of APAP is converted to NAPQI and the products of NAPQI reaction with GSH can be readily excreted in the bile or urine as a mixture of GSH, cysteine, and mercapturate conjugates. Since most of the drug is excreted in the urine and since cholestyramine protects against toxicity, it is likely that some of the conjugates undergo enterohepatic cycling (56, 57). With overdose there is saturation of the glucuronidation and sulfation pathways, allowing more APAP to be activated by cytochrome P450. Thus, more NAPQI can form conjugates with GSH and other reactive nucleophilic sites on cellular macromolecules to initiate toxicity (4, 39, 42, 58). Finally, the relative rates of APAP conversion to a reactive metabolite, as reflected in mercapturic acid excretion, correlated with species differences in susceptibility to APAP-induced toxicity (9).

The chemical and biochemical mechanisms of APAP activation by cytochrome P450 have recently been reviewed (59), and the early suggestion that NAPQI formation involved an intermediate N-hydroxylation of APAP has been rejected (49, 60, 61). The responsible cytochrome P450 (CYP) isoforms vary among species, with APAP activation mediated by CYPs 1A2 and 2E1 in rabbit liver (62) and CYP1A1 in rat liver (63). CYPs 1A2, 2E1, and 3A4 are the major contributors to APAP bioactivation in human liver (64–66).

Increased cytochrome P450-dependent biotransformation of APAP increases susceptibility to hepatotoxicity. For example, 3-methylcholanthrene, an inducer of CYPs 1A1 and 1A2, increased APAP covalent binding to microsomal proteins (46, 67, 68), urinary excretion of mercapturate (9, 69), biliary excretion of APAP-GSH conjugates (70), and increased APAP toxicity (67, 71). Acetone and diabetes, which increase CYP2E1, increase APAP toxicity (72). Ethanol, which greatly increases susceptibility to APAP in animals and humans (73, 74), increased microsomal activation and covalent binding of APAP in vitro (75) and increased APAP-dependent GSH depletion and covalent binding in association with increased CYP2E1 and CYP3A (76, 77). Phenobarbital also increases APAP induced hepatotoxicity for mice and rats in vivo and hepatocytes in culture (43, 78, 79). Phenobarbital pretreatment caused a corresponding increase of APAP covalent binding in vivo and in vitro (45, 46) and of the urinary excretion of mercapturates (69) and biliary excretion of APAP GSH conjugates (80, 81). By contrast, phenobarbital does not enhance APAP covalent binding or toxicity in hamsters (67, 68, 82, 83). Neither did it increase the hamster's formation in vitro or excretion in vivo of APAP-GSH conjugates (9, 70, 83). Caffeine modulation of APAP biotransformation and toxicity also varies with species and induction state. Coadministration of caffeine increased APAP toxicity in rats (84) but decreased it in mice (85), whereas 3-day pretreatment with caffeine increased APAP toxicity in mice (85). Subsequent studies suggest that caffeine may activate the phenobarbital-inducible forms of cytochrome P450 and thereby increase APAP bioactivation and toxicity, but with 3-methylcholanthrene-induced forms of P450 the caffeine inhibits APAP bioactivation and toxicity (86, 87). Also, HepG2 cells that lack CYP2E1 are generally resistant to APAP binding and toxicity, but when transfected with CYP2E1 these cells respond to APAP with covalent binding and toxicity (88).

Compounds that inhibit cytochrome P450–mediated biotransformation of APAP prevent its toxicity. Thus, cobaltous chloride (89) or piperonyl butoxide pretreatment prevented APAP-induced toxicity in mice (7, 38) and rats (7), and piperonyl butoxide caused a corresponding diminution in APAP covalent binding both in vivo (38, 45) and in vitro (46). Interestingly, piperonyl butoxide (38) and methoxsalen (90) also diminished toxicity when administered after APAP, at a time when APAP activation and binding are already maximized, if not near complete. This suggests that the later protection may have occurred by a mechanism other than prevention of APAP activation. Dimethyl sulfoxide prevented APAP hepatotoxicity in mice and decreased APAP covalent binding both in vivo and in vitro (91). Garlic and its active component, diallyl sulfide, also prevent APAP hepatotoxicity, and this too has been attributed to diminished P450-dependent activation of APAP (92, 93). Similarly, the H_2-receptor antagonist cimetidine inhibits APAP oxidation by rat and human microsomes in vitro (94) and correspondingly prevents toxicity in rats (94–97), mice (98), and humans (99). Finally, simultaneous exposure to ethanol can antagonize APAP toxicity in contrast to the toxic interaction mentioned above (100). Thus, a wide variety of compounds capable of enhancing or interfering with bioactivation cause corresponding enhancements or blockade of APAP covalent binding, GSH depletion, and toxicity. This strongly supports a key initiating role for cytochrome P450–dependent bioactivation in APAP-induced toxicity.

In addition to the large body of evidence supporting a role for the cytochromes P450 in APAP bioactivation with formation of NAPQI, there are reports of alternative activation mechanisms. APAP is also metabolized by horseradish peroxidase to a reactive species postulated to be a semiquinone imine radical that becomes covalently bound to protein or GSH (101). However, the contribution of this reaction to APAP toxicity is not widely supported (102). Several studies have demonstrated APAP activation by prostaglandin synthetase (63, 103, 104). Most were conducted in vitro, and the relevance of such reactions to APAP-induced hepatotoxicity is not certain. However, stimulation or inhibition of prostaglandin synthesis increased and decreased APAP toxicity in mice, respectively (105), suggesting that hepatic cyclooxygenase activity may also contribute to APAP activation and hepatotoxicity.

As noted above, glucuronidation and sulfation play an important role in clearing APAP from the body. During overdose these pathways become saturated and more drug is shunted through the P450 "initiation" pathway. Therefore, one might predict that increases or decreases in either pathway might, under the appropriate conditions, alter the metabolic balance and either increase or decrease the amount of APAP that undergoes bioactivation to NAPQI. Glucuronidation of APAP was increased in mice by both oleanolic acid and butylated hydroxyanisole, and both prevented APAP toxicity (106, 107), with a corresponding diminution of binding in mice treated with the latter compound (106). Both oltipraz (108) and pregnenolone-16α-carbonitrile (109) increased glucuronidation and prevented APAP toxicity in hamsters. Finally, the Gunn rat is deficient in UDP-glucuronosyltransferase activity and exhibits a high susceptibility to APAP-induced toxicity (110), and this suggest that patients with Gilbert's syndrome may experience greater sensitivity to APAP-induced hepatotoxicity (111).

Hepatic GSH plays a key role in protecting cells against reactive electrophiles both through conjugation and through its antioxidant function. The tripeptide GSH (L-γ-glutamyl-L-cysteinyl-glycine) is present in millimolar concentrations and is the main nonprotein thiol in mammalian cells that can readily form conjugates through its nucleophilic cysteinyl SH (112). Early studies demonstrated the importance of hepatic GSH in determining the toxicity threshold with APAP (42). This has been widely acknowledged and led to the development of N-acetyl cysteine (NAC) as the popular antidote for APAP overdose (39). Agents or conditions that alter hepatic GSH content will usually cause a corresponding change in APAP toxicity. For example, phenylpropanolamine and diethyl maleate decrease hepatic GSH and increase APAP toxicity in mice (42, 113). By contrast, zinc administration before APAP challenge enhanced hepatic GSH levels and decreased toxicity in mice (114). Cysteine restores depleted GSH (115) and decreases APAP covalent binding and toxicity in mice (42, 43). Protection also occurs when cysteine is given up to 4 hr after APAP (115), when maximal depletion of GSH and peak covalent binding have occurred (43). Similarly, cysteamine also partially repleted GSH after APAP and prevented protein arylation in microsomes (116) and hepatotoxicity in mice (115). Methionine, which can restore depleted GSH in vivo, also prevents APAP-induced toxicity (117). Finally, the peroxisome proliferator, clofibrate, prevented APAP toxicity and covalent binding in association with elevated hepatic GSH and increased early excretion of APAP-GSH conjugates in bile (118, 119).

Hepatic GSH content in control and GSH-depleted animals was increased by NAC (120, 121), and NAC treatment diminished APAP-induced GSH depletion (69), covalent binding (122, 123), and toxicity in mice (124–126), rats (96), and humans (44, 127) and, in vitro, in rat (128) and mouse hepatocytes (120, 121, 129). Inhibition of GSH biosynthesis with buthionine sulfoximine prevents NAC antagonism of APAP toxicity, suggesting that NAC antidotal action is mediated by GSH repletion (69, 130), but in rats NAC also increased APAP sulfation (131). In addition to its role in repleting GSH and trapping electrophile, NAC may have another antidotal action. Thus, NAC also diminished APAP toxicity when added to hepatocytes in culture after APAP had been removed. Associated with this protection was increased degradation of APAP-arylated proteins (129).

The distribution of GSH and P450s varies across the hepatic lobule. GSH is most concentrated in the periportal region (132), while P450s are concentrated in the centrizonal region. This is consistent with the centrizonal localization of APAP-induced necrosis. Recent immunochemical studies have demonstrated the colocation of CYP 2E1 and bound APAP in the hepatic centrizonal parenchymal cells, which ultimately become necrotic during APAP toxicity (133).

Overall, the general view is that, with overdose, APAP glucuronidation and sulfation pathways become saturated, allowing more cytochrome P450–dependent activation of APAP to NAPQI. NAPQI then reacts with and depletes GSH. The threshold for toxicity is passed when the amount of NAPQI generated greatly exceeds that which can be inactivated by GSH and is thus free to react with proteins and other macromolecules. These metabolic relationships are depicted in Fig. 1 and have generally stood the test of time (59, 102, 134–136). Current research emphasizes identification of targets for covalent binding and clarifying the mechanistic roles of binding and other APAP actions in toxicity.

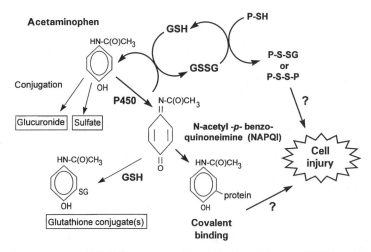

FIG. 1. Acetaminophen (APAP) biotransformation. At therapeutic doses APAP is predominantly cleared by glucuronidation and sulfation, with a small portion of the dose being metabolized by cytochrome P450 to NAPQI. NAPQI is detoxified by reaction with glutathione (GSH). In overdose the primary conjugation pathways become saturated, greater amounts of NAPQI are formed, and GSH becomes depleted. Excess NAPQI is free to increasingly react with cellular constituents, e.g., protein covalent binding, which may play a critical initiating role in toxicity. Alternatively, NAPQI may react with GSH to form oxidized GSH (GSSG), which can, in turn, react with protein sulfhydryls (PSH) to form protein disulfides (PSSP) or protein-mixed disulfides (PSSG), which may play an equally important role in the toxicity. Finally, it is also possible that NAPQI may directly oxidize PSH without the GSSG intermediate step (not shown).

COVALENT BINDING

Early studies with radiolabeled APAP documented that covalent binding increased significantly when GSH was depleted and that a variety of treatments that modulated toxicity were accompanied by a corresponding change in protein arylation, which suggests a mechanistic role for the binding in APAP-induced toxicity (10, 43, 45). Covalent binding may also be viewed solely as an indicator of reactive intermediate presence and, as such, may have no direct role in the resultant toxicity (137). There are many studies in hepatocytes and intact animals that show prevention of APAP toxicity without a corresponding decrease in covalent binding and thus purport to challenge the strong association between binding and toxicity documented above (128, 138–144). Since the majority of the protective agents were antioxidant in nature, e.g., dithiothreitol, superoxide dismutase, 3-methyl(+)catechin, deferoxamine, α-tocopherol, many of the cited papers suggested that oxidative damage rather than binding mediated the hepatotoxicity. However, APAP toxicity has not been documented in the absence of covalent binding. If the toxicity were a multistage process involving both initiation and progression events (41), arylation of specific targets that may be critical to cell vitality might still occur and initiate toxicity, but progression would be blocked by the intervening antioxidant. Finally, not all covalent binding may be of equal significance. Other targets could be electrophile scavengers or sensors that might inactivate electrophiles or serve in a detection mode to "warn" the cell of their presence (145). Recent reviews describe the active research efforts to address the potential mechanistic importance of metabolite covalent binding for APAP and a variety of other toxicants (59, 134–136, 146).

Previous studies with radioactive APAP did not readily permit identification of individual protein targets. Recently, antibodies that recognize bound APAP have been developed and characterized (15, 147–150). Western blot analysis of liver proteins from APAP-dosed mice has revealed that APAP protein arylation is not random but highly selective and that the relative intensity of the immunochemical staining was not reflective of the relative amount of the individual proteins (147, 151). Selective protein arylation by APAP as detected with immunochemical techniques is better correlated with target organ toxicity than is total protein arylation as detected by radioisotopic methods (17, 152) and is closely associated with APAP toxicity in general (79, 147, 151, 153–155). The immunochemical approach has proven valuable for the identification of proteins that become arylated by APAP (see below). One major concern with this approach is the possibility that some adducts may go undetected, perhaps as a result of unique differences in antigenicity. This has recently been addressed for APAP, with excellent agreement reported between immunochemical and phosphorimage detection of APAP adducts (156). Immunochemical approaches have facilitated the determination of the dose and time course of selective protein arylation, the distribution of binding among tissues and organelles, the immunohistochemical localization of adducts (15, 18, 79, 133, 147, 153–155, 157, 158), and the documentation of adduct formation in humans after APAP overdosage (155, 159). However, it remains possible that a small percentage of adducts may go undetected. For example, given the epitope specificity of the anti-APAP antibodies developed to date, it is unlikely that they would detect adducts from which the N-acetyl moiety had been removed, e.g., p-benzoquinoneimine (55). It is has also been postulated that NAPQI may form unstable *ipso* adducts with protein thiols in the initial phase of GSH depletion (59). It is similarly unlikely that such *ipso* adducts of APAP, if they are formed, will be recognized by anti-APAP. Similar, reversible *ipso* adducts have been postulated for reaction of NAPQI with GSH and have been suggested to provide a mechanism for transport of the reactive NAPQI to sites beyond its formation in the endoplasmic reticulum (160).

Western blot analysis of subcellular fractions of livers from APAP-treated mice revealed selective protein arylation in several organelles (148, 151, 161). The greatest binding was in the cytosolic fraction, with the most prominent adduct being a protein of approximately 56–58 kDa (147, 157). Another prominent target detected in cytosol was a 44-kDa protein that was first detectably arylated in the microsomal fraction (162). Subsequent studies revealed that upon arylation, this protein was released from the endoplasmic reticulum to the cytosol (162). APAP-protein adducts were also detectable in the plasma of mice after toxic APAP treatments and may reflect leakage from damaged cells or an early cellular clearance of adducted proteins (15, 153).

The 56–58 and the 44-kDa proteins and five other proteins that are prominent targets for APAP binding in vivo have now been identified (Table 1). Five of these

TABLE 1. *Identification of acetaminophen binding proteins*

Fraction	Molecular mass (kDa)	Protein	Reference
Cytosol	55–58	Selenium binding protein (169) or acetaminophen binding protein (170)	(154, 163)
Cytosol	100	N10-formyl tetrahydrofolate dehydrogenase	(164)
Microsomes	44	Glutamine synthetase	(40)
Mitochondria	50	Glutamate dehydrogenase	(165)
Mitochondria	54	Aldehyde dehydrogenase	(166)
Mitochondria	130	Carbamylphosphate synthetase I	(167)
Nucleus	74–75	Lamin-A	(168)

proteins have known enzymatic activity that becomes decreased in association with APAP binding prior to any overt liver damage. The collective loss of these, and possibly other, enzyme activities may play a critical role in the onset of APAP toxicity. Thus, glutamine synthetase (40), glutamate dehydrogenase (163), and carbamyl phosphate synthetase (164) are involved in trapping ammonia in the liver, which could alter pH (165, 166). Plasma ammonia accumulates after APAP (164), and interestingly, elevated intracellular pH may contribute to the altered calcium homeostasis (167, 168), which likely also contributes to APAP cytotoxicity (169). Diminution of mitochondrial aldehyde and glutamate dehydrogenase activities (165, 166) may influence the NAD:NADH ratio, disrupt oxidative phosphorylation, and contribute to early structural and functional changes in mitochondria after APAP (11, 170–176). In addition, it has been reported that the activity of glyceraldehyde-3-phosphate dehydrogenase, which may form adducts with APAP in mice, is also inhibited by APAP (59). This important glycolytic enzyme not only is involved with ATP formation but also is a major determinant of the NAD:NADH ratio in the cytosol. Tetrahydrofolate dehydrogenase (177) is involved in transmethylation reactions and detoxification of formaldehyde (178). The role of its arylation and inhibition by APAP has not been established. However, dehydrogenases protect the liver against toxic aldehydes (179), and this function would be diminished during inhibition. Overall, there is to date no direct evidence to support these postulated links between protein arylation, enzyme inhibition, and APAP-induced hepatotoxicity, but given the many enzymes that are inhibited in association with early protein arylation, it is likely that the multiple inhibitions collectively contribute to toxicity as initiating events.

Two arylated proteins in the nucleus have been identified (180). The first is 58-ABP, which is discussed below. The second is a major nuclear structural protein, lamin A, one of three intermediate filaments that form the nuclear lamina that anchors interphase chromatin to the inner nuclear membrane (181). Arylation of lamin A may contribute to the detachment of chromatin from the inner nuclear membrane early after APAP and to the later blebbing of the outer nuclear membrane (180). Such changes may contribute to APAP-induced alterations of nuclear function (182, 183). Covalent binding to calreticulin, an intraluminal endoplasmic reticulum calcium-binding protein, and Q5, a thiol:protein disulfide oxidoreductase, has been detected from in vitro incubations of APAP with fortified microsomes (184). These proteins have not been detected as targets of APAP after in vivo exposure, and their arylation may be an artifact of the in vitro system. This remains to be clarified. Several other APAP arylated proteins have also been detected but have not yet been identified (151, 153, 155, 161, 185, 186, 187).

The cytosolic 56–58 kDa APAP-binding protein (58-ABP), as the most prominent target detected during APAP toxicity in mice (154, 188) and humans (155), was the first arylated protein to be purified and identified. It shows sequence identity with a selenium binding protein (189, 190) whose function is unknown. Polyclonal anti-58-ABP prepared against purified mouse liver protein also reacts with proteins of approximately 58 kDa in livers from humans (154). Arylation of the 58 kDa ABP is detected within 30–60 min after APAP administration and is closely correlated with APAP toxicity (17, 79, 147, 151–155, 158). The 2,6-dimethylated analogue of APAP depleted GSH with minimal formation of oxidized GSH (GSSG) and was not hepatotoxic (191–193). However, for this analogue covalent binding could be greatly increased and toxicity could be induced by prior treatment with diethyl maleate or phenobarbital (79, 193). With phenobarbital induction, hepatocyte toxicity after 2,6-dimethyl APAP was accompanied by a large increase in arylation of a 58-kDa cytosolic protein that is likely 58-ABP. However, the mere presence of adducted protein does not guarantee cell injury (147, 194), and there is no direct evidence of a critical initiating role for 58-ABP arylation. Instead, it may act as a scavenger to protect cells from reactive electrophiles. The cysteine residues of 58-ABP can form mixed disulfides with glutathione under oxidative conditions (195) and could readily bind with NAPQI or other electrophiles when GSH reserves become depleted. Interestingly, the 58-ABP appears to be preferentially targeted relative to other cytosolic proteins (187). Recent evidence suggests that electrophilic metabolites of 2,6-dimethyl APAP (155), 3-OH acetanilide (AMAP) (156), 3-methyl indole (196), and bromobenzene (197) also target a cytosolic protein of approximately 56–58 kDa.

The 58-ABP also moves into the nucleus when bound by NAPQI, suggesting that it may serve a surveillance function for detection of electrophiles and signaling their presence to the nucleus or, perhaps, delivering them to the nucleus. In control liver the 58-ABP is detected only in cytosol. However, within 1 hr after APAP, an arylated 58-kDa protein target was detected in nuclear fractions (180). Western blot analysis of two-dimensional gels and immunogold electron microscopy with anti-58-ABP each confirmed that 58-ABP had moved into the nucleus shortly after APAP treatment. Selective washing, extraction, and digestion procedures indicated that the translocated protein is chromatin-associated (180). Other cytosolic markers were not concomitantly detected in the purified nuclear extracts, suggesting that 58-ABP translocation is unlikely to be due to an APAP-induced leakiness of nuclear membranes. Treatments that increased or prevented APAP toxicity caused corresponding changes in 58-ABP translocation, and translocation was also evident after a toxic dose of bromobenzene (198) but not after nontoxic AMAP (168), both of which likely bind to 58-ABP (156, 197). Furthermore, on two-dimensional gels, 58-ABP can be separated into four isoforms, and the relative temporal appearance of the isoforms within the nucleus reflected their relative arylation after APAP rather than their relative abundance in control cytosol. This suggests that arylation initiated the translocation of 58-ABP into the nucleus and would be consistent with a novel role postulated for the 58-ABP as a sensor for the presence of electrophiles (145). Once in the nucleus, the arylated 58-ABP could interact with chromatin to alter transcriptional or replicative events appropriate to the homeostatic needs of the cell, e.g., induction of stress proteins (199), initiate destruction of APAP-injured cells (200), promote tissue repair (201, 202). These relationships are highly speculative at this point; the toxicologic significance of 58-ABP translocation subsequent to arylation remains to be determined.

MITOCHONDRIAL INJURY

One of the early morphologic manifestation of APAP toxicity is a disruption of mitochondrial integrity. Within 1–2 hr after APAP the mitochondria appear to have lost portions of their double limiting membranes and are swollen and distorted (11–13). This altered morphology is coincident with functional damage to the mitochondrial respiratory apparatus (171, 174, 175, 203). In isolated mouse hepatocytes respiration at site 2 was most sensitive to APAP and was decreased by 47% after 1 hr; respiration at the NADH-linked site 1 was inhibited to a lesser extent, while site-3 respiration was not altered (174). The loss of mitochondrial respiration was accompanied by a decrease in ATP levels and ATP:ADP ratios (energy charge) of the cytosol and was preceded by a loss of GSH in both the cytosol and the mitochondria (204). It is of interest that even depletion of cellular ATP levels is considered necessary, but not by itself sufficient, to mediate APAP toxicity (205).

Studies with AMAP, the positional isomer of APAP, provide additional evidence for the importance of mitochondrial changes. Thus, AMAP covalently binds to hepatic proteins in the absence of toxicity or a large decrease in GSH (206–209). Its reactive metabolite, like NAPQI, may form arylthioether adducts (210–212) and is equipotent to NAPQI in vitro (209). Clearance of adducts is more rapid for AMAP than for APAP (208), and adducts derived from AMAP appear to be less stable than those from APAP (156). Protein arylation and GSH depletion in mitochondria are more rapid and extensive after toxic APAP than nontoxic AMAP (156, 213), but buthionine sulfoximine–pretreated mice are sensitive to AMAP-induced hepatotoxicity, and in such mice mitochondrial AMAP binding and depletion of mitochondrial GSH was significantly increased compared to AMAP-challenged controls (214). These observations indicate that protein arylation in mitochondria and depletion of mitochondrial GSH may be very important determinants of toxicity. Given the importance of the mitochondria in maintaining cellular redox balance and calcium homeostasis (see below), these findings and recent temporal studies of the effect of APAP on mitochondrial function (203), along with electron microscopic evidence mentioned earlier, suggest that mitochondrial insult may be very important early in APAP toxicity. Thus, the binding to and functional inhibition of individual mitochondrial proteins, as described above, may contribute mechanistically to the initiation of such insult.

OXIDATIVE DAMAGE

The arylation of proteins by APAP may be necessary but not sufficient for the development of the hepatocellular injury. Some antioxidants can protect against liver damage caused by APAP or NAPQI without markedly affecting covalent binding. Research into the mechanism of oxidative cell injury is shifting away from the central association of cytosolic calcium with lethal cell injury to focus on the adverse effects of oxidants on cellular macromolecules. Oxidative stress occurs in cells when there is disruption of the cellular redox balance. It may contribute to the lipid peroxidation, oxidation of protein thiols, altered calcium homeostasis, and altered mitochondrial permeability and function, which have been associated with APAP toxicity (215, 216). Cellular defenses against this include superoxide dismutase, glutathione peroxidase, catalase, and vitamins C and E (217–221).

The 3,5-dimethyl analogue of APAP depleted GSH with formation of GSSG and oxidation of protein sulfhydryls in association with toxicity, but there was no detectable covalent binding (191–193). Toxicity was prevented by the reducing agent, dithiothreitol (193), and this is consistent with 3,5-dimethyl APAP causing a significant oxidative stress. Similarly, oxidative stress likely contributes to APAP toxicity (191). APAP actually exhibits some antioxidant activity in vitro (222, 223), which would seem inconsistent with oxidant stress. However, it has been suggested that NAPQI may oxidize protein sulfhydryls to form mixed disulfides with GSH (59). In addition, reactive oxygen may originate from the P450 cycle during APAP biotransformation (224–227). Some inhibitors of cytochrome P450 diminish APAP toxicity even when given after most APAP activation and binding is complete (38, 90), and this would be consistent with a role for cytochrome P450-derived reactive oxygen species as contributors to the progression events in the toxicity. There is substantial evidence, both in vivo and in vitro, that supports a role for oxidative stress in APAP hepatotoxicity. For example, lipid peroxidation has been observed in isolated hepatocytes exposed to APAP (140, 228). Ethane exhalation, indicating lipid peroxidation, was detected in APAP-dosed mice and correlated with toxicity (229, 230). Inhibition of GSH reductase with BCNU (1,3-bis(chloroethyl)-1-nitrosourea) increased GSH oxidation and GSSG excretion in isolated hepatocytes exposed to APAP (231, 232) and increased APAP toxicity in vivo and in vitro (128, 231–235). Similarly, modulation of GSH peroxidase activity with ebselen protects hepatocytes from APAP-induced toxicity (232, 236), while selenium- or vitamin E-deficient diets or inhibition of GSH peroxidase with gold thioglucose increases APAP toxicity in vivo and in vitro (31, 235). Protein sulfhydryl oxidation occurs with APAP treatment and can be prevented with dithiothreitol (141, 191, 231, 237), and a wide variety of antagonists to oxidative stress can correspondingly diminish APAP toxicity both in vivo and in vitro. Examples include deferoxamine, superoxide dismutase, N,N'-diphenylphenylene-diamine, catalase, α-tocopherol, promethazine, and β-scymnol (128, 142, 143, 228, 232, 233, 238). Collectively these studies link oxidative stress with APAP toxicity. However, agents that protected against lipid peroxidation did not prevent APAP toxicity (239). Also, examination of bile from APAP-dosed rats did not yield evidence of oxidative stress, although such evidence is found after diquat, whose hepatotoxicity is mediated by oxidative stress (240, 241). Careful temporal investigations in vivo suggest that oxidative events may be involved in the progression of toxicity rather than its initiation (242, 243) and suggest that in vitro systems may be more susceptible to redox manipulation than in vivo systems (240). Thus, there is little direct evidence to support generalized oxidative damage as the initiating event in APAP toxicity in vivo. However, it remains possible that early oxidation of sulfhydryls on critical proteins may also alter protein function and contribute to the initiation of toxicity.

CALCIUM HOMEOSTASIS

Oxidative stress can also initiate permeability transition of the inner mitochondrial membrane and result in mitochondrial swelling, uncoupling of oxidative phosphorylation, and collapse of the mitochondrial membrane potential with consequent disruption of calcium homeostasis (244). An increase in the intracellular concentration of calcium has been suggested as the final common pathway to toxic cell death produced in the liver and other organs by drugs and chemicals (169, 245–250). Normally, the concentration of free intracellular calcium is four orders of magnitude less than the extracellular level. This concentration is maintained by specific plasma membrane ATPases that transport calcium out of the cell or by sequestration within mitochondria and the endoplasmic reticulum. Xenobiotic-induced disruption of calcium homeostasis can lead to a number of detrimental cellular processes. These include disruption of the cytoskeleton (251); activation of catabolic enzymes, e.g., phospholipases (252) and proteases (253); and endonucleases (169); and the loss of mitochondrial ATP production (254).

APAP treatment increases intracellular calcium both in vitro and in vivo (213, 255, 256). This was not simply due to APAP induced GSH depletion, since equivalent depletion by buthionine sulfoximine did not similarly elevate intracellular calcium levels (257). Altered calcium homeostasis may result from increased influx of extracellular calcium (258) due to decreased calcium-ATPase activity (256), and early APAP binding to the plasma membrane (259). On the other hand, intracellular compartments can also be the source of the free calcium. Thus, oxidation of sulfhydryl groups on ATPase or other critical enzymes in mitochondria or the endoplasmic reticulum by APAP metabolites may impair thiol metabolizing enzymes and lead to decreased sequestration of calcium (247, 254), and this is consistent with the suggestion that the rise in free calcium results from an APAP- or NAPQI-induced disruption of mitochondrial function, redox state, and permeability (213, 260, 261).

Recent temporal studies suggest that the rise in intracellular calcium, like oxidative stress, is unlikely to be an initiating event in APAP-induced hepatotoxicity (244, 262). Most of the evidence that a rise in free calcium causes the cell injury has relied on indirect indicators of calcium, such as measurement of phosphorylase *a* activity (256) or use of indicator dyes such as Quin-2 (263). However, phosphorylase *a* activity can be increased without increased calcium (244), and Quin-2 is inherently toxic and may also be cytoprotective through sequestration of Fe^{2+} (264, 265). When calcium was measured more directly in single mouse hepatocytes using digital imaging fluorescence microscopy, the increase in free calcium occurred only in the late stage of toxicity well after the initiation of irreversible cell damage. At that time neither chelators of calcium nor inhibitors of phospholipases or proteases protect the cell from injury (258). It is thus unlikely that a rise in cytosolic calcium plays a central role in initiating cell injury (244). However, calcium perturbations likely play a very important role as progression events in APAP-induced hepatotoxicity.

DNA DAMAGE

APAP and NAPQI bind covalently to DNA both in vitro and in vivo at levels that are 1/100th of that observed for protein binding (183, 266–268). While binding of NAPQI to other vital macromolecules may be more critical to cell survival (269), binding to DNA may be responsible for the increased single strand breaks that occur in mouse liver after an hepatotoxic dose of APAP (183). Also, relatively low concentrations of APAP (0.1–1.0 mM) inhibit DNA synthesis and cell replication in mammalian cell lines that lack cytochrome P450 (88, 270, 271). APAP blockage of V79 cell replication at the G_1 phase could be reversed with ascorbate, suggesting an oxidative process (270). Indeed, APAP-related oxidation of a tyrosyl residue at the active site of ribonucleotide reductase may be responsible for the inhibition of DNA synthesis (182).

DNA damage has also been implicated in the acute pathogenesis of APAP toxicity. Administration of toxic doses of APAP to mice results in increased levels of nuclear calcium and DNA fragmentation and "laddering" prior to cell death. This suggests that activation of a calcium-dependent endonuclease may be involved in hepatotoxicity (272, 273). Antagonism of nuclear calcium accumulation by blocking calcium-calmodulin with chlorpromazine, or calcium channels with verapamil, prevented DNA fragmentation and decreased APAP toxicity (200, 274). In addition, aurintricarboxylic acid, a calcium endonuclease inhibitor, decreased DNA fragmentation and toxicity in mouse hepatocytes exposed to APAP (275). Since inhibitors of DNA polymerase a (aphidicolin, myricetin), DNA ligase (ethidium bromide), or DNA repair enzymes (doxorubicin) potentiate APAP-induced cell death (276), these data collectively suggest that DNA damage is a critical event that may also contribute to APAP toxicity. Whether such effects are involved in initiation or progression remains to be determined.

KUPFFER CELLS

Inflammatory responses are not prominent early in APAP toxicity in humans or mice, but such a response was evident in livers from rats given APAP (277) and likely resulted from recruitment and activation of macrophages by factors released from hepatocytes exposed to APAP (278). Subsequent studies demonstrated that agents that enhance or diminish macrophage activity similarly modulated APAP toxicity (279–281). Recent evidence (282) supports the hypothesis that injured hepatocytes release cellular factors that activate macrophages, and these, in turn, may release reactive oxygen species as well as mediators that exacerbate the damage initiated by APAP (277, 283). The proinflammatory cytokines, TNF-α and IL-1α, are produced in Kupffer cells activated after APAP (284), and selective neutralization of either cytokine by antibodies alters the hepatic pathophysiologic response to APAP intoxication (285). Recent studies in mice with both methyl palmitate and gadolinium chloride reported decreased Kupffer cell phagocytic activity, and this was associated with protection from APAP-induced hepatotoxicity (286, 287). Thus, Kupffer cells likely contribute to the progression phase of APAP-induced hepatotoxicity.

SUMMARY

More than 20 years have passed since the first reports of acute hepatotoxicity with APAP overdose. During that period investigative research to discover the "mechanism" underlying the toxicity has been conducted in many species and strains of intact animals as well as in a variety of in vitro and culture systems. Such work has demonstrated the primary role of biotransformation and led to the development of antidotes for the treatment of acute poisoning. It has also shed significant light on the biochemical and cellular events that accompany the histopathologic changes. However, it has not as yet revealed a unique mechanism that is universally accepted. It is apparent that the concept of a multistage process involving both initiation and progression events (41) best describes APAP toxicity. Thus, we should no longer be seeking a single initiating event. Rather, a number of such "events" likely occur very early after toxic overdosage and collectively set in motion and perpetuate the biochemical, cellular, and molecular processes that determine outcome for the hepatocyte and the whole organ (Fig. 2). This is consistent with the thesis put forth by Mourelle and coworkers that toxicity results from NAPQI attack upon several points of cell function (288).

Whether protein arylation, protein oxidation, or both mediates the initiating event is not readily resolved. It is clear that APAP can initiate both processes and that each is independently capable of altering protein function. Thus, both arylation and oxidation of cell macromolecules likely contribute to the initiation of APAP toxicity. Selective experimental blockade of different cellular processes can modulate APAP toxicity. However, many studies that utilize "unique" tools of molecular and cell biology to alter toxicity do not verify that those tools had no effect on APAP biotransformation and pharmacokinetics and thus may be inconclusive. In spite of this caution, the weight of evidence suggests that APAP toxicity is the result of multiple processes, likely initiated by arylation and oxidation, that act in concert to bring about cell death. Continued investigation of these processes and the interplay among them will advance our understanding of cellular responses to potentially lethal toxicant insult.

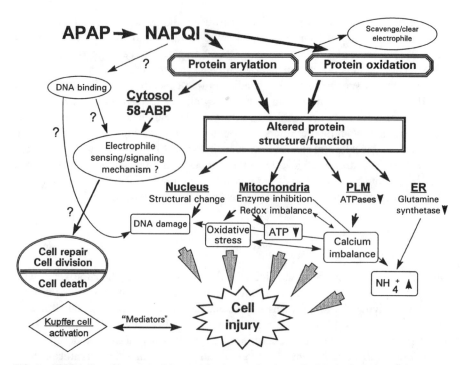

FIG. 2. APAP-induced hepatotoxicity-contributing mechanisms. Toxicity is depicted as consisting of both initiation and progression events (41). Initiation (large bold arrows) involves biotransformation of APAP to NAPQI, arylation or oxidation of several important proteins, and alteration of protein structure and function. The immediate consequence of the alterations is detectable in several organelles (small dark arrows) and these may represent multiple initiating events, each of which is, by itself, inadequate to drive the progression events. Rather, these many processes are depicted as acting in concert (large arrowheads) to cause cell injury. DNA binding and arylation of cytosolic 58-ABP are also implicated as possible signaling mechanisms for determining outcome. See text for details.

ACKNOWLEDGMENTS

The authors' research was supported in part through grants from the National Institutes of Health (General Medical Sciences 31460 and Environmental Health Sciences 07163) and from the University of Connecticut Center for Biochemical Toxicology and the University of Connecticut Research Foundation. Dr. Hoivik was supported by a Boehringer Ingelheim Predoctoral Fellowship in Toxicology.

REFERENCES

1. Clissold SP. Paracetamol and phenacetin. *Drugs* 1986;32:46–59.
2. Vane, JR. Inhibition of prostaglandin synthesis as a mechanism of action for aspirin-like drugs. *Nature New Biol* 1971;231:232–234.

3. Thomas SHL. Paracetamol (acetaminophen) poisoning. *Pharmacol Ther* 1993;50:91–120.
4. Anker AJ, Smilkstein MJ. Acetaminophen: concepts and controversies. *Emerg Med Clin North Am* 1994;12:335–349.
5. Savides MC, Oehme FW, Nash SL, Leipold HW. The toxicity and biotransformation of single doses of acetaminophen in dogs and cats. *Toxicol Appl Pharmacol* 1984;74:26–34.
6. Miller DJ, Hickman R, Fratter CMR, Terblance J, Saunders SJ. An animal model of fulminant hepatic failure: a feasibility study. *Gastroenterology* 1976;71:109–113.
7. Mitchell JR, Jollow DJ, Potter WZ, Davis DC, Gillette JR, Brodie BB. Acetaminophen-induced hepatic necrosis. I. Role of drug metabolism. *J Pharmacol Exp Ther* 1973;187:185–194.
8. Davis DC, Potter WZ, Jollow DJ, Mitchell JR. Species differences in hepatic glutathione depletion, covalent binding and hepatic necrosis after acetaminophen. *Life Sci* 1974;14:2099–2109.
9. Jollow DJ, Thorgeirsson SS, Potter WZ, Hashimoto M, Mitchell JR. Acetaminophen-induced hepatic necrosis. VI. Metabolic disposition of toxic and nontoxic doses of acetaminophen. *Pharmacology* 1974;12:251–271.
10. Potter WZ, Thorgeirsson SS, Jollow DJ, Mitchell JR. Acetaminophen-induced hepatic necrosis. V. Correlation of hepatic necrosis, covalent binding and glutathione depletion in hamsters. *Pharmacology* 1974;12:129–143.
11. Placke ME, Ginsberg GL, Wyand DS, Cohen SD. Ultrastructural changes during acute acetaminophen-induced hepatotoxicity in the mouse: a time and dose study. *Toxicol Pathol* 1987;15:431–438.
12. Walker RM, Racz WJ, McElligott TF. Acetaminophen-induced hepatotoxicity in mice. *Lab Invest* 1980;42:81–189.
13. Dixon MF, Dixon B, Aparicio SR, Lowey DP. Experimental paracetamol-induced hepatic necrosis: a light and electron-microscope, and histochemical study. *J Pathol* 1975;116:17–29.
14. Chiu S, Bhakthan NMG. Experimental acetaminophen-induced hepatic necrosis: biochemical and electron microscopic study of cysteamine protection. *Lab Invest* 1978;39:193–203
15. Pumford NR, Hinson JA, Potter DW, Rowland KL, Benson RW, Roberts DW. Immunochemical quantitation of 3-(cystein-S-yl)acetaminophen adducts in serum and liver proteins of acetaminophen-treated mice. *J Pharmacol Exp Ther* 1989;248:190–196.
16. Corcoran GB, Racz WJ, Smith CV, Mitchell JR. Effects of N-acetylcysteine on acetaminophen covalent binding and hepatic necrosis in mice. *J Pharmacol Exp Ther* 1984;232:864–872.
17. Beierschmitt WP, Brady JT, Bartolone JB, Wyand DS, Khairallah EA, Cohen SD. Selective protein arylation and the age dependency of acetaminophen hepatotoxicity in mice. *Toxicol Appl Pharmacol* 1989;98:517–529.
18. Roberts DW, Bucci TJ, Benson RW, Warbritton AR, McRae TA, Pumford NR, Hinson JA. Immuno-histochemical localization and quantification of the 3-(cystein-S-yl)-acetaminophen protein adduct in acetaminophen hepatotoxicity. *Am J Pathol* 1991;138:359–371.
19. Nebert DW, Jensen NM. The Ah locus:genetic regulation of the metabolism of carcinogens, drugs and other environmental chemicals by cytochrome P450-mediated monooxygenases. *Crit Rev Biochem* 1979;6:401–437.
20. Hart JG, Timbrell JA. The effect of age on paracetamol hepatotoxicity in mice. *Biochem Pharmacol* 1979;28:3015–3017.
21. Adamson GM, Papadimitriou JM, Harman AW. Postnatal mice have low susceptibility to paracetamol toxicity. *Pediatr Res* 1991;29:496–499.
22. Munoz FG, Fearon Z. Sex related differences in acetaminophen toxicity in the mouse. *Clin Toxicol* 1984;22:149–156.
23. Raheja KL, Linscheer WG, Cho C. Hepatotoxicity and metabolism of acetaminophen in male and female rats. *J Toxicol Environ Health* 1983;12:143–158.
24. Green MD, Shires TK, Fischer LJ. Hepatotoxicity of acetaminophen in neonatal and young rats. I. Age-related changes in susceptibility. *Toxicol Appl Pharmacol* 1984;74:116–124.
25. Rikans LE, Moore DR. Acetaminophen hepatotoxicity in aging rats. *Drug Chem Toxicol* 1988;11: 237–247.
26. Price VF, Jollow DJ. Strain differences in susceptibility of normal and diabetic rats to acetaminophen hepatotoxicity. *Biochem Pharmacol* 1986;35:687–695.
27. Nelson, EB. Method and composition for reducing the toxicity of acetaminophen. *United States Patent 4.307.073* issued Dec. 22, 1981.
28. Hughes RD, Gove CD, Williams R. Protective effects of propylene glycol, a solvent used pharmaceutically, against paracetamol-induced liver injury in mice. *Biochem Pharmacol* 1991;42:710–713.

29. Schnell RC, Bozigian HP, Davies MH, Merrick A, Park JS, MacMillan DA. Factors influencing circadian rhythms in acetaminophen lethality. *Pharmacology* 1984;29:149–157.
30. Martinelli ALC, Meneghelli UG, Zucoloto S, Lima SO. Effect on the intake of an exclusive sucrose diet on acetaminophen hepatotoxicity in rats. *Brazilian J Med Biol Res* 1989;22:1381–1387.
31. Peterson FJ, Lindemann NJ, Duquette PH, Holtzman JL. Potentiation of acute acetaminophen lethality by selenium and vitamin E deficiency in mice. *J Nutr* 1992;122:74–81.
32. Pessayre D, Dolder A, Artigou JY, Wandscheer JC, Descatoire V, Degott C, Benhamou JP. Effect of fasting on metabolite-mediated hepatotoxicity in the rat. *Gastroenterology* 1979;77:264–271.
33. Hong RW, Rounds RD, Helton WS, Robinson MK, Wilmore DW. Glutamine preserves liver glutathione after lethal hepatic injury. *Ann Surg* 1992;215:114–119.
34. Kroger H, Klewer M, Gratz R, Dietrich A, Ehrlich W, Altrichter S, Kurpisz M, Miesel R. Influence of diet free of NAD-precursors on acetaminophen hepatotoxicity in mice. *Gen Pharmacol* 1996;27:79–82.
35. Ishida K, Hanada T, Sakai T, Doi K. Effects of fructose-induced hypertriglyceridemia on hepatorenal toxicity of acetaminophen in rats. *Exp Toxicol Pathol* 1995;47:509–516.
36. Miller MG, Price VF, Jollow DJ. Anomalous susceptibility of the fasted hamster to acetaminophen hepatotoxicity. *Biochem Pharmacol* 1986;35:817–825.
37. Baranowitz SA, Maderson PFA. Acetaminophen toxicity is substantially reduced by beta carotene in mice. *Internat J Vit Nutr Res* 1995;65:175–180.
38. Brady JT, Montelius DA, Beierschmitt WP, Wyand DS, Khairallah EA, Cohen SD. Effect of piperonyl butoxide post-treatment on acetaminophen hepatotoxicity. *Biochem Pharmacol* 1988;37:2097–2099.
39. Meredith TJ, Jacobsen D, Haines JA, Berger, JC. *Antidotes for poisoning by paracetamol.* Cambridge: Cambridge University Press, 1995:1–30.
40. Bulera SJ, Birge RB, Cohen SD, Khairallah EA. Identification of the mouse liver 44-kDa acetaminophen-binding protein as a subunit of glutamine synthetase. *Toxicol Appl Pharmacol* 1995;134:313–320.
41. Trump BF, Berezesky IK, Smith MW, Phelps PC, Elliget KA. The relationship between cellular ion deregulation and acute and chronic toxicity. *Toxicol Appl Pharmacol* 1989;91:6–22.
42. Mitchell JR, Jollow DJ, Potter WZ, Gillette JR, Brodie BB. Acetaminophen-induced hepatic necrosis. IV. Protective role of glutathione. *J Pharmacol Exp Ther* 1973;187:211–217.
43. Mitchell JR, Jollow DJ, Gillette JR, Brodie BB. Drug metabolism as a cause of drug toxicity. *Drug Metab Dispos* 1973;1;418–423.
44. Mitchell JR, Thorgeirsson SS, Potter WZ, Jollow DJ, Keiser H. Acetaminophen induced hepatic injury: protective role of glutathione in man and rationale for therapy. *Clin Pharmacol Ther* 1974;16:676–684.
45. Jollow DJ, Mitchell JR, Potter WZ, Davis DC, Gillette JR, Brodie BB. Acetaminophen-induced hepatic necrosis. II. Role of covalent binding *in vivo*. *J Pharmacol Exp Ther* 1973;187:195–202.
46. Potter WZ, Davis DC, Mitchell JR, Jollow DJ, Gillette JR, Brodie BB. Acetaminophen-induced hepatic necrosis. III. Cytochrome P450 mediated covalent binding *in vitro*. *J Pharmacol Exp Ther* 1973;187:203–210.
47. Dahlin DC, Miwa GT, Lu AYH, Nelson SD. N-acetyl-*p*-benzoquinone imine: a cytochrome P450-mediated oxidation product of acetaminophen. *Proc Nat Acad Sci USA* 1984;81:1327–1331.
48. Dahlin DC, Nelson SD. Synthesis, decomposition kinetics and preliminary toxicological studies on pure N-acetyl-*p*-benzoquinone imine, a proposed toxic metabolite of acetaminophen. *J Med Chem* 1982;25:885–886.
49. Holme JA, Dahlin DC, Nelson SD, Dybing E. Cytotoxic effects of N-acetyl-*p*-benzoquinone imine, a common arylating intermediate of paracetamol and N-hydroxy-paracetamol. *Biochem Pharmacol* 1984;33:401–406.
50. Harvison PJ, Guengerich FP, Rashed MS, Nelson SD. Cytochrome P450 isozyme selectivity in the oxidation of acetaminophen. *Chem Res Toxicol* 1988;1:47–52.
51. Streeter AJ, Dahlin DC, Nelson SD, Baillie TA. The covalent binding of acetaminophen to protein, evidence for cysteine residues as major sites of arylation in vitro. *Chem Biol Interactions* 1984;48:349–366.
52. Hoffman KJ, Streeter AJ, Axworthy DB, Baillie TA. Identification of the major covalent adduct formed in vitro and in vivo between acetaminophen and mouse liver proteins. *Mol Pharmacol* 1985;27:566–573.
53. Moldeus P. Paracetamol metabolism and toxicity in isolated hepatocytes from rat and mouse. *Biochem Pharmacol* 1978;27:2859–2963.

54. Forte AJ, Wilson JM, Slattery JT, Nelson SD. The formation and toxicity of catechol metabolites of acetaminophen in mice. *Drug Metab Dispos* 1984;12:484–491.
55. Pascoe GA, Calleman CJ, Baille TA. Identification of S-(2,5-dihydroxyphenyl)-N-acetyl-cysteine as urinary metabolites of acetaminophen in the mouse. Evidence for *p*-benzoquinone as a reactive intermediate in acetaminophen metabolism. *Chem Biol Interact* 1988;68:85–98.
56. Siegers CP, Rozman K, and Klaassen CD. Biliary excretion and enterohepatic circulation of paracetamol in the rat. *Xenobiotica* 1983;13:591–596.
57. Siegers CP, Moller-Hartmann W. Cholestyramine as an antidote against paracetamol-induced hepato- and nephrotoxicity in the rat. *Toxicol Lett* 1989;47:179–184.
58. Hjelle JJ, Hazelton GA, Klaassen CD. Acetaminophen decreases adenosine 3'-phosphate 5'-phosphosulfate and uridine diphospate glucuronic acid in rat liver. *Drug Metab Dispos* 1985;13:35–41.
59. Nelson SD. Mechanisms of the formation and disposition of reactive metabolites that can cause acute liver injury. *Drug Metab Rev* 1995;27:147–177.
60. Corcoran GB, Mitchell JR, Vaishnav YN, Horning EC. Evidence that acetaminophen and N-hydroxyacetaminophen form a common arylating intermediate, N-acetyl-*p*-benzoquinoneimine. *Molec Pharmacol* 1980;18:536–542.
61. Nelson EB. The pharmacology and toxicology of meta-substituted acetanilid: acute toxicity of 3-hydroxyacetanilide in mice. *Res Commun Chem Pathol Pharmacol* 1980;28:447–456.
62. Morgan ET, Koop DR, Coon MJ. Comparison of six rabbit liver cytochrome P450 isoenzymes in formation of a reactive metabolite of acetaminophen. *Biochem Biophys Res Commun* 1983;112:8–13.
63. Harvison PJ, Egan RW, Gale PH, Christian GD, Hill BS, Nelson SD. Acetaminophen and analogs as cosubstrates and inhibitors of prostaglandin H synthase. *Chem Biol Interactions* 1988;64:251–266.
64. Patten CL, Thomas PE, Guy RL, Lee M, Gonzalez FJ, Guengerich P, Yang CS. Cytochrome P450 enzymes involved in acetaminophen activation by rat and human liver microsomes and their kinetics. *Chem Res Toxicol* 1993;6:511–518.
65. Raucy JL, Lasker JM, Lieber CS, Black M. Acetaminophen activation by human liver cytochrome P450 2E1 and P450 1A2. *Arch Biochem Biophys* 1989;271:270–283.
66. Thummel KE, Lee CA, Kunze KL, Nelson SD, Slattery JT. Oxidation of acetaminophen to N-acetyl-*p*-aminobenzoquinone imine by human CYP3A4. *Biochem Pharmacol* 1993;45:1563–1569.
67. Hinson JA, Nelson SD, Mitchell JR. Studies on the microsomal formation of arylating metabolites of acetaminophen and phenacetin. *Mol Pharmacol* 1977;13:625–633.
68. Ioannides C, Steele CM, Parke DV. Species variation in the metabolic activation of paracetamol to toxic intermediates: role of cytochromes P450 and P448. *Toxicol Lett* 1983;16:55–61.
69. Miners JO, Drew R, Birkett DJ. Mechanism of action of paracetamol protective agents in mice in vivo. *Biochem Pharmacol* 1984;33:2995–3000.
70. Madhu C, Gregus Z, Klaassen CD. Biliary excretion of acetaminophen-glutathione as an index of toxic activation of acetaminophen: effect of chemicals that alter acetaminophen hepatotoxicity. *J Pharmacol Exp Ther* 1989;248:1069–1077.
71. Holme JA, Søderlund EJ. Species differences in cytotoxic and genotoxic effects of phenacetin and paracetamol on primary monolayer cultures of hepatocytes. *Mutation Res* 1986;164:167–175.
72. Jeffery EH, Arndt K, Haschek WM. The role of cytochrome P4502E1 in bioactivation of acetaminophen in diabetic and acetone treated mice. *Adv Exp Med Biol* 1991;283:249–251.
73. Zimmerman HJ, Maddrey WC. Acetaminophen (paracetamol) hepatotoxicity with regular intake of alcohol: analysis of instances of therapeutic misadventure. *Hepatology* 1995;22:767–773.
74. Peterson FJ, Holloway DE, Erickson RR, Duquette PHM, McClain CJ, Holtzman JL. Ethanol induction of acetaminophen toxicity and metabolism. *Life Sci* 1980;27:1705–1711.
75. Prasad JS, Chen NQ, Lui YX, Goon DJ, Holtzman JL. Effects of ethanol and inhibitors on the binding and metabolism of acetaminophen and N-acetyl-*p*-benzoquinone imine by hepatic microsomes from control and ethanol-treated rats. *Biochem Pharmacol* 1990;40:1989–1995.
76. Kostrubsky VE, Wood SG, Bush MD, Szakacs J, Bement WJ, Sinclair PR, Jeffery EH, Sinclair JF. Acute hepatotoxicity of acetaminophen in rats treated with ethanol plus isopentanol. *Biochem Pharmacol* 1995;50:1743–1748.
77. Kostrubsky VE, Strom SC, Wood SG, Wrighton SA, Sinclair PR, Sinclair JF. Ethanol and isopentanol increase CYP3A and CYP2E in primary cultures of human hepatocytes. *Arch Biochem Biophys* 1995;322:516–520.
78. Hayes MA, Roberts E, Roomi MW, Safe SH, Farber E, Cameron RG. Comparative influences of different Pb type and 3-MC type polychlorinated biphenyl-induced phenotypes on cytocidal hepatotoxicity of bromobenzene and acetaminophen. *Toxicol Appl Pharmacol* 1984;76:118–127.

79. Birge RB, Bartolone JB, McCann DJ, Mangold JB, Cohen SD, Khairallah EA. Selective arylation by acetaminophen and 2,6-dimethylacetaminophen in cultured hepatocytes from phenobarbital-induced and uninduced mice: relationship to cytotoxicity. *Biochem Pharmacol* 1989;38:4429–4438.
80. Gregus Z, Madhu C, Klaassen CD. Effect of microsomal enzyme inducers on biliary and urinary excretion of acetaminophen metabolites in rats: decreased hepatobiliary and increased hepatovascular transport of acetaminophen-glucuronide after microsomal enzyme induction. *Drug Metab Dispos* 1990;8:10–19.
81. Loeser W, Siegers CP. Effects of phenobarbital, phorone and carbon tetrachloride pretreatment on the biliary excretion of acetaminophen in rats. *Arch Int Pharmacodyn Ther* 1985;275:180–188.
82. Jollow DJ, Roberts S, Price V, Longacre S, Smith C. Pharmacokinetic considerations in toxicity testing. *Drug Metab Rev* 1982;13:983–1007.
83. Lupo S, Yodis LA, Mico BA, Rush GF. In vivo and in vitro hepatotoxicity and metabolism of acetaminophen in Syrian hamsters. *Toxicology* 1987;44:229–239.
84. Sato C, Izumi N, Nouchi T, Hasumura Y, Takeuchi J. Increased hepatotoxicity of acetaminophen by concomitant administration of caffeine in the rat. *Toxicology* 1985;34:95–101.
85. Gale GR, Atkins LM, Smith AB, Walker EM. Effects of caffeine on acetaminophen-induced hepatotoxicity and cadmium redistribution in mice. *Res Commun Chem Pathol Pharmacol* 1986;51:337–349.
86. Kalhorn TF, Lee CA, Slattery JT, Nelson SD. Effect of methylxanthines on acetaminophen hepatotoxicity in various induction states. *J Pharmacol Exp Ther* 1990;252:112–116.
87. Jaw SJ, Jeffery EH. Interaction of caffeine with acetaminophen. *Biochem Pharmacol* 1993;46:493–501.
88. Dai Y, Cederbaum AI. Cytotoxicity of acetaminophen in human cytochrome P4502E1-transfected HepG cells. *J Pharmacol Exp Ther* 1995;273:1497–1505.
89. Roberts SA, Price VF, Jollow DJ. The mechanisms of cobalt chloride-induced protection against acetaminophen hepatotoxicity. *Drug Metab Dispos* 1986;14:25–33.
90. Letteron PL, Descatoire V, Larrey D, Geneve J, Pessayre D. Pre- or post-treatment with methoxsalen prevents the hepatotoxicity of acetaminophen in mice. *J Pharmacol Exp Ther* 1986;239:559–567.
91. Park Y, Smith RD, Combs AB, Kehrer JP. Prevention of acetaminophen-induced hepatotoxicity by dimethyl sulfoxide. *Toxicology* 1988;52:165–175.
92. Brady JF, Wang M-H, Hong J-Y, Xiao F, Li Y, Yoo JS, Ning SM, Lee MJ, Fukuto JM, Gapac JM, Yang CS. Modulation of rat hepatic microsomal monoxygenase activities and cytotoxicity by diallyl sulfide. *Toxicol Appl Pharmacol* 1991;108:342–354.
93. Wang E-J, Li Y, Lin M, Chen L, Stein AP, Reuhl KR, Yang CS. Protective effects of garlic and related organosulfur compounds on acetaminophen-induced hepatotoxicity in mice. *Toxicol Appl Pharmacol* 1996;136:146–154.
94. Mitchell MC, Schenker S, Speeg KV. Selective inhibition of acetaminophen oxidation and toxicity by cimetidine and other H$_2$-receptor antagonists *in vivo* and *in vitro* in the rat and in man. *J Clin Invest* 1984;73:383–391.
95. Jackson CH, MacDonald NC, Cornett JW. Acetaminophen: a practical pharmacologic overview. *Canadian Medical Assoc Journal* 1984;131:25–32.
96. Mitchell MC, Schenker S, Avant GR, Speeg KV. Cimetidine protects against acetaminophen hepatotoxicity in rats. *Gastroenterology* 1991;81:1052–1060.
97. Speeg KV, Mitchell MC, Maldanado AL. Additive protection of cimetidine and N-acetylcysteine treatment against acetaminophen-induced hepatic necrosis in the rat. *J Pharmacol Exp Ther* 1985;234:550–554.
98. Peterson FJ, Knodell RG, Lindemann NJ, Steele NM. Prevention of acetaminophen and cocaine hepatotoxicity in mice by cimetidine treatment. *Gastroenterology* 1983;85:122–129.
99. Burkhart KK, Janco N, Kulig KW, Rumack BH. Cimetidine as adjunctive treatment for acetaminophen overdose. *Hum Exp Toxicol* 1995;3:299–304.
100. Sato C, Nakano M, Lieber CS. Prevention of acetaminophen-induced hepatotoxicity by acute ethanol administration in the rat: comparison with carbon tetrachloride-induced hepatotoxicity. *J Pharmacol Exp Ther* 1981;218:805–810.
101. Nelson SD, Dahlin DC, Rauckman EJ, Rosen GM. Peroxidase-mediated formation of reactive metabolites of acetaminophen. *Mol Pharmacol* 1981;20:195–199.
102. Vermeulen NPE, Bessems JGM, Van De Straat R. Molecular aspects of paracetamol-induced hepatotoxicity and its mechanism-based prevention. *Drug Metab Rev* 1992;24:367–407.

103. Moldéus P, Rahimtula A. Metabolism of paracetamol to a glutathione conjugate catalyzed by prostaglandin synthetase. *Biochem Biophys Res Commun* 1980;96:496–475.
104. Moldéus P, Andersson B, Rahimtula A, Berggren M. Prostaglandin synthetase catalyzed activation of paracetamol. *Biochem Pharmacol* 1982;31:1363–1368.
105. Ben-Zvi Z, Weissman-Teitellman B, Katz S, Danon A. Acetaminophen hepatotoxicity: is there a role for prostaglandin synthesis? *Arch Toxicol* 1990;64:299–304.
106. Hazelton GA, Hjelle JJ, Klaassen CD. Effect of butylate hydroxyanisole on acetaminophen hepatotoxicity and glucuronidation *in vivo*. *Toxicol Appl Pharmacol* 1986;83:474–485.
107. Liu J, Liu Y, Madhu C, Klaassen CD. Protective effects of oleanolic acid on acetaminophen-induced hepatotoxicity in mice. *J Pharmacol Exp Ther* 1993;266:1607–1613.
108. Davies MH, Schnell RC. Oltipraz-induced amelioration of acetaminophen hepatotoxicity in hamsters. II. Competitive shunt in metabolism *via* glucuronidation. *Toxicol Appl Pharmacol* 1991;109:29–40.
109. Madhu C, Klaassen CD. Protective effect of pregnenolone-16-α-carbonitrile on acetaminophen-induced hepatotoxicity in hamsters. *Toxicol Appl Pharmacol* 1991;109:305–313.
110. DeMorais SMF, Chow SYM, Wells PG. Biotransformation and toxicity of acetaminophen in congenic RHA rats with or without a hereditary deficiency in bilirubin UDP-glucuronosyltransferase. *Toxicol Appl Pharmacol* 1992;117:81–87.
111. DeMorais SMF, Uetrecht JP, Wells PG. Decreased glucuronidation and increased bioactivation of acetaminophen in Gilbert's syndrome. *Gastroenterology* 1992;102:577–586.
112. DeLeve LD, Kaplowitz N. Glutathione metabolism and its role in hepatotoxicity. *Pharmacol Ther* 1991;52:287–305.
113. James RC, Harbison RD, Roberts SM. Phenylpropanolamine potentiation of acetaminophen-induced hepatotoxicity: evidence for a glutathione-dependent mechanism. *Toxicol Appl Pharmacol* 1993;118:159–168.
114. Szymańska JA, Świetlicka EA, Piotrowski JK. Protective effect of zinc in the hepatotoxicity of bromobenzene and acetaminophen. *Toxicology* 1991;66:81–91.
115. Strubelt O, Siegers CP, Schött A. The curative effects of cysteamine, cysteine and dithiocarb in experimental paracetamol poisoning. *Arch Toxicol* 1974;33:55–64.
116. Buckpitt AR, Rollins DE, Mitchell JR. Varying effects of sulfhydryl nucleophiles on acetaminophen oxidation and sulfhydryl adduct formation. *Biochem Pharmacol* 1979;28:2941–2946.
117. McLean AE, Day PA. The effect of diet on the toxicity of paracetamol and the safety of paracetamol-methionine mixtures. *Biochem Pharmacol* 1975;24:37–42.
118. Manautou JE, Tveit A, Hoivik DJ, Khairallah EA, Cohen SD. Clofibrate pretreatment diminishes acetaminophen (APAP) selective covalent binding and hepatotoxicity. *Toxical Appl Pharmacol* 1994;129:252–263.
119. Manautou JE, Tveit A, Hoivik DJ, Khairallah EA, Cohen SD. Protection by clofibrate against acetaminophen hepatotoxicity in male CD-1 mice is associated with enhanced biliary clearance of acetaminophen-glutathione adducts. *Toxical Appl Pharmacol* 1996;140:30–38.
120. Harman AW, Self G. Comparison of the protective effects of N-acetylcysteine, 2-mercaptopropionglycine and dithiothreitol against acetaminophen toxicity in mouse hepatocytes. *Toxicology* 1986;41:83–93.
121. Massey TE, Racz WJ. Effects of N-acetylcysteine on metabolism, covalent binding, and toxicity of acetaminophen in isolated mouse hepatocytes. *Toxical Appl Pharmacol* 1981;60:220–228.
122. Corcoran GB, Racz WJ, Mitchell JR. Inhibition by N-acetylcysteine of acetaminophen covalent binding and liver injury. *The Pharmacologist* 1978;20:259.
123. Piperno E, Berssenbruegge DA. Reversal of experimental toxicosis with N-acetylcysteine. *Lancet* 1976;2:738–739.
124. Piperno E, Mosher AH, Berssenbruegge DA, Winkler JD, Smith RB. Pathophysiology of acetaminophen overdosage toxicity: implications for management. *Pediatrics* 1978;62:880–889.
125. Corcoran GB, Wong BK. Role of glutathione in prevention of acetaminophen-induced hepatotoxicity by N-acetyl-L-cysteine in vivo: studies with N-acetyl-D-cysteine in mice. *J Pharmacol Exp Ther* 1986;238:54–61.
126. Hazelton GA, Hjelle JJ, Klaassen CD. Effects of cysteine prodrugs on acetaminophen-induced hepatotoxicity. *J Pharmacol Exp Ther* 1986;237:341–349.
127. Smilkstein MJ, Knapp GL, Kulig KW. Efficacy of oral N-acetylcysteine in the treatment of acetaminphen overdose: analysis of the national multicenter study (1976-1985). *N Engl J Med* 1988;319:1557–1562.

128. Gerson RJ, Casini A, Gilfor D, Serroni A, Farber JL. Oxygen-mediated cell injury in the killing of cultured hepatocytes by acetaminophen. *Biochem Biophys Res Commun* 1985;126:1129–1137.
129. Bruno MK, Cohen SD, Khairallah EA. Antidotal effectiveness of N-acetylcysteine in reversing acetaminophen-induced hepatotoxicity. *Biochem Pharmacol* 1988;37:4319–4325.
130. Drew R, Miners JO. The effects of buthionine sulphoximine (BSO) on glutathione depletion and xenobiotic biotransformation. *Biochem Pharmacol* 1984;33:2989–2994.
131. Galinsky RE, Levy G. Effect of N-acetylcysteine on the pharmacokinetics of acetaminophen in rats. *Life Sci* 1979;25:693–700.
132. Gebhart R. Metabolic zonation of the liver: regulation and implications for liver function. *Pharmacol Thery* 1992;53:275–354.
133. Emeigh-Hart SG, Cartun RW, Wyand DS, Khairallah EA, Cohen SD. Immunohistochemical localization of acetaminophen in target tissues of the CD-1 mouse: correspondence of covalent binding with toxicity. *Fundam Appl Toxicol* 1995;24:260–274.
134. Nelson SD, Pearson PG. Covalent and noncovalent interactions in acute lethal cell injury caused by chemicals. *Annu Rev Pharmacol Toxicol* 1990;30:169–195.
135. Holtzman JL. The role of covalent binding to microsomal proteins in hepatotoxicity of acetaminophen. *Drug Metab Rev* 1995;27:277–297.
136. Boelsterli UA. Specific targets of covalent drug-protein interactions in hepatocytes and their toxicological significance in drug-induced liver injury. *Drug Metab Rev* 1993;25:395–451.
137. Gillette JR. A perspective on the role of chemically reactive metabolites of foreign compounds in toxicity. I. Correlation of changes in covalent binding of reactive metabolites with changes in the incidence and severity of toxicity. *Biochem Pharmacol* 1974;23:2785–2794.
138. Labadarios D, Davis M, Portmann B, Williams R. Paracetamol-induced hepatic necrosis in the mouse-relationship between covalent binding, hepatic glutathione depletion and the protective effect of alpha-mercaptopropionylglycine. *Biochem Pharmacol* 1977;26:31–35.
139. Gerber JG, MacDonald ZJS, Harbison RD, Villeneuve JP, Wood AJ, Nies AS. Effect of N-acetylcysteine on hepatic covalent binding of paracetamol. *Lancet* 1977;8012:657–658.
140. Albano E, Poli G, Chiarpotto E, Blasi F, Dianzani MU. Paracetamol-stimulated lipid peroxidation in isolated rat and mouse hepatocytes. *Chem Biol Interact* 1983;47:249–263.
141. Tee LB, Boobis AR, Huggett AC, Davies DS. Reversal of acetaminophen toxicity in isolated hamster hepatocytes by dithiothreitol. *Toxicol Appl Phamacol* 1986;83:294–314.
142. Nakae D, Yamamoto K, Hitoshi Y, Kinugasa T, Maruyama H, Farber JL, Konishi Y. Liposome-encapsulated dismutase prevents liver necrosis induced by acetaminophen. *Am J Pathol* 1990;136:787–795.
143. Lucas AM, Hoivik DJ, Manautou JE, Khairallah EA, Macrides TA, Cohen SD. 5-β scymnol (5βS) decreases acetaminophen (APAP) toxicity but not covalent binding. *The Toxicologist* 1995;15:152.
144. Devalia JL, Ogilvie RC, McLean AEM. Dissociation of cell death from covalent binding of paracetamol by flavones in a hepatocyte stystem. *Biochem Pharmacol* 1982;31:3745–3749.
145. Khairallah EA, Bruno MK, Hong M, Cohen SD. Cellular consequences of protein adduct formation. *The Toxicologist* 1995;15:86.
146. Hinson JA, Pumford NR, Roberts DW. Mechanisms of acetaminophen toxicity: immunochemical detection of drug-protein adducts. *Drug Metab Rev* 1995;27:73–92.
147. Bartolone JB, Sparks K, Cohen SD, Khairallah EA. Immunochemical detection of acetaminophen-bound liver proteins. *Biochem Pharmacol* 1987;36:1193–1196.
148. Bartolone JB, Birge RB, Sparks K, Cohen SD, Khairallah EA. Immunochemical analysis of acetaminophen covalent binding to proteins:partial characterization of the major acetaminophen-binding liver proteins. *Biochem Pharmacol* 1988;37:4763–4774.
149. Roberts DW, Pumford NR, Potter DW, Benson RW, Hinson JA. A sensitive immunochemical assay for acetaminophen-protein adducts. *J Pharmacol Exp Ther* 1991;241:527–533.
150. Potter DW, Pumford NR, Hinson JA, Benson RW, Roberts DW. Epitope characterization of acetaminophen bound to protein and nonprotein sulfhydryl groups by an enzyme-linked immunosorbent assay. *J Pharmacol Exp Ther* 1989;248:182–189.
151. Pumford NR, Hinson JA, Benson RW, Roberts DW. Immunoblot analysis of protein containing 3-(cystein-S-yl)acetaminophen adducts in serum and subcellular liver fractions from acetaminophen-treated mice. *Toxical Appl Pharmacol* 1990;104:521–532.
152. Brady JT, Birge RB, Khairallah EA, Cohen SD. Post-treatment protection with piperonyl butoxide against acetaminophen hepatotoxicity is associated with changes in selective but not total covalent binding. In: Witmer CM, Snyder RR, Jollow DJ, Kalf GF, Kocsis JJ, Sipes IG, eds. *Biological reactive intermediates IV.* New York: Plenum Press, 1990:685–688.

153. Bartolone JB, Beierschmitt WP, Birge RB, Hart SGE, Wyand S, Cohen SD, Khairallah EA. Selective acetaminophen metabolite binding to hepatic and extrahepatic proteins: an *in vivo* and *in vitro* analysis. *Toxicol Appl Pharmacol* 1989;99:240–249.
154. Bartolone JB, Birge RB, Bulera SJ, Bruno MK, Nishanian EV, Cohen SD, Khairallah EA. Purification, antibody production, and partial amino acid sequence of the 58-kDa acetaminophen-binding liver proteins. *Toxicol Appl Pharmacol* 1992;113:19–29.
155. Birge RB, Bartolone JB, Hart SGE, Nishanian EV, Tyson CA, Khairallah EA, Cohen SD. Acetaminophen hepatotoxicity: correspondence of selective protein arylation in human and mouse liver *in vitro*, in culture and *in vivo*. *Toxicol Appl Pharmacol* 1990;105:472–482.
156. Myers TG, Dietz EC, Anderson NL, Khairallah EA, Cohen SD, Nelson SD. A comparative study of mouse liver proteins arylated by reactive metabolites of acetaminophen and its nonhepatotoxic regioisomer, 3'-hydroxyacetanilide. *Chem Res Toxicol* 1995;8:403–413.
157. Pumford NR, Roberts DW, Benson RW, Hinson JA. Immunochemical quantitation of 3-(cystein-S-yl)acetaminophen protein adducts in subcellular liver fractions following a hepatotoxic dose of acetaminophen. *Biochem Pharmacol* 1990;40:573–579.
158. Bartolone JB, Cohen SD, Khairallah EA. Immunohistochemical localization of acetaminophen-bound liver proteins. *Fundam Appl Toxicol* 1989;13:859–862.
159. Hinson JA, Roberts DW, Benson RW, Dalhoff K, Loft S, Poulsen HE. Regarding the mechanism of paracetamol toxicity in humans. *Lancet* 1990;332:732.
160. Baillie TA, Slatter JG. Glutathione: a vehicle for the transport of chemically reactive metabolites *in vivo*. *Acc Chem Res* 1991;24: 264–270.
161. Mathews AM, Pumford NR, Roberts DW, Benson RW, Hinson JA. A novel procedure for production of antibodies to acetaminophen-protein adducts. *The Toxicologist* 1994;14: 426.
162. Birge RB, Bulera SJ, Bartolone JB, Ginsberg GL, Cohen SD, Khairallah EA. The arylation of microsomal membrane proteins by acetaminophen is associated with the release of a 44 kDa acetaminophen-binding mouse liver protein complex into the cytosol. *Toxicol Appl Pharmacol* 1991;109:443–454.
163. Halmes NC, Hinson JA, Martin BM, Pumford N. Glutamate dehydrogenase covalently binds to a reactive metabolite of acetaminophen. *Chem Res Toxicol* 1996;9:541–546.
164. Gupta S, Rogers LK, Smith CV. Biliary excretion of lysosomal enzymes, iron, and oxidized protein in Fischer-344 and Sprague-Dawley rats and the effects of diquat and acetaminophen. *Toxicol Appl Pharmacol* 1994;125:42–50.
165. Cooper AJL. Glutamine synthetase. In: Kvamme E, ed. *Glutamine and glutamate in mammals*, vol. 1. Boca Raton: CRC Press, 1988:7–31.
166. Tate SS, Meister A. Glutamine synthetase of mammalian liver and brain. In: Prusiner S, Statman ER, eds. *The enzymes of glutamine metabolism*. New York: Academic Press, 1973:77–127.
167. Gores GJ, Nieminen AL, Wray BE, Herman B, Lemasters JL. Intracellular pH during "chemical hypoxia" in cultured rat hepatocytes: protection by intracellular acidosis against the onset of cell death. *J Clin Invest* 1979;83:386–396.
168. Herman B, Gores GJ, Niemeine AL, Kawanishi A, Harman A, Lemaster JL. Calcium and pH in anoxic injury. *Crit Rev Toxicol* 1990;21:127–148.
169. Nicotera P, Bellomo G, Orrenius S. Calcium-mediated mechanisms in chemically induced cell death. *Annu Rev Pharmacol Toxicol* 1992;32:449–470.
170. Porter KE, Dawson AG. Inhibition of respiration and gluconeogenesis by paracetamol in rat kidney preparations. *Biochem Pharmacol* 1979;28:3057–3062.
171. Esterline R, Ji S. Metabolic alterations resulting from the inhibition of mitochondrial respiration by acetaminophen in vivo. *Biochem Pharmacol* 1989;38:2390–2392.
172. Burcham PC, Harman AW. Effect of acetaminophen hepatotoxicity on hepatic mitochondrial and microsomal calcium contents in mice. *Toxicol Lett* 1988;44:91–99.
173. Burcham PC, Harman AW. Mitochondrial dysfunction in paracetamol hepatotoxicity: in vitro studies in isolated mouse hepatocytes. *Toxicol Lett* 1990;50:37–48.
174. Burcham PC, Harman AW. Acetaminophen toxicity results in site-specific mitochondrial damage in isolated mouse hepatocytes. *J Biol Chem* 1991;266:5049–5054.
175. Meyers LL, Beierschmitt WP, Khairallah EA, Cohen SD. Acetaminophen-induced inhibition of hepatic mitochondrial respiration in mice. *Toxicol Appl Pharmacol* 1988;93:378–387.
176. Nazareth WM, Sethi JK, McLean AE. Effect of paracetamol on mitochondrial membrane function in rat liver slices. *Biochem Pharmacol* 1991;42:931–936.

177. Pumford NR, Halmes NC, Martin BM, Hinson JA. Covalent binding to N-10-formyltetrahydrofolate dehydrogenase following a hepatotoxic dose of acetaminophen. *The Toxicologist* 1994;14:426.
178. Cook RJ, Lloyd RS, Wagner C. Isolation and characterization of c-DNA clones for rat liver 10-formyltetrahydrofolate dehydrogenase. *J Biol Chem* 1991;266:4965–4973.
179. Weiner H. Aldehyde dehydrogenase: Mechanism of action and possible physiological roles. In: Majckrowicz EI, ed. *Biochemistry and pharmacology of ethanol*, vol. 1. New York: Plenum, 1979:107–124.
180. Hong M, Cohen SD, Khairallah EA. Translocation of the major cytosolic acetaminophen (APAP) protein adducts into the nucleus. *The Toxicologist* 1994;14:427.
181. Spector DL. Macromolecular domains within the cell nucleus. *Ann Rev Cell Biol* 1993;9:265–316.
182. Hongslo JK, Bjørge C, Schwarze PE, Brøgger A, Mann G, Thelander l, Holme JA. Paracetamol inhibits replicative DNA synthesis and induces sister chromatid exchange and chromosomal aberations by inhibition of ribonucleotide reductase. *Mutagenesis* 1990;5:475–482.
183. Hongslo JK, Smith CV, Brunborg G, Söderlund EJ, Holme JA. Genotoxicity of paracetamol in mice and rats. *Mutagenesis* 1994;9:93–100.
184. Zhou LX, Srivastava SP, Holtzman JL. Binding of 14C-acetaminophen (AC) to mouse, hepatic, microsomal proteins. *The Toxicologist* 1995;34:150.
185. Landin JS, Cohen SD, Khairallah EA. Redox and the covalent binding of acetaminophen (APAP) to mitochondrial aldehyde dehydrogenase. *Fundam Appl Toxicol* 1996;30S:278.
186. Halmes NC, Hinson JA, Pumford NR. Purification of a 67 kDa hepatic mitochondrial protein which covalently binds to a metabolite of acetaminophen. *The Toxicologist* 1994;14:426.
187. Hoivik DJ, Manautou JE, Tveit A, Mankowski DC, Khairallah EA, Cohen SD. Evidence suggesting the 58-kDa acetaminophen binding protein is a preferential target for acetaminophen electrophile. *Fund Appl Toxicol* 1996;32:79–86.
188. Pumford NR, Martin BM, Hinson JA. A metabolite of acetaminophen covalently binds to the 56 kDa selenium binding protein. *Biochem Biophys Res Comm* 1992;182:1348–1355.
189. Bansal MP, Mukhopadhyay T, Scott J, Cook RG, Muchopadhyah R, Medina D. DNA sequencing of a mouse liver protein that binds selenium: implications for selenium's mechanism of action in cancer prevention. *Carcinogenesis* 1990;11:2071–2073.
190. Lanfear J, Fleming J, Walker M, Harrison P. Different patterns of regulation of the genes encoding the closely related 56 kDa selenium- and acetaminophen-binding proteins in normal tissues and during carcinogenesis. *Carcinogenesis* 1993;14:335–340.
191. Birge RB, Bartolone JB, Nishanian EV, Bruno MK, Mangold JB, Cohen SD, Khairallah EA. Dissociation of covalent binding from the oxidative effects of acetaminophen: studies using dimethylated acetaminophen derivatives. *Biochem Pharmacol* 1988;37:3383–3393.
192. Rosen GM, Rauckman EJ, Ellington SP, Dahlin DC, Christie JL, Nelson SD. Reduction and glutathione conjugation reactions of N-acetyl-*p*-benzoquinone imine and two dimethylated analogues. *Mol Pharmacol* 1984;25:151–157.
193. Porubek DJ, Rundgren M, Harvison PJ, Nelson SD, Moldéus P. Investigation of mechanisms of acetaminophen toxicity in isolated rat hepatocytes with the acetaminophen analogs 3,5-dimethylacetaminophen and 2,6-dimethylacetaminophen. *Mol Pharmacol* 1987;31:647–653.
194. Tveit A, Leung CY, Emeigh Hart SG, Wyand DS, Khairallah EA, Cohen SD. Repeated acetaminophen dosing results in selective arylation to hepatic and renal proteins without toxicity in the CD-1 mouse. *The Toxicologist* 1992;12:254.
195. Birge RB, Bartolone JB, Cohen SD, Khairallah EA, Smolin LA. A comparison of proteins S-thiolated by glutathione to those arylated by acetaminophen. *Biochem Pharmacol* 1991;42:S197–S207.
196. Kaster JK, Yost GS. Targets of 3-methylindole reactive intermediate are characterized by a selective antibody. *The Toxicologist* 1996;30:283.
197. Manautou JE, Khairallah EA, Cohen SD. Evidence for common binding of acetaminophen and bromobenzene to the 58 kDa acetaminophen binding protein. *J Toxicol Environ Health* 1995;46:263–269.
198. Sanghani M, Hong M, Bruno MK, Cohen SD, Khairallah EA. Model hepatotoxicants induce the translocation of the cytosolic 58 kDa acetaminophen binding protein into the nucleus. *FASEB J* 1995;9:A695.
199. Bruno MK, Cohen SD, Khairallah EA. Selective alterations in the patterns of newly synthesized proteins by acetaminophen and its dimethylated analogues in primary cultures of mouse hepatocytes. *Toxicol Appl Pharmacol* 1992;112:282–290.

200. Ray SD, Kamendulis LM, Gurule MW, Yorkin RD, Corcoran GB. Ca^{2+} antagonists inhibit DNA fragmentation and toxic cell death induced by acetaminophen. *FASEB J* 1993;7:453–463.

201. Mehendale HM, Thakore KN, Rao CV. Autoprotection: stimulated tissue repair permits recovery from injury. *J Biochem Toxicol* 1994;9:131–139.

202. Chanda S, Mangipudy RS, Warbritton A, Bucci TJ, Mehendale HM. Stimulated hepatic tissue repair underlies heteroprotection by thioacetamide against acetaminophen-induced lethality. *Hepatology* 1995;21:477–486.

203. Donnelly PJ, Walker RM, Racz WJ. Inhibition of mitochondrial respiration in vivo is an early event in acetaminophen-induced hepatotoxicity. *Arch Toxicol* 1994;68:110–118.

204. Andersson BS, Rundgren R, Nelson SD, Harder S. N-acetyl-p-benzoquinone imine-induced changes in the energy metabolism in hepatocytes. *Chem Biol Interactions* 1998;75:201–221.

205. Martin FL, McLean AEM. Adenosine triphosphate (ATP) levels in paracetamol-induced cell injury in the rat in vivo and in vitro. *Toxicology* 1995;104:91–97.

206. Roberts SA, Jollow DJ. Acetaminophen structure-toxicity relationships: why is 3-hydroxyacetanilide not hepatotoxic? *The Pharmacologist* 1978;20:574.

207. Nelson SD, Forte AJ, Dahlin DC. Lack of evidence for the involvement of N-hydroxyacetaminophen as a reactive metabolite of acetaminophen *in vitro*. *Biochem Pharmacol* 1980;29:1617–1620.

208. Rashed MS, Myers TG, Nelson SD. Hepatic protein arylation, glutathione depletion, and metabolite profiles of acetaminophen and a non-hepatotoxic regioisomer, 3'-hydroxyacetanilide, in the mouse. *Drug Metab Dispos* 1990;18:765–770.

209. Holme JA, Hongslo JK, Bjørhge C, Nelson SD. Comparative cytotoxic effects of acetaminophen (N-acetyl-p-aminophenol), a non-hepatotoxic regioisomer acetyl-m-aminophenol and their postulated reactive hydroquinone and quinone metabolites in monolayer cultures of mouse hepatocytes. *Biochem Pharmacol* 1991;42:1137–1142.

210. Streeter AJ, Bjorge SM, Axworthy DB, Nelson SD, Baillie TA. The microsomal metabolism and site of covalent binding to protein of 3'-hydroxyacetanilide, a nonhepatotoxic positional isomer of acetaminophen. *Drug Metab Dispos* 1984;12:565–576.

211. Hamilton M, Kissinger PT. The metabolism of 2- and 3-hydroxyacetanilide: determination of metabolic products by liquid chromatography/electrochemistry. *Drug Metab Dispos* 1986;14:5–12.

212. Rashed MS, Nelson SD. Characterization of glutathione conjugates of reactive metabolites of 3'-hydroxyacetanilide, a nonhepatotoxic positional isomer of acetaminophen. *Chem Res Toxicol* 1989;2:41–45.

213. Tirmenstein MA, Nelson SD. Subcellular binding and effects on calcium homeostasis produced by acetaminophen and a nonhepatotoxic regioisomer, 3'-hydroxyacetanilide, in mouse liver. *J Biol Chem* 1989;264:9814–9819.

214. Tirmenstein MA, Nelson SD. Hepatotoxicity after 3'-hydroxyacetanilide administration to buthionine sulfoximine pretreated mice. *Chem Res Toxicol* 1991;4:214–217.

215. Brent JA, Rumack BH. Role of free radicals in toxic hepatic injury. I. Free radical biochemistry. *Clin Toxicol* 1993;31:139–171.

216. Brent AJ, Rumack BH. Role of free radicals in toxic hepatic injury. II. Are free radicals the cause of toxin-induced liver injury? *Clin Toxicol* 1993;31:173–196.

217. Sies H. Strategies of antioxidant defense. *Eur J Biochem* 1993;215:213–219.

218. Sunde RA, Hoekstra WG. Structure, synthesis, and function of glutathione peroxidase. *Nutr Rev* 1980;38:265–273.

219. Reed DJ. Regulation of reductive processes by glutathione. *Biochem Pharmacol* 1986;35:7–13.

220. Oshino N, Chance B. Properties of glutathione release observed during reduction of organic hydroperoxide, demethylation of aminopyrine and oxidation of some substances in perfused rat liver, and their implications for the physiological function of catalase. *Biochem J* 1977;162:509–525.

221. Bascetta E, Gunstone FD, Walton JC. Electron spin resonance study of the role of vitamin E and vitamin C in the inhibition of fatty acid oxidation in a model membrane. *Chem Phys Lipids* 1983;33:207–210.

222. Dubois RN, Hill KE, Burk RF. Antioxidant effect of acetaminophen in rat liver. *Biochem Pharmacol* 1983;32:2621–2622.

223. Van de Straat R, Bijloo GJ, Vermeulen NPE. Paracetamol, 3-monoalkyl- and 3,5-dialkyl-substituted derivatives: antioxidant activity and relationship between lipid peroxidation and cytotoxicity. *Biochem Pharmacol* 1988;37:3473–3476.

224. Gillette JR, Brodie BB, LaDu BN. Oxidation of drugs by liver microsomes: on the role of TPNH and oxygen. *J Pharmacol Exp Ther* 1957;119:532–540.
225. Nordblom GD, Coon MJ. Hydrogen peroxide formation and stoichiometry of hydroxylation reactions catalyzed by highly purified liver microsomal cytochrome P450. *Arch Biochem Biophys* 1977;180:343–347.
226. Rosen GM, Singletary WV, Raukman EJ, Killenberg PG. Acetaminophen hepatotoxicity: an alternative mechanism. *Biochem Pharmacol* 1983;32:2053–2059.
227. Van de Straat R, De Vries J, Vermeulen NPE. Role of hepatic microsomal and purified cytochrome P450 in one-electron reduction of two quinone imines and concomitant reduction of molecular oxygen. *Biochem Pharmacol* 1987;36:613–619.
228. Kyle ME, Miccadei S, Nakae D, Farber JL. Superoxide dismutase and catalase protect cultured hepatocytes from the cytotoxicity of acetaminophen. *Biochem Biophys Res Commun.* 1987;149:889–896.
229. Wendel A, Feuerstein S. Drug-induced lipid peroxidation in mice. I. Modulation by monooxygenase activity, glutathione and selenium status. *Biochem Pharmacol* 1981;30:2513–2520.
230. Wendel A, Jaeschke H. Drug-induced lipid peroxidation in mice. II. Protection against paracetamol-induced liver necrosis by intravenous liposomally entrapped glutathione. *Biochem Pharmacol* 1982; 31:3601–3605.
231. Albano E, Rundgren M, Harvison PJ, Nelson SD, Moldeus P. Mechanisms of N-acetyl-p-benzoquinone imine cytotoxicity. *Mol Pharmacol* 1985;28:306–311.
232. Harman AW, Adamson GM, Shaw SG. Protection from oxidative damage in mouse liver cells. *Toxicol Lett* 1992;64:581–587.
233. Kyle ME, Nakae D, Serroni A, Farber JL. 1,3-(2-chloroethyl)-1-nitrosurea potentiates the toxicity of acetaminophen both in phenobarbital-induced rat and in hepatocytes cultured from such animals. *Mol Pharmacol* 1988;34:584–589.
234. Harman AW, Kyle ME, Serroni A, Farber JL. The killing of cultured hepatocytes by N-acetyl-p-benzoquinone imine (NAPQI) as a model of the cytotoxicity of acetaminophen. *Biochem Pharmacol* 1991;41:1111–1117.
235. Adamson GM, Harman AW. A role for the glutathione peroxidase/reductase enzyme system in the protection from paracetamol toxicity in isolated mouse hepatocytes. *Biochem Pharmacol* 1989;38:3323–3330.
236. Li QJ, Bessems JGMM, Commandeur JNM, Adams B, Vermeulen NPE. Mechanisms of protection of ebselen against paracetamol-induced toxicity in rat hepatocytes. *Biochem Pharmacol* 1994;48:1631–1640.
237. Prechek D, Birge RB, Tonidandell W, Bruno MK, Cohen SD, Khairallah EA. The protective effects of dithiothreitol (DTT) on acetaminophen hepatotoxicity are associated with a decreased capacity of a cell to rid itself of arylated protein. *The Toxicologist* 1992;12:964.
238. Harman AW. The effectiveness of antioxidants in reducing paracetamol-induced damage subsequent to paracetamol activation. *Res Comm Chem Path Pharmacol* 1985;49:215–228.
239. Kamiyama T, Sato C, Liu J, Tajin K, Miyakawa H, Marumo F. Role of lipid peroxidation in acetaminophen-induced hepatotoxicity: comparison with carbon tetrachloride. *Toxicol Lett* 1993;66:7–12.
240. Smith CV, Mitchell JR. Acetaminophen hepatotoxcity *in vivo* is not accompanied by oxidative stress. *Biochem Biophys Res Comm* 1989;133:329–336.
241. Gupta S, Rogers LK, Smith CV. Inhibition of carbamyl phosphate synthetase (CPS1) by hepatotoxic doses of acetaminophen (AP) in mice. *The Toxicologist* 1995;15:53.
242. Mitchell DB, Acosta D, Bruckner JV. Role of glutathione depletion in the cytotoxicity of acetaminophen in a primary culture system of rat hepatocytes. *Toxicology* 1995;37:127–146.
243. Jaeschke H. Glutathione disulfide formation and oxidative stress during acetaminophen-induced hepatotoxicity in mice in vivo: the protective effect of allopurinol. *J Pharmacol Exp Ther* 1990;255:935–941.
244. Harman AW, Maxwell MJ. An evaluation of the role of calcium in cell injury. *Ann Rev Pharmacol Toxicol* 1995;35:129–144.
245. Schanne FAX, Kane AB, Young EE, Farber JL. Calcium dependence on toxic cell death: a final common pathway. *Science* 1979;206:700–702.
246. Trump BF, Berezesky IK. Calcium-mediated cell injury and cell death. *FASEB J* 1995;9:219–228.
247. Orrenius S, McConkey DJ, Bellomo G, Nicotera P. Role of calcium in toxic cell killing. *Trends Pharmacol Sci* 1989;10:281–285.
248. Reed DJ. Review of the current status of calcium and thiols in cellular injury. *Chem Res Toxicol* 1990;3:495–502.
249. Farber JL. The role of calcium in lethal cell injury. *Chem Res Toxicol* 1990;3;503–16.

250. Fawthrop DJ, Boobis AR, Davies DS. Mechanisms of cell death. *Arch Toxicol* 1991;65:437–444.

251. Jewell SA, Bellomo G, Thor H, Orrenius S. Bleb formation in hepatocytes during drug metabolism is caused by disturbances in thiol and calcium ion heomeostasis. *Science* 1982;217:1257–1259.

252. Chien KR, Pfau RG, Farber JL. Ischemic myocardial cell injury:prevention by chlorpromazine of an accelerated degradation and associated membrane dysfunction. *Am J Pathol* 1979;97:505–530.

253. Nicotera P, Hartzell P, Baldi C, Svensson SA, Bellomo G, Orrenius S. *J Biol Chem* 1986;261:14628–14635.

254. Moore M, Thor H, Moore G, Nelson SD, Moldéus P, Orrenius S. The toxicity of acetaminophen and N-acetyl-benzoquinone imine in isolated hepatocytes is associated with thiol depletion and increased cytosolic Ca^{2+}. *J Biol Chem* 1985;260:13035–13040.

255. Long RM, Moore L. Evaluation of the calcium mobilizing action in acetaminophen and bromobenzene in rat hepatocyte culture. *J Biochem Toxicol* 1988;3:353–362.

256. Tsokos-Kuhn JO. Evidence in vivo for elevation of intracellular free calcium in the liver after diquat. *Biochem Pharmacol* 1989;38:3061–3065.

257. Corcoran GB, Bauer JA, Lau TWD. Immediate rise in intracellular calcium and glycogen phosphory-lase a activities upon acetaminophen covalent binding leading to hepatotoxicity in mice. *Toxicology* 1988;50:151–167.

258. Harman AW, Mahar SO, Burcham PC, Madsen BW. Level of cytosolic free calcium during acetaminophen toxicity. *Mol Pharmacol* 1992;1:655–667.

259. Tsokos-Kuhn JO, Hughes H, Smith CV, Mitchell JR. Alkylation of the liver plasma membrane and inhibition of the Ca^{2+} ATPase by acetaminophen. *Biochem Pharmacol* 1988;37:2125–2131.

260. Tirmenstein MA, Nelson SD. Acetaminophen-induced oxidation of protein thiols: contribution of impaired thiol metabolizing enzymes and the breakdown of adenine nucleotides. *J Biol Chem* 1990;265:3059–3065.

261. Weis M, Moore GA, Cotgreave IA, Nelson SD, Moldeus P. Quinone imine-induced Ca^{2+} release from isolated rat liver mitochondria. *Chem Biol Interactions* 1990;76:227–240.

262. Grewal KK, Racz WJ. Intracellular calcium disruption as a secondary event in acetaminophen-induced hepatotoxicity. *Can J Physiol Pharmacol* 1993;71:26–33.

263. Boobis AR, Seddon CE, Nasseri-Sina P, Davies DS. Evidence for a direct role of intracellular calcium in paracetamol toxicity. *Biochem Pharmacol* 1990;39:1277–1281.

264. Carpenter-Deyo L, Reed DJ. Involvement of calcium and iron in quin-2 toxicity to isolated hepatocytes. *J Pharmacol Exp Ther* 1991;258:747–752.

265. Schnellman RG. Intracellular calcium chelators and oxidant-induced renal proximal tubule cell death. *J Biochem Toxicol* 1991;6:209–303.

266. Smith CV, Mitchell JR, Horning EC. Covalent binding of reactive metabolites of acetaminophen and furosemide to hepatic DNA, RNA and protein *in vivo*. *The Pharmacologist* 1978;20:258.

267. Dybing E, Holme JA, Gordon WP, Siderlund EJ, Dahlin DC, Nelson SD. Genotoxicity studies with paracetamol. *Mutation Res* 1984;138:21–32.

268. Rogers LK, Smith CV. Acetaminophen (AP) at therapeutic doses (for humans) covalently binds to DNA in mice. *Fundam Appl Toxicol* 1996;31:282.

269. Rannug U, Holme JA, Hongslo JK, Srám R. An evaluation of the genetic toxicity of paracetamol. *Mutation Res* 1995;327:179–200.

270. Hongslo JK, Bjørnstad C, Schwarze PE, Holme JA. Inhibition of replicative DNA synthesis by paracetamol in V79 Chinese hamster cells. *Toxicol In Vitro* 1989;3:13–20.

271. Navarro C, Cohen SD, Khairallah EA. Acetaminophen administration alters rate of cell replication in hepatoma cells without activation of drug by cytochrome P450. *FASEB J* 1994;8:A1468.

272. Ray SD, Sorge CL, Raucy JL, Corcoran GB. Early loss of large genomic DNA *in vivo* with accumu-lation of Ca^{2+} in the nucleus during acetaminophen-induced liver injury. *Toxicol Appl Pharmacol* 1990;106:346–351.

273. Shen W, Kamendulis LM, Ray SD, Corcoran GB. Acetaminophen-induced cytotoxicity in cultured mouse hepatocytes: correlation of nuclear Ca^{2+} accumulation and early DNA fragmentation and cell death. *Toxicol Appl Pharmacol* 1991;111:242–254.

274. Harris SR, Hamrick ME. Antagonism of acetaminophen hepatotoxicity by phospholipase A2 inhibitors. *Res Commun Chem Pathol Pharmacol* 1993;79:23–44.

275. Shen W, Kamendulis LM, Ray SD, Corcoran GB. Acetaminophen-induced cytotoxicity in cultured mouse hepatocytes: effects of Ca^{2+}-endonuclease, DNA repair, and glutathione depletion inhibitors on DNA fragmentation and cell death. *Toxicol Appl Pharmacol* 1992;112:32–40.

276. Kamendulis LM, Corcoran GB. Further evidence that DNA is a critical target in toxic cell death: Effects of DNA repair inhibitors on acetaminophen toxicity in cultured mouse hepatocytes. *ISSX Pro* 1993;4:154.
277. Laskin DL, Pilaro AM. Potential role of activated macrophages in acetaminophen hepatotoxicity. I. Isolation and characterization of activated macrophages from rat liver. *Toxicol Appl Pharmacol* 1986;86:204–215.
278. Laskin DL, Pilaro AM, Ji S. Potential role of activated macrophages in acetaminophen hepatotoxicity. II. Mechanism of macrophage accumulation and activation. *Toxicol Appl Pharmacol* 1986;86:216–226.
279. Laskin DL, Gardner CR, Todaro JA, Price V, Jollow D. Modulation of macrophage functioning abrogates the acute hepatotoxicity of acetaminophen. *Hepatology* 1995;21:1045–1050.
280. El Sisi AE, Earnest DL, Sipes IG. Vitamin A potentiation of carbon tetrachloride hepatotoxicity: role of liver macrophages and active oxygen species. *Toxicol Appl Pharmacol* 1993;119:295–301.
281. Rosengren RJ, Sauer JM, Hooser SB, Sipes IG. The interactions between retinol and five different hepatotoxicants in the Swiss Webster Mouse. *Fundam Appl Toxicol* 1995;25:281–292.
282. Takada H, Mawet E, Shiratori Y, Hikiba Y, Nakata R, Yoshida H, Okano K, Kamii K, Omata M. Chemotactic factors released from hepatocytes exposed to acetaminophen. *Dig Dis Sci* 1995;40:1831–1836.
283. Laskin DL. Nonparenchymal cells and hepatotoxicity. *Semin Liver Dis* 1990;10:293–304.
284. Blaszka ME, Wilmer JL, Holladay SD, Wilson RE, Luster MI. Role of proinflamatory cytokines in acetaminophen hepatotoxicity. *Toxicol Appl Pharmacol* 1995;133:43–52.
285. Blaszka ME, Elwell MR, Holladay SD, Wilson RE, Luster MI. Histopathology of acetaminophen-induced liver changes: role of interleukin 1α and tumor necrosis factor α. *Toxicol Pathol* 1996;24:181–189.
286. Bailie MB, Scozzaro AJ, Jean PA, Ganey PE, Roth RA. Gadolinium chloride attenuates acetaminophen hepatotoxicity in mice. *The Toxicologist* 1995;15:219.
287. Best WS, Hoivik DJ, Manautou JE, Hart SGE, Khairallah EA, Cohen SD. Methyl palmitate (MP) diminishes selective protein arylation and protects against acetaminophen (APAP) hepatotoxicity in male CD-1 mice. *Fundam Appl Toxicol* 1996;30:280.
288. Mourelle M, Beales D, McLean AE. Electron transport and protection of liver slices in the late stage of paracetamol injury. *Biochem Pharmacol* 1990;40:2023–2028.

Toxicology of the Liver, 2nd ed.,
Edited by Gabriel L. Plaa and William R. Hewitt
Copyright © 1998 Taylor & Francis

6

Evaluation of Chemical-Induced Oxidative Stress as a Mechanism of Hepatocyte Death

Donald J. Reed

Oregon State University, Corvallis, OR 97331

- **Oxidative Stress**
  - Aerobic Metabolism: Endogenous Oxidative Stress
  - Redox Cycling of Chemicals
  - Hepatocellular Injury by Redox Cycling
- **Glutathione as a Cellular Protective Agent**
  - Role of Glutathione
  - Cysteine Biosynthesis via the Cystathionine Pathway
  - Organelle Glutathione
  - Mitochondria as Targets of Oxidants
- **Chemical Depletion of Glutathione**
  - Depletion of Glutathione by Fasting
  - Glutathione Compartmentation and Chemical-Induced Injury
  - Glutathione Reductase and Glutathione Peroxidase
  - Glutathione Redox Cycle
- **Cellular Changes During Chemical-Induced Injury**
- **Mitochondrial Permeability Transition**
  - Mitochondrial Glutathione as Marker
  - Induction Within Cells
- **Chemical-Induced Apoptosis**
- **Evaluation of Oxidative Stress**
- **Conclusions**
- **References**

In this chapter we will evaluate the contribution of chemical-induced oxidative stress as a mechanism of hepatocyte death. The hypothesis we will discuss here is that chemical-induced cell injury in part is the result of oxidative stress related to the effects of chemicals on the metabolism of molecular oxygen. Oxygen is metabolized to oxygen-containing reactive intermediates, many of which can undergo a cycling process between oxidation and reduction. This process is known as redox cycling and causes a form of oxidative stress in cells. Such oxidative stress can cause oxidation of cellular constituents such as low-molecular-weight thiol-containing compounds including glutathione, protein thiols, and other functional groups on macromolecules and peroxidation of lipids and other susceptible cellular constituents. It is now known that many chemicals can undergo both bioactivation to form biologic reactive intermediates that bind to macromolecules and also enhance the formation of oxygen radicals with a concomitant oxidative stress. Covalent binding of biologic reactive intermediates to cellular molecules to form stable adducts is a dominant mechanism for loss of control of genetic functions and expression. Therefore, the evolution of bioactivation processes that form biologic reactive intermediates is thought to have necessitated the concomitant evolution of cellular protection systems for cell survival in an oxygen-containing atmosphere. Cellular injury processes have reversible and irreversible features that are a consequence of the interplay of bioactivation and oxidative stress with the cellular protective systems that prevent or limit cellular injury and possibly repair. Reversible injury occurs even with chemicals known as "safe" chemicals. Dose is the determining factor of whether any chemical causes irreversible injury. Such irreversible injury may cause cell death regardless of what antidotal or preventive measures are taken after exposure of cell or tissues to a sufficient dose of the toxic chemical. The actual time of death of a cell is difficult to assess, but, in general terms, it can include death being at the time that loss of cellular integrity occurred to such a degree that free exchange between the intracellular constituents and the surrounding milieu prevents cell survival. We review here oxidative stress and the mechanisms by which cells are protected by preventing or limiting cellular damage.

Any model of cell death should include a role for calcium ions; whether calcium ions are important initiators of cell death is uncertain. Assuming that chemical-induced injury must occur initially, then the potential for alteration of calcium ion homeostasis to contribute to cell death is very great. Almost every aspect of cell function is associated in some manner with the status and functions of calcium ions. Again, what is much less certain is the role of the various major compartments for calcium ion sequestration in the events associated with cell injury. For example, with normal physiologic conditions, liver mitochondria do not appear to have a major role in the control of intracellular calcium ion concentrations. However, under pathologic conditions, the loss of calcium storage ability by other sites in the cell will cause the mitochondria to become highly involved in the uptake of calcium ions and may even initiate calcium recycling. Whether calcium ion recycling occurs or not, the ability of mitochondria to take up calcium ions is enormous and has the potential of major alterations in not only the inner membrane potential but also the availability of a protonmotive force for ATP synthesis, ion homeostasis, and other functions. Of course, loss of cellular integrity has the potential of allowing even greater amounts of calcium to be available from exogenous sources and can eliminate the ability of the cell to cope with the total amount of calcium ion that must be regulated by sequestration. Overall, the effects of oxidative stress include the potential loss of homeostasis of cellular thiols and free calcium ion regulation.

OXIDATIVE STRESS

The production of oxygen free radicals was not of biologic consequence until 1969, when McCord and Fridovich (1) discovered that superoxide dismutase exists in essentially every mammalian cell, suggesting ubiquitous superoxide formation in vivo. Later, oxygen free radicals were linked to inflammatory disease states, and the imbalance between proxidants and antioxidants was defined as oxidative stress (2).

A major concept developed during the past 10 years is that a mechanism for chemical-induced hepatocyte death could be based upon oxidative stress. This advance in our knowledge is in part due to the many new findings that have been reported about reactive oxygen intermediates (ROIs) and cell defenses. Targets of oxidants have been identified and intracellular events described in detail. Inflammation that is based on cytokines and stress responses has added dimensions to various types of liver injury, nonhepatic diseases, immune function, and HIV. A major discovery has been the oxidative events associated with ischemia and reperfusion. Liver diseases including alcoholic liver disease, metal storage diseases, and chloestatic liver disease have been described in terms of an oxidative stress component. Therefore, an appropriate theme for this chapter is the description of chemical-induced hepatocyte injury and death involving a mechanism based on the pathologic effects of oxidative stress.

The occurrence of reactive oxygen species in normal metabolism of mammalian organs was first demonstrated in the liver (3). Rates of hydrogen peroxide production of 50–100 nmol/min per gram of liver under normal conditions could be enhanced up to sevenfold in the presence of substrates for peroxisomal oxidases (4, 5). Subsequently, it was shown that oxidative stress-induced hepatocyte injury may accompany metabolism of chemicals to biologic reactive intermediates. From these studies came the concept that a disbalance in the prooxidant/antioxidant steady state, potentially leading to damage, is termed *oxidative stress* (2). The loss of control of endogenous oxidative events related to the use of molecular oxygen by the cell is the major factor in oxidative stress injury. Such a process, which is known as chemical-induced oxidative stress, may occur to an extent that ranges from a minor to a major contribution to overall toxicity. For example, chemicals that are known to undergo redox cycling cause exogenous oxidative stress to such a degree that they play a major role in chemical-induced cell injury. In addition, some of these chemicals are known to form adducts with cellular constituents, particularly proteins that are necessary for protection against oxygen toxicity. However, as indicated above, all tissues and cells contain systems for detoxification of biologic reactive intermediates and antioxidants and antioxidant enzyme systems to prevent or limit cellular damage due to oxidative stress events.

Normal fluxes of prooxidants serve useful functions at the cellular and whole-organism levels and therefore need to be balanced with sufficient antioxidant defense to maintain a biologic steady state. For example, the continual formation of reactive oxygen species is a physiologic necessity and an unavoidable consequence of oxygen metabolism. When reactive oxygen species are generated in excess, they can be toxic, particularly in the presence of transition metal ions such as iron or copper (6). However, defense systems are present and functioning under normal conditions Therefore, endogenous free radicals do not necessarily place biologic tissues and

TABLE 1. *Factors responsible for oxidative stress*

Superoxide and hydrogen peroxide production in mitochondria.
Redox cycling agent production of superoxide.
Transition metal activation of oxygen species.
Loss of calcium homeostasis leading to calcium recycling.
Stimulation of production of arachidonic acid and prostaglandins.

cells at risk. Chemical exposures can cause these defense systems to be overwhelmed during various pathologic conditions, including anoxia, radiation, and loss of control of both intracellular and extracellular constituents such as calcium (Table 1).

It is estimated that nearly 90% of the total O_2 consumed by mammalian species is delivered to mitochondria, where a four-electron reduction to H_2O by the respiratory chain is coupled to ATP synthesis (5, 7). Nearly 4% of mitochondrial O_2 is incompletely reduced by leakage of electrons along the respiratory chain, especially at ubiquinone, forming reactive oxygen species such as superoxide ($O_2^{\bullet}$), hydrogen peroxide (H_2O_2), singlet oxygen, and hydroxyl radical ($HO^{\bullet}$) (5, 7). Richter (8) calculated that during normal metabolism, one rat liver mitochondrion produces 3×10^7 superoxide radicals per day. Specific sources of reactive oxygen species are listed in Table 2. It is estimated that superoxide and hydrogen peroxide steady state concentrations are in the picomolar and nanomolar range, respectively (9). Jones et al. (10) estimated the hepatocyte steady state H_2O_2 concentration to be up to 25 μM. These events are thought to contribute over 85% of the free radical production in mammalian species. Sohal (11) has concluded that there is a variation in the sites of superoxide or hydrogen peroxide generation among mitochondria from different tissues and species. This is a result of the rate of mitochondrial superoxide production being dependent on at least three variables: (1) ambient oxygen concentration; (2) levels of autoxidizable respiratory carriers, especially ubiquinone; and (3) the redox state of the autoxidizable carriers (5, 9, 11–13).

Aerobic Metabolism: Endogenous Oxidative Stress

If endogenously formed H_2O_2 is not detoxified to H_2O, formation of the $HO^{\bullet}$ by a metal (iron)-catalyzed Haber Weiss or Fenton reaction can occur (Equations 1A

TABLE 2. *Specific sources of reactive oxygen species involved in pathogenic oxidative stress in the liver*

Mitochondrial electron transport system.
Stimulated phagocytic cells.
Nonphagocytic cells being promoted during metabolism of xenobiotics.
Induction of prooxidant enzymes including xanthine oxidase.
Ubiquinone semiquinone and other redox cycling agents.
Induction of fatty acid CoA oxidases by peroxisome proliferators.
Ischemia/reperfusion.
Inhibition of antioxidant enzymes.
Loss of homeostasis of calcium and transition metals.
Ionizing radiation.

and 1B) (14). The HO• species is one of the most reactive and short-lived biologic radicals and has the potential to initiate lipid peroxidation of biologic membranes (14, 15), although not as effectively as other radicals including the ROO• radical (16). Unless termination reactions occur, the process of lipid peroxidation will propagate, resulting in potentially high levels of oxidative stress. Therefore, detoxification of endogenously produced H_2O_2 is critical for redox maintenance of mitochondrial as well as cellular homeostasis.

Haber Weiss reaction

$$O_2^{\bullet} + H_2O_2 + Fe^{+3} \rightarrow Fe^{2+} + O_2 + OH^- + HO^{\bullet} \tag{1A}$$

Fenton reaction

$$H_2O_2 + Fe^{+2} \rightarrow Fe^{+3} + HO^{\bullet} \tag{1B}$$

Other reactive oxygen species of biologic relevance include singlet oxygen ($^1O_2$), hypochlorous acid (HOCl), and nitric oxide (NO). Thus, several reactive oxygen species can be formed by one-electron step reductions of molecular oxygen and spontaneous reactions with nitric oxide, including the formation of the oxidant peroxynitrite (Fig. 1).

Redox Cycling of Chemicals

Toxicity by hepatotoxic chemicals can be classified as either direct or indirect, with direct-acting agents displaying dose-dependent damage based on inherent toxicity. Indirect-acting agents would, for example, alter immune function (18). Direct-acting agents generally undergo one or two electron changes during metabolism and may

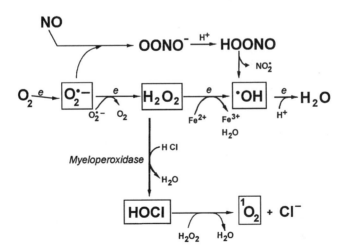

FIG. 1. Reactive oxygen species formed by one-electron reductions of molecular oxygen. Adapted from Jaeschke (17).

cause oxidative stress as a component of their toxicity. Examples of such chemicals are bromobenzene, carbon tetrachloride, ethanol, paraquat, diquat, menadione, and iron loading (19). Drugs that can undergo redox cycling include anthracyclines such as adriamycin, mitomycin C, bleomycin, β-lapachone, alloxan, acetaminophen, and the radiosensitizers, e.g., misonidazole and metronidazole (20). It is now known that activation of oxygen by reduction can play an important role in the toxicity of these drugs and chemicals. In general, they are enzymatically reduced or oxidized by a one-electron transfer. After a one-electron redox reaction, the intermediate formed then transfers the extra one electron to molecular oxygen to yield the superoxide anion radical and the parent drug or chemical, which can undergo repeated one-electron reduction or oxidation to then provide one electron to molecular oxygen. This process of generation of reactive oxygen species, termed *redox cycling*, is involved in the toxicity of many hydroquinones, quinones, metal chelates, nitro compounds, amines, and azo compounds (20).

In general, chemical toxicity compromises the ability of cellular processes to detoxify endogenous oxidative events related to oxygen metabolism. Further, the inherent toxicity of many chemicals includes the ability to produce additional oxidative stress, which can then become a dominant component of the overall toxicity.

Hepatocellular Injury by Redox Cycling

The evolution of bioactivation processes that form biologic reactive intermediates, both free radical and ionic, probably necessitated the concomitant evolution of cellular defense and repair systems for cell survival. All tissues and cells contain defense systems for detoxification of biologic reactive intermediates and to prevent or limit cellular damage. Formation of hydrogen peroxide leads to the consumption of reduced glutathione (GSH) as glutathione peroxidase activity transforms the hydrogen peroxide to water and GSH to glutathione disulfide (GSSG), which is then reduced by an NADPH (reduced nicotinamide adenine dinucleotide phosphate)-dependent enzyme, glutathione reductase. Whether certain chemicals may cause both reactive intermediate effects such as covalent binding and redox cycling stress is being examined in some detail with the classes of compounds mentioned above.

Diquat (DQ), a bipyridyl herbicide that is hepatotoxic, is a model compound for redox cycling. It generates large amounts of superoxide anion radical hydrogen peroxide within cells. Jaeschke and Benzick (21) reported that isolated perfused rat liver when treated with diquat (200 μM) in the perfusate could generate 1 μmole/min per gram of liver of superoxide. These workers observed that only after depletion of GSH (10% of control) with phorone pretreatment (200 mg/kg body weight) and either ferrous sulfate (100 mg/kg) or BCNU (40 mg/kg) was it possible to significantly increase the diquat-induced liver injury. These findings support other evidence of the protective role of the glutathione redox cycle in the toxicity of diquat in vivo and in vitro. Since diquat toxicity is mediated by redox cycling, it is greatly enhanced by prior treatment with BCNU (22), an inhibitor of glutathione reductase

(23). Ebselen, a synthetic compound possessing glutathione peroxidaselike activity, protects against diquat cytotoxicity when extracellular glutathione is present in the medium (24). Superoxide, which can reduce ferric iron to ferrous iron, is produced during diquat toxicity. Desferrioxamine, which chelates intracellular iron in the ferric state with an affinity constant of 10^{31} (25), provides considerable protection against diquat-induced toxicity. Therefore, hydrogen peroxide and transition metals have been suggested as major contributors to diquat toxicity (25). Even though the hydroxyl radical or a related species seems the most likely ultimate toxic product of the hydrogen peroxide/ferrous iron interaction, scavengers of hydroxyl radical afford only minimal protection (25). The high degree of reactivity of hydroxyl radicals assures, however, that the site of interaction with cellular components is within close proximity (a few angstroms) of the site of generation of the radical. Much remains to be understood about the mechanism of cytotoxicity by the various redox cycling agents including the quinones, menadione, and adriamycin, which are discussed in more detail below.

Menadione has been studied as a redox cycling agent for the generation of oxidative stress in vivo and in vitro. Fischer-Nielsen and coworkers (26) have reported that isolated rat hepatocytes undergo profound glutathione depletion with 25–400 μM menadione but that the oxidative stress induced DNA fragmentation as demonstrated by a ladder of DNA fragments on agarose gel electrophoresis was not accompanied by increased 8-oxodG formation. These results support apoptotic cell injury and death with the depletion of glutathione as an early event.

During their metabolism, many drugs and other chemicals involve the cellular production of radical oxygen species that participate in lipid peroxidation. For example, nonsteroidal antiinflammatory drugs including naproxen and acetaminophen have been shown to undergo metabolism that causes a decrease in glutathione, enhanced lipid peroxidation and alteration of cellular proteins. A major question is whether the events of cell injury and death include apoptotic processes that limit the necrotic features of cell death.

t-Butylhydroperoxide (TBH) is widely utilized to investigate the mechanisms of cell injury initiated by oxidative stress. Although the mechanism remains unknown, lipid peroxidation and altered thiol status are implicated as components (2, 27–30). Evidence has been presented that supports the hypothesis that the mitochondrial permeability transition can occur under conditions of oxidative stress and contribute to the mechanism of cell death (29). Importantly, cyclosporin A (CsA), a high-activity inhibitor of the transition, prolongs survival of hepatocytes treated with TBH under conditions where extensive lipid peroxidation is prevented (29). Nieminen et al. (30) have concluded that during oxidative stress induced by TBH treatment cultured hepatocytes displayed the characteristics of permeability transition, which quickly lead to mitochondrial depolarization and cell death.

The mechanism of acetaminophen-induced hepatotoxicity involves contributions by covalent binding and oxidative stress as indicated by the protective role of glutathione (31) (Fig. 2). The toxicity of acetaminophen in vitro and in vivo is with GSH depletion and formation of GSSG due to the bioactivation of acetaminophen

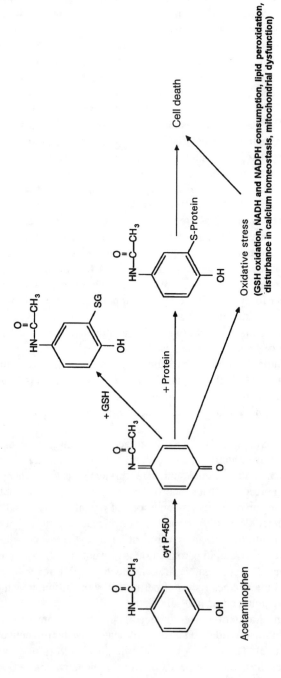

FIG. 2. Proposed mechanisms for the hepatotoxicity induced by the reactive metabolite of acetaminophen.

to the reactive metabolite N-acetyl-p-benzoquinone imine, which is both an electrophile and an oxidizing agent (32). Although recent evidence indicates acetaminophen covalent binding is the primary mechanism of toxicity (33), ample evidence supports an oxidative stress mechanism that is accompanied by lipid peroxidation-associated hepatic injury (34–36). Acetaminophen (500 mg/kg intraperitoneally) increased the mitochondrial GSSG content from 2% in controls to greater than 20% in treated animals. It is known that GSSG does not efflux from mitochondria and must be reduced back to GSH by mitochondria-derived reducing equivalents (37). Therefore, if levels of GSSG approach 20% in treated animals, then the ability to maintain mitochondrial integrity is in question as loss of calcium regulation potentiates the mitochondria for undergoing permeability transition (38). BCNU (1,3-bis(2-chloroethyl)-1-nitrosourea) increases the susceptibility of hepatocytes to oxidative stress (23) and increased both the formation of GSSG and cell killing produced by acetaminophen (36).

These findings strongly support the concept that oxidative stress is an important mechanism that can be the basis for chemical-induced hepatocyte injury and death. Although exposure to many chemicals causes enhanced hydrogen peroxide production by hepatocytes, especially after GSH depletion, it is not known whether the enhanced hydrogen peroxide exerts its toxicity by promoting lipid peroxidation or eliminating the reducing equivalents that modulate calcium effects (39). Only by an adequate antioxidant defense can such effects be either limited or prevented. Glutathione is a major component in antioxidant defense and is described below.

GLUTATHIONE AS A CELLULAR PROTECTIVE AGENT

Role of Glutathione

All living organisms have evolved protective systems to minimize injurious events that result from bioactivation of chemicals including xenobiotics (40) and oxidative products of cellular metabolism of molecular oxygen (41) (Fig. 3). The major protective system is dependent upon the unique tripeptide, glutathione (GSH) (42). GSH acts as both a nucleophilic scavenger of numerous compounds and their metabolites, via enzymatic and chemical mechanisms, converting electrophilic centers to thioether bonds, and as a cofactor in the GSH peroxidase-mediated destruction of hydroperoxides. GSH depletion to about 15–20% of total glutathione levels can impair the cell's defense against the toxic actions of such compounds and may lead to cell injury and death (41, 43–45). The key to the evaluation of oxidative stress as a mechanism for chemical-induced hepatocyte death is that the consumption of oxygen even during normal environmental conditions requires a considerable amount of cellular resources on a constant basis to detoxify toxic oxygen metabolites. If not reduced, these metabolites can lead to the formation of very reactive radicals including the hydroxyl radical and cause the formation of lipid hydroperoxides that can damage membranes, nucleic acids, proteins, and their functions. Failure to provide or maintain

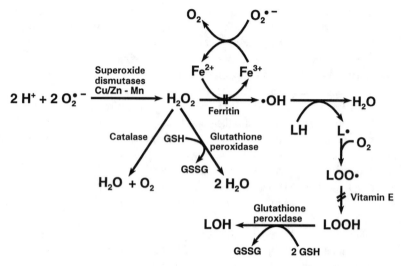

FIG. 3. Cellular defense systems for the metabolism and inactivation of reactive oxygen species (ROS).

the cellular protective systems is now known to cause serious human diseases that can be greatly exacerbated by exposures to toxic chemicals.

Depending on the cell type, the intracellular concentration of glutathione is maintained in the range of 0.5–10 mM (46). Concentrations in the liver are 4–8 mM. Nearly all the glutathione is present as GSH. Less than 5% of the total is present as GSSG. This is so because of the redox status of glutathione that is maintained by intracellular GSH reductase and NADPH. Continual endogenous production of reduced oxygen species, including hydrogen peroxide and lipid hydroperoxides, causes constant production of some GSSG, however. The GSH content of various organs and tissues represents at least 90% of the total nonprotein, low-molecular-weight thiols. The liver content of GSH is nearly twice that found in kidney and testes and over threefold greater than in the lung. The importance of hepatic GSH for protection against reactive intermediates has been reviewed extensively (47, 48). However, additional information about the status of GSH in mammalian tissues continues to be reported. The high concentration (up to 7–8 mM) of GSH in the glandular tissue of the stomach, as compared with the squamous portion or other portions of the gastrointestinal tract, has been suggested to account for the resistance of the glandular portion of the stomach to certain carcinogens as compared with the squamous portion, which is highly susceptible to induction of tumors by polycylic aromatic hydrocarbons (49).

Cysteine Biosynthesis via the Cystathionine Pathway

Cysteine has a sparing effect on the requirement of the essential amino acid methionine in the rat (50). This observation is in agreement with the unidirectional process of transsulfuration, in which methionine sulfur and serine carbon are utilized in cysteine biosynthesis via the cystathionine pathway (47, 51).

The cystathionine pathway is of major importance to pathways of drug metabolism that involve GSH or cysteine or both (Fig. 4). Depletion of GSH by rapid conjugation can increase synthesis of GSH to rates as high as 2–3 μmoles/hr per gram of wet liver tissue (52). The cysteine pool in the liver, which is about 0.2 μmole/g, has an estimated half-life of 2–3 min at such high rates of synthesis of GSH (47). Although the cystathionine pathway appears to be highly responsive to the need for cysteine biosynthesis in the liver, the organ distribution of the pathway may be limited. Evidence indicates that in mammals, such as rats, the liver is the main site of cysteine biosynthesis, which occurs via the cystathionine pathway. Maintenance of high concentrations of GSH in the liver, in association with high rates of secretion into plasma and extensive extracellular degradation of GSH and GSSG, supports the concept that liver GSH is a physiologic reservoir of cysteine. This idea was proposed originally by Tateishi et al. (53) and Higashi et al. (54).

The concentration of GSH in the liver is altered in rats by diurnal or circadian variations and by starvation. The diurnal variation in hepatic GSH results in the highest levels of GSH at night and early morning and the lowest levels in the late afternoon. The maximum variation is as much as 25–30% (49, 55, 56). Starvation limits the availability of methionine for synthesis of GSH in the liver and decreases the concentration of GSH by about 50% of the level in fed animals (55, 57, 58). Assuming GSH is a physiologic reservoir for plasma cysteine (54), efflux of GSH from liver will continue during starvation, and the released cysteine will help maintain levels of GSH in other organs, including the kidney.

In vivo treatment of rats with an inhibitor of γ-glutamyltransferase, L-(α5, 5δ)-α-amino-3-chloro-4, 5-dihydro-5-isoxazoleacetic acid (AT-125) prevents degradation of GSH in plasma leading to massive urinary excretion of GSH (59). This treatment also lowers the hepatic content of GSH because it inhibits recycling of cysteine to the liver (60). A physiologic decrease in interorgan recycling of cysteine to the liver for synthesis of GSH also may account in part for the decrease of hepatic GSH during starvation and for the marked diurnal variation in concentration of GSH in liver. As mentioned, the nadir occurs in the late afternoon, whereas the early morning peak occurs shortly after the animals are fed (55, 57, 58).

The efflux of liver GSH and metabolism of the resulting plasma GSH and GSSG appear to help insure a continuous supply of plasma cysteine. This cysteine pool should in turn minimize the degree of fluctuation of GSH concentrations within the various body organs and cell types that require cysteine or cystine, or both, rather than methionine for synthesis of GSH.

Organelle Glutathione

Compartmentation of glutathione has been demonstrated in that a separate pool of glutathione exist in the cytoplasm from that in the mitochondria (Fig. 4). A separate pool has been proposed for the nucleus; however, that finding is in dispute. Mitochondrial

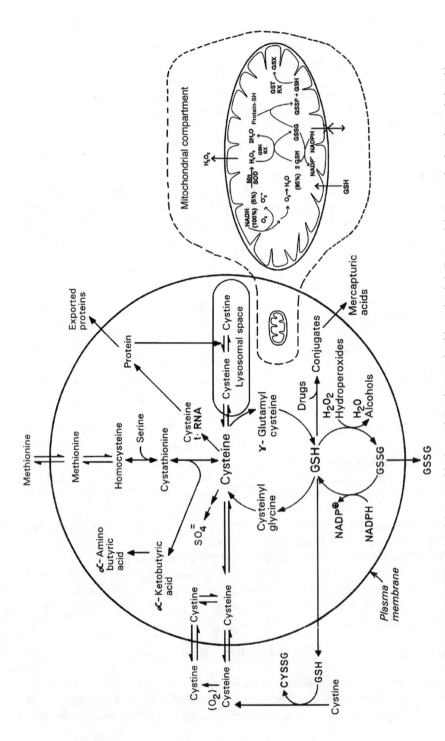

FIG. 4. Glutathione biosynthesis and the cystathionine pathway for cysteine biosynthesis in liver and the protective functions of glutathione.

198

glutathione is a separate physiologic pool of glutathione in agreement with the observation that the liver has two pools of GSH. One has a fast (2-hr) and the other a slow (30-hr) turnover (54, 61). Meredith and Reed (60) observed that in freshly isolated rat hepatocytes the mitochondrial pool of GSH (about 10% of the total cellular pool) had a half-life of 30 hr while the half-life of the cytoplasmic pool was 2 hr and concluded that the mitochondrial pool might represent the stable pool of GSH observed in whole animals.

Mitochondrial GSH functions as a discrete pool separate from cytosolic GSH. A report by Jocelyn (62) demonstrated that mitochondrial GSH is impermeable to the inner membrane following isolation of mitochondria, and Wahlländer et al. (63) reported that the concentration of mitochondrial GSH (10 mM) is higher than that of cytosolic GSH (7 mM). Studies by Meredith and Reed (60) demonstrated different rates of GSH turnover in the cytosol and mitochondria, confirming the existence of separate intracellular GSH pools. The ratio of GSH:GSSG in mitochondria is approximately 10:1 under normal (untreated) conditions. Unlike cytosolic GSSG, mitochondrial GSSG is not effluxed from the matrix compartment as reported by Olafsdottir and Reed (37). This study demonstrated that during oxidative stress induced with t-butylhydroperoxide, GSSG is accumulated in the mitochondrial matrix and eventually reduced back to GSH. However, as the redox state of the mitochondria increased, an increase in protein-mixed disulfides was also observed. This study concluded that mitochondria are more sensitive to redox changes in GSH:GSSG than the cytosol and that mitochondria may therefore be more susceptible to the damaging effects of oxidative stress. These findings suggest that under certain experimental conditions, irreversible cell injury due to oxidative challenge may result from irreversible changes in mitochondrial function.

Since rat liver mitochondria contain the enzymes and cofactors necessary for the GSH/GSSG redox cycle (64) (Fig. 5) but do not contain catalase (65), we may assume that a primary function of mitochondrial glutathione (GSH) is for the detoxification of endogenously produced H_2O_2. This redox cycle requires the enzymes GSH peroxidase (selenium-containing) and GSSG reductase along with the cofactors GSH and NADPH. In addition to detoxifying H_2O_2, GSH also protects protein sulfhydryls from oxidation (66).

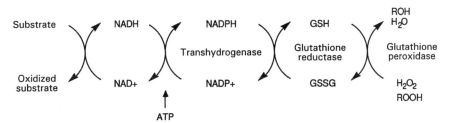

FIG. 5. Mitochondrial glutathione redox cycle and oxidative stress.

Mitochondria as Targets of Oxidants

Studies addressing mitochondria as target organelles of certain types of irreversible cell injury, as related to oxidative stress as well as disrupted Ca^{2+} homeostasis, represent an area of intense investigation (67–71). GSH-dependent protection against lipid peroxidation has been demonstrated in mitochondria, nuclei, microsomes, and cytosol of rat liver. Lipid peroxidation induced in mitochondria is inhibited by respiratory substrates such as succinate, which leads indirectly to reduction of ubiquinone to ubiquinol. The latter is a potent antioxidant (72, 73). The essential factor in preventing accumulation of lipid peroxides and lysis of membranes in mitochondria, however, is glutathione peroxidase (64). Although the prevention of free radical attack on membrane lipids may occur by an electron shuttle that utilizes vitamin E and GSH in microsomes, similar activity may not be capable of inhibiting peroxidation in mitochondria (74, 75). Instead, mitochondrial GSH transferase(s) may prevent lipid peroxidation in mitochondria by a nonselenium glutathione-dependent peroxidase activity. Three GSH transferases have been isolated from the mitochondrial matrix (76), and nearly 5% of the mitochondrial outer membrane protein consists of microsomal glutathione transferase (77). GSH transferase in the outer mitochondrial membrane could provide the GSH-dependent protection of mitochondria by scavenging lipid radicals by a mechanism that requires vitamin E and is abolished by bromosulfophthalein (77).

A very important discovery is a previously unrecognized effect of mitochondrial oxidative stress and mitochondrial GSH defense on transcription factor activation (39). Not only can oxidant stress in mitochondria promote the loss of mitochondrial GSH and mitochondrial functions, it can promote extramitochondrial activation of NF-κB and therefore may affect nuclear gene expression.

Since there is growing experimental evidence that oxidative stress is a factor in the neuropathology of several adult neurodegenerative disorders, many studies are being directed toward understanding the mitochondrial oxidative stress associated with these diseases (78). For example, Adams et al. (79) examined brain oxidative stress induced by t-butylhydroperoxide and concluded from studies with 2- and 8-month-old mice that aging makes the brain more susceptible to oxidative damage.

CHEMICAL DEPLETION OF GLUTATHIONE

Depletion of hepatocyte glutathione has been widely studied with hundreds of chemicals, including acetaminophen (32) and bromobenzene (80–82). These studies demonstrated very clearly that bioactivation followed by glutathione adduct formation causes depletion of cytosolic glutathione and oxidative stress as shown by indicators including enhanced levels of GSSG, lipid peroxidation, and loss of membrane integrity. The mechanism of acetaminophen-induced hepatotoxicity involves glutathione depletion followed by covalent binding and oxidative stress as indicated by the protective role of glutathione (31). The bioactivation of acetaminophen in vitro and in vivo is associated with GSH depletion and formation of GSSG due to the formation of the reactive metabolite N-acetyl-p-benzoquinone imine, which is both an electrophile and an oxidizing agent (32). Loss of glutathione and protein thiol homeostasis and in mitochondria could contribute to mitochondrial dysfunction and increase the potential for cell death via a mechanism involving oxidative stress.

Depletion of Glutathione by Fasting

Fasting enhances the hepatotoxicity of many chemicals. One of the earliest studies of this phenomenon compared the effects of fasting and various diets on chloroform induced hepatotoxicity (83). Increased hepatotoxicity in association with fasting occurs with chemicals that are capable of depleting GSH, including carbon tetrachloride (84–89), 1,1-dichloroethylene (90), acetaminophen (89, 91, 92), bromobenzene (89, 91), and many others. Because fasting decreases the hepatic concentration of GSH in mice (89) and rats (90–93), such a decrease could account for the enhanced toxicity of many of these chemicals in fasted animals. After depletion of GSH in the liver with diethyl maleate, acetaminophen, bromobenzene, carbon tetrachloride, and anthracyclines showed increased hepatotoxicity (94, 95). Interestingly, the hepatotoxicity of thioacetamide, a substrate for the flavin-dependent monooxygenase present in microsomes (96), is enhanced after fasting (89) but not after pretreatment with diethyl maleate (95).

The enhancement of hepatotoxicity by depletion of GSH has been noted during the metabolism of bromobenzene (80–82). When hepatocytes were pretreated with diethyl maleate, which reduced intracellular levels of GSH by about 70%, added bromobenzene caused levels of GSH to fall to 5% of initial levels, and cell death (75% by 5 hr) was noted. The addition of cysteine, methionine, or N-acetylcysteine prevented bromobenzene-induced toxicity (97) but did not prevent depletion of GSH. Bromobenzene, in the presence of a cysteine source, reduced initial levels of GSH to about 40% of control (81). The presence of metyrapone, an inhibitor of cytochrome P450–dependent monooxygenase reactions, eliminated bromobenzene-induced toxicity. These data are consistent with a requirement for bromobenzene activation prior to GSH conjugation. They do not indicate significant oxidative stress due to redox cycling of a metabolite of bromobenzene.

Glutathione Compartmentation and Chemical-Induced Injury

Since the depletion of hepatocellular GSH by diethyl maleate (DEM) does not exceed 90–95% of total cell GSH except at very high doses of DEM, a pool of GSH appears unavailable to conjugate with DEM. Hepatocytes, thus depleted, can remain viable for several hours, eventually resynthesizing the original complement of GSH. Without additional stress, such as acetaminophen (98) or ADP•Fe^{3+} (99), lipid peroxidation and cell death are not observed. Studies in this laboratory (100) have shown that no formation of malondialdehyde above control levels was noted during 5 hr of incubation in hepatocytes partially depleted of GSH by 1,3-bis(2-chloroethyl)-1-nitrosourea (BCNU). If adriamycin were included to enhance oxidative stress by redox cycling of adriamycin, however, GSH levels were decreased to less than 10% by 3 hr, coincident with a dramatic increase in production of malondialdehyde and leakage of lactate dehydrogenase from the cells. Additional studies have shown that there is a pool of GSH that is unaffected by treatment with diethyl maleate or BCNU, or both, and that this pool is sequestered within the mitochondria (60, 101). However, accessibility of BCNU to the mitochondrial matrix was shown by inhibition of the mitochondrial glutathione reductase. In contrast to the effects of BCNU on mitochondrial GSH depletion of the mitochondrial pool of GSH, a GSH S-transferase–dependent reaction with ethacrynic acid occurred in association with a rapid leakage of lactate dehydrogenase (101). Thus, alterations of chemical hepatotoxicity (or the lack thereof) by either fasting or pretreatment with diethyl maleate and related changes in the amounts of GSH should be considered from the standpoint of compartmentalization of intracellular GSH. Chemical-induced lipid peroxidation, in some instances, correlates better with depletion of GSH in the mitochondrial compartment than with cytosolic GSH (60, 101). Time course studies by Gonzalez-Flecha et al. (102) of oxidative stress and tissue damage to zonal liver during ischemia-reperfusion in rat liver in vivo provides additional evidence that mitochondria are the major source of hydrogen peroxide in control and in reperfused liver. The uncoupler carbonylcyanide p-(trifluoromethoxy)phenylhydrazone provided almost complete inhibition of hydrogen peroxide production, whereas antimycin in liver slices increased the production. These workers concluded that increased rates of oxyradical production by inhibited mitochondria appear as the initial cause of oxidative stress and liver damage during early reperfusion in rat liver. These findings support the conclusion that alterations in mitochondrial functions greatly enhance cell injury and death by a mechanism involving permeability transition.

The mitochondrial pool of GSH, as stated already, has a half-life of about 30 hr (60). It is expected, therefore, that fasting will not deplete this pool of GSH. Fasting, in fact, does not increase the spontaneous rates or carbon tetrachloride-induced rates of lipid peroxidation. Hence, it may be that lipid peroxidation events are related to the size of the mitochondrial pool of GSH in liver. Moreover, perhaps certain "antioxidant" proteins in the mitochondria participate with GSH in preventing lipid peroxidation.

A controversial approach to assessing the potential for chemicals to cause lipid peroxidation in vivo is to treat an intact animal with a chemical or chemical combination and subsequently to measure products of lipid peroxidation in microsomes. In this manner, the depletion of glutathione in vivo with agents that form glutathione conjugates enhances subsequent lipid peroxidation in vitro. Results from such experiments show consistently that an in vivo threshold of 1 μmol GSH/g of liver is associated with spontaneous lipid peroxidation in microsomes (103). This critical value of GSH is about 20% of the initial concentration of GSH. Addition of exogenous GSH inhibited the lipid peroxidation in vitro in a concentration-dependent manner; 1 μM GSH yielded 50% inhibition. Strong enhancement of spontaneous lipid peroxidation in phenobarbital-induced rats also is observed.

Glutathione Reductase and Glutathione Peroxidase

Glutathione reductase, which is important in the regulation of the bioreductive activation of chemicals by GSH, is itself regulated by the redox status of the cell. Being similar to other reductases such as nitrate, nitrite, and $NADP^+$ reductase, GSH reductase is inactivated upon reduction by its own electron donor, NADPH. It has been proposed that this autoinactivation of glutathione reductase by NADPH and the protection as well as reactivation by GSSG regulates the enzyme in vivo (104). The activity of glutathione reductase may reflect the physiologic needs of the cell especially during oxidative stress. For example, 40–50 μM intracellular NADPH inactivates glutathione reductase in the absence of GSSG and decreases glucose metabolism via the hexose monophosphate pathway. The physiologic ratio of GSSG:GSH should provide sufficient GSSG at this level of NADPH to permit retention of significant glutathione reductase activity by preventing inactivation (104).

Glutathione Redox Cycle

It is apparent that a major protective role against the reactive chemical intermediates, which are generated by bioreduction and cause oxidative stress by redox cycling, is provided by the ubiquitous glutathione redox cycle. This cycle utilizes NADPH- and, indirectly, NADH-reducing equivalents in the mitochondrial matrix as well as the cytoplasm to provide GSH by the glutathione reductase-catalyzed reduction of GSSG (Fig. 5). The rates of NADPH consumption in liver by the various NADPH dependent enzymes indicate that glutathione reductase has by far the highest rate to detoxify the reactive oxygen species generated by the various sources (Table 2).

Hillesheim et al. (105) determined that with a rat liver perfusion system, extra production of 70 nmol/min per gram of liver of GSSG could occur before GSSG was excreted into the bile as a result of t-butylhydroperoxide in the perfusate. These findings suggest that liver glutathione could be oxidized to GSSG and reduced back to GSH over 10 times per minute prior to exceeding the reducing capacity of the liver. These and other studies including Jaeschke and Benzick (21), lead to the conclusion that the liver possesses high resistance to intracellular reactive oxygen formation that is dependent upon the glutathione redox cycle system. Therefore, when the glutathione redox cycle is functioning at maximum capacity to eliminate hydrogen peroxide, a major regulatory effect is imposed on other NADPH-dependent pathways. The ability of the glutathione redox cycle to consume major quantities of reducing equivalents (NADPH) is further evidence that oxidative stress is a mechanism for injury and cell death since loss of this redox cycle potentiates hepatocyte death, as clearly shown by many studies including that of Babson et al. (100).

The mitochondrial glutathione redox cycle has a role in regulating mitochondrial oxidations in liver. Various oxidants decrease O_2 uptake by isolated mitochondria and cause a complete turnover of GSH via glutathione peroxidase every 10 min (106). It appears that a continuous flow of reducing equivalents through the glutathione redox cycle is balanced by continuous formation of mitochondrial NADPH, which is needed for glutathione reductase activity. In addition, metabolism of hydrogen peroxide in mitochondria poses a regulatory function in regard to the oxidation of substrates by lipoamide-dependent ketoacid oxidases (106), which generate NADPH-reducing equivalents. The entire NADPH:NADP$^+$ pool may turn over at least once every minute during a maximum oxidant challenge (106).

CELLULAR CHANGES DURING CHEMICAL-INDUCED INJURY

Blebbing of the cell surface has been described as an early consequence of hypoxic and toxic injury to cells (107–111). Since a rise in cytosolic free calcium has been suggested as the stimulus for bleb formation (109, 111, 112) and the final common pathway to irreversible cell injury (111, 113–115), individual hepatocytes in culture have been monitored for "chemical hypoxia" induced by cyanide and iodoacetate (116). During chemical hypoxia, free calcium in the cytosol compartment did not change with bleb formation or before loss of cell viability. Cell death appears to be precipitated by a sudden breakdown of the permeability of the plasma membrane barrier, as would occur by rupture of a surface bleb (116). The only change observed to accompany bleb formation was a fall of the mitochondrial membrane potential (116). Andersson et al. (117) reported, however, the persistence of the mitochondrial membrane potential during anoxia in suspensions of isolated hepatocytes, which may be essential for the maintenance of calcium homeostasis. An important question remaining is whether there is a trigger in calcium homeostasis that determines when the mitochondria will begin to become actively involved in regulation of intracellular calcium. Calcium cycling due to low calcium levels created by calcium omission from the media may be one of the best examples to date. Elucidation of the pathologic conditions that can initiate similar responses may be central to resolving the nature of the proximate mechanism of cell injury and death (Fig. 6).

Changes in cell morphology can also be expressed by changes in the cytoskeleton during cell injury when that injury is related to oxidative stress. An example of such injury is that generated by stimulated polymorphonuclear leukocytes in areas of inflammation associated with tissue injury. These cells produce superoxide anion radicals and hydrogen peroxide as major oxidants and cause cell lysis within a few hours after exposure (118–123). Oxidant production causes oxidation of GSH, loss of NAD (124–127) concomitant with activation of poly-ADP ribose polymerase and single-stranded breaks in DNA (126), loss of cellular ATP, and elevation of intracellular free calcium. Cells that are injured and are dying display morphologic changes that include swelling of the volume of cytoplasm and blebbing of the plasma membrane (128). Membrane blebbing is associated with alteration in

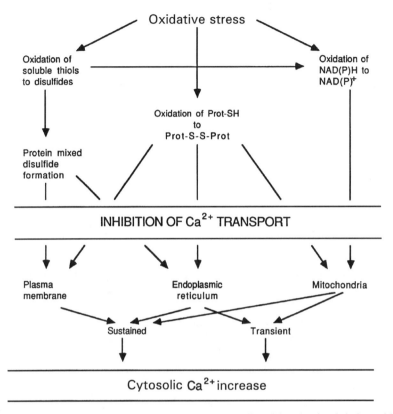

FIG. 6. Mechanisms contributing to the increase in cytosolic calcium ion level during oxidative stress in hepatocytes. Redrawn from Bellomo and Orrenius (113).

the redox state of GSH and intracellular homeostasis of calcium, which perturbs normal cytoskeletal organization. Since such alterations can be caused in hepatocytes as well as in other cell types by two well-known cytoskeletal toxins, cytochalasin B and phalloidin, considerable effort is being focussed on determination of the mechanisms of such cell injury. A variety of drugs, including alkylating agents, induce the formation of blebbing in different cell types (111, 129–131). One mechanism implicates redistribution of cellular filamentous (F) actin in cells with blebs and changes in the G-actin/F-actin ratio (132–134). These effects include considerable swelling of mitochondria and subcellular organelles within 2 hr of oxidant injury. Side-to-side aggregation of F-actin bundles (microfilaments) developed during this time. The injury also produced a marked increase in F-actin, associated rearrangement of the microfilaments, and simultaneous changes in the plasma membrane prior to cell death (131, 133, 134). Thus, cytoskeletal changes during oxidant injury may have considerable importance for both the organization of subcellular organelles and the plasma membrane.

MITOCHONDRIAL PERMEABILITY TRANSITION

Several decades of studies with isolated mitochondria from a variety of tissues indicate that under certain experimental conditions, the mitochondrial inner membrane, which is normally impermeable to solutes, becomes permeable (135–137). Although the mechanism by which this occurs remains controversial, this process is frequently referred to as mitochondrial permeability transition (137, 138). The permeability transition is characterized as a nonspecific and as a specific (139) Ca^{2+}-dependent inner membrane pore that presents itself in mitochondria following treatment with Ca^{2+} and a second agent, termed an *inducing agent*. Many inducing agents have been identified and vary greatly in both structure and function (137). It is thought that these agents, in the presence of Ca^{2+}, act through a common mechanism during the permeability transition. Examples of inducing agents include inorganic phosphate, cytosolic factor, fatty acids, heavy metals, organic sulfhydryl reagents, and oxidants such as t-butylhydroperoxide (137).

Several identifiable events of the permeability transition have been characterized in the last several years. These include inner membrane permeability to small ions and solutes with molecular weights <1500 Da, large-amplitude swelling, loss of coupled functions, and sensitivity to cyclosporin A (CsA) (140–143). In addition, loss of matrix proteins via the inner membrane pore has also been reported (144). During permeability transition, Ca^{2+} and other ions are rapidly released from the mitochondrial matrix, presumably via the inner membrane pore. Following inner membrane permeability and the release of matrix solutes, a colloidal osmotic pressure arises in the mitochondrial matrix due to the high concentration of proteins that are slow to equilibrate (137). In order to correct the osmotic imbalance, the entrance of H_2O results in massive swelling of the mitochondria (137).

Mitochondrial swelling under these conditions is termed *large-amplitude swelling*. Although secondary to inner membrane permeability and solute release, large-amplitude swelling occurs within a short time (3–10 min) and is easily detected by monitoring light scatter of mitochondrial suspensions at 540 nm. Monitoring of mitochondrial swelling is a simple assay and is often utilized as an indicator of permeability transition. Different experimental conditions result, however, in different patterns and times of swelling, some with shorter or longer lag periods (143). Studies by Fournier et al. (145) showed with isolated mitochondria that CsA treatment promoted retention of accumulated Ca^{2+}. Subsequent studies by Crompton et al. (142) were designed to examine the effect of CsA on pore opening since the loss of Ca^{2+} observed by Fournier et al. (145) was possibly due to pore opening. This study revealed that CsA is a potent inhibitor of the permeability transition when the inducing agents inorganic phosphate or t-butylhydroperoxide were added in the presence of Ca^{2+}. Broekemeier et al. (143) tested CsA as an inhibitor of the inner membrane pore in the presence of several different inducing agents and found that very low concentrations of CsA protected against permeability transition. These studies demonstrated the potency of CsA in preventing the permeability transition, as inhibition of inner membrane permeability is observed with concentrations as low as 100 pmoles of CsA per milligram of mitochondrial protein.

A study by Halestrap and Davidson (146) focused on the mechanism of pore formation and proposed that the adenine nucleotide translocase is the putative pore structure. They hypothesize that the "m" conformation of this inner-membrane protein is modified to the "c" conformation by the binding of negative effectors such as Ca^{2+}, cyclophilin, and inducing agents resulting in a protein conformation that can no longer function as an adenine nucleotide translocase but as a nonspecific pore. Atractyloside and bongkrekic acid are known modifiers of the translocase and have been helpful in proposing this mechanism. This study also demonstrates that both ATP and ADP are positive effectors of the putative permeability transition pore.

Richter et al. (139) propose that pore formation is not required for Ca^{2+} release and suggest that ADP-ribosylation of inner membrane proteins is the responsible mechanism of permeability transition. They hypothesize that uptake of Ca^{2+} and the consequent recycling of Ca^{2+} results in NAD(P)H oxidation followed by the hydrolysis of NAD^+ forming a nicotinamide and an ADP-ribose moiety. Subsequent ADP-ribosylation of critical proteins results in inner membrane permeability allowing the specific release of Ca^{2+}.

The present understanding of permeability transition is that the pore structure is an allosteric inner-membrane protein, perhaps the adenine nucleotide translocase, with several different regulatory sites affected by Ca^{2+}, inorganic phosphate (Pi), oxidants, sulfhydryl reagents, heavy metals, cyclophilin, ADP, ATP, atractyloside, and bongkrekic acid. Depending upon which sites are modified may determine whether permeability transition occurs. It is hypothesized that inhibition of permeability transition with CsA results from the binding of cyclophilin, a matrix protein cis-trans isomerase thought to be involved with protein folding (147). Whether the process of permeability transition is physiologic remains an intriguing question.

Several methods are available to detect and measure mitochondrial permeability transition in isolated mitochondria. Crompton and Costi (148) developed a method that exploits two aspects of the permeability transition: the entry of radiolabled sucrose into the mitochondrial matrix, a normally impermeable solute to the mitochondrial inner membrane, and the reversible nature of the pore. By adding a chelator of Ca^{2+}, such as EDTA or CsA (a potent pore inhibitor), the inner membrane nonspecific pore can be closed. This allows for the entrapment of sucrose into the matrix, which can then be quantified. Release of added Ca^{2+} or other ions from mitochondria and its inhibition by CsA are also indicative of permeability transition (137, 143). As previously discussed, loss of absorbance at 540 nm of mitochondrial suspensions is frequently used as an indicator of permeability transition in isolated mitochondria. However, since large amplitude swelling is a secondary event that does not always accompany permeability transition (149), monitoring of solute movement may be a more sensitive parameter of permeability changes.

Mitochondrial Glutathione as Marker

Mitochondrial GSH (307 Da) release may be a useful and sensitive endogenous indicator of permeability transition under the conditions we have examined (38, 150).

s from the Reed laboratory with rat liver mitochondria have shown that during
eability transition induced with 70 μM Ca^{2+} and 3 mM Pi, mitochondrial GSH
is rapidly and completely released from the matrix and recovered extramitochon-
drially as GSH (150) (Fig. 2). This release is completely prevented by addition of
0.5 μM CsA, indicating that release occurs via the Ca^{2+}-dependent, CsA-sensitive
inner-membrane pore (150). GSH release under these conditions parallel Ca^{2+} release
in that both of these molecules are nearly completely released during a 5-min incubation. Mitochondrial swelling, a secondary process, is somewhat slower; however, this
process results in a substantial loss of mitochondrial density that is prevented by the
addition of CsA. An interesting finding is that 3 mM Pi alone induces a permeability transition by a CsA-sensitive mechanism. Mitochondria undergo large-amplitude
swelling with Pi alone, although not as extensive as in mitochondria treated with both
Ca^{2+} and Pi. However, complete GSH release occurs with Pi treatment alone, although
at a slower rate than with the addition of both Ca^{2+} and Pi. This release and swelling
is due to the presence of 6–10 nmoles of Ca^{2+} per miligram of protein in the mitochondrial preps (149). The effect of Pi is abolished following the addition of EGTA.
Although monitoring of swelling indicates that permeability transition is occurring,
the finding suggests permeability transition is not as extensive relative to Ca^{2+} and
Pi treatment. However, without exogenously added Ca^{2+}, monitoring of Ca^{2+} release
is not a sensitive indicator of permeability transition, as endogenous Ca^{2+} levels are
very low and therefore a significant change in Ca^{2+} levels is not observed (38, 149).

Although swelling is detected when Pi is added alone, it is less than maximal
swelling detected by light scatter in the presence of 70 μM Ca^{2+} and 3 mM Pi.
However, electron microscopy of samples treated with Pi alone or Pi plus Ca^{2+} reveals
an indistinguishable level of large-amplitude swelling, with varied times (38). This
evidence, combined with biochemical data, show that monitoring of Ca^{2+} release or
swelling is not always a sensitive indicator of the degree of permeability transition
(149). Monitoring release of a highly concentrated endogenous solute, such as GSH
release by a CsA-sensitive mechanism, may be a sensitive indicator of inner membrane
permeability transition.

More recent studies have supported this finding (38). Mitochondria treated with
Ca^{2+} and Pi in the presence of metabolic inhibitors of electron transport or ATP synthesis prevented mitochondrial large-amplitude swelling as detected by light scatter
and electron microscopy. However, monitoring of matrix GSH indicates that GSH
is released from the matrix into the extramitochondrial environment. Treatment with
0.5 μM CsA prevents this release of GSH, suggesting that release occurred via the
Ca^{2+}-dependent inner-membrane pore (38). The rate and extent of GSH release vary
with the different conditions; however, release of this endogenous molecule may be
a useful marker of mitochondrial permeability transition.

Induction Within Cells

The pathogenesis of chemical-induced hepatocyte injury and death during oxidative stress may be caused by calcium ion–induced permeability transition of the

mitochondrial inner membrane that initiates cell death. A feature of oxidative stress-induced cell injury is morphologic and functional changes in mitochondria (151–153). Mitochondrial dysfunction, a critical event in anoxia/reoxygenation injury of liver sinusoidal endothelial cells, appears due to the permeability transition since acidosis protects against lethal oxidative injury (154), as does a combination of CsA plus trifluoperazine (155).

CHEMICAL-INDUCED APOPTOSIS

Apoptosis, or programmed cell death, is a mode of cell death with a defined set of characteristics that distinguish apoptotic cells from cells dying by other means: shrinkage, membrane blebbing, chromatin condensation, internucleosomal DNA cleavage, cytoplasmic compaction with preservation of mitochondrial structure, and cell fragmentation (156–162). Martin and Green (163) have reviewed protease activation during apoptosis and concluded that events are better described as a collapse of the cell. Their analogy is the manner in which a large tent collapses if lines are cut and the tent remains erect until a sudden crashing down of the structure. One of the main questions is whether this sudden collapse is closely associated with the loss of mitochondria structure and function—loss of energy production and the status of cytoplasmic or mitochondrial glutathione. Therefore, the sequence of mitochondrial events associated with death of hepatocytes that have different concentrations of glutathione due to exposure to chemicals that undergo bioactivation could be the key to chemical-induced cell death.

Apoptosis has been found to display within the mitochondria the characteristics of mitochondrial permeability transitions (MPT) of the inner mitochondrial membrane. As discussed above, these include the decrease of transmembrane potential, $\Delta\Psi m$, permeability to low-molecular-weight (<1500 Da) solutes, and loss of coupled functions (143, 164–166). MPT occurs when mitochondria are treated with Ca^{2+} in the presence of an inducing agent, of which several structurally and mechanistically different compounds have been identified. Examples include inorganic phosphate, hydroperoxides, some heavy metals, and sulfhydryl reagents. The increased permeability is thought to occur through a Ca^{2+}-dependent nonspecific inner-membrane pore through which ions and small molecules can diffuse very quickly from, and into, the mitochondrial matrix (143, 164–166). Cyclosporin A (CsA), an immunosuppressive cyclic peptide, that inhibits apoptosis in lymphocytes (161), is a potent inhibitor of the permeability transition and solute movement via this nonspecific pore (142, 143). Petronilli et al. (167) have concluded that the oxidation-reduction state of vicinal thiols has a role in the opening of the MPT pore.

Oxidants including menadione, diamide, arsenite, and t-butylhydroperoxide can cause cell death by one or more mechanisms that are responsive to the effects of CsA to prevent such cell death, presumably via mitochondrial permeability transition. These workers have concluded that oxidants cause vicinal thiols to form a protein disulfide to enhance pore opening, which can be reversed by thiols such as DTT. Connern and Halestrap (168) demonstrated the recruitment of mitochondrial cyclophilin to the mitochondrial inner membrane under conditions of oxidative stress that enhance the opening of a Ca^{2+}-sensitive nonspecific channel. Cyclophilin binding was prevented by 5 μM CsA but not reversed by CsA treatment of the membranes. These workers concluded that the function of cyclophilins may be to interact with integral membrane proteins to modulate their function in response to an appropriate signal (168). It is not known if the binding of either cyclophilin or CsA alters accessibility to the dithiols (167) that enhance MPT when oxidized by TBH, diamide, menadione, or arsenite anion and limit MPT when reduced or prevented from oxidizing by NEM. In agreement with the participation of protein dithiols with MPT is the work of Vercesi et al. (169) and Valle et al. (170) that indicates the induction of MPT with protein thiol cross linking. Evidence for the participation of MPT in loss of cell viability during exposure to toxic agents is numerous (41, 45, 171). Since overexpression of the Bcl-2 oncogen protects cells from apoptotic and oxidative cell death (159), an intriguing possibility suggested by Petronilli et al. (167) is that some type of link exists between Bcl-2 expression and MPT regulation—a suggestion that is supported by Kroemer et al. (161). They proposed that MPT and its regulation by Bcl-2 is responsible for the effector phase of apoptosis.

An important aspect of MPT is the effect of modulation of glutathione status on the induction of apoptosis by MPT-mediated $\Delta\Psi$m. Inhibitors of MPT have been shown to interfere with the disruption of the $\Delta\Psi$m during apoptosis (172). These workers concluded that $\Delta\Psi$m disruption appears to be the earliest alteration of cellular biochemistry that constitutes a constant feature of pre-apoptotic cells. Therefore, since considerable evidence supports the participation of protein dithiols in MPT, the status of glutathione has an important indirect effect on apoptosis. Inability to sustain normal levels of glutathione in vivo and in vitro indicates that the self-amplificatory properties of MPT are enhanced by a decrease in glutathione levels by electrophilic chemicals. This occurs with many chemicals upon bioactivation with self-amplificatory properties that include loss of matrix calcium and glutathione, depolarization of the inner membrane, loss of oxidized pyridine nucleotides and adenine nucleotides, and increased oxidation of thiols, all of which result from chemical-induced MPT and increase the MPT gating potential (38, 141, 173). Richter and coworkers (174) reported that changes in $\Delta\Psi$m are paralleled by movement of Ca^{2+} across the inner mitochondrial membrane and speculated that the reversible release of Ca^{2+} from mitochondria could constitute a cellular signal.

Because the thiol status of cells is closely associated with bioactivation of chemicals, Ca^{2+} homeostasis, and reactive oxygen species (ROS) generation, it is important to understand better the role of chemical exposure to the possible effects of glutathione modulation on MPT and the sequential reduction of $\Delta\Psi$m and generation of reaction oxygen species in cell death. Zamzami et al. (175, 176) have observed a sequential disregulation of mitochondrial function that precedes cell shrinkage and nuclear fragmentation. This disregulation consists of an initial CsA-inhibitable step of ongoing apoptosis that is characterized as a reduction of $\Delta\Psi$m followed by generation of ROS upon a short-term in vitro culture. ROS generation is inhibitable by rotenone and ruthenium red but is not affected by CsA (175, 176). Inhibitors of MPT have

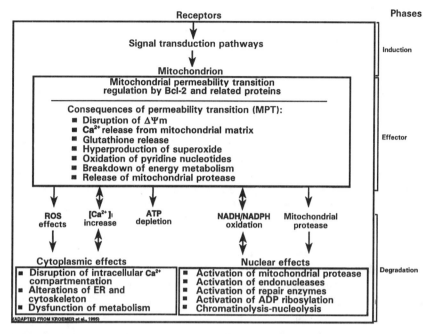

FIG. 7. Mitochondrion as an effector for apoptosis and associated oxidative stress. Redrawn from Kroemer et al. (161).

been shown to interfere with the disruption of the $\Delta\Psi$m during apoptosis (172). As evidence, CsA, N-methyl-Val-4-CsA, and bongkrekic acid, have been shown both to inhibit the disruption of MPT-mediated $\Delta\Psi$m and to prevent apoptotic chromatinolysis. The self-amplificatory properties of MPT are expected to be enhanced by a decrease in glutathione levels. Kroemer et al. (161) have concluded that experimental evidence exists to support the suggestion that a sequential mitochondrial dysfunction expressed as loss of $\Delta\Psi$m followed by enhanced superoxide generation is implicated in apoptosis (Fig. 7). It is known that MPT has self-amplificatory properties including loss of matrix Ca^{2+}, glutathione, depolarization of the inner membrane, and increased oxidation of thiols that are contributors to a point of no return in the apoptosis process.

Alterations of mitochondrial functions before cell death could be reflected in changes in the mitochondrial glutathione status, especially during the ROS generation phase. It is important to point out that measurement of total glutathione does not reflect change in glutathione status in the mitochondria, as mitochondria are expected to contain only about 10% of the total intracellular glutathione. Because of the importance of the status of mitochondrial glutathione in hepatocytes, the depletion of hepatocyte GSH with DEM (177) is of interest. It was important to know the amount of GSH that could be depleted prior to cell injury. Diethyl maleate under the conditions used is known not to deplete hepatocyte mitochondrial GSH (60). Rat hepatocytes were depleted of 50% of their total GSH by 0.4 mM diethyl maleate in

135 min without observable injury. Additional GSH depletion initiated cell injury that increased with increasing depletion of GSH (177, 178). These findings suggest that less than 50% of the total GSH was required to prevent cell injury during in vitro incubation (178). Further, after depletion, [^{35}S]cysteine was incorporated into newly synthesized GSH, with the resulting radiospecific activity of the repleted GSH being 28% of that of the precursor [^{35}S]cysteine (178).

Gunter and coworkers (171) suggest that mitochondrial Ca^{2+} transport may have evolved to protect the cytosol against damage from high Ca^{2+} concentration. Questions about the dynamics of thiol homeostasis, especially with respect to glutathione, the rate of energy consumption for cellular processes related to such homeostasis during pathologic conditions, and the fate of glutathione during MPT and apoptosis are major areas of interest as they relate very closely to many human diseases.

Kinetic analysis of the chronology of toxic agent–induced cytotoxicity in vitro has given significant information concerning the multicomponent events associated with chemical-induced cell death that have an associated oxidative stress. Barhoumi and Burghardt (179) have described vital fluorescence bioassays that provided a chronology of cellular injury caused by patulin and gossypol. With patulin the chronology was simultaneous suppression of gap junction–mediated intercellular communication (GJIC) and GSH depletion $\longrightarrow$ reactive oxygen species (ROS) $\longrightarrow$ mitochondrial membrane depolarization $\longrightarrow$ simultaneous increase in [Ca^{2+}]i and cytoplasmic acidification $\longrightarrow$ depolarization of plasma membrane. In contrast, with gossypol the chronology of cellular injury was simultaneous suppression of GJIC and generation of ROS $\longrightarrow$ cytoplasmic acidification $\longrightarrow$ simultaneous elevation of [Ca^{2+}]i and partial depletion of GSH $\longrightarrow$ mitochondrial membrane depolarization $\longrightarrow$ depolarization of plasma membrane. Although, many chemicals are known to induce apoptotic cell death, many difficulties remain concerning distinguishing the differences between apoptotic and necrotic cell death. These differences have been described by several recent reviews (180–182). Kinetic analysis of the events of chemical-induced cytotoxicity with hepatocytes that posses varying levels of glutathione such as those we can establish with GGT-deficient mice and PPG treatment will need to be investigated. Thus, it is appropriate to continue to seek to understand better those events that are characteristic of either necrotic or apoptotic or both types of cell death.

EVALUATION OF OXIDATIVE STRESS

Evidence continues to support the concept that hepatocytes possess very efficient antioxidant defense systems that have a capacity to consume a significant amount of the cellular energy for the purpose of elimination of oxidant-induced oxygen-reactive species (183). As discussed, glutathione is the major source of antioxidant capacity, and depletion of cellular glutathione compromises the prevention of oxidative events including peroxidation of lipids and other susceptible cellular constituents. Further, oxidant-induced stress alone can cause alteration in cellular functions resulting in loss of calcium homeostasis and mitochondrial dysfunction. These events can be lethal for hepatocytes if allowed to progress too far. Chemical-induced hepatocyte cell death is always accompanied by an oxidative stress component. The reason for this appears to be due to the impact chemicals have upon the balance between prooxidants and antioxidants. Any loss of cellular ability to detoxify reactive oxygen species enhances the prooxidant stress on the cell. This in turn has a multitude of responses, some of which remain poorly understood, e.g., the ability of alterations in oxidant stress to change gene expression and programmed cell death or apoptosis.

CONCLUSIONS

Cell death resulting from chemical exposure with few exception involves an early challenge to the cellular defense systems based on glutathione. Glutathione adduct formation or formation of GSSG limits the ability of the cell to detoxify reactive oxygen species and in turn loss of regulation of other cellular processes, including calcium homeostasis. These events participate in chemical-induced oxidative stress as a mechanism for hepatocyte death. Evidence suggests that apoptosis could be involved in a mechanism of cell death with an early involvement of generation of reactive oxygen species.

REFERENCES

1. McCord JM, Fridovich I. The utility of superoxide dismutase in studying free radical reactions. I. Radicals generated by the interaction of sulfite, dimethyl sulfoxide, and oxygen. *J Biol Chem* 1969;244:6056–6063.
2. Sies H. Introduction. In: Sies H, ed. *Oxidative stress*. Orlando: Academic Press, 1985:1–7.
3. Sies H, Chance B. The steady state level of catalase compound I in isolated hemoglobin-free perfused rat liver. *FEBS Lett* 1970;11:172–176.
4. Oshino N, Chance B, Sies H, Bucher T. The role of H_2O_2 generation in perfused rat liver and the reaction of caralase compound I and hydrogen donors. *Arch Biochem Biophys* 1973;154:117–131.
5. Chance B, Sies H, Boveris A. Hydroperoxide metabolism in mammalian organs. *Physiol Rev* 1979;59:527–605.
6. Halliwell B, Gutteridge JMC. Role of free radicals and catalytic metal ions in human disease: an overview. In: Packer L, Glazer AN, eds. *Methods in enzymology*, vol. 186(B). San Diego: Academic Press, 1990:1–85.
7. Cadenas E. Biochemistry of oxygen toxicity. *Annu Rev Biochem* 1989;58:79–110.
8. Richter C. Do mitochondrial DNA fragments promote cancer and aging? *FEBS Lett* 1988;241:1–5.
9. Forman HJ, Boveris A. Superoxide radical and hydrogen peroxide in mitochondria. In: Pryor WA, ed. *Free radicals in biology*, vol. 5. New York: Academic Press, 1982.
10. Jones DP, Eklow L, Thor H, Orrenius S. Metabolism of hydrogen peroxide in isolated hepatocytes: relative contributions of catalase and glutathione peroxidase in decomposition of endogenously generated H_2O_2. *Arch Biochem Biophys* 1981;210:505–516.
11. Sohal RS. Aging, cytochrome oxidase activity, and hydrogen peroxide release by mitochondria. *Free Rad Biol Med* 1993;14:583–588.
12. Turrens JF, McCord JM. Mitochondrial generation of reactive oxygen species. In: Paulet AC, Douste-Blazy L, Paoletti R, eds. *Free radicals, lipoproteins, and membrane lipids*. New York: Plenum Press, 1990:203–212.
13. Boveris A, Cadenas E. Production of superoxide in mitochondria. In: Oberley LW, ed. *Superoxide dismutase II*. Boca Raton: CRC Press, 1982:15–30.

14. Pryor WA. Oxy-radicals and related species: their formation, lifetimes, and reactions. *Annu Rev Physiol* 1986;48:657–667.
15. Bindoli A. Lipid peroxidation in mitochondria. *Free Rad Biol Med* 1988;5:247–261.
16. Dix TA, Aikens J. Mechanisms and biological relevance of lipid peroxidation initiation. *Chem Res Toxicol* 1993;6:2–18.
17. Jaeschke H. Mechanisms of oxidant stress-induced acute tissue injury. *Drug Metab Res* 1995;209:104–111.
18. Zimmerman HJ. Experimental hepatotoxicity. In: Eichler O, ed. *Handbook of experimental pharmacology*, vol. 16, part 5. New York: Springer-Verlag, 1976:1–120.
19. Tribble DL, Aw TY, Jones DP. The pathophysiological significance of lipid peroxidation in oxidative cell injury. *Hepatology* 1987;7:377–386.
20. Kappus H, Sies H. Toxic drug effects associated with oxygen metabolism: redox cycling and lipid peroxidation. *Experientia* 1981;37:1233–1241.
21. Jaeschke H, Benzick AE. Pathophysiological consequences of enhanced intracellular superoxide formation in isolated perfused rat liver. *Chem Biol Interact* 1992;84:55–68.
22. Sandy MS, Moldéus P, Ross D, et al. Cytotoxicity of the redox cycling compound diquat in isolated hepatocytes: involvement of hydrogen peroxide and transition metals. *Arch Biochem Biophys* 1987;259:29–37.
23. Reed DJ. Nitrosoureas. In: Sies H, ed. *Oxidative stress*. London: Academic Press, 1985:115–130.
24. Muller A, Cadenas E, Graf P, et al. A novel biologically active seleno-organic compound. I. Glutathione peroxidase-like activity in vitro and antioxidant capacity of PZ 51 (Ebselen). *Biochem Pharmacol* 1984;33:3235–3239.
25. Keberle H. The biochemistry of desferrioxamine and its relation to iron metabolism. *Annu NY Acad Sci* 1964;119:758–768.
26. Fischer-Nielsen A, Corcoran GB, Poulsen HE, Kamendulis LM, Loft S. Menadione-induced DNA fragmentation without 8-oxo-2″-deoxyguanosine formation in isolated rat hepatocytes. *Biochem Pharmacol* 1995;49:1469–1474.
27. Thomas CE, Reed DJ. Current status of calcium in hepatocellular injury. *Hepatology* 1989;10:375–384.
28. Orrenius S, Thor H, Bellomo G. Alterations in thiol and calcium ion homeostasis during hydroperoxide and drug metabolism. *Biochem Soc Trans* 1984;12:23–28.
29. Broekemeier KM, Carpenter-Deyo L, Reed DJ, Pfeiffer DR. Cyclosporin A protects hepatocytes subjected to high Ca^{2+} and oxidative stress. *FEBS Lett* 1992;304:192–194.
30. Nieminen AL, Saylor AK, Tesfai SA, Herman B, Lemaster JJ. Contribution of the mitochondrial permeability transition to lethal injury after exposure of hepatocytes to t-butylhydroperoxide. *Biochem J* 1995;307:99–106.
31. Mitchell JR, Jollow DJ, Potter WZ, et al. Acetaminophen-induced hepatic necrosis. IV. Protective role of glutathione. *J Pharmacol Exp Ther* 1973;187:185–194.
32. Hinson JA, Pumford NR, Roberts DW. Mechanisms of acetaminophen toxicity: immunochemical detections of drug-protein adducts. *Drug Metab Rev* 1995;27:73–92.
33. Gibson JD, Pumford NR, Samokyszn VM, Hinson JA. Mechanism of acetaminophen-induced hepatotoxicity: covalent binding versus oxidative stress. *Chem Res Toxicol* 1996;9:580–585.
34. Amimoto T, Matsura T, Koyama SY, Nakanishi T, Yamada K, Kajiyama G. Acetaminophen-induced hepatic injury in mice: the role of lipid peroxidation and effects of pretreatment with coenzyme Q10 and alpha-tocopherol. *Free Rad Biol Med* 1995;19:169–176.
35. Lores Arnaiz S, Llesuy S, Cutrin JC, Boveris A. Oxidative stress by acute acetaminophen administration in mouse liver. *Free Rad Biol Med* 1995;19:303–310.
36. Adamson G, Harman AW. Oxidative stress in cultured hepatocytes exposed to acetaminophen. *Biochem Pharmacol* 1993;45:2289–2294.
37. Olafsdottir K, Reed DJ. Retention of oxidized glutathione by isolated rat liver mitochondria during hydroperoxide treatment. *Biochim Biophys Acta* 1988;964:377–382.
38. Reed DJ, Savage MK. Oxidative stress and mitochondrial permeability transition. In: Davies KJA, Ursini F, eds. *The oxygen paradox*. Padova, Italy: CLEUP University Press, 1995:487–502.
39. Garcia-Ruiz C, Colell A, Morales A, Kaplowitz N, Fernández-Checa JC. Role of oxidative stress generated from the mitochondrial electron transport chain and mitochondrial glutathione status in loss of mitochondrial function and activation of transcription factor nuclear factor-κB: studies with isolated mitochondria and rat hepatocytes. *Mol Pharmacol* 1995;48:825–834.
40. Reed DJ. Cellular defense mechanisms against reactive metabolites. In: Anders MW, ed. *Bioactivation of foreign compounds*. Orlando: Academic Press, 1985:71–108.

41. Reed DJ. Toxicity of oxygen. In: De Matteis F, Smith LL, eds. *Molecular and cellular mechanisms of toxicity.* Boca Raton: CRC Press, 1995:35–68.
42. Reed DJ. Glutathione: toxicological implications. *Annu Rev Pharmacol Toxicol* 1990;30:603–631.
43. Reed DJ, Fariss MW. Glutathione depletion and susceptibility. *Pharmacol Rev* 1984;36:25S–33S.
44. Reed DJ, Olafsdottir K. The role of glutathione in mitochondria. In: Taniguchi N, Higashi T, Sakamoto Y, Meister A, eds. *Glutathione centennial: molecular perspectives and clinical implications.* San Diego: Academic Press, 1989:35–55.
45. Reed DJ. Oxidative stress and mitochondrial permeability transition. In: Packer L, Cadenas E, eds. *Biothiols in health and disease.* New York: Marcel Dekker, 1995:231–263.
46. Kosower NS, Kosower E. Glutathione status of cells. *Int Rev Cytol* 1979;54:109–160.
47. Reed DJ, Beatty PW. Biosynthesis and regulation of glutathione: toxicological implications. In: Hodgson E, Bend JR, Philpot RM, eds. *Reviews in biochemical toxicology.* New York: Elsevier Press, 1980:213–241.
48. Reed DJ. Regulation and function of glutathione in cells. In: Nygaard OF, Simic MG, eds. *First conference on radioprotectors and anticarcinogens.* New York: Academic Press, 1983;153–168.
49. Boyd SC, Sasame HA, Boyd MR. High concentrations of glutathione in glandular stomach: possible implications for carcinogenesis. *Science* 1979;205:1010–1012.
50. Womack M, Kremmer KS, Rose WC. The relation of cysteine and methionine to growth. *J Biol Chem* 1937;121:403–410.
51. Reed DJ. Cystathionine. In: Packer L, ed. *Methods in enzymology.* San Diego: Academic Press, 1995:92–102.
52. White INH. Role of liver glutathione in acute toxicity of retrorsine to rats. *Chem Biol Interact* 1976;13:333–342.
53. Tateishi N, Higashi T, Naruse A, et al. Rat-liver glutathione: possible role as a reservoir of cysteine. *J Nutr* 1977;107:51–60.
54. Higashi T, Tateishi N, Naruse A, et al. Novel physiological role of liver glutathione as a reservoir of L-cysteine. *J Biochem* 1977;82:117–124.
55. Beck LV, Riecls VD, Duncan B. Diurnal variation in mouse and rat liver sulfhydryl. *Proc Soc Exp Biol Med* 1958;97:229–231.
56. Calcutt G, Ting M. Diurnal variations in the rat tissue disulphide levels. *Naturwissenschaften* 1969;56:419–420.
57. Jaeger RJ, Connolly RB, Murphy SD. Diurnal-variation of hepatic glutathione concentration and its correlation with 1,1-dichloroethylene inhalation toxicity in rats. *Res Commun Chem Pathol Pharmacol* 1973;6:465–471.
58. Lauterburg BH, Vaishnov Y, Stillwell WG, et al. The effects of age and glutathione depletion on hepatic glutathione turnover in vivo determined by acetaminophen probe analysis. *J Pharmacol Exp Ther* 1980;213:54–58.
59. Reed DJ, Ellis WW. Influence of γ-glutamyl transpeptidase inactivation on the status of extracellular glutathione and glutathione conjugates. In: Snyder R, Parke CV, Kocsis JJ, et al., eds. *Biological reactive intermediates, IIA.* New York: Plenum Press, 1982:75–86.
60. Meredith MJ, Reed DJ. Status of the mitochondrial pool of glutathione in the isolated hepatocyte. *J Biol Chem* 1982;257:3747–3753.
61. Cho ES, Sahyoun N, Stegink LD. Tissue glutathione as a cyst(e)ine reservoir during fasting and refeeding of rats. *J Nutr* 1981;111:914–922.
62. Jocelyn PC. Some properties of mitochondrial glutathione. *Biochim Biophys Acta* 1975;396:427–436.
63. Wahlländer A, Sobell S, Sies H, Linke I, Müller M. Hepatic mitochondrial and cytosolic glutathione content and the subcellular distribution of GSH-S-transferases. *FEBS Lett* 1979;97:138–140.
64. Flohe L, Schlegel W. Glutathione peroxidase. IV. Intracellular distribution of the glutathione peroxidase system in the rat liver. *Hoppe Seylers Z Physiol Chem* 1971;352:1401–1410.
65. Neubert D, Wojtszak AB, Lehninger AL. Purification and enzymatic identity of mitochondrial contraction factors I and II. *Proc Natl Acad Sci USA* 1962;48:1651–1658.
66. Vignais PM, Vignais PV. Fuscin, an inhibitor of mitochondrial SH-dependent transport-linked functions. *Biochim Biophys Acta* 1973;325:357–374.
67. Nohl H, deSilva D, Summer KH. 2,3,7,8,-tetrachlorodibenzo-p-dioxin induces oxygen activation associated with cell respiration. *Free Rad Biol Med* 1989;6:369–374.
68. Chacon E, Acosta D. Mitochondrial regulation of superoxide by Ca^{2+}: an alternate mechanism for the cardiotoxicity of doxorubicin. *Toxicol Appl Pharmacol* 1991;107:117–128.

69. Turrens JF, Beconi M, Barilla J, Chavez UB, McCord JM. Mitochondrial generation of oxygen radicals during reoxygenation of ischemic tissues. *Free Rad Res Commun* 1991;12-13:681–689.
70. Cleeter MW, Cooper JM, Schapira AH. Irreversible inhibition of mitochondrial complex I by 1-methyl-4-phenylpyridinium: evidence for free radical involvement. *J Neurochem* 1992;58:786–789.
71. Schulze-Osthoff K, Bakker AC, Vanhaesebroeck B, Beyaert R, Jacob WA, Fiers W. Cytotoxic activity of tumor necrosis factor is mediated by early damage of mitochondrial functions: evidence for the involvement of mitochondrial radical generation. *J Biol Chem* 1992;267:5317–5323.
72. Takayanagi R, Takeshige K, Minakami S. NADH- and NADPH-dependent lipid peroxidation in bovine heart submitochondrial particles: dependence on the rate of electron flow in the respiratory chain and an antioxidant role of ubiquinol. *Biochem J* 1980;192:853–860.
73. Mészaros L, Tihanyi K, Horvath I. Mitochondrial substrate oxidation-dependent protection against lipid peroxidation. *Biochim Biophys Acta* 1982;731:675–677.
74. Reddy CC, Sholz WW, Thomas CB, et al. Vitamin E-dependent reduced glutathione inhibition of rat liver microsomal lipid peroxidation. *Life Sci* 1982;31:571–576.
75. McCray PB, Gibson DD, Fong KL, et al. Effect of glutathione peroxidase activity on lipid peroxidation in biological membranes. *Biochim Biophys Acta* 1976;431:459–468.
76. Kraus P. Resolution, purification and some properties of three glutathione transferases from rat liver mitochondria. *Hoppe Seylers Z Physiol Chem* 1980;361:9–15.
77. Morgenstern R, Lundqvist G, Andersson G, et al. The distribution of microsomal glutathione transferase among different organelles, different organs, and different organisms. *Biochem Pharmacol* 1984;33:3609–3614.
78. Coyle JT, Puttfarcken P. Oxidative stress, glutamate, and neuro-degenerative disorders. *Science* 1993;262:689–695.
79. Adams JD Jr, Wang B, Klaidman LK, LeBel CP, Odunze IN, Shah D. New aspects of brain oxidative stress induced by *tert*-butylhydroperoxide. *Free Rad Biol Med* 1993;15:195–202.
80. Thor H, Moldéus P, Högberg J, et al. Toxicological aspects of food safety. *Arch Toxicol Suppl* 1978;1:107–114.
81. Thor H, Moldéus P, Kristofersson A, et al. Metabolic activation and hepatotoxicity. Metabolism of bromobenzene in isolated hepatocytes. *Arch Biochem Biophys* 1978;188:114–122.
82. Thor H, Moldéus P, Hermanson R, et al. Metabolic activation and hepatotoxicity. Toxicity of bromobenzene in hepatocytes isolated from phenobarbital-treated and diethylmaleate-treated rats. *Arch Biochem Biophys* 1978;188:122–129.
83. Davis N, Whipple C. The influence of fasting and various diets on the liver injury effected by chloroform anesthesia. *Arch Intern Med* 1919;23:612–635.
84. Davis NC. The influence of diet upon liver injury produced by carbon tetrachloride. *J Med Res* 1924;44:601–614.
85. Krishnan N, Stenger RJ. Effects of starvation on the hepatotoxicity of carbon tetrachloride. *Amer J Pathol* 1966;49:239–255.
86. McLean AEM, McLean EK. Effect of diet and 1,1,1-tetrachloro-2,2-bis-(p-chlorophenyl)ethane (DDT) on microsomal hydroxylating enzymes and on sensitivity of rats to carbon tetrachloride poisoning. *Biochem J* 1966;100:564–571.
87. Highman B, Cyr WH, Streett RP Jr. Effect of x-irradiation and fasting on hepatotoxicity of carbon tetrachloride in rats. *Radiat Res* 1973;54:444–452.
88. Diaz Gomez MI, DeCastro CR, DeFerreyra EC, et al. Mechanistic studies on carbon tetrachloride hepatotoxicity in fasted and fed rats. *Toxicol Appl Pharmacol* 1975;32:101–108.
89. Strubelt O, Dost-Kempf E, Siegers CP, et al. The influence of fasting on the susceptibility of mice to hepatotoxic injury. *Toxicol Appl Pharmacol* 1981;60:66–77.
90. Jaeger RJ, Connolly RB, Murphy SD. Effect of 18 hr fast and glutathione depletion on 1,1-dichloroethylene-induced hepatotoxicity and lethality in rats. *Exp Mol Pathol* 1974;20:187–198.
91. Pessayre D, Dolder A, Artigou JY, et al. Effect of fasting on metabolite-mediated hepatotoxicity in the rat. *Gastroenterology* 1979;77:264–271.
92. Pessayre D, Wanscheer JC, Corbert B, et al. Additive effects of inducers and fasting on acetaminophen hepatotoxicity. *Biochem Pharmacol* 1980;29:2219–2223.
93. Maruyama E, Kojuma J, Higashi T, et al. Effect of diet on liver glutathione and glutathione reductase. *J Biochem* 1968;63:398–399.
94. Mitchell JR, Jollow DJ, Potter WZ, et al. Acetaminophen-induced hepatic necrosis. 1. Role of drug-metabolism. *J Pharmacol Exp Ther* 1973;187:211–217.

95. Siegers CP, Schütt A, Strubelt O. Influence of some hepatotoxic agents on hepatic glutathione levels in mice. *Proc Eur Soc Toxicol* 1977;18:160–162.
96. Vadi HV, Neal RA. Microsomal activation of thioacetamide-S-oxide to a metabolite(s) that covalently binds to calf thymus DNA and other polynucleotides. *Chem Biol Interact* 1981;35:25–38.
97. Thor H, Moldéus P, Orrenius S. Metabolic activation and hepatotoxicity: effect of cysteine, N-acetylcysteine, and methionine on glutathione biosynthesis and bromobenzene toxicity in isolated rat hepatocytes. *Arch Biochem Biophys* 1979;192:405–413.
98. Högberg J, Kristofersson A. Correlation between glutathione levels and cellular damage in isolated hepatocytes. *Eur J Biochem* 1977;74:77–82.
99. Högberg J, Orrenius S, Larson R. Lipid peroxidation in isolated hepatocytes. *Eur J Biochem* 1975;50:595–602.
100. Babson JR, Abell NS, Reed DJ. Protective role of the glutathione redox cycle against adriamycin-mediated toxicity in isolated hepatocytes. *Biochem Pharmacol* 1981;30:2299–2304.
101. Meredith MJ, Reed DJ. Depletion in vitro of mitochondrial glutathione in rat hepatocytes and enhancement of lipid peroxidation by adriamycin and 1,3-bis(2-chloroethyl)-1-nitrosourea (BCNU). *Biochem Pharmacol* 1983;32:1383–1388.
102. Gonzalez-Flecha B, Cutrin JC, Boveris A. Time course and mechanism of oxidative stress and tissue damage in rat liver subjected to in vivo ischemia-reperfusion. *J Clin Invest* 1993;91:456–464.
103. Younes M, Siegers CP. Mechanistic aspects of enhanced lipid peroxidation following glutathione depletion in vivo. *Chem Biol Interact* 1981;34:257–266.
104. Lopez-Barea J, Lee CY. Mouse-liver glutathione reductase: purification, kinetics, and regulation. *Eur J Biochem* 1979;98:487–499.
105. Hillesheim W, Jaeschke H, Neumann HG. Cytotoxicity of aromatic amines in rat liver and oxidative stress. *Chem Biol Interact* 1995;98:85–95.
106. Sies H, Moss KM. A role of mitochondrial glutathione peroxidase in modulating mitochondrial oxidations in liver. *Eur J Biochem* 1978;84:377–383.
107. Trump BF, Pentilla A, Berezesky IK. Studies on cell surface conformation following injury. *Virchows Arch B Cell Pathol* 1979;29:281–296.
108. Lemasters JJ, Ji S, Thurman RG. Centrilobular injury following hypoxia in isolated, perfused rat liver. *Science* 1981;213:661–663.
109. Lemasters JJ, Stemkowski CJ, Ji S, et al. Cell surface changes and enzyme release during hypoxia and reoxygenation in the isolated, perfused rat liver. *J Cell Biol* 1983;97:778–786.
110. Thor H, Hartzell P, Svensson SA, et al. On the role of thiol groups in the inhibition of liver microsomal Ca^{2+} sequestration by toxic agents. *Biochem Pharmacol* 1985;34:3717–3723.
111. Jewell SA, Bellomo G, Thor H, et al. Bleb formation in hepatocytes during drug metabolism is caused by disturbances in thiol and calcium ion homeostasis. *Science* 1982;217:1257–1259.
112. Moore M, Thor H, Moore G, et al. The toxicity of acetaminophen and N-acetyl-p-benzoquinone imine in isolated hepatocytes is associated with thiol depletion and increased cytosolic Ca^{2+}. *J Biol Chem* 1985;260:13035–13040.
113. Bellomo G, Orrenius S. Altered thiol and calcium homeostasis in oxidative hepatocellular injury. *Hepatology* 1985;5:876–882.
114. Schanne FAX, Kane AB, Young EE, et al. Calcium dependence of toxic cell death: a final common pathway. *Science* 1979;206:700–702.
115. Farber JL. Biology of disease: membrane injury and calcium homeostasis in the pathogenesis of coagulative necrosis. *Lab Invest* 1982;47:114–123.
116. Lemasters JJ, DiGuiseppi J, Nieminen AL, et al. Blebbing, free Ca^{2+} and mitochondrial membrane potential preceding cell death in hepatocytes. *Nature* 1987;325:78–81.
117. Andersson BS, Aw TY, Jones DP. Mitochondrial transmembrane potential and pH gradient during anoxia. *Am J Physiol* 1985;252:C349–C355.
118. Nathan CF, Silverstein SC, Breckner LH, et al. Extracellular cytolysis by activated macrophages and granulocytes. II. Hydrogen peroxide as a mediator of cytotoxicity. *J Exp Med* 1979;149:100–113.
119. Simon RH, Scoggin CH, Patterson D. Hydrogen peroxide causes the fatal injury to human fibroblasts exposed to oxygen radicals. *J Biol Chem* 1981;256:7181–7186.
120. Weiss SJ, Young J, LoBuglio AF, et al. Role of hydrogen peroxide in neutrophil-mediated destruction of cultured endothelial cells. *J Clin Invest* 1981;68:714–721.
121. Sacks T, Moldow CF, Craddock PR, et al. Oxygen radicals mediate endothelial cell damage by complement-stimulated granulocytes: an in vitro model of immune vascular damage. *J Clin Invest* 1978;61:1161–1167.

122. Martin WJ II. Neutrophils kill pulmonary endothelial cells by a hydrogen peroxide dependent pathway. *Am Rev Respir Dis* 1984;130:209–213.
123. Hinshaw DB, Sklar LA, Bohl B, et al. Cytoskeletal and morphologic impact of cellular oxidant injury. *Am J Pathol* 1986;123:454–464.
124. Spragg RG, Hinshaw CB, Hyslop PA, et al. Alteractions in adenosine triphosphate and energy change in cultured endothelial and P388D1 cells following oxidant injury. *J Clin Invest* 1985;76:1471–1476.
125. Schraufstatter IU, Hinshaw CB, Hyslop PA, et al. Glutathione cycle activity and pyridine nucleotide levels in oxidant induced injury of cells. *J Clin Invest* 1985;76:1131–1139.
126. Schraufstatter IU, Hinshaw DB, Hyslop PA, et al. Oxidant injury of cells: DNA strand breaks activate polyadenosine diphosphate-ribose polymerase and lead to depletion of nicotinamide adenine dinucleotide. *J Clin Invest* 1986;77:1312–1320.
127. Bellomo G, Jewell SA, Thor H, et al. Regulation of intracellular calcium compartmentation: studies with isolated hepatocytes and t-butyl hydroperoxide. *Proc Natl Acad Sci USA* 1982;79:6842–6846.
128. Trump BF, Mergner WJ. The inflammatory process. In: Zweifach BW, et al., eds. *Cell Injury*, vol. 1. New York: Academic Press, 1974:115–257.
129. Scott RE. Plasma membrane vesiculation: a new technique for isolation of plasma membranes. *Science* 1976;194:743–745.
130. Scott RE, Perkins RG, Axchunke MA, et al. Plasma membrane vesiculation in 3T3 and SV 3T3 cells. I. Morphological and biochemical characterization. *J Cell Sci* 1979;35:229–243.
131. Kinn SR, Allen TD. Conversion of blebs to microvilli: cell surface reorganization after trypsin. *Differentiation* 1981;20:168–173.
132. Wu E, Tank DW, Webb WW. Unconstrained lateral diffusion of concanavalin A receptors on bulbous lymphocytes. *Proc Natl Acad Sci USA* 1982;79:4962–4967.
133. Tank DW, Wu E, Webb W. Enhanced molecular diffusibility in muscle membrane blebs: release of lateral constraints. *J Cell Biol* 1982;92:207–212.
134. Dang CV, Bell WR, Kaiser D, et al. Disorganization of cultured vascular endothelial cell monolayers by fibrinogen fragment D. *Science* 1985;227:1487–1490.
135. Malamed S, Recknagel RO. The osmotic behavior of the sucrose-inaccessible space of mitochondrial pellets from rat liver. *J Biol Chem* 1959;234:3027–3030.
136. Lehninger AL. Water uptake and extrusion by mitochondria in relation to oxidative phosphorylation. *Phys Rev* 1962;42:467–517.
137. Gunter TE, Pfeiffer DR. Mechanisms by which mitochondria transport calcium. *Am J Physiol* 1990;258:C755–C786.
138. Szabö I, Zoratti M. The mitochondrial megachannel is the permeability transition pore. *J Bioenerg Biomembr* 1992;24:111–117.
139. Richter C, Theus M, Schlegel J. Cyclosporine A inhibits mitochondrial pyridine nucleotide hydrolysis and calcium release. *Biochem Pharmacol* 1990;40:779–782.
140. Al-Nasser I, Crompton M. The reversible Ca^{2+}-induced permeabilization of rat liver mitochondria. *Biochem J* 1986;239:19–29.
141. Petronilli V, Cola C, Bernardi P. Modulation of the mitochondrial cyclosporin A-sensitive permeability transition pore. II. The minimal requirements for pore induction underscore a key role for transmembrane electrical potential, matrix pH, and matrix Ca^{2+}. *J Biol Chem* 1993;268:1011–1016.
142. Crompton M, Ellinger H, Costi A. Inhibition by cyclosporin A of a Ca^{2+}-dependent pore in heart mitochondria activated by inorganic phosphate and oxidative stress. *Biochem J* 1988;255:357–360.
143. Broekemeier KM, Dempsey ME, Pfeiffer DR. Cyclosporin A is a potent inhibitor of the inner membrane permeability transition in liver mitochondria. *J Biol Chem* 1989;264:7826–7830.
144. Igbavboa U, Zwizinski CW, Pfeiffer DR. Release of mitochondrial matrix proteins through a Ca^{2+}-requiring, cyclosporin-sensitive pathway. *Biochem Biophys Res Commun* 1989;161:619–625.
145. Fournier N, Ducet G, Crevat A. Action of cyclosporine on mitochondrial calcium fluxes. *J Bioenerg Biomembr* 1987;19:297–303.
146. Halestrap AP, Davidson AM. Inhibition of Ca^{2+}-induced large amplitude swelling of liver and heart mitochondria by cyclosporin is probably caused by the inhibitor binding to mitochondrial-matrix peptidyl-prolyl cis-trans isomerase and preventing it interacting with the adenine nucleotide translocase. *Biochem J* 1990;268:153–160.
147. Griffiths EJ, Halestrap AP. Further evidence that cyclosporin A protects mitochondria from calcium overload by inhibiting a matrix peptidyl-prolyl cis-trans isomerase: implications for the immunosuppressive and toxic effects of cyclosporin. *Biochem J* 1991;274:611–614.
148. Crompton M, Costi A. Kinetic evidence for a heart mitochondrial pore activated by Ca^{2+}, inorganic

phosphate and oxidative stress: a potential mechanism for mitochondrial dysfunction during cellular Ca^{2+} overload. *Eur J Biochem* 1988;178:489–501.

149. Savage MK, Reed DJ. Release of mitochondrial glutathione and calcium by a cyclosporin A-sensitive mechanism occurs without large amplitude swelling. *Arch Biochem Biophys* 1994;315:142–152.

150. Savage MK, Jones DP, Reed DJ. Calcium- and phosphate-dependent release and loading of glutathione by liver mitochondria. *Arch Biochem Biophys* 1991;290:51–56.

151. Takeyama N, Matsuo N, Tanaka T. Oxidative damage to mitochondria is mediated by the Ca^{2+}-dependent inner membrane permeability transition. *Biochem J* 1993;294:719–725.

152. Carini R, Parola M, Dianzani MU, Albano E. Mitochondrial damage and its role in causing hepatocyte injury during stimulation of lipid peroxidation by iron nitriloacetate. *Arch Biochem Biophys* 1992;297:110–118.

153. Masaki N, Kyle ME, Serroni A, Farber JL. Mitochondrial damage as a mechanism of cell injury in the killing of cultured hepatocytes by tert-butyl hydroperoxide. *Arch Biochem Biophys* 1989;270:672–680.

154. Bronk SF, Gores GJ. Acidosis protects against lethal oxidative injury of liver sinusoidal endothelial cells. *Hepatology* 1991;14:150–157.

155. Fujii Y, Johnson ME, Gores GJ. Mitochondrial dysfunction during anoxia/reoxygenation injury of liver endothelial cells, *Hepatology* 1994;20:177–185.

156. Martin DP, Schmidt RE, Distefan PS, Lowry OH, Carter JG, Johnson EM. Inhibitors of protein synthesis and RNA synthesis prevent neuronal death caused by nerve growth factor deprivation. *J Cell Biol* 1988;106:829–844.

157. Arends MJ, Morris RG, Wyllie AH. Apoptosis: the role of the endonuclease. *Am J Pathol* 1990;136:593–608.

158. Koury MJ, Bondurant MC. Erythroprotein retards DNA breakdown and prevents programmed cell death in erythroid progenitor cells. *Science* 1990;248:378–381.

159. Hockenbery DM, Oltval Z, Yin M, Milliman CL, Korsmeyer SJ. Bcl-2 functions in an antioxidant pathway to prevent apoptosis. *Cell* 1993;75:241–251.

160. Lavin M, Watters D, eds. *Programmed cell death.* Langhorne, PA: Harwood Academic Publishers. 1993:1–331.

161. Kroemer G, Petit P, Zamzami N, Vayssiere JC, Mignotte B. The biochemistry of programmed cell death. *FASEB J* 1995;9:1277–1287.

162. Ashkenas J, Werb Z. Proteolysis and the biochemistry of life-or-death decisions. *J Exp Med* 1996;183:1947–1951.

163. Martin SJ, Green DR. Protease activation during apoptosis: death by a thousand cuts? *Cell* 1995;82:349–352.

164. Beatrice MC, Palmer JW, Pfeiffer DR. The relationship between mitochondrial membrane permeability, membrane potential, and retention of Ca^{2+} by mitochondria. *J Biol Chem* 1980;255:8663–8671.

165. Beatrice MC, Stiers DL, Pfeiffer DR. Increased permeability of mitochondria during calcium release induced by t-butyl hydroperoxide oroxaloacetate: the effect of ruthenium red. *J Biol Chem* 1982;257:7161–7171.

166. Beatrice MC, Stiers DL, Pfeiffer DR. The role of glutathione in the retention of calcium by liver mitochondria. *J Biol Chem* 1984;259:1279–1287.

167. Petronilli V, Costantini P, Scorrano L, Colonna R, Passamonti S, Bernardi P. The voltage sensor of the mitochondrial permeability transition pore is tuned by the oxidation-reduction state of vicinal thiols. *J Biol Chem* 1994;269:16638–16642.

168. Connern CP, Halestrap AP. Recruitment of mitochondrial cyclophilin to the mitochondrial inner membrane under conditions of oxidative stress that enhance the opening of a calcium-sensitive nonspecific channel. *Biochem J* 1994;302:321–324.

169. Vercesi AE, Castilho RF, Meinicke AR, Valle VGR, Hermes-Lima M, Bechara EJH. Oxidative damage of mitochondria induced by 5-aminolevulinic acid: role of Ca^{2+} and membrane protein thiols. *Biochim Biophys Acta* 1994;1188:86–92.

170. Valle VG, Fagian MM, Parentoni LS, Meinicke AR, Vercesi AE. The participation of reactive oxygen species and protein thiols in the mechanism of mitochondrial inner membrane permeabilization by calcium plus prooxidants. *Arch Biochem Biophys* 1993;307:1–7.

171. Gunter TE, Gunter KK, Sheu SS, Gavin CE. Mitochondrial calcium transport: physiology and pathological relevance. *Am J Physiol* 1994;267:C313–C339.

172. Zamzami N, Marchetti P, Castedo M, Hirsch T, Susin SA, Masse B, Kroemer G. Inhibitors of permeability transition interfere with the disruption of the mitochondrial transmembrane potential during apoptosis. *FEBS Lett* 1996;384:53–57.

173. Bernardi P. Modulation of the mitochondrial cyclosporin A-sensitive permeability transition pore by the proton electrochemical gradient. *J Biol Chem* 1992;267:8834–8839.
174. Richter C, Gogvadze V, Laffranchi R, et al. Oxidants in mitochondria: from physiology to diseases. *Biochim Biophys Acta* 1995;1271:67–74.
175. Zamzami N, Marchetti P, Castedo M, et al. Sequential reduction of mitochondrial transmembrane potential and generation of reactive oxygen species in early programmed cell death. *J Exp Med* 1995;182:367–377.
176. Zamzami N, Marchetti P, Castedo M, et al. Reduction in mitochondrial potential constitutes an early irreversible step of programmed lymphocyte death in vivo. *J Exp Med* 1995;181:1661–1672.
177. Brodie AE, Potter J, Reed DJ. Unique characteristics of rat spleen lymphocyte, L1210 lymphoma and HeLa cels in glutathione biosynthesis from sulfur-containing amino acids. *Eur J Biochem* 1982;123:159–164.
178. Reed DJ, Brodie AE, Meredith MJ. Cellular heterogeneity in the status and functions of cysteine and glutathione. In: Larsson A, Orrenius S, Holmgren A, Mannervik B, eds. *Functions of glutathione. biochemical, physiological, toxicological, and clinical aspects*. New York: Raven Press, 1983:39–49.
179. Barhoumi R, Burghardt RC. Kinetic analysis of the chronology of patulin- and gossypol-induced cytotoxicity in vitro. *Fund Appl Toxicol* 1996;30:290–297.
180. Uchiyama Y. Apoptosis: the history and trends of its study. *Arch Histol Cytol* 1995;58:127–137.
181. Columbano A. Cell death: current difficulties in discriminating apoptosis from necrosis in the context of pathological process in vivo. *J Cell Biochem* 1995;58:181–190.
182. Farber E. Programmed cell death: necrosis versus apoptosis. *Mod Pathol* 1994;7:605–609.
183. Reed DJ. Regulation of reductive processes by glutathione, *Biochem Pharmacol* 1986;35:7–13.

Toxicology of the Liver, 2nd ed.,
Edited by Gabriel L. Plaa and William R. Hewitt
Copyright © 1998 Taylor & Francis

7

Lipid Peroxidation as a Mediator of Chemical-Induced Hepatocyte Death

Mario Comporti

*Instituto di Patologia Generale, Universita di Siena,
Via del Laterino, 8, 1-53100 Siena, Italy*

A current problem in pathology is that related to the formation of free radicals and to the molecular lesions produced by them. This problem implies the question of how free radicals are generated in the living cell and of which are the consequences of their production.

Oxygen is undispensable for the life of aerobic organisms and acts as terminal oxidant in the mitochondrial respiratory chain. However, the univalent reduction of oxygen leads to the formation of one of the reactive oxygen species, the superoxide anion ($O_2^{\bullet-}$). In the mitochondrial electron transport chain, and particularly in the transfer of electrons from reduced cytochrome c to molecular oxygen, about 95% of the consumed oxygen undergoes the cytochrome oxidase-catalyzed tetravalent reduction to H_2O, but over 5% of the consumed oxygen is released in the form of reactive species, such as $O_2^{\bullet-}$ and hydrogen peroxide (1–3). Thus, reactive oxygen species are produced even in the normal respiratory chain. It will be shown below that oxygen species are also formed in the microsomal electron transport chain.

Iron is necessary for life too, being an essential component of vital enzymes, such as cytochromes, cytochrome oxidase, and catalase, and equally vital iron complexes, such as hemoglobin and myoglobin. However, when released from these complexes in a free form, as will be seen below, iron can react with oxygen species or with molecular oxygen itself to yield additional oxyradicals (Fenton reaction) or reactive iron-oxygen complexes. Iron is therefore potentially toxic to biologic structures.

Similar considerations are true for cytochrome P450. This enzyme is a key component of the mixed function oxidase system, expecially expressed in liver endoplasmic reticulum, and is basically involved in a wide variety of reactions concerned with detoxification of xenobiotics. Yet cytochrome P450 activity can result in adverse effects, since a large number of xenobiotics are not toxic per se but elicit their toxic effects only after their activation to radical species or electrophilic intermediates by the cytochrome P450 mixed function oxidase system. In summary, free radicals can originate from both oxygen and xenobiotics.

With the appearance of oxygen on the earth crust, several defense mechanisms have been developed by aerobic organisms against oxygen species. The functional components of these systems are called antioxidants, and according to their functions, they are generally divided into three categories (4): preventive antioxidants, radical scavenging antioxidants, and repair compounds. Preventive antioxidants are those that reduce the rate of chain initiation by suppressing free radical generation by decomposing lipid hydroperoxides or hydrogen peroxide without generating free radicals (glutathione [GSH] peroxidase, phospholipid hydroperoxide GSH peroxidase [5], catalase, GSH-S-transferase); by quenching or dismutating active oxygen species (superoxide dismutase [SOD], carotenoids); or by sequestering metal ions (apoferritin, transferrin, lactoferrin, ceruloplasmin). Radical scavenging antioxidants are those that inhibit chain initiation and break chain propagation (vitamin E, vitamin C, ubiquinol, carotenoids, uric acid, bilirubin). Compounds with repair mechanisms are those that repair the damage and reconstitute the membrane (phospholipase A_2 [6], protease [7]). In addition to these defense systems, adaptation mechanisms should be also considered, i.e., the mechanisms operating in inducing formation of oxidative stress proteins that play a role in protecting cells against oxidative stress (8, 9).

The mechanisms of free-radical–induced cell injury have been reviewed by several authors (10, 11). In summary, they include reactions with nucleic acids, nucleotides, polysaccharides, protein and nonprotein thiols (thiol oxidation); covalent binding to membrane components (proteins, lipids, enzymes, receptors, and transport systems); and initiation of lipid peroxidation. Thus, the production of free radicals triggers an expanding network of multifarious disturbances.

Lipid peroxidation of cellular membranes has been suggested as a common mechanism in a large number of pathologic conditions and, more recently, even in many clinical diseases. Yet, up to some decades ago lipid peroxidation was known only in the chemistry of oil and fat rancidity, and its interest was confined mainly to the field of food technology. The possible importance of lipid peroxidation in biology as damaging process to cellular membranes was first suggested in the field of radiation injury (12, 13), as a consequence of the formation of free radicals from water ionization, and in the field of nutrition, as a consequence of vitamin E deficiency (14). Thus, at the beginning of the 1960s, the only knowledge available on lipid peroxidation was that liver homogenates (or subcellular fractions) from vitamin E–deficient animals would produce, upon incubation, a higher amount of malonaldehyde with respect to controls. Thus vitamin E could act as a natural antioxidant (14). The condition of vitamin E deficiency was limited, however, to animals maintained on particular diets. The spreading out of interest in lipid peroxidation in the field of pathology in the 1960s was mainly due to the knowledge that lipid peroxidation can be linked to the electron transport chain of drug metabolism (15); the recognition that the metabolism of the model hepatotoxic molecule, carbon tetrachloride, yields alloalkane free radicals (16, 17); and the observation that CCl_4 greatly stimulates the peroxidation of liver microsomal lipids (18, 19). This and other information led to the assumption that lipid peroxidation could be a basic mechanism of toxicity for a wide variety of chemicals.

Today it is well established that lipid peroxidation is only one of the reactions set into motion as a consequence of the formation of free radicals in cells and tissues. It was one of the first aspects of abnormal oxidative reactions to be recognized in cell pathology, probably because it represents the most prominent phenomenon of uncontrolled oxidative stress. With the discovery of SOD (20) and with the consequent acquisition that oxyradicals can be easily produced in the living tissues, a much more complex spectrum of pathologic oxidations has been progressively recognized, so that the term *oxidative stress* has been introduced (21) to signify any condition in which the prooxidant–antioxidant balance is shifted in favor of oxidations.

LIPID PEROXIDATION IN CELLULAR MEMBRANES

Although the chemistry of lipid peroxidation, which has been extensively reviewed elsewhere (11, 17, 22–26), is not the purpose of this chapter, the general mechanism of the process with particular regard to the initiation in cellular membranes (a simplified scheme is reported in Fig. 1) will be briefly summarized.

Lipid peroxidation is commonly divided into three phases, namely, initiation, propagation, and termination. The initiation step is the interaction of free radicals with polyenoic fatty acids of membrane phospholipids. Such an attack occurs at the allylic hydrogens on a carbon atom between two double bonds because of the relatively low bond dissociation energy (75 kcal/mol) that renders these hydrogens particularly susceptible to the attack (27). A fatty acid radical is thus formed. Carbon-centered radicals can initiate the process, e.g., the trichloromethyl radical ($CCl_3^•$) resulting from CCl_4 metabolism. Oxygen-centered radicals can also initiate lipid peroxidation, but very likely the presence of catalytically active iron (or other transition metals) is also required. Superoxide ($O_2^•$), hydrogen peroxide (H_2O_2), and hydroxyl radical ($OH^•$) can in principle take part in the initiation step, but the exact mechanisms are not known

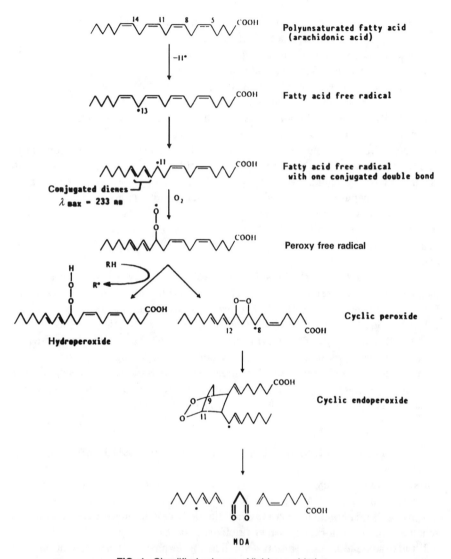

FIG. 1. Simplified scheme of lipid peroxidation.

with certainty (11, 28). Iron (II) ions can take part in electron transfer reactions with molecular oxygen:

$$Fe^{2+} + O_2 \rightleftarrows (Fe^{2+} - O_2 \longleftrightarrow Fe^{3+} - O_2^{\bullet-}) \rightleftarrows Fe^{3+} + O_2^{\bullet-}$$

Superoxide probably is not reactive enough to abstract hydrogen from lipids, while its protonated form $HO_2^{\bullet}$ is more reactive and, being uncharged, would enter membranes fairly easily. In addition, superoxide can dismutate (via SOD) to form H_2O_2, and OH$^\bullet$ is produced via the Fenton reaction:

$$O_2^{\bullet-} + Fe^{3+} \rightarrow O_2 + Fe^{2+}$$

$$Fe^{2+} + H_2O_2 \rightarrow Fe^{3+} + OH^- + OH^\bullet \text{ (Fenton reaction)}$$

$$\text{net reaction } \overline{O_2^{\bullet-} + H_2O_2 \rightarrow O_2 + OH^- + OH^\bullet} \text{ (Haber-Weiss reaction)}$$

The hydroxyl radical has certainly the capacity of abstracting hydrogen from polyenoic fatty acids, but because of its extreme reactivity, it is unlikely that it can migrate from its site of origin to fatty acid molecules in cellular membranes. Direct participation of OH$^\bullet$ radicals in the initiation has been questioned (29, 30). As is known, the addition of iron (II) to unsaturated fatty acids, liver microsomes, or liposomes initiates lipid peroxidation, but in most of these studies the OH$^\bullet$ scavengers do not inhibit the reaction. Yet OH$^\bullet$ radicals can be detected in these systems, and their formation is inhibited by the scavengers. It seems, therefore, that OH$^\bullet$ formation is not required for the initiation, even if the possibility exists that, as suggested by Halliwell and Gutteridge (11, 31), membrane-bound iron ions catalyze a site-specific generation of OH$^\bullet$; the latter would react immediately with membrane lipids before being scavenged. A number of studies (29, 30) led to the hypothesis that an iron–oxygen complex, rather than OH$^\bullet$, is required for the initiation. Such a complex could be ferryl iron (FeO^{2+}) (32) or perferryl ion (Fe^{2+}O$_2 \leftrightarrow$ Fe^{3+}O$_2^{\bullet-}$) (29, 33), but it seems that the latter is not sufficiently reactive to initiate the reaction (11). Recently it has been proposed (34) that the active oxidant is a Fe^{3+}–O$_2$–Fe^{2+} complex (Fe^{3+}/Fe^{2+} ratio = 1), but its precise nature has not been established. In any case, in the cellular environment, iron must be available in a free, redox active form, which implies the presence of a free iron pool in equilibrium with iron bound to macromolecular complexes. As will be seen below, the problem of iron delocalization (30, 31) is central to oxidative stress.

In the fatty acid radical initially formed, resonance of the free radical electron results in the shift of a double bond and formation of conjugated dienes. Detection of the latter, which absorb intensely at 233 nm, has been widely used to detect lipid peroxidation in vitro and in vivo.

Carbon-centered radicals, such as the fatty acid radicals, easily react with oxygen to form oxygen-centered lipid peroxy radicals (LOO$^\bullet$). These can abstract hydrogen from neighboring polyunsaturated fatty acids (PUFA) and form the corresponding lipid hydroperoxides. Propagation is the reaction of a peroxyl radical with another PUFA to yield hydroperoxide and a new lipid radical, thus conserving the number of radicals in the reaction sequence. Decomposition of hydroperoxides catalyzed by iron or other transition metals yields alkoxy and peroxy radicals and amplifies propagation, since such a secondary generation of free radicals can initiate new chains of lipid hydroperoxide formation.

$$LOOH + Fe^{2+} \rightarrow LO^\bullet + Fe^{3+} + OH^- \text{ reductive decomposition}$$

$$LOOH + Fe^{3+} \rightarrow LOO^\bullet + Fe^{2+} + H^+ \text{ oxidative decomposition}$$

Decomposition of the peroxidized fatty acid involving breakdown of the molecule (scission of C–C bonds) yields a variety of end products. Decomposition of fatty acid endoperoxides yields malonaldehyde (MDA), the most commonly measured lipid peroxidation product. A large number of other aldehydes (alkanals, alkenals, 4-hydroxyalkenals, alkadienals, etc.) are also formed (see below). Other decomposition products are small-chain hydrocarbons, such as ethane (from omega-6 fatty acids) and penthane (from omega-3 fatty acids) (24), the detection of which in the expired air has represented a noninvasive method for lipid peroxidation in vivo (35, 36).

The reaction chain can be terminated through the combination of two radicals to yield a nonradical product. In biologic membranes, abnormal lipid–lipid or lipid–protein interactions can occur. The latter are due to the fact that lipid radicals can abstract hydrogen from proteins, which results in lipid–protein cross linking (37).

The effects of lipid peroxidation in cellular membranes have been widely reported and can be summarized as follows: decrease in membrane fluidity; formation of hydrophilic centers (peroxide and carbonyl groups) in the hydrophobic regions of phospholipids, with increase in membrane permeability (passive swelling of mitochondria, vesciculation of endoplasmic reticulum, lysis of red blood cells, leakage of enzymes, etc.); and loss of the normal lipid–lipid and lipid–protein interaction, with consequent impairment of enzyme function. In addition to the loss of membrane structure, lipid peroxidation can also result in the release of toxic products, particularly aldehydes.

FORMATION AND REACTIVITY OF ALDEHYDES DERIVED FROM LIPID PEROXIDATION

The aldehyde products of lipid peroxidation have been of particular interest in food chemistry, because they are mainly responsible for flavor changes in the process of rancidity. Nevertheless, up to some decades ago relatively few aldehydes, such as malonaldehyde (MDA) and other dicarbonyl compounds, had been identified. It was then demonstrated (38) that the autoxidation of methyl linoleate leads to the formation of 4-hydroxyoctenal, a prototype of a new class of aldehydes, namely 4-hydroxyalkenals. These aldehydes proved to exhibit a number of biologic effects (39).

It was subsequently shown in our laboratory (40, 41) that hydroxyalkenals are formed during lipid peroxidation occurring in a well-known biologic condition such as that represented by the NADPH oxidation by liver microsomes in the absence of an electron-accepting terminal substrate. In particular, the thin-layer chromatography analysis of an ether extract of a dialysate obtained from peroxidizing microsomes showed the presence of a band (40) that contained almost entirely (more than 95%) 4-hydroxy-2,3 trans-nonenal (4-hydroxynonenal, 4-HNE).

The structure was ascertained by means of ultraviolet, infrared, and mass spectrometry (41).

The kinetics of formation of 4-HNE in peroxidizing liver microsomes is similar to that of MDA. The ratio between 4-HNE and MDA production is about 1:10/1:20 on a molar basis (42). The whole pattern of carbonyls originating from the ADP-Fe^{2+}–stimulated peroxidation of liver microsomal lipids includes alkanals (mostly hexanal and propanal), alk-2-enals (mostly oct-2-enal) and 4-hydroxyalkenals (mostly 4-HNE) (43).

In contrast to alkanals, 2-alkenals and 4-hydroxyalkenals are highly reactive products. The biologic effects depend mostly on their reactivity with -SH groups of low-molecular-weight thiols (GSH, cysteine, coenzyme A), proteins, and enzymes (39). Under physiologic conditions the main reaction is the Michael addition, in which the α-β unsaturated aldehyde binds with C_3 to the -SH group by a thioether linkage. 4-Hydroxyalkenals react about five times faster than 2-alkenals, and the adducts formed are about 500 times more stable (44). Alkenals and 4-hydroxyalkenals can also react with amino groups of amino acids, proteins, phospholipids, and nucleic acids to give Schiff's bases, as do saturated aldehydes (alkanals), but the reactivity with amino groups is two to three orders of magnitude lower than that with -SH groups (39). However, the reaction of 4-HNE with the ε-amino group of a lysine residue (45) or with histidine (46) is well documented.

Since the discovery of 4-hydroxyalkenals, in particular 4-HNE, which has been assumed as a model molecule of oxidative stress, extensive studies have been carried out on the effects of these aldehydes on biologic systems. Most of these effects, which have been extensively reviewed (47–50), are detrimental for a large number of biologic functions. Therefore, 4-HNE and related aldehydes have been proposed as mediators of the damage induced by chemicals that promote lipid peroxidation (see below).

In addition to the cytotoxic effects, physiologic or pathophysiologic activities too have been proposed for aldehydes derived from oxidation of phospholipids and either released from or still attached to the latter ones (51–54). This topic, however, is beyond the purpose of this chapter.

FORMATION OF F_2-ISOPROSTANES FROM PEROXIDATION OF ARACHIDONIC ACID

An important advance in the field of oxidative stress appears to be the recent discovery of a series of bioactive prostaglandin F_2-like compounds (F_2-isoprostanes[1]), which are produced by free radical–catalyzed peroxidation of arachidonic acid, independent of cyclooxygenase enzyme pathway (55, 56). The formation of these compounds proceeds through intermediates composed of four positional peroxyl radical isomers of arachidonic acid that undergo endocyclization to yield bicyclic endoperoxide PGG_2-like compounds (Fig. 2). The latter are then reduced to PGF_2-like compounds (55, 56). F_2-isoprostanes are initially formed *in situ* on phospholipids, from which they are subsequently released into the circulation, presumably by phospholipases (57). Therefore, unlike cyclooxygenase-derived prostanoids, F_2-isoprostanes are not formed from free arachidonic acid (57).

---

[1]The term isoprostane has been sanctioned by a special committee on eicosanoid nomenclature.

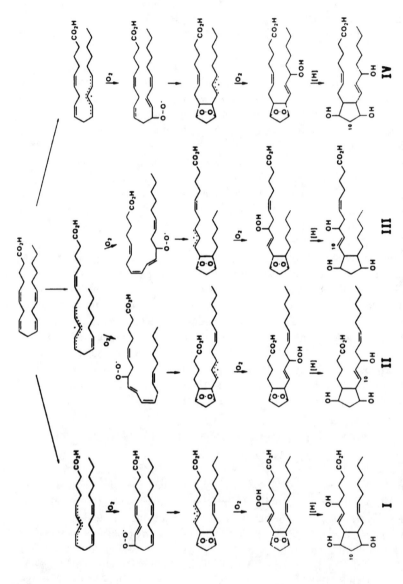

FIG. 2. Proposed mechanism for noncyclooxygenase oxidative formation of PGF$_2$ compounds (F$_2$-isoprostanes). This pathway leads to the formation of four regioisomers of PGF$_2$(I–IV). For simplicity, stereochemical orientation is not indicated in the figure. Each regioisomer theoretically is composed of a mixture of eight racemic diastereomers Reproduced from Morrow et al. (55), with permission.

228

After intoxication of rats with CCl_4 the plasma level of F_2-isoprostanes are increased over 50-fold by 4 hr (58). The level decreases thereafter, but at 24 hr it is still elevated over 20-fold, indicating continuing lipid peroxidation. Pretreatment of the animals with phenobarbital or SKF-525A increased or decreased F_2-isoprostane formation, respectively (58). Increased F_2-isoprostanes esterified to lipids have been found, besides in liver, also in kidney and lung (58).

F_2-isoprostane metabolites have been also identified in plasma and urine with the advantage of being able to handle more stable products than the unmetabolized parent compounds (59). Such metabolites appear to be tetranor, dicarboxylic acid compounds containing one double bond, *cis*-cyclopentane ring hydroxyls, and one keto group similar in structure to the major urinary metabolite of prostaglandin D_2 (9α, 11β-dihydroxy-15-oxo-2,3,18,19-tetranorprost-5-ene-1, 20-dioic acid).

This series of studies has apparently afforded a number of important contributions to the field of oxidative stress. First, the measure of F_2-isoprostanes seems to represent a method to detect lipid peroxidation in vivo with good reliability and with a sensitivity several orders of magnitude higher than that of the previously used methods (60). For instance, it is possible to detect lipid peroxidation in vivo in several tissues in vitamin E and selenium deficiency (61), a condition in which only a higher susceptibility to lipid peroxidation had been previously appreciated by most studies. Since F_2-isoprostanes or their metabolites can be found in plasma and urine, quantification of these products may provide a new and noninvasive tool for the assessment of oxidative stress in humans. Second, formation of F_2-isoprostanes itself may contribute to oxidative damage. On the one hand, molecular modeling of F_2-isoprostane–containing phospholipids reveals them to be remarkably distorted molecules (57), which may contribute to alterations in membrane fluidity and other physicochemical characters. On the other hand, free F_2-isoprostanes exhibit biologic activities (56, 62). Therefore, the idea that mediators of the damage may originate from oxidation of membrane lipids is still emerging. Such an idea has dominated other research, which suggested that the generation of eicosanoids could play an important role as a secondary mechanism leading to cell damage (see below).

LIPID PEROXIDATION AND TOXIC LIVER INJURY: GENERAL CONSIDERATIONS

Before reviewing the most studied examples of hepatotoxicant-induced lipid peroxidation, it is helpful to consider what evidence is needed, in the opinion of this reviewer, to assess the occurrence of lipid peroxidation and its role in the mechanism of toxicity of a given compound. With in vitro systems lipid peroxidation can be assessed using a variety of methods (thiobarbituric acid [TBA] test for MDA, detection of conjugated dienes and many others [63–65]), which show in general good agreement among themselves. In addition, there is in general a good correlation between the extent of lipid peroxidation and the degree of functional membrane damage (e.g., alterations of the enzymatic activities, transport systems, etc.). The somewhat diffuse skepticism on similar methods used to assess lipid peroxidation in vivo can be obviated if various methods used give similar indications (66) (the use of one methods only, e.g., TBA test, may be unreliable for many reasons [26, 67, 68]) or the results of the in vivo studies agree with those of in vitro studies, carried out on appropriate systems. In addition, as previously mentioned, the determination of F_2-isoprostanes represents a new and very promising method for the detection of lipid peroxidation in vivo.

Another fact that has generated confusion as to the assessment of lipid peroxidation in vivo has been the assumption that lipid peroxidation must occur whenever the toxic effects are ameliorated by prior administration of antioxidants. The effectiveness of antioxidants in vivo may be only a circumstantial indication of the involvement of free radical processes—not necessarily lipid peroxidation—under certain conditions. Induction of lipid peroxidation in cell membranes must be proved and not indirectly deduced.

Finally, the claim that lipid peroxidation may be the consequence rather than the cause of cell death (69–71) has been discussed elsewhere (72, 73). In my opinion, at least in some well-studied models of toxic cell injury, lipid peroxidation cannot be considered as the consequence of cell death. Rather, lipid peroxidation has been detected well before cell death (18, 19, 58, 74–76), and when the latter is increasing, the various indices of lipid peroxidation are, on the contrary, decreasing. In other cases, however, lipid peroxidation, even if occurring, does not appear to be the primary cause of cell death, as will be discussed below.

Another consideration that must be added is that in many instances lipid peroxidation probably is not the sole cause of cell death. Rather, the initial peroxidative damage in cell membranes is the trigger for a subsequent cascade of pathologic events finally resulting in cell death. Nevertheless, lipid peroxidation may play a critical role as a link between the metabolism of a certain toxicant and the subsequent events. In other cases lipid peroxidation can be induced as the consequence of particular imbalances and disorders created in the cell by the toxic insult. It could be argued that such disturbances can produce cell death even in the absence of lipid peroxidation, but, according to our experience, in such cases prevention of lipid peroxidation largely prevents cell death.

PROTOTYPES OF TOXIC MOLECULES IMPLICATED IN THE INDUCTION OF LIPID PEROXIDATION

Since most chemicals are metabolized in the liver, the hepatocyte is the cell where a free radical attack resulting in lipid peroxidation is most likely to occur. The toxicants that can induce lipid peroxidation in the liver cell fall broadly into the following groups (77): those that are metabolized to reactive free radicals which promote directly peroxidation of membrane lipids; those that are metabolized to electrophilic intermediates which readily conjugate with GSH, thus producing extensive GSH depletion; and those that are converted to intermediates generating active oxygen species by redox cycling. As will be discussed, many redox cycling compounds can also produce GSH depletion, but their toxicity seems more directly connected with their ability to form oxyradicals.

Carbon Tetrachloride and Monobromotrichloromethane

With regard to the first group of agents, prototypes such as CCl_4 and the more potent analog $CBrCl_3$ must be considered. They are metabolized by the microsomal mixed function oxidase system utilizing the NADPH-cytochrome P450 electron transport chain. It is generally accepted (17, 78–80) that the reaction involved in the metabolism is a one-electron reduction catalyzed by cytochrome P450, the latter being maintained in the reduced form by NADPH:

$$CCl_4 + e^- \rightarrow CCl_3^{\bullet} + Cl^-$$

A specific isoenzyme of cytochrome P450, CYP1A2 (in the rat), is involved, whereas other isoenzymes, such as P4501A1, are not. The trichloromethyl radical is thus generated, which, in the presence of molecular oxygen, can form the trichloromethyl peroxy radical. These radicals, whose formation has been demonstrated in vitro and in vivo (81–85), can act both directly by covalently binding to membrane lipids and proteins (in particular to those of the endoplasmic reticulum) and indirectly through interaction with membrane unsaturated lipids and consequent promotion of lipid peroxidation. Both possibilities have been demonstrated (lipid peroxidation has been detected with all the methods available to date) and occur immediately (few minutes) after the in vivo intoxication (71, 86). Therefore, a debated question has been for some time whether the CCl_4-induced liver injury is due to covalent binding of CCl_4 radicals to cellular components (87–89) or whether lipid peroxidation is involved as an intermediate pathway between the metabolism of CCl_4 and the cellular alterations. The topic has been extensively reviewed elsewhere (77, 78, 90). Briefly, studies from our laboratory (91) and other laboratories (92) have shown that at least some effects of CCl_4, such as the inactivation of microsomal glucose-6-phosphatase (G-6-Pase, assumed as a test membrane enzyme) are mediated by lipid peroxidation rather than by covalent binding. In fact, the incubation of liver microsomes with CCl_4 (and NADPH) under anaerobic conditions that suppressed lipid peroxidation resulted in no decrease of the enzyme activity, in spite of a relatively high covalent binding of CCl_4 radicals to microsomal lipids and proteins. CCl_4 is in fact metabolized even under anaerobic conditions, the metabolism depending on an electron transfer from NADPH to CCl_4 itself. G-6-Pase was, on the contrary, completely destroyed under aerobic conditions, in which lipid peroxidation maximally developed. Additional studies of ours (93) suggested that also the CCl_4-induced decrease in cytochrome P450 is hardly accounted for by the mere covalent binding of CCl_4 radicals (73, 94). It was also shown (91–95) that the alterations of microsomal lipids seen after CCl_4 in vivo (formation of branched chain fatty acids, i.e., binding of CCl_4 radicals to double bonds of unsaturated fatty acids, and formation of conjugated dienes) are reproduced in the anaerobic in vitro system with microsomes and CCl_4. Since

G-6-Pase is not affected in anaerobiosis, as already stated, it seemed (91) that some product downstream with respect to conjugated dienes in the peroxidative cascade and originating from the oxidative breakdown of unsaturated fatty acids could be responsible for the enzyme inactivation.

These and other results (96, 97) led to the hypothesis that toxic products originate from the peroxidation of cellular membranes, diffuse from the locus in which lipid peroxidation is set into motion, and act at distant *loci* both in the membrane and at cellular sites removed from the membrane itself. Therefore, a number of studies were devoted to the search of lipid peroxidation products that could represent the second toxicologic messengers of the damage and explain the so-called action at a distance (96), which is the spreading of the damage from the locus of CCl_4 activation (cytochrome P450 *locus* in the endoplasmic reticulum) throughout the cell. It was in fact difficult to imagine that the short-lived CCl_4 radicals could travel from their site of origin and act at a distance. In this line of research we showed (98) that products originating from the peroxidation of liver microsomal lipids were capable of inducing cytopathologic effects (hemolysis, inhibition of microsomal enzymes, etc.) in target systems (erythrocytes, liver microsomes) that were separated from the peroxidizing system by a dialysis membrane. Thus, we had to deal with metastable products (much more stable than the CCl_4 radicals), capable of crossing a dialysis membrane to induce pathologic effects at a distance. In further studies (40) some of these toxic products derived from lipid peroxidation were separated from the dialysate and characterized. As already mentioned, of particular importance was the identification of 4-HNE (41), an aldehyde of the 4-hydroxyalkenal class.

In other studies we showed that aldehydes derived from lipid peroxidation are actually formed in vivo in the livers of animals intoxicated with various agents that promote lipid peroxidation. In a first set of studies (99) evidence was forwarded for alkenals bound to the liver microsomal protein of rats intoxicated with CCl_4 or $BrCCl_3$. In subsequent studies (100–102), 4-HNE and other aldehydes were found even in a free form in the livers of animals intoxicated with CCl_4, $BrCCl_3$, bromobenzene, and allyl alcohol.

It has been questioned (103, 104) whether toxic aldehydes could be generated from peroxidation of membrane lipids in amounts sufficient to induce cytopathologic effects, such as inhibition of enzymes of the endoplasmic reticulum. The fact that 4-HNE has been detected in the free form in the liver despite its reactivity seems to indicate that it is produced in significant amounts. Furthermore, an approximate estimation reported elsewhere (90) led to the conclusion that 4-HNE and other alkenals are indeed generated in sufficient amounts to produce damaging effects in membranes, in which they can diffuse laterally and reach a number of possible targets. Nevertheless, the hypothesis that these aldehydes represent the toxicologic second messengers linking lipid peroxidation in the membranes to pathologic consequences at distant cellular sites presents several conceptual difficulties. As previously stated, 4-hydroxyalkenals react readily with GSH, whose concentration in the liver cytoplasm is 5–10 mM. Also, the reaction is catalyzed by cytosolic GSH-S-transferases, of which 4-HNE is a good substrate (105, 106). In addition, a cytosolic alcohol dehydrogenase can reduce 4-HNE to the corresponding alcohol (107). It seems therefore that the cell is provided with specific defense systems against the formation of 4-HNE and other toxic aldehydes. Even if the half-life of these aldehydes is certainly several orders of magnitude higher than that of free radicals, it is difficult to imagine that these molecules can traverse the soluble cytoplasm and produce all the alterations spread throughout the cell.

Thus it is now acknowledged that the lipid peroxidation–induced loss of membrane structure and formation of toxic products, although of great importance in the damage to endoplasmic reticulum and probably to plasma membranes (108), are only early events that trigger secondary pathologic consequences.

One consequence that has been thoroughly studied is the perturbation of intracellular calcium homeostasis (109–111). Briefly, alteration of intracellular calcium distribution would represent the trigger for the final common pathway leading to cell death in many types of cell injury. The initial pathologic events in the membrane (lipid peroxidation, covalent binding, loss of protein thiols, etc.) lead to a disturbance in the mechanisms that regulate the concentration of free cytosolic calcium. In particular, it has been shown (112–116) that CCl_4 and $CBrCl_3$ cause, as a consequence of their metabolism in vitro and in vivo, a marked inhibition of the microsomal calcium sequestering activity. When the microsomal calcium pump is impaired, a sustained rise in cytosolic Ca^{2+} can be anticipated. This would cause a number of pathologic consequences, such as activation of phospholipases (117) and lytic enzymes (118), and, in particular, collapse of mitochondrial membrane potential, with consequent ATP depletion (119). The latter would presumably affect, among many other functions, plasma membrane calcium pumps and Na/K-ATPase (120). The critical level of cytosolic Ca^{2+} capable of producing a collapse of mitochondrial membrane potential would be reached when, in addition to inhibition of microsomal Ca^{2+} sequestration activity, a severe disturbance of plasma membrane Ca^{2+} pumps is also produced (120).

The mechanism of action of carbon tetrachloride can be considered now as a model for the explanation of the hepatotoxic effects of several other halogenated aliphatic hydrocarbons such as bromoform ($CHBr_3$), iodoform (CHI_3), vinyl chloride (CH_2=$CHCl$), halothane (CF_3—$CHBrCl$), and ethrane (77, 121). The available data suggest that the toxicity is inversely related to the dissociation energy of the carbon–halogen bond ($CBrCl_3$ has the lowest dissociation energy and the highest toxicity, followed by $CCl_4 > CH_3Cl > CHCl_3$).

Possible Role of Eicosanoids in Toxic Liver Cell Injury

The formation of prostaglandin—like substances (F_2-isoprostanes) in CCl_4 hepatotoxicity has been mentioned. Here we will also cite the studies on the possible involvment of eicosanoids in toxic liver injury. These studies started from the observation (122) that some prostagandins (PGs) protect the gastric mucosa against necrotizing agents that do not act *via* stimulation of gastric acid secretion. It was subsequently shown (123–128) that such a cytoprotective effect also occurs in the case of the liver injury induced by a number of toxicants such as CCl_4, bromobenzene, acetaminophen, ethanol, galactosamine, aflatoxin, and α-naphthylisothiocyanate. Particularly studied was a derivative of PGE_2 (16,16-dimethyl PGE_2), which produced remarkable protective effects in vivo (123–125, 128) and in vitro (isolated hepatocytes incubated with CCl_4 [127]). The fact that the protective effect occurs in such a wide variety of toxic injuries, with widely different biochemical mechanisms of cell damage, implies that PGs interfere with some phenomenon occurring late in the sequence of events leading from the initial insult to the ultimate irreversible cell injury. The same conclusion was also reached in studies (129) in which prostacyclin (PGI_2) and two of its derivatives were tested for the protective effects against the CCl_4-induced liver injury.

Recent studies (130–133) have shown that eicosanoids (prostaglandins, prostacyclin, and tromboxanes) are produced during the response of the liver to a number of toxicants. The observation that PGI_2 exhibits cytoprotective activity (127, 129, 130, 134) and that, on the contrary, tromboxanes (TXA_2, TXB_2) show cytotoxic potential (130–133, 135) has generated the idea that a natural $PGI_2 \leftrightarrow TX$ balance may exist, in which the cytoprotective action of PGI_2 acts as a counterweight to the cytotoxic activity of tromboxanes. In particular, it has been shown (130) that liver homogenates from acetaminophen-intoxicated animals produce, upon incubation, far higher amounts of PGE_2, PGI_2, and TXB_2 than do controls. The selective tromboxane inhibitor, OKI 1581, inhibits TXB_2 formation and increases production of PGI_2 (130). Both PGI_2 and OKI 1581 given in vivo decrease acetaminophen-induced liver necrosis to a great extent. On the contrary, indomethacin alone or in conjunction with OKI 1581 has no effect (130). These studies thus suggest that modulation of eicosanoid response can result in modulation of acetaminophen toxicity. The cyclooxygenase pathway of arachidonic acid leads to the endoperoxide PGH_2, which is the common precursor of various PGs, PGI_2, and TX. The TX inhibitor, OKI 1581, by blocking the conversion of PGH_2 to TX, increases the availability of PGH_2 for alternative routes. Therefore, selective inhibition of TX synthesis may, besides decreasing TX levels, increase PGI_2 production. Under these conditions liver necrosis is decreased. It seems therefore that acetaminophen toxicity can upset a natural $PGI_2 \leftrightarrow TX$ balance, in which TX is cytotoxic while PGI_2 is cytoprotective. Indomethacin, which inhibits the cyclooxygenase pathway, inhibits the whole eicosanoid response (including PGI_2 synthesis), and therefore the toxicity is not affected.

The origin of eicosanoids in liver injury has been the object of several investigations. In part they can originate in the hepatocytes (their production has been observed with isolated cells); in part they may derive from blood cells (leucocytes and platelets) leaving the sinusoids and accumulating in the space of Disse. It has been shown (136) that in peritoneal leukocytes incubated with CCl_4, an activation of phospholipase A_2 occurs with generation of TXB_2 and, to a lower extent, of PGE_2, PGI_2, and leukotriene B_4.

Activation of phospholipase A_2 is another important topic concerning eicosanoids, production, and toxic liver injury. The subject, which has been reviewed elsewhere (111, 137), will be not treated here because it is only marginally related to lipid peroxidation.

Glutathione-Depleting Agents

The second group of toxicants that can promote lipid peroxidation in cellular membranes is represented by chemicals that are metabolized to electrophilic intermediates readily conjugating with GSH and giving extensive GSH depletion. They include aryl halides, such as bromobenzene and other halobenzenes, acetaminophen (paracetamol), alcohols such as allyl alcohol, halogenated aliphatic hydrocarbons such as 1,2-dibromoethane (ethylene dibromide), 1,1-dichloroethylene (vinylidene chloride), 1,1,2-trichloroethylene (trielin, etc.), diethylmaleate and many other substances (72, 77). The most studied molecules are bromobenzene and acetaminophen.

Bromobenzene is an industrial solvent that causes centrilobular hepatic necrosis in experimental animals. The route of bromobenzene metabolism thought to be mainly associated with hepatotoxicity is the microsomal monooxygenase catalyzed formation of 3,4-bromobenzene epoxide (138). The latter can covalently bind to cellular macromolecules but can also be converted to other products. The epoxide in fact can be rearranged to form 4-bromophenol, can be converted to a dihydrodiol (by an epoxide hydrolase) or can react with GSH to give a glutathionyl conjugate (139). The latter reaction, catalyzed by GSH-S-transferases, represents the main pathway, and the conjugate is excreted in urine as a mercapturic acid. The result is a marked decrease in hepatic GSH level. The covalent binding of bromobenzene metabolites to protein markedly increases after the GSH stores of the liver cell have been depleted (138). Pretreatment of rats with phenobarbital or with SKF-525A increases or decreases, respectively, both covalent binding and liver necrosis (140–143). Similar results were reported for acetaminophen (144). Thus, it appeared that the liver injury induced by these aromatic hydrocarbon derivatives was caused by the covalent binding of their reactive metabolites to cellular macromolecules (140) and that the fundamental role of GSH was to protect essential thiols and other nucleophilic groups in cellular macromolecules from the electrophilic reactants formed from the metabolism of a number of xenobiotics. There is no doubt that one of the protective effects of GSH is to scavenge electrophiles by GSH-S-transferases present in large amounts in liver cytosol. However, a number of studies (72, 77, 124) showed a dissociation of cell death from covalent binding. Most of these studies demonstrated that the treatment of animals or isolated hepatocytes with substances that prevent the liver cell injury induced by some of these chemicals do not significantly modify the extent of covalent binding of the respective metabolites to liver protein. The concept therefore was developed that when the GSH level is severely decreased, the liver cell becomes more susceptible to the development of lipid peroxidation. The latter was detected in several studies in vitro (isolated hepatocytes treated with chloracetamide, chloramine T, etc. [145] or with bromobenzene [146]) and in vivo (mice intoxicated with acetaminophen [147]). We found (148) that the intoxication of starved mice with bromobenzene and iodobenzene results in a sharp decrease in liver GSH level within the first hours. Subsequently (14–18 hr) severe lipid peroxidation develops and is accompanied by a likewise severe liver necrosis (serum transaminases). The plot of the individual values for lipid peroxidation and for liver necrosis against the corresponding hepatic GSH levels showed that the two phenomena develop only when the hepatic GSH depletion has reached critical or threshold values (approximately 10% of the control value). The treatment of the animals, after the intoxication, with the antioxidant Trolox C[2] (a lower homolog of vitamin E) completely prevents both lipid peroxidation and liver necrosis while not changing at all the extent of covalent binding of bromobenzene metabolites to liver protein (148). Also, the hepatotoxicity of 1,2-dibromoethane has been related to lipid peroxidation rather than to covalent binding in both in vitro (149) and in vivo (150) studies.

The agreement between the results obtained in vitro and in vivo supports the view that covalent binding, at least as measured usually, is not directly related to cell injury and that the liver damage produced by many GSH depleting agents is mediated by events, such as lipid peroxidation and probably many others, which are more strictly related to the oxidative stress imposed by GSH depletion. It must be considered, however, that in the case of bromobenzene, different types of metabolites are involved in covalent binding. In addition to the 3,4-epoxide, the 2,3-epoxide is also formed (151). Both epoxides covalently bind to hepatic proteins (152), but the two epoxides may have different reactivity and may bind to different proteins and to different groups in proteins (152). Accordingly, they may have different toxicities, the 3,4-epoxide being thought to be more toxic than the 2,3-epoxide (153). The former, although reactive, would be provided with sufficient stability to leave the endoplasmic reticulum where it is formed and react with macromolecules in various parts of the cell. This possibility could be one of the reasonable explanations for some results (154) we obtained with the use of desferrioxamine (DFO) given after bromobenzene intoxication. While at 15 hr all the animals were protected against lipid peroxidation and liver necrosis, at later times (24 hr) some animals (25–30%) showed elevated transaminases in the absence of lipid peroxidation. Based on these results and others (146) obtained with cultured hepatocytes, two mechanisms of toxicity were proposed: one, the most frequent, responsible for liver cell death during the first phase (14–18 hr) and based on lipid peroxidation; and another one, operating at later times and unrelated to lipid peroxidation. During the phase between the massive loss of GSH (2–3 hr) and the appearance of cell death (14–18 hr), an uncoupling of oxidative phosphorylation was observed in mitochondria, probably due to the phenolic metabolites of bromobenzene, particularly 4-bromophenol derived from the 3,4-epoxide (155).

Another example in which a severe GSH depletion is accompanied by lipid peroxidation is that of allyl alcohol intoxication. As is known, the main metabolic pathway of allyl alcohol is the cytosolic alcohol dehydrogenase-catalyzed reduction to acrolein. The latter, which is a strong electrophile, reacts immediately with nucleophiles such as GSH, which is almost completely lost within the first minutes after the intoxication (77). When the capacity of the GSH defense system is overwhelmed, allyl alcohol metabolites will bind to protein (156), possibly producing damage. As in the case of bromobenzene, an alternative or complementary mechanism is lipid peroxidation. The latter has been shown in in vitro (157, 158) and in vivo (159) studies. In our

---

[2] 6-Hydroxy-2,5,5,8-tetramethylchroman-2-carboxylic acid.

experiments (160) lipid peroxidation was increased when no or minor liver necrosis (serum transaminases) occurred. The treatment of the animal with DFO protected against lipid peroxidation and liver cell damage (159, 161). Other studies (162–164), however, reported that in isolated hepatocytes suppression of lipid peroxidation was not associated with prevention of cell death. Probably under conditions in which lipid peroxidation is hindered, covalent binding of acrolein to cellular macromolecules is an important factor for cell death. However, under normal conditions in which lipid peroxidation is free to develop, the latter process may be the predominant mechanism.

Possible Mechanisms of Induction of Lipid Peroxidation

Recently it has been proposed (165) that allyl alcohol toxicity depends, at least in part, on the release of iron in a free form from hepatic ferritin. As is known, iron is normally transported and stored in specific proteins (transferrin, ferritin, heme proteins, etc.) that prevent its reaction with reduced oxygen species. Thus, to be redox cycling, active iron has to be released from these complexes. The release of iron from ferritin has been widely investigated (166–168). It occurs following a reductive stress with consequent reduction of Fe(III) to Fe(II). Conversely, iron can be released from hemoglobin as a result of an oxidative stress that leads to methemoglobin (Fe III) formation (169–171).

In the liver cell actively metabolizing allyl alcohol, the NAD/NADH ratio is shifted toward the reduced form (reductive stress). In an in vitro system NADH was able to release small amounts of iron from ferritin (165). Catalytic concentrations of flavine mononucleotide greatly enhanced the NADH-induced reductive release of ferritin-bound iron (reduced flavins themselves can mobilize iron from ferritin [172]). NADH effectively reduced ferric iron in solution (165). Moreover a mixture of NADH and ferritin induced lipid peroxidation in liver microsomes (165). These results provide a rationale for allyl alcohol-induced lipid peroxidation. They can also contribute to the explanation of lipid peroxidation in ethanol toxicity (see below), since generation of NADH during ethanol metabolism can likewise mobilize iron from ferritin (173). Very recently it has been shown (174) that the administration of the GSH depleting agent phorone to rats results in an increased free iron pool.

While the mechanism of induction of lipid peroxidation is becoming more clear in some cases, in many others equally concerned with GSH depleting agents, the source of oxidative stress responsible for lipid peroxidation is still under investigation. Briefly, lipid peroxidation could be due to either the formation of active species from the metabolism of the toxicants or the depletion of hepatic GSH. A reasonable way to discriminate between these two possibilities was to study the effects of the administration of drugs, such as diethylmaleate, that are mainly conjugated with GSH by GSH-S-transferases without previous metabolism. We found (148) that about 45% of the animals given diethylmaleate and sacrificed 15–20 hr later showed liver necrosis and lipid peroxidation, which mostly occurred below the same threshold level of hepatic GSH as seen with bromobenzene and iodobenzene. These findings could lead to the idea that the effects of diethylmaleate were entirely the result of its

GSH-depleting activity; this would imply the assumption that lipid peroxidation and accompanying cell damage are the consequence of a constitutive oxidative stress in a hepatocyte depleted of GSH. Diethylmaleate may have, however, as yet unknown effects that relate to the induction of lipid peroxidation other than simply the depletion of GSH. Furthermore, for chemicals that are metabolized in the monooxygenase system, alternative or additional explanations must be considered. Active turnover of the cytochrome P450 system during mixed function oxidation involves the production of active oxygen species. It has been shown (175–178), in fact, that part of the oxygen consumed by microsomal drug oxidation is released in the form of H_2O_2. The superoxide anion released from the oxy-complex of cytochrome P450 would be the precursor, yielding H_2O_2 (179–181) by dismutation, either spontaneously or catalyzed by SOD. These oxygen species and others possibly produced by their interaction could interact with polyunsaturated fatty acids of membrane phospholipids; in a cell whose antioxidant defenses are compromised by a dramatic loss of GSH, lipid peroxidation would ensue. This sequence of events is strongly suggested by a number of in vivo and in vitro studies (182–184) that reported that, when the antioxidant systems centered on GSH are eliminated, lipid peroxidation can be induced by drugs such as aminopyrine, ethylmorphine, and ethoxycoumarin, which are normally metabolized by the cytochrome P450 system without giving GSH conjugates and covalent binding.

Relationships Among the Various Antioxidant Systems of the Liver Cell

In recent studies (185) we have investigated the changes in the antioxidant systems, α-tocopherol (vitamin E) and ascorbic acid (vitamin C), during the development of the liver injury induced by the GSH-depleting agents considered above. It was in fact conceivable that an abrupt loss of the antioxidant system based on GSH can affect other antioxidant defense systems. Both GSH and ascorbic acid, in fact, have been implicated in the continuous regeneration of α-tocopherol (186–189), i.e., in the continuous reduction of the oxidized forms of tocopherol (it must be considered that in the membranes α-tocopherol is present in a molar ratio with unsaturated fatty acids of 1:1000 or less, and therefore a continuous regeneration of tocopherol must occur).

We found (185) that in the case of bromobenzene intoxication, the hepatic level of vitamin E is decreased at 9–12 hr, prior to the development of lipid peroxidation. A further decrease occurs as lipid peroxidation markedly increases. Ascorbic acid is increased during the first hours of the intoxication, while it is decreased at the latest time (18 hr). Dehydroascorbic acid (the double oxidized form of ascorbic acid) is markedly increased in the first hours after the intoxication, when a severe GSH depletion occurs but lipid peroxidation has not yet started. The ascorbic: dehydroascorbic acid ratio shows a marked decrease throughout the intoxication period. Somewhat similar results have been obtained (185) with the two other GSH-depleting agents studied, diethylmaleate and allyl alcohol. Again, the ascorbic:dehydroascorbic acid ratio is dramatically decreased. Thus, the decrease in the reduced:oxidized ascorbic acid ratio can be regarded as an index of oxidative stress occurring with GSH depletion even before the appearance of lipid peroxidation.

Finally, we have studied (185) the effects of GSH depletion under conditions of different availability of tocopherol in the liver cell, to clarify the role of vitamin E in the defense mechanisms against oxidative stress induced by GSH-depleting agents. To this end the intoxications with the three GSH-depleting agents considered were performed in animals maintained on either a vitamin E-deficient diet or the same diet supplemented with different levels of tocopherol (35 and 65 mg/kg). On the whole these studies showed that vitamin E affects to a great extent the expression of the hepatotoxicity of GSH-depleting agents. In fact, in the animals fed the vitamin E–deficient diet, lipid peroxidation and liver necrosis were greatly accelerated and more severe, while in the animals fed the vitamin E–rich diet (65 mg/kg) the three toxicants had only minor effects, in spite of a quite comparable GSH depletion. Similar results were obtained with isolated hepatocytes prepared from the vitamin E–deficient or vitamine E–supplemented animals (190).

In summary, these and many other studies have stressed the relevance of the antioxidant potential to the cell life. GSH is certainly important in the defense lines against oxidative stress. However, when GSH is virtually lost, the tocopherol level in the membrane appears to be the determinant of the fate of the cell. A hepatic level of vitamin E approximately double that obtained with a commercial standard diet can prevent the pathologic phenomena occurring as a consequence of GSH depletion (185).

Additional studies performed with isolated hepatocytes incubated with a number of prooxidants (allyl alcohol, diethylmaleate, CCl_4 [190], and diquat [191]) have further clarified the antioxidant ability of ascorbic acid. The latter seems to play a vital role in maintaining α-tocopherol levels in the membranes, especially when GSH is depleted (191). Therefore, cellular systems capable of reducing the oxidized forms of ascorbic acid are of particular importance to restore the antioxidant potential of vitamin C. In a series of our studies on the enzymatic systems capable of reducing the double-oxidized form of ascorbic acid (dehydroascorbic acid), two dehydroascorbate reductases have been isolated in a pure form from rat liver cytosol: one is GSH-dependent, (192) and the other is NADPH-dependent (193). Microsequence analysis of the two enzymatic proteins has shown that the GSH-dependent enzyme is a novel enzyme (192), while the NADPH-dependent one is a member of the aldo-keto reductase superfamily and corresponds to 3α-hydroxysteroid dehydrogenase (193). The implications of these enzymes in the defenses against oxidative stress is under investigation.

Redox Cycling Compounds

The third group of toxicants that can induce oxidative stress and possibly lipid peroxidation is represented by substances that, after metabolism, yield nonalkylating metabolites that interact with oxygen and generate reactive oxygen species. Paraquat, diquat, menadione, and anthracyclines such as adriamycin and nitrofurantoin are the most studied molecules. Paraquat (1,1-dimethyl-4,4-bipyridilium ion; methyl violo-gen) and diquat (1,1'-ethylene-2,2'-bipyridilium ion) are quaternary bipyridyl com-pounds used as herbicides. The toxicity of many of these compounds is expressed mainly in organs other than the liver (paraquat is toxic for the lung, where it accu-mulates, adriamycin is toxic for the heart, etc.), and therefore the discussion will be limited to general mechanisms that can be studied with suitable models, the most used of which are represented by isolated hepatocytes. This does not mean that the liver cell is necessarily affected in vivo; for instance, menadione is toxic in vitro for hepatocytes, even if in vivo it has no effects on the liver.

The general mechanism of toxicity of redox cycling compounds involves the one electron reduction pathway, catalyzed by the flavoprotein H-cytochrome P450 reduc-tase. This pathway yields the corresponding free radicals, which, in the presence of dioxygen, are rapidly reoxidized to the parent compounds, with concomitant forma-tion of superoxide anions. Dismutation of O_2^- by SOD produces H_2O_2. More potent oxidants ($OH^\bullet$) can be produced by the Fenton reaction.

The prototype of these molecules is paraquat. The formation of the paraquat rad-ical following a single electron reduction of paraquat was demonstrated many years ago (194). Later studies (195) showed that the paraquat radical, generated by pulse radiolysis of an aqueous aerobic solution of paraquat, reacts rapidly with oxygen, gen-erating O_2^-. It was then realized that biologic systems are also capable of catalyzing the cyclic reduction-oxidation of paraquat. When paraquat is incubated with liver micro-somes and NADPH under anaerobic conditions, a stable, blue-colored, radical cation is formed (196). Under aerobic conditions, O_2 uptake and NADPH oxidation occur. Paraquat acts as an uncoupler of the microsomal electron transport chain by receiving electrons from the flavoprotein NADPH-cytochrome P450 reductase. The electron is then transferred to oxygen, giving rise to superoxide. The same redox cycling of paraquat is catalyzed by rat lung microsomes (197) and by nonmammalian systems, such as plants and bacteria, and this underlies the herbicide and bactericide activities.

There is no doubt that paraquat-induced lung toxicity is due to the formation of active oxygen species. What is controversial is whether lipid peroxidation, possibly induced by oxyradicals, is also involved. With liver microsomes conflicting results have been obtained (25, 77). Also controversial are the results of studies attempting to detect lipid peroxidation in the lung in vivo (25, 77). The difficulty probably derives also from the fact that paraquat toxicity is restricted to alveolar epithelial type I and II cells, which together constitute only a small percentage of the total cell population of the lung. In other studies (25, 77) the occurrence of lipid peroxidation was only indirectly inferred by the effects obtained by modulating the antioxidant potential.

In our opinion the oxyradicals generated by many of these compounds can directly produce cell and membrane damage, all the more when the GSH level is severely decreased mainly by the H_2O_2 metabolism. Lipid peroxidation, even if occurring, probably is not the primary or the necessary mechanism of cell death. For instance, it is well documented (190, 198, 199) that menadione added to isolated hepatocytes produces cell death in the absence of lipid peroxidation. In the case of adriamycin, however, the drug can form complexes with iron and ADP-iron, and the ferrous form of these complexes may initiate lipid peroxidation (200).

A number of studies carried out with menadione, other quinones or t-butylhydroperoxide have shown (201, 202) the relevance of the thiol status to the cell life. The one-electron reduction pathway of the quinone leads to the semiquinone radical, which in the presence of dioxygen is rapidly reoxidized to the parent quinone with concomitant formation of superoxide. The latter is dismutated to H_2O_2, which is reduced by GSH peroxidase, and the GSSG formed is reduced back to GSH by the NADPH-linked GSH reductase. When regeneration of NADPH becomes rate-limiting, GSSG accumulates and is actively excreted. Thus, when the rate of redox cycling of menadione exceeds the capacity of detoxifying enzymes, cytotoxicity occurs. GSH depletion is mainly produced by GSH oxidation, while in the case of the GSH-depleting agents (bromobenzene, allyl alcohol, diethylmaleate) GSH is lost through the formation of glutathionyl conjugates with the reactive metabolites. In addition to GSH depletion a marked decrease in protein thiols occurs in hepatocytes as a result of menadione metabolism. Such a decrease is mainly due to oxidation, while arylation accounts for a minor pathway. The redox transition of protein sulfhydryl groups has been reported to affect or modulate a variety of cellular processes including enzyme activities and transport of small solutes and ions across membranes (203–205). According to Orrenius and coworkers (201, 206) alterations in normal thiol homeostasis are associated with severe cellular damage, the link being represented by perturbation of intracellular calcium homeostasis.

ETHANOL

Even if it is well known that ethanol metabolism is accompanied by a decrease in liver GSH (conjugation of GSH with acetaldehyde), in this chapter ethanol is not treated in conjunction with GSH-depleting agents, because the loss of GSH (20–30%) is by far smaller than that occurring with many GSH depletors (bromobenzene, allyl alcohol, etc.) and cannot account by itself for the induction of lipid peroxidation.

Since the initial reports of increased lipid peroxidation in ethanol toxicity (207, 208), the occurrence of this process in acute and chronic ethanol intoxication has been the object of a long debate (90, 209, 210). More recent studies have conclusively shown that an oxidative stress is imposed on the liver cell as a result of ethanol metabolism (211). The sources of such an oxidative stress are various. First of all, ethanol oxidation results in the production of free radicals, which can derive from both oxygen and ethanol itself. Oxygen radicals can originate as follows: microsomal NADPH-cytochrome c reductase and cytochrome P450, which are components of the microsomal ethanol oxidizing system (MEOS) (212), can generate O_2^- and H_2O_2 (175–178, 213, 214); the same oxygen species can be produced by aldehyde oxidase and xanthine oxidase (215), both involved in the metabolism of ethanol-derived acetaldehyde; O_2^- and H_2O_2 can also be generated by microsomal NADPH oxidase, which has been shown to be increased after acute (216) or chronic (217–220) ethanol administration; during NADPH oxidation liver microsomes produce significant amount of OH$^\bullet$ (being H_2O_2 the precursor), which in turn appears to be required for ethanol oxidation (221–223).

With regard to ethanol-derived radicals, it has been shown (224, 225) that ethanol is activated to a free radical intermediate by the ethanol inducible form of cytochrome P450, i.e., the specific isoenzymatic form involved in MEOS, CYP2E1. With the use of electron spin resonance (ESR) spectroscopy in combination with the spin trapping agent 4-pyridyl-1-oxo-t-butyl nitrone (4-POBN), it has been demonstrated (224, 225) that rat liver microsomes incubated with ethanol and NADPH can produce a free radical intermediate, identified as α-hydroxyethyl radical. Free radical intermediates are also produced by liver microsomes during the metabolism of various aliphatic alcohols (1-propanol, 2-propanol, 1-butanol, 2-butanol, and 1-pentanol), indicating the existence of a common activating pathway for these compounds (225–226). The formation of radical intermediates has been confirmed in the whole animal in vivo with the use of 4-POBN (227–229). The generation of ethanol radicals would occur during the process of univalent reduction of dioxygen and possibly would be carried out by ferric cytochrome P450 oxy-complex (P450–$Fe^{3+}O_2^{\bullet}$) formed during the reduction of heme-oxygen. In such a state, cytochrome would be sufficiently reactive to abstract a proton from the α-carbon of ethanol, yielding a carbon-centered radical and H_2O_2 (230). Alternatively, hydroxyethyl radicals could be produced by the addition to ethanol of OH$^\bullet$ radicals generated from liver microsomes (231). However generated, hydroxyethyl radicals bind to microsomal protein (232) and probably play an important role in the induction of lipid peroxidation (233). The binding of alcohol radical to protein represents another mechanism of hepatic protein alkylation in addition to that operated by acetaldehyde (234) and known to contribute to overall liver cell damage. Furthermore, hydroxyethyl radical-derived protein adducts are immunogenic and give rise to antibodies different from those generated by acetaldehyde-derived protein adducts (235). Chronic alcohol feeding of rats leads to the production of antibodies that recognize hydroxyethyl rat serum albumin but do not recognize rat serum albumin (235). Moreover, sera of alcoholic cirrhotic patients contain IgG and IgA antibodies that recognize proteins modified by hydroxyethyl radicals (236). Such antibodies may play an important role in the immunologic reactions triggered by ethanol and due to antibodies against liver cells found in the serum of patients with alcoholic liver injury (237).

An additional source of oxidative stress in ethanol toxicity is the release of iron from hepatic ferritin. As previously mentioned, the shift of the NAD:NADH ratio toward the reduced form, which occurs during ethanol metabolism, results in the reduction of ferric iron present in the ferritin molecule. In the reduced form iron is released from ferritin and, if maintained in redox active form, can promote lipid peroxidation. This sequence of events has been reported (174) after acute ethanol administration. In in vitro systems iron is mobilized from ferritin when ethanol is oxidized by alcohol dehydrogenase or when acetaldehyde is oxidized by xanthine oxidase (174). Acetaldehyde oxidation by xanthine oxidase can produce superoxide (215), and xanthine oxidase-generated superoxide can mobilize iron from ferritin acting as a reductant and promote lipid peroxidation (177).

GSH decrease, even if not the cause of lipid peroxidation by itself, may contribute to the overall oxidative stress.

Lipid peroxidation has been recently detected (238) in alcoholic liver disease by the measurement of plasma isoprostanes, the novel method for lipid peroxidation in vivo discussed above.

HEPATIC IRON OVERLOAD

Excess iron deposited chronically in liver parenchymal cells is associated with hepatic injury, fibrosis, and ultimately cirrhosis (239). These pathologic changes occur in both hereditary hemochromatosis and in the various forms of secondary hemochromatosis. Among the various mechanisms responsible for the liver cell injury, lipid peroxidation has been considered in view of its possible induction by the deposited iron. An increased hepatic content of MDA was reported many years ago (240); more recently, lipid peroxidation has been measured (conjugated dienes) in mitochondrial and microsomal lipid of rats treated with ferric nitrilotriacetate (FeNTA) or fed a diet supplemented with carbonyl iron (241). Lipid peroxidation did not occur until the hepatic iron concentration exceeded 1000 $\mu g/g$. Above this level it was detectable in mitochrondria, and only at concentrations higher than 4000 $\mu g/g$ in microsomes (241). Both mitochondria and microsomes showed functional damage (241). Under the same conditions of hepatic iron overload, lipid peroxidation has also been detected by the measurement of F_2-isoprostanes in the liver (242). After a single dose of FeNTA, lipid peroxidation has also been found in kidney (76) by both biochemical (TBA–reactive substances and 4-HNE) and immunohistochemical means (see below).

It is likely that under conditions of severe iron overload the ability of the hepatocyte to maintain iron in the nontoxic, protein-bound ferric state is exceeded, resulting in an increased level of so-called free iron, i.e., redox active iron probably present as low-molecular-weight chelates. In a model of endogenously induced hepatic iron overload, obtained by six daily injections of the hemolytic drug phenylhydrazine (0.1 mmol/kg body weight subcutaneously), we found (243, 244) that a relatively small increase in hepatic total iron concentration (181.5 ± 17.9 compared to $23.0 \pm 5.9 \mu g/g$ in controls) is accompanied by an approximately 10-fold increase in free iron. The hepatic DNA appears markedly fragmented on agarose-gel electrophoresis, and this damage is attributable to free iron rather than to the hepatic metabolism of phenylhydrazine.

LIPID PEROXIDATION AND HEPATIC FIBROSIS

The pathway leading from liver cell damage to liver cirrhosis has been the object of many investigations. Recently it has been reported (245, 246) that in the model of chronic carbon tetrachloride hepatotoxicity, the treatment of the intoxicated rats with α-tocopherol, which decreased lipid peroxidation (245), also blocks, at both the mRNA and protein level, the synthesis of the transforming growth factor-$\beta 1$ (TGF-

β1), which is a major mediator of liver fibrogenesis (247). The secretion of TGF-β1 by activated macrophages can, in fact, induce the transformation of perisinusoidal fat-storing cells (Ito cells) into myofibroblasts, thus triggering collagen production in the liver (247). One possibility is that lipid peroxidation products play a role in the activation of Kupffer cells leading to secretion of TGF-β1, which in turn promotes the transformation of Ito cells. An alternative mechanism by which lipid peroxidation can promote collagen deposition has been proposed by Chojkier and coworkers (248–250), who reported that the induction of lipid peroxidation in cultured fibroblasts can act as a direct stimulus for collagen synthesis. Consistent with this mechanism, stimulation of lipid peroxidation in cultured human Ito cells can increase the expression of procollagen α_1 (I) gene expression (251) by about four times.

HISTOCHEMICAL DETECTION OF LIPID PEROXIDATION

As previously discussed, sophisticated and sensitive biochemical procedures are now available for the determination of even minimal levels of oxidative stress in vivo, as well as in isolated cells or cellular subfractions. However, such approaches do not generally allow the gathering of information concerning the distribution of phenomena in situ, while this aspect is of great potential importance for the understanding of oxidative mechanisms involved in cell injury, especially in the case of tissues with a heterogeneous cell composition, such as brain, lung, or kidney.

In a few laboratories, including ours, the issue has been dealt with from a histochemical point of view. Thus, the possibility has been evaluated to develop procedures provided with high sensitivity and specificity in order to directly reveal the effects of oxidative stress on sections of tissue or cellular smears to discriminate areas, cellular types and—possibly—subcellular sites being involved in these processes. To this aim, several biochemical changes introduced by oxidative stress in tissues can be exploited. Production of superoxide anion, as an example, can be revealed in living tissues and isolated cells preloaded with 2′,7′-dichlorofluoresceine diacetate, a compound whose fluorescence is sharply increased in the presence of oxygen radical species (252, 253). Others could demonstrate the production of superoxide anions at the endothelial surface of cardiac vessels, during the first moments of reperfusion following a period of anoxia, by using a modified manganese–diaminobenzidine reaction (254).

Our attention was originally directed to lipid peroxidation, by developing methods aimed at revealing aldehyde and carbonyl products. In fact, in the case of alkenals, the binding to -SH groups of proteins leaves the aldehyde grouping free for the reaction with aldehyde reactants (39, 77, 90). The same reaction could also involve the carbonyl functions present, as previously shown (255) in acyl residues of membrane phospholipids and formed as a consequence of the peroxidative breakdown of unsaturated fatty acids. We first used the direct Schiff reaction for the visualization of small foci with decreased sensitivity to induction of lipid peroxidation in vitro, in cryostat sections obtained from the liver of rats treated with a carcinogen (256). Subsequently, the same procedure was applied to the detection of hepatic lipid peroxidation in vivo

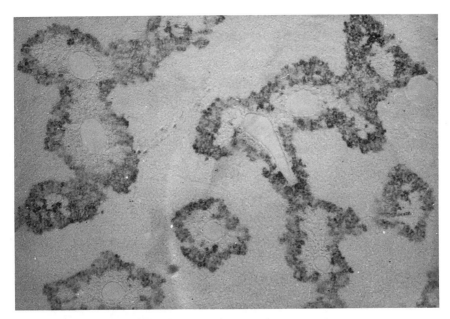

FIG. 3. Cryostat liver section obtained from a bromobenzene-intoxicated mouse. The section was processed by the direct Schiff reaction for the histochemical detection of aldehyde functions derived from lipid peroxidation. The mid-lobular distribution of the process can be appreciated. x 40. (Reproduced from Pompella et al. [257], with permission).

following bromobenzene intoxication (257). Figure 3 illustrates the distribution of the reaction in the liver of bromobenzene-treated mice. At low, initial levels of lipid peroxidation, as assessed by biochemical methods on adjacent tissue specimens, the histochemistry of lipid-derived aldehydes revealed a mid-lobular distribution, which then spreads to involve the remaining parenchyma.

Direct Schiff reaction was subsequently employed with success in other experimental conditions, allowing the demonstration of the selective involvement of the substantia nigra during in vitro iron-induced lipid peroxidation (258) and of rat tubular proximal epithelium during kidney lipid peroxidation induced in vivo by the kidney carcinogen iron nitrilotriacetate (259). Very interesting results were obtained by Masuda and Yamamori, who studied the distribution of lipid peroxidation in relationship to that of cell injury, in rat livers subjected to anterograde versus retrograde perfusion with different prooxidant toxins and different oxygen tension condition (260).

Our subsequent efforts were focused on the development of procedures provided with sensitivity and reproducibility higher than those of the Schiff reaction. Good results were obtained by using a reaction based on 3-hydroxy-2-naphthoic acid hydrazide (NAH) followed by coupling with a tetrazolium salt (261). As well as in the case of the direct Schiff reaction (257), the reliability of the NAH reaction was assessed by means of microspectrophotometric analysis of tissue sections, with a comparison with data provided by biochemical determination of lipid peroxidation in the same specimens (261). The use of the NAH reaction allowed us to visualize the regions first involved by lipid peroxidation in vivo, following the intoxication with haloalkanes; such lipid peroxidation had proved smaller than the detection limits offered by the direct Schiff reaction (261). NAH reaction also avoids the lack of specificity of the Schiff reaction in tissues other than the liver, thus allowing selective visualization of cells involved by lipid peroxidation in lung or kidney tissue (261).

A further improvement in histochemistry of lipid peroxidation is offered by the employment of fluorescent reagents for lipid peroxidation-derived carbonyls in tissues and isolated cells, with an appreciable increase in the sensitivity of detection, and the possibility of analysis by means of confocal laser scanning fluorescence microscopy with image videoanalysis. We obtained interesting results with these procedures by exploiting the fluorescence of the NAH reagent itself. Plate I shows the selective involvement of the first rows of pericentral hepatocytes by lipid peroxidation induced in vivo in the rat intoxicated with carbon tetrachloride. The results obtained in isolated cells are illustrated in Plate II, showing increasing levels of lipid peroxidation in isolated rat hepatocytes incubated in vitro with carbon tetrachloride.

An elegant improvement of the approach employing fluorescent derivativization of cellular carbonyls followed by confocal laser scanning microscopy has been recently published by others, using a biotin-labeled hydrazide coupled with fluorescent-conjugated streptavidin (263). An alternative approach is the one exploiting the naturally fluorescent fatty acid, cis-parinaric acid, which is readily consumed during lipid peroxidation. Once preloaded in cells, cis-parinaric acid can thus allow the detection of the lipid peroxidation process in the form of a decreased fluorescence in viable cells, as successfully employed in, for example, flow cytometry (264).

Several recent studies dedicated to the visualization of lipid peroxidation in tissues have used an immunohistochemical approach based on the fact that some important lipid peroxidation-derived product—malonaldehyde and 4-hydroxyalkenals in the first place—can easily react with cellular macromolecules, thus leading to the appearance of recognizable epitopes in proteins. This approach has produced important results such as the revelation of MDA-modified proteins in collagen-producing fibroblasts (248, 250) and in the liver of human alcoholics (265) as well as the localization of 4-HNE–modified proteins in arterial wall during experimental atherosclerosis (266) and in renal carcinogenesis (267).

ACKNOWLEDGMENTS

I wish to thank Dr. A. Pompella for helpul discussions, especially concerned with the section "Histochemical Detection of Lipid Peoxidation." The unpublished experimental work reported here was supported by the Italian CNR (Finalized Project A.C.R.O. and Strategic Project "Stress Ossidativo e Stress Cellulare in Biopatologia").

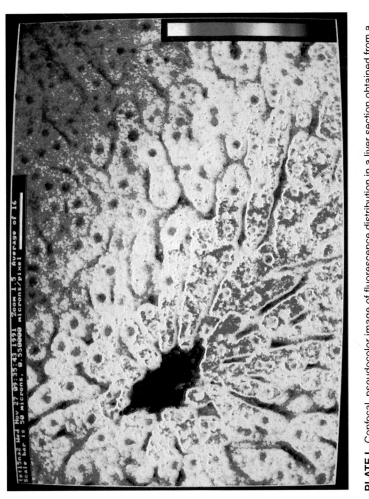

PLATE I. Confocal, pseudocolor image of fluorescence distribution in a liver section obtained from a rat intoxicated with carbon tetrachloride (250 μmol/100 g of body weight, 1 hr). False colors represent lower to higher fluorescence intensities (see scale bar). Hydroxynaphthoic hydrazide reaction of tissue carbonyls deriving from lipid peroxidation. An involvement of the first rows of hepatocytes around the central vein can be appreciated. Reproduced from Pompella and Comporti (262), with permission.

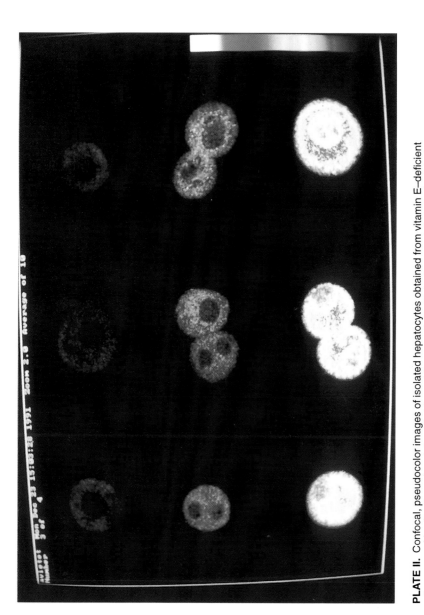

PLATE II. Confocal, pseudocolor images of isolated hepatocytes obtained from vitamin E–deficient rats, exposed in vitro to carbon tetrachloride and then reacted with hydroxynaphthoic hydrazide for the detection of cellular carbonyls deriving from lipid peroxidation. Top row, controls (0 time); middle, 5 min of exposure (MDA content, 172 pmol/10⁶ cells); bottom, 10 min of exposure (MDA content, 340 pmol/10⁶ cells). Reproduced from Pompella and Comporti (262), with permission.

REFERENCES

1. Chance B, Sies H, Boveris A. Hydroperoxide metabolism in mammalian organs. *Physiol Rev* 1989;59:527–605.
2. Boveris A, Chance B. The cellular production of hydrogen peroxide. *Biochem J* 1973;128:617–630.
3. Nohl H. Formation of reactive oxygen species associated with mitochondrial respiration. In: Davies KJA, ed. *Oxidative damage and repair: chemical, biological and medical aspects.* Oxford: Pergamon Press, 1991:108–116.
4. Niki E. Antioxidant compounds. In: Davies KJA, ed. *Oxidative damage and repair: chemical, biological and medical aspects.* Oxford: Pergamon Press, 1991:57–64.
5. Ursini F, Maiorino M, Valente M, Ferri L, Gregolin C. Purification from pig liver of a protein which protects liposomes and biomembranes from peroxidative degradation and exhibits glutathione peroxidase activity on phosphatidyl-cholin liposomes. *Biochim Biophys Acta* 1982;710:197–211.
6. Sevanian A. Phospholiphase and lipid peroxidation. In: Chow C-K, ed. *Cellular antioxidant defense mechanisms.* Boca Raton, FL: CRC Press, 1988:2:77–95.
7. Pacifici RE, Salo DC, Davies KJA. Macroxyproteinase, M.O.P.: a 670 kDa proteinase complex that degrades oxidatively denatured proteins in red blood cells. *Free Rad Biol Med* 1989;7:521–536.
8. Spitz DR, Dewey WC, Li GC. Hydrogen peroxide or heat shock induce resistance to hydrogen peroxide in Chinese hamster fibroblasts. *J Cell Physiol* 1987;131:364–373.
9. Christman MF, Morgan RW, Jacobson FS, Ames BN. Positive control of a regulon for defenses against oxidative stress and some heat shock proteins in *Salmonella typhimurium. Cell* 1985;41:755–762.
10. Slater TF. Free-radical mechanisms in tissue injury. *Biochem J* 1984;222:1–15.
11. Halliwell B, Gutteridge JMC. *Free radicals in biology and medicine,* 2nd ed., Oxford: Clarendon Press, 1989.
12. Horgan VJ, Philpot JS. Attempted estimation of organic peroxides in X-irradiated mice. *Br J Radiol NS* 1954;27:63–72.
13. Bernheim F, Ottolenghi A, Wilbur M. Studies on bone marrow lipid in normal and irradiated rabbits. *Radiat Res* 1956;4:132–138.
14. Tappel AL. Vitamin E as the biological lipid antioxidant. *Vitam Horm* 1962;20:493–510.
15. Hochstein P, Ernster L. ADP-activated lipid peroxidation coupled to the TNPH oxidase system of microsomes. *Biochem Biophys Res Commun* 1963;12:388–394.
16. Recknagel RO. Carbon tetrachloride hepatotoxicity. *Pharmacol Rev* 1967;19:145–208.
17. Slater TF. *Free radical mechanisms in tissue injury.* London: Pion Limited, 1972.
18. Comporti M, Saccocci C, Dianzani MU. Effect of CCl_4 in vitro and in vivo on lipid peroxidation of rat liver homogenates and subcellular fractions. *Enzymologia* 1965;29:185–204.
19. Recknagel RO, Ghoshal AK. Lipoperoxidation as a vector in carbon tetrachloride hepatotoxicity. *Lab Invest* 1966;15:132–146.
20. McCord JM, Fridovich I. Superoxide dismutase: an enzymic function for erythrocuprein (hemocuprein). *J Biol Chem* 1969;244:6049–6057.
21. Sies H, ed. *Oxidative stress.* London: Academic Press, 1985:1–8.
22. Porter NA. Chemistry of lipid peroxidation. *Methods Enzymol* 1984;105:273–282.
23. Kanner J, German JB, Kinsella JE. Initiation of lipid peroxidation in biological systems. *CRC Crit Rev Food Sci Nutr* 1987;25:317–364.
24. Kappus H. Lipid peroxidation: mechanisms, analysis, enzymology and biological relevance. In: Sies H, ed. *Oxidative stress.* London: Academic Press, 1985:273–310.
25. Horton AA, Fairhurst S. Lipid peroxidation and mechanisms of toxicity. *CRC Crit Rev Toxicol* 1987;18:27–79.
26. Girotti AW. Mechanisms of lipid peroxidation. *J Free Rad Biol Med* 1985;1:87–95.
27. Egger KW, Cocks AT. Homopolar and heteropolar bond dissociation energies and heats of formation of radicals and ions in the gas phase. I. Data on organic molecules. *Helv Chim Acta* 1973;56:1516–1536.
28. Gutteridge JMC, Halliwell B. The measurement and mechanism of lipid peroxidation in biological systems. *Trends Biochem Sci* 1990;15:129–135.
29. Aust SD, Svingen BA. The role of iron in enzymatic lipid peroxidation. In: Pryor WA, ed. *Free radicals in biology.* New York: Academic Press, 1982;5:1–28.
30. Aust SD, Morehouse LA, Thomas CE. Role of metals in oxygen radical reactions. *J Free Rad Biol Med* 1985;1:3–25.
31. Halliwell B, Gutteridge JMC. Oxygen toxicity, oxygen radicals, transition metals and disease. *Biochem J* 1984;219:1–14.

32. Gutteridge JMC. The role of superoxide and hydroxyl radicals in phospholipid peroxidation catalysed by iron salts. *FEBS Lett* 1982;150:454–458.
33. Kornbrust DL, Mavis RD. Microsomal lipid peroxidation. I. Characterization of the role of iron and NADPH. *Mol Pharmacol* 1980;17:400–407.
34. Minotti G, Aust SD. The role of iron in oxygen radical mediated lipid peroxidation. *Chem Biol Interact* 1989;71:1–19.
35. Riely CA, Cohen G, Lieberman M. Ethane evolution: a new index of lipid peroxidation. *Science* 1974;183:208–210.
36. Tappel AL. Measurement and protection from in vivo lipid peroxidation. In: Pryor WA, ed. *Free radicals in biology*. New York: Academic Press, 1980;4:1–47.
37. Roubal WT, Tappel AL. Polymerization of proteins induced by free-radical lipid peroxidation. *Arch Biochem Biophys* 1966;113:150–155.
38. Schauenstein E. Autoxidation of polyunsaturated esters in water: chemical structure and biological activity of the products. *J Lipid Res* 1967;8:417–428.
39. Schauenstein E, Esterbauer H, Zollner H. *Aldehydes in biological systems*. London: Pion Limited, 1977.
40. Benedetti A, Casini AF, Ferrali M, Comporti M. Extraction and partial characterization of dialysable products originating from the peroxidation of liver microsomal lipids and inhibiting microsomal glucose 6-phosphatase activity. *Biochem Pharmacol* 1979;28:2909–2918.
41. Benedetti A, Comporti M, Esterbauer H. Identification of 4-hydroxynonenal as a cytotoxic product originating from the peroxidation of liver microsomal lipids. *Biochim Biophys Acta* 1980;620:281–296.
42. Benedetti A, Comporti M. Formation, reactions and toxicity of aldehydes produced in the course of lipid peroxidation in cellular membranes. *Bioelectrochem Bioenerg* 1987;18:187–202.
43. Esterbauer H, Cheeseman KH, Dianzani MU, Poli G, Slater TF. Separation and characterization of the aldehydic products of lipid peroxidation stimulated by ADP-Fe^{2+} in rat liver microsomes. *Biochem J* 1982;208:129–140.
44. Esterbauer H, Zollner H, Scholz N. Reaction of glutathione with conjugated carbonyls. *Z Naturforsch* [C] 1975;30:466–473.
45. Szweda LI, Uchida K, Tsai L, Stadtman ER. Inactivation of glucose-6-phosphate dehydrogenase by 4-hydroxy-2-nonenal. *J Biol Chem* 1993;268:3342–3347.
46. Uchida K, Szweda LI, Chae H-Z, Stadtman ER. Immunochemical detection of 4-hydroxynonenal protein adducts in oxidized hepatocytes. *Proc Natl Acad Sci USA* 1993;90:8742–8746.
47. Dianzani MU. Biochemical effects of saturated and unsaturated aldehydes. In: McBrien DCH, Slater TF, ed. *Free radicals, lipid peroxidation and cancer*. New York: Academic Press, 1982:129–158.
48. Brambilla G, Sciaba L, Faggin P, Maura A, Marinari UM, Ferro M, Esterbauer H. Cytotoxicity, DNA fragmentation and sister-chromatid exchange in chinese hamster ovary cells exposed to the lipid peroxidation product 4-hydroxynonenal and homologous aldehydes. *Mutation Res* 1986;171:169–176.
49. Cajone F, Salina M, Bernelli-Zazzera A. 4-hydroxynonenal induces DNA-binding protein similar to the heat-shock factor. *Biochem J* 1989;262:977–979.
50. Esterbauer H, Schaur RJ, Zollner H. Chemistry and biochemistry of 4-hydroxynonenal, malonaldehyde and related aldehydes. *Free Rad Biol Med* 1991;11:81–128.
51. Pereira A, Brackman J-C, Dumont E, Boeynaems J-M. Identification of a major iodolipid from the horse thyroid gland as 2-iodohexadecanal. *J Biol Chem* 1990;265:17018–17025.
52. Tanaka T, Minamino H, Unezaki S, Tsukatani H, Tokumura A. Formation of platelet-activating factor-like phospholipids by Fe^{2+}/ascorbate/EDTA-induced lipid peroxidation. *Biochim Biophys Acta* 1993;1166:264–274.
53. Stremler KE, Stafforini DM, Prescott SM, Zimmerman GA, McIntyre TM. An oxidized derivative of phosphatidylcholine is a substrate for the platelet activating factor acetylhydrolase from human plasma. *J Biol Chem* 1989;264:5331–5334.
54. Dianzani MU. Lipid peroxidation and cancer. *Crit Rev Oncol Hematol* 1993;15:125–147.
55. Morrow JD, Harris TM, Jackson Roberts L II. Noncyclooxygenase oxidative formation of a series of novel prostaglandins: analytical ramifications for measurement of eicosanoids. *Anal Biochem* 1990;184:1–10.
56. Morrow JD, Hill KE, Burk RF, Nammour TM, Badr KF, Jackson Roberts L II. A series of prostaglandin F_2-like compounds are produced in vivo in humans by a non-cyclooxygenase, free radical-catalyzed mechanism. *Proc Natl Acad Sci USA* 1990;87:9383–9387.

57. Morrow JD, Awad JA, Boss HJ, Blair IA, Jackson Roberts L II. Non-cyclooxygenase-derived prostanoids (F_2-isoprostanes) are formed in situ on phospholipids. *Proc Natl Acad Sci USA* 1992;89:10721–10725.
58. Morrow JD, Awad JA, Kato T, Takahashi K, Badr KF, Jackson Roberts L II, Burk RF. Formation of novel non-cyclooxygenase-derived prostanoids (F_2-isoprostanes) in carbon tetrachloride hepatotoxicity: an animal model of lipid peroxidation. *J Clin Invest* 1992;90:2502–2507.
59. Awad JA, Morrow JD, Takahashi K, Jackson Roberts L II. Identification of non-cyclooxygenase-derived prostanoid (F_2-isoprostane) metabolites in human urine and plasma. *J Biol Chem* 1993; 268:4161–4169.
60. Longmire AW, Swift LL, Jackson Roberts L II, Awad JA, Burk RF, Morrow JD. Effect of oxygen tension on the generation of F_2-isoprostanes and malondialdehyde in peroxidizing rat liver microsomes. *Biochem Pharmacol* 1994;47:1173–1177.
61. Awad JA, Morrow JD, Hill KE, Jackson Roberts L II, Burk RF. Detection and localization of lipid peroxidation in selenium- and vitamin E-deficient rats using F_2-isoprostanes. *J Nutr* 1994;124:810–816.
62. Morrow JD, Minton TA, Mukundan CR, Campbell MD, Zackert WE, Daniel VC, Badr KF, Blair IA, Roberts II LJ. Free radical-induced generation of isoprostanes in vivo. Evidence for the formation of D-ring and E-ring isoprostanes. *J Biol Chem* 1994;269:4317–4326.
63. Slater TF. Overview of methods used for detecting lipid peroxidation. *Methods Enzymol* 1984;105: 283–293.
64. Pryor VA. On the detection of lipid hydroperoxides in biological samples. *Free Rad Biol Med* 1989;7:177–178.
65. van Ginkel G, Sevanian A. Lipid peroxidation-induced membrane structural alterations. *Methods Enzymol* 1994;233:273–288.
66. Pompella A, Maellaro E, Casini AF, Ferrali M, Ciccoli L, Comporti M. Measurement of lipid peroxidation in vivo: a comparison of different procedures. *Lipids* 1987;22:206–211.
67. Gutteridge JMC, Halliwell B. The measurement and mechanism of lipid peroxidation in biological systems. *Trends Bioch Sci* 1990;15:129–135.
68. Kirkpatrick DT, Guth DJ, Mavis RD. Detection of in vivo lipid peroxidation using the thiobarbituric acid assay for lipid hydroperoxides. *J Biochem Toxicol* 1986;1:93–104.
69. Smith MT, Thor H, Hartzell P, Orrenius S. The measurement of lipid peroxidation in isolated hepatocytes. *Biochem Pharmacol* 1982;31:19–26.
70. Smith MT, Thor H, Orrenius S. The role of lipid peroxidation in the toxicity of foreign compounds to liver cells. *Biochem Pharmacol* 1983;32:763–764.
71. Halliwell B. Oxidants and human disease: some new concepts. *FASEB J* 1987;1:358–364.
72. Comporti M. Glutathione depleting agents and lipid peroxidation. *Chem Phys Lipids* 1987;45:143–169.
73. Comporti M, Pompella A. Toxicological significance of free radical. In: Nohl H, Esterbauer H, Rice Evans C, eds. *Free radicals in environment, medicine and toxicology*. London: Richelieu Press, 1994:97–117.
74. Rao KS, Recknagel RO. Early onset of lipoperoxidation in rat liver after carbon tetrachloride administration. *Exp Mol Pathol* 1968;9:271–278.
75. Jose PJ, Slater TF. Increased concentration of malonaldehyde in the livers of rats treated with carbon tetrachloride. *Biochem J* 1972;128:141P.
76. Toyokuni S, Uchida K, Okamoto K, Hattori-Nakakuki Y, Hiai H, Stadtman ER. Formation of 4-hydroxy-2-nonenal-modified proteins in the renal proximal tubules of rats treated with a renal carcinogen, ferric nitrilotriacetate. *Proc Natl Acad Sci USA* 1994;91:2616–2620.
77. Comporti M. Three models of free radical-induced cell injury. *Chem Biol Interact* 1989;72:1–56.
78. Recknagel RO, Glende EA Jr. Carbon tetrachloride hepatotoxicity: an example of lethal cleavage. *CRC Crit Rev Toxicol* 1973;2:263–297.
79. Recknagel RO, Glende EA Jr, Hruszkewycz AM. Chemical mechanisms in carbon tetrachloride toxicity. In: Pryor WA, ed. *Free radical in biology*. New York: Academic Press, 1977:97–132.
80. Recknagel RO, Glende EA Jr, Dolak JA, Waller RL. Mechanisms of carbon tetrachloride toxicity. *Pharmacol Ther* 1989;43:139–154.
81. Poyer JL, Floyd RA, McCay PB, Janzen EG, Davis ER. Spin-trapping of the trichloromethyl radical produced during enzymic NADPH oxidation in the presence of carbon tetrachloride or bromotrichloromethane. *Biochim Biophys Acta* 1978;539:402–409.

82. Lai EK, McCay PB, Noguchi T, Fong K-L. In vivo spin-trapping of trichloromethyl radicals formed from CCl₄. *Biochem Pharmacol* 1979;28:2231–2235.

83. McCay PB, Lai EK, Poyer JL, DuBose CM, Janzen EG. Oxygen- and carbon-centered free radical formation during carbon tetrachloride metabolism. *J Biol Chem* 1984;259:2135–2143.

84. Packer JE, Slater TF, Willson RL. Reaction of the carbon tetrachloride-related peroxy free radical (CCl₃O₂⁻) with amino acids: pulse radiolysis evidence. *Life Sci* 1978;23:2617–2620.

85. Albano E, Lott KAK, Slater TF, Stier A, Symons MCR, Tomasi A. Spin-trapping studies on the free-radical products formed by metabolic activation of carbon tetrachloride in rat liver microsomal fractions isolated hepatocytes and in vivo in the rat. *Biochem J* 1982;204:593–603.

86. Rao KS, Recknagel RO. Early incorporation of carbon-labeled carbon tetrachloride into rat liver particulate lipids and proteins. *Exp Mol Pathol* 1969;10:219–228.

87. Castro JA, Cignoli EV, de Castro CR, de Fenos OM. Prevention by cystamine of liver necrosis and early biochemical alterations induced by carbon tetrachloride. *Biochem Pharmacol* 1972;21:49–57.

88. Cignoli EV, Castro JA. Effect of inhibitors of drug metabolizing enzymes on carbon tetrachloride hepatotoxicity. *Toxicol Appl Pharmacol* 1971;18:625–637.

89. McLean AEM. The effect of diet and vitamin E on liver injury due to carbon tetrachloride. *Br J Exp Pathol* 1967;48:632–636.

90. Comporti M. Lipid peroxidation and cellular damage in toxic liver injury. *Lab Invest* 1985;53:599–623.

91. Benedetti A, Casini AF, Ferrali M, Comporti M. Studies on the relationships between carbon tetrachloride-induced alterations of liver microsomal lipids and impairment of glucose-6-phosphatase activity. *Exp Mol Pathol* 1977;27:309–323.

92. Glende EA Jr, Hruszkewycz AM, Recknagel RO. Critical role of lipid peroxidation in carbon tetrachloride-induced loss of aminopyrine demethylase, cytochrome P-450 and glucose-6-phosphatase. *Biochem Pharmacol* 1976;25:2163–2170.

93. Ferrali M, Comporti M. On the mechanisms of the CCl₄-induced inhibition of liver cytochrome P-450. *Res Commun Chem Pathol Pharmacol* 1987;56:375–386.

94. De Groot H, Haas W. O₂-independent damage of cytochrome P450 by CCl₄-metabolites in hepatic microsomes. *FEBS Lett* 1980;115:253–256.

95. Benedetti A, Casini AF, Ferrali M, Comporti M. Early alterations induced by carbon tetrachloride in the lipids of the membranes of the endoplasmic reticulum of the liver cell. I. Separation and partial characterization of altered lipids. *Chem-Biol Interact* 1977;17:151–166.

96. Roders MK, Glende EA Jr, Recknagel RO. NADPH-dependent microsomal lipid peroxidation and the problem of pathological action at a distance: new data on induction of red cell damage. *Biochem Pharmacol* 1978;27:437–443.

97. Roders MK, Glende EA Jr, Recknagel RO. Prelytic damage of red cells in filtrates from peroxidizing microsomes. *Science* 1977;196:1221–1222.

98. Benedetti A, Casini AF, Ferrali M, Comporti M. Effects of diffusible products of peroxidation of rat liver microsomal lipids. *Biochem J* 1979;180:303–312.

99. Benedetti A, Esterbauer H, Ferrali M, Fulceri R, Comporti M. Evidence for aldehydes bound to liver microsomal protein following CCl₄ or BrCCl₃ poisoning. *Biochim Biophys Acta* 1982;711:345–356.

100. Goldring C, Casini AF, Maellaro E, Del Bello B, Comporti M. Determination of 4-hydroxynonenal by high-performance liquid chromatography with electrochemical detection. *Lipids* 1993;28:141–145.

101. Benedetti A, Pompella A, Fulceri R, Romani A, Comporti M. Detection of 4-hydroxynonenal and other lipid peroxidation products in the liver of bromobenzene-poisoned mice *Biochim Biophys Acta* 1986;876:658-666.

102. Pompella A, Romani A, Fulceri R, Benedetti A, Comporti M. 4-Hydroxynonenal and other lipid peroxidation products are formed in mouse liver following intoxication with allyl alcohol. *Biochim Biophys Acta* 1988;961:293–298.

103. Recknagel RO. Carbon tetrachloride hepatotoxicity: status quo and future prospects. *Trends Pharmacol Sci* 1983;4:129–131.

104. Recknagel RO. A new direction in the study of carbon tetrachloride hepatotoxicity. *Life Sci* 1983;33:401–408.

105. Danielson AUH, Mannervik B. 4-hydroxyalk-2-enals are substrates for glutathione transferase. *FEBS Lett* 1985;179:267–270.

106. Ishikawa T, Esterbauer H, Sies H. Role of cardiac glutathione transferase and of the glutathione S-conjugate export system in biotransformation of 4-hydroxynonenal in the heart. *J Biol Chem* 1986;261:1576–1581.

107. Esterbauer H, Zollner H, Lang J. Metabolism of the lipid peroxidation product 4-hydroxynonenal by isolated hepatocytes and by liver cytosolic fractions. *Biochem J* 1985;228:363–373.
108. Paradisi L, Panagini C, Parola M, Barrera G, Dianzani MU. Effect of 4-hydroxynonenal on adenylate cyclase and 5′-nucleotidase activities in rat liver plasma membrane. *Chem-Biol Interact* 1985;53:209–217.
109. Recknagel RO, Glende EA Jr. The carbon tetrachloride hepatotoxicity model: free radicals and calcium homeostasis. In: Miquel J, Quintanilha AT, Weber H, ed. *Handbook of free radicals and antioxidants in biomedicine*. Boca Raton, FL: CRC Press, 1989;3:3–16.
110. Recknagel RO, Glende EA Jr. Effect of carbon tetrachloride on liver cell calcium homeostasis. In: Heilmann C, ed. *Calcium-dependent processes in the liver*. Falk Symposium 48, Lancaster (U.K.): MTP Press Ltd, 1987:229–236.
111. Recknagel RO, Glende EA Jr. Calcium, Phospholipase A₂, and eicosanoids in toxigenic liver cell injury. In: Csomós G, Fehér J, ed. *Free radicals and the liver*. Berlin: Springer-Verlag, 1992:43–62.
112. Moore L, Davenport GR, Landon EJ. Calcium uptake of a rat liver microsomal subcellular fraction in response to in vivo administration of carbon tetrachloride. *J Biol Chem* 1976;251:1197–1201.
113. Moore L. Inhibition of liver-microsome calcium pump by in vivo administration of CCl₄, CHCl₃ and 1,1-dichloroethylene (vinylidene chloride). *Biochem Pharmacol* 1980;29:2505–2511.
114. Lowrey K, Glende EA Jr, Recknagel RO. Destruction of liver microsomal calcium pump activity by carbon tetrachloride and bromotrichloromethane. *Biochem Pharmacol* 1981;30:135–140.
115. Lowrey K, Glende EA Jr, Recknagel RO. Rapid depression of rat liver microsomal calcium pump activity after administration of carbon tetrachloride or bromotrichloromethane and lack of effect after ethanol. *Toxicol Appl Pharmacol* 1981;59:389–394.
116. Waller RL, Glende EA Jr, Recknagel RO. Carbon tetrachloride and bromotrichloromethane toxicity: dual role of covalent binding of metabolic cleavage products and lipid peroxidation in depression of microsomal calcium sequestration. *Biochem Pharmacol* 1983;32:1613–1617.
117. Glende EA Jr, Pushpendran CK. Activation of phospholipase A₂ by carbon tetrachloride in isolated rat hepatocytes. *Biochem Pharmacol* 1986;35:3301–3307.
118. Nicotera P, Bellomo G, Orrenius S. Calcium-mediated mechanisms in chemically induced cell death. *Annu Rev Pharmacol Toxicol* 1992;32:449–470.
119. Orrenius S, McConkey DJ, Bellomo G, Nicotera P. Role of Ca²⁺ in toxic cell killing. *Trends Pharmacol Sci* 1989;10:281–285.
120. Bellomo G, Fulceri, R, Albano E, Gamberucci A, Pompella A, Parola M, Benedetti A. Ca²⁺-dependent and -independent mitochondrial damage in hepatocellular injury. *Cell Calcium* 1991;12:335–341.
121. Koch RR, Glende EA, Recknagel RO. Hepatotoxicity of bromotrichloromethane: bond dissociation energy and lipoperoxidation. *Biochem Pharmacol* 1974;23:2907–2915.
122. Robert A. Current hystory of cytoprotection. *Prostaglandins* 1981;21(suppl):89–96.
123. Ruwart MJ, Rush BD, Friedle NM, Piper RC, Kolaja GJ. Protective effects of 16,16-dimethyl PGE₂ on the liver and kidney. *Prostaglandins* 1981;21:97–102.
124. Funck-Brentano C, Tinel M, DeGroot C, Letteron P, Babany G, Pessayre D. Protective effect of 16,16-dimethyl prostaglandin E₂ on the hepatotoxicity of bromobenzene in mice. *Biochem Pharmacol* 1984;33:89–96.
125. Stachura J, Tarnawski A, Ivey JJ, et al. 16,16-dimethyl PGE₂ protection of rat liver against acute injury by galactosamine, acetaminophen, ethanol and ANIT(Abstr.). *Gastroenterol* 1981;80:1349.
126. Nodu Y, Hughes RD, Williams R. Effect of prostacyclin and a prostaglandin analogue BW245C on galactosamine-induced hepatic necrosis. *J Hepatol* 1986;2:58–64.
127. Guarner F, Fremont-Smith M, Prieto J. Cytoprotective effects of prostaglandins on isolated liver cells. *Liver* 1985;5:35–39.
128. Rush BD, Wilkinson KF, Nichols NM, Ochoa R, Brunden MN, Ruwart MJ. Hepatic protection by 16,16-dimethyl PGE₂ (DMPG) against acute aflatoxin B₁-induced injury in the rat. *Prostaglandins* 1989;37:683–692.
129. Divald A, Ujhelyi E, Jeney A, Lapis K, Institoris L. Hepatoprotective effects of prostacyclins on CCl₄-induced liver injury in rats. *Exp Mol Pathol* 1985;42:163–166.
130. Guarner F, Boughton-Smith NK, Blackwell GJ, Moncada S. Reduction by prostacyclin of acetaminophen-induced liver toxicity in the mouse. *Hepatology* 1988;8:248–253.
131. Horton AA, Wood JM. Effect of inhibitors of phospholipase A₂, cyclooxygenase and thromboxane synthetase on paracetamol hepatotoxicity in the rat. *Eicosanoids* 1989;2:123–129.
132. Nagai H, Shimazawa T, Yakuo I, Aoki M, Koda A, Kasahara M. The role of thromboxane A₂ [TXA₂] in liver injury in mice. *Prostanglandins* 1989;38:439–446.

133. Marinovich M, Flaminio LM, Papagni M, Galli CL. Stimulation of arachidonic acid metabolism by CCl4 in isolated rat hepatocytes. *Prostaglandins* 1989;37:23–30.
134. Marinovich M, Flaminio LM, Papagni M, Galli CL. Evaluation of the cytoprotective effect of natural and synthetic prostaglandins in CCl4 -induced liver cell damage. *Adv Prostaglan Thromb Leucotriene Res* 1987;17:1094–1097.
135. Horton AA, Wood JM. Prevention of thromboxane B2-induced hepatocyte plasma membrane bleb formation by certain prostaglandins and a proteinase inhibitor. *Biochim Biophys Acta* 1990;1022:319–324.
136. Lynch TJ, Blackwell GJ, Moncada S. Carbon tetrachloride-induced eicosanoid synthesis and release from rat peritoneal leucocytes. *Biochem Pharmacol* 1985;34:1515–1522.
137. Ungemach FR. Pathobiological mechanisms of hepatocellular damage following lipid peroxidation. *Chem Phys Lipids* 1987;45:171–205.
138. Jollow DJ, Mitchell JR, Zampaglione N, Gillette JR. Bromobenzene-induced liver necrosis: protective role of glutathione and evidence for 3,4-bromobenzene oxide as the hepatotoxic metabolite. *Pharmacology* 1974;11:151–169.
139. Brodie BB, Reid WD, Cho AK, Sipes G, Krishna G, Gillette JR. Possible mechanism of liver necrosis caused by aromatic organic compounds. *Proc Natl Acad Sci USA* 1971;68:160–164.
140. Reid WD, Krishna G. Centrolobular hepatic necrosis related to covalent binding of metabolites of halogenated aromatic hydrocarbons. *Exp Mol Pathol* 1973;18:80–99.
141. Reid WD, Christie B, Krishna G, Mitchell JR, Moskowitz J, Brodie BB. Bromobenzene metabolism and hepatic necrosis. *Pharmacology* 1971;6:41–55.
142. Zampaglione N, Jollow DJ, Mitchell JR, Stripp B, Hamrich M, Gillette JR. Role of detoxifying enzymes in bromobenzene-induced liver necrosis. *J Pharmacol Exp Ther* 1973;187:218–227.
143. Mitchell JR, Reid WD, Christie B, Moskowitz J, Krishna G, Brodie BB. Bromobenzene-induced hepatic necrosis: species differences and protection by SKF 525-A. *Res Commun Chem Pathol Pharmacol* 1971;2:877–888.
144. Jollow DJ, Mitchell JR, Potter WZ, Davis DC, Gillette JR, Brodie BB. Acetaminophen-induced hepatic necrosis. II. Role of covalent binding in vivo. *J Pharmacol Exp Ther* 1973;187:195–202.
145. Anundi I, Högberg J, Stead AH. Glutathione depletion in isolated hepatocytes: its relation to lipid peroxidation and cell damage. *Acta Pharmacol Toxicol* 1979;45:45–51.
146. Casini A, Giorli M, Hyland RJ, Serroni A, Gilfor D, Farber JL. Mechanisms of cell injury in the killing of cultured hepatocytes by bromobenzene. *J Biol Chem* 1982;257:6721–6728.
147. Wendel A, Feuerstein S, Konz K-H. Acute paracetamol intoxication of starved mice leads to lipid peroxidation in vivo. *Biochem Pharmacol* 1979;28:2051–2055.
148. Casini AF, Pompella A, Comporti M. Liver glutathione depletion induced by bromobenzene, iodobenzene, and diethylmaleate poisoning and its relation to lipid peroxidation and necrosis. *Am J Pathol* 1985;118:225–237.
149. Albano E, Poli G, Tomasi A, Bini A, Vannini V, Dianzani MU. Toxicity of 1,2-dibromoethane in isolated hepatocytes: role of lipid peroxidation. *Chem-Biol Interact* 1984;50:255–265.
150. Nachtomi E, Alumot E. Comparison of ethylene dibromide and carbon tetrachloride toxicity in rats and chicks: blood and liver levels, lipid peroxidation. *Exp Mol Pathol* 1972;16:71–78.
151. Lau SS, Zannoni VG. Hepatic microsomal epoxidation of bromobenzene to phenols and its toxicological implication. *Toxicol Appl Pharmacol* 1979;50:309–318.
152. Lau SS, Zannoni VG. Bromobenzene epoxidation leading to binding on macromolecular protein sites. *J Pharmacol Exp Ther* 1981;219:563–572.
153. Lau SS, Abrams GD, Zannoni VG. Metabolic activation and detoxification of bromobenzene leading to cytotoxicity. *J Pharmacol Exp Ther* 1980;214:703–708.
154. Casini AF, Maellaro E, Pompella A, Ferrali M, Comporti M. Lipid peroxidation, protein thiols and calcium homeostasis in bromobenzene-induced liver damage. *Biochem Pharmacol* 1987;36:3689–3695.
155. Maellaro E, Del Bello B, Casini AF, Comporti M, Ceccarelli D, Muscatello U, Masini A. Early mitochondrial disfunction in bromobenzene treated mice: a possible factor of liver injury. *Biochem Pharmacol* 1990;40:1491–1497.
156. Reid WD. Mechanism of allyl alcohol-induced hepatic necrosis. *Experimentia* 1972;28:1058–1061.
157. Zitting A, Heinonen T. Decrease of reduced glutathione in isolated rat hepatocytes caused by acrolein, acrylonitrile, and the thermal degradation products of styrene copolymers. *Toxicology* 1980;17:333–341.
158. Dawson JR, Norbeck K, Anundi I, Moldéus P. The effectiveness of N-acetyl-cysteine in isolated hepatocytes, against the toxicity of paracetamol, acrolein and paraquat. *Arch Toxicol* 1984;55:11–15.

159. Jaeschke H, Kleinwaechter C, Wendel A. The role of acrolein in allyl alcohol-induced lipid peroxidation and liver cell damage in mice. *Biochem Pharmacol* 1987;36:51–58.
160. Pompella A, Romani A, Fulceri R, Maellaro E, Benedetti A, Comporti M. In: Nigam S, McBrien D, Slater TF, eds. Detection of 4-hydroxynonenal and other lipid peroxidation products in the liver of allyl alcohol-intoxicated mice. *Eicosanoids, lipid peroxidation and cancer.* Heidelberg: Springer Verlag 1988:253–263.
161. Pompella A, Romani A, Benedetti A, Comporti M. Loss of membrane protein thiols and lipid peroxidation in allyl alcohol hepatotoxicity. *Biochem Pharmacol* 1991;41:1255–1259.
162. Dogterom P, Nagelkerke JF, van Stevenink J, Mulder GJ. Inhibition of lipid peroxidation by disulfiram and diethyldithiocarbamate does not prevent hepatotoxin-induced cell death in isolated rat hepatocytes. *Chem-Biol Interact* 1988;66:251–265.
163. Haenen GRMM, Vermeulen NPE, Tai Tin Tsoi JNL, Ragetli HMN, Timmerman H, Bast A. Activation of the microsomal glutathione-*S*-transferase and reduction of the glutathione dependent protection against lipid peroxidation by acrolein. *Biochem Pharmacol* 1988;37:1933–1938.
164. Hormann VA, Moore DR, Rikans L. Relative contributions of protein sulfhydryl loss and lipid peroxidation to allyl alcohol-induced cytotoxicity in isolated rat hepatocytes. *Toxicol Appl Pharmacol* 1989;98:375–384.
165. Jaeschke H, Kleinwaechter C, Wendel A. NADH-dependent reductive stress and ferritin-bound iron in allyl alcohol-induced lipid peroxidation in vivo: the protective effect of vitamin E. *Chem-Biol Interact* 1992;81:57–68.
166. Thomas CE, Morehouse LA, Aust SD. Ferritin and superoxide-dependent lipid peroxidation. *J Biol Chem* 1985;260:3275–3280.
167. Thomas CE, Aust SD. Release of iron from ferritin by cardiotoxic anthracycline antibiotics. *Arch Biochem Biophys* 1986;248:684–689.
168. Crichton RR, Roman F, Roland F. Iron mobilization from ferritin by chelating agents. *J Inorganic Biochem* 1980;13:305–316.
169. Gutteridge JMC. Iron promoters of the Fenton reaction and lipid peroxidation can be released from haemoglobin by peroxides. *FEBS Lett* 1986;201:291–295.
170. Puppo A, Halliwell B. Formation of hydroxyl radicals from hydrogen peroxide in the presence of iron. *Biochem J* 1988;249:185–190.
171. Ferrali M, Signorini C, Ciccoli L, Comporti M. Iron release and membrane damage in erythrocytes exposed to oxidizing agents, phenylhydrazine, divicine and isouramil. *Biochem J* 1992;285:295–301.
172. Sirivech S, Frieden E, Osaki S. The release of iron from horse spleen ferritin by reduced flavins. *Biochem J* 1974;143:311–315.
173. Shaw S, Jayatilleke E, Lieber CS. Lipid peroxidation as a mechanism of alcoholic liver injury: role of iron mobilization and microsomal induction. *Alcohol* 1988;5:135–140.
174. Cairo C, Tacchini L, Pogliaghi G, Anzon E, Tomasi A, Bernelli-Zazzera A. Induction of ferritin synthesis by oxidative stress: transcriptional and post-transcriptional regulation by expansion of the "free" iron pool. *J Biol Chem* 1995;270:300–303.
175. Hildebrandt AG, Speck M, Roots I. Possible control of hydrogen peroxide production and degradation in microsomes during mixed function oxidase reaction. *Biochem Biophys Res Commun* 1973;54:968–975.
176. Hildebrandt AG, Roots I. Reduced nicotinamide adenine dinucleotide phosphate (NADPH)-dependent formation and breakdown of hydrogen peroxide during mixed function oxidation reactions in liver microsomes. *Arch Biochem Biophys* 1975;171:385–397.
177. Nordblom GD, Coon MJ. Hydrogen peroxide formation and stoichiometry of hydroxylation reactions catalyzed by highly purified liver microsomal cytochrome P-450. *Arch Biochem Biophys* 1977;180:343–347.
178. White RE, Coon MJ. Oxygen activation by cytochrome P-450. *Annu Rev Biochem* 1980;49:325–356.
179. Strobel HW, Coon MJ. Effect of superoxide generation and dismutation on hydroxylation reactions catalyzed by liver microsomal cytochrome P-450. *J Biol Chem* 1971;246:7826–7829.
180. Richter C, Azzi A, Weser U, Wendel A. Hepatic microsomal dealkylation: inhibition by a tyrosine copper (II) complex provided with superoxide dismutase activity. *J Biol Chem* 1977;252:5061–5066.
181. Kuthan H, Tsuji H, Graf H, Ullrich V, Werringloer J, Estabrook RW. Generation of superoxide anion as a source of hydrogen peroxide in a reconstituted monooxygenase system. *FEBS Lett* 1978;91:343–345.
182. Wendel A, Feuerstein S. Drug-induced lipid peroxidation in mice. I. Modulation by monooxygenase activity, glutathione and selenium status. *Biochem Pharmacol* 1981;30:2513–2520.

183. Gerson RJ, Serroni A, Gilfor D, Ellen JM, Farber JL. Killing of cultured hepatocytes by the mixed-function oxidation of ethoxycoumarin. *Biochem Pharmacol* 1986;35:4311–4319.
184. Kloss MW, Rosen GM, Rauckman E. Cocaine-mediated hepatotoxicity. *Biochem Pharmacol* 1984;33:169–173.
185. Maellaro E, Casini AF, Del Bello B, Comporti M. Lipid peroxidation and antioxidant systems in the liver injury produced by glutathione depleting agents. *Biochem Pharmacol* 1990;39:1513–1521.
186. McCay PB, Lai EK, Powell SR. Vitamin E functions as an electron shuttle for glutathione-dependent "free radical reductase" activity in biological membranes. *Fed Proc* 1986;45:451.
187. Packer IE, Slater TF, Willson RL. Direct observation of free radical interaction between vitamin E and vitamin C. *Nature* 1979;278:737–738.
188. Scarpa M, Rigo A, Maiorino M, Ursini F, Gregolin C. Formation of α-tocopherol radical and recycling of α-tocopherol by ascorbate during peroxidation of phosphatidylcholine liposomes: an electron paramagnetic resonance study. *Biochim Biophys Acta* 1984;801:215–219.
189. Wefers H, Sies H. The protection by ascorbate and glutathione against microsomal lipid peroxidation is dependent on vitamin E. *Eur J Biochem* 1988;174:353–357.
190. Maellaro E, Del Bello B, Sugherini L, Pompella A, Casini AF, Comporti M. Protection by ascorbic acid against oxidative injury of isolated hepatocytes. *Xenobiotica* 1994;24:281–289.
191. Nakagawa Y, Cotgreave IA, Moldéus P. Relationships between ascorbic acid and α-tocopherol during diquat-induced redox cycling in isolated rat hepatocytes. *Biochem Pharmacol* 1991;42:883–888.
192. Maellaro E, Del Bello B, Sugherini L, Santucci A, Comporti M, Casini AF. Purification and characterization of glutathione-dependent dehydroascorbate reductase from rat liver. *Biochem J* 1994;301:471–476.
193. Del Bello B, Maellaro E, Sugherini L, Santucci A, Comporti M, Casini AF. Purification of NADPH-dependent dehydroascorbate reductase from rat liver and its identification with 3α-hydroxysteroid dehydrogenase. *Biochem J* 1994;304:385–390.
194. Michaelis L, Hill ES. Potentiometric studies on semiquinones. *J Am Chem Soc* 1933;55:1481–1494.
195. Farrington JA, Ebert M, Land EJ, Fletcher K. Bipyridylium quaternary salts and related compounds. V. Pulse radiolysis studies of the reaction of paraquat radical with oxygen: implications for the mode of action of bipyridyl herbicides. *Biochim Biophys Acta* 1973;314:372–381.
196. Gage JC. The action of paraquat and diquat on the respiration of liver cell fractions. *Biochem J* 1968;109:757–761.
197. Montgomery MM. Interaction of paraquat with the pulmonary microsomal fatty acid desaturase system. *Toxicol Appl Pharmacol* 1976;36:543–554.
198. Thor H, Smith MT, Hartzell P, Bellomo G, Jewell SA, Orrenius S. The metabolism of menadione (2-methyl-1,4-naphthoquinone) by isolated hepatocytes. *J Biol Chem* 1982;257:12419–12425.
199. Bellomo G, Thor H, Mirabelli F, Richelmi P, Finardi G, Orrenius S. Alterations in hepatocyte cytoskeleton during the metabolism of quinones. In: Poli G, Cheeseman KH, Dianzani MU, Slater TF, eds. *Free radicals in the pathogenesis of liver injury.* Oxford: Pergamon Press, 1988:21–35.
200. Sugioka K, Nagano H, Nagano M, Tero-Kubota S, Igekami Y. Generation of hydroxyl radicals during the enzymatic reductions of the Fe^{3+}-ADP-phosphate-adriamycin and Fe^{3+}-ADP-EDTA systems: less involvment of hydroxyl radical and a great importance of proposed perferryl ion complexes in lipid peroxidation. *Biochim Biophys Acta* 1983;753:411–421.
201. Bellomo G, Orrenius S. Altered thiol and calcium homeostasis in oxidative hepatocellular injury. *Hepatology* 1985;5:876–882.
202. Orrenius S, Bellomo G. Toxicological implications of perturbation of Ca^{2+} homeostasis in hepatocytes. In: Cheung WJ, ed. *Calcium and cell functions.* New York: Academic Press, 1986;6:186–208.
203. Gilbert HF. Biological disulfides: the third messenger? Modulation of phosphofructokinase activity by thiol/disulfide exchange. *J Biol Chem* 1982;257:12086–12091.
204. Rasmussen H, Goodman DBP, Freidman N, Allen JA, Korekawz L. Ionic control of metabolism. In: Aurbach GD, ed. *Handbook of physiology.* Washington: American Physiology Society, 1976;7:225–264.
205. Rubin E. *Calcium in secretory processes.* New York: Plenum Press, 1974.
206. Bellomo G, Jewell SA, Smith MT, Thor H, Orrenius S. Perturbation of Ca^{2+} homeostasis during hepatocyte injury. In: Keppler D, Popper H, Bianchi L, Reutter W, eds. *Mechanisms of hepatocyte injury and death.* Lancaster: MTP Press Ltd, 1984:119–128.
207. Kalish GH, Di Luzio NR. Peroxidation of liver lipids in the pathogenesis of the ethanol-induced fatty liver. *Science* 1966;152:1390–1392.

208. Comporti M, Hartman A, Di Luzio NR. Effect of in vivo and in vitro ethanol administration on liver lipid peroxidation. *Lab Invest* 1967;16:616–624.
209. Dianzani MU. Lipid peroxidation in ethanol poisoning: a critical reconsideration. *Alcohol Alcoholism* 1985;20:161–173.
210. Albano E, Ingelman-Sundberg M, Tomasi A, Poli G. Free radical mediated reactions and ethanol toxicity: some considerations on the methodological approaches. In: Palmer TN, ed. *Alcoholism: a molecular perspective*. New York: Plenum Press, 1991:45–56.
211. Nordmann R, Ribière C, Rouach H. Implication of free radical mechanisms in ethanol-induced cellular injury. *Free Rad Biol Med* 1992;12:219–240.
212. Lieber CS, De Carli LM. Hepatic microsomal ethanol-oxidizing system: in vitro characteristics and adaptative properties in vivo. *J Biol Chem* 1970;245:2505–2512.
213. Lai CS, Grover TA, Piette LH. Hydroxyl radical production in a purified NADPH-cytochrome c (P-450) reductase system. *Arch Biochem Biophys* 1979;193:373–378.
214. Mishin V, Pokrovsky A, Lyakhovich VV. Interactions of some acceptors with superoxide anion radicals formed by the NADPH-specific flavoprotein in rat liver microsomal fractions. *Biochem J* 1976;154:307–310.
215. Massey V, Strickland S, Mayhew SG, Hawell LG, Engel PC, Matthews RG, Schuman M, Sullivan PA. The production of superoxide anion radicals in the reaction of reduced flavins and flavoproteins with molecular oxygen. *Biochem Biophys Res Commun* 1969;36:891–897.
216. Valenzuela A, Fernandez N, Fernandez V, Ugarte G, Videla LA, Guerra R, Villanueva A. Effect of acute ethanol ingestion on lipoperoxidation and on the activity of the enzymes related to peroxide metabolism in rat liver. *FEBS Lett* 1980;111:11–13.
217. Lieber CS, De Carli LM. Reduced nicotinamide-adenine dinucleotide phosphate oxidase: activity enhanced by ethanol consumption. *Science* 1970;170:78–80.
218. Reitz RC. A possible mechanism for the peroxidation of lipids due to chronic ethanol ingestion. *Biochim Biophys Acta* 1975;380:145–154.
219. Thurman RG. Induction of hepatic microsomal reduced nicotinamide adenine dinucleotide phosphate-dependent production of hydrogen peroxide by chronic prior treatment with ethanol. *Mol Pharmacol* 1973;9:670–675.
220. Videla L, Bernstein J, Israel I. Metabolic alterations produced in the liver by chronic ethanol administration: increased oxidative capacity. *Biochem J* 1973;134:507–514.
221. Cederbaum AI, Dicker E, Cohen G. Effect of hydroxyl radical scavengers on microsomal oxidation of alcohols and associated microsomal reactions. *Biochemistry* 1978;17:3058–3064.
222. Cederbaum AI, Dicker E. Inhibition of microsomal oxidation of alcohols and of hydroxyl-radical-scavenging agents by the iron-chelating agent desferrioxamine. *Biochem J* 1983;210:107–113.
223. Ingelman-Sundberg M, Johanson I. Mechanisms of hydroxyl radical formation and ethanol oxidation by ethanol inducible and other forms of rabbit liver microsomal cytochromes P450. *J Biol Chem* 1984;259:6447–6458.
224. Albano E, Tomasi A, Goria-Gatti L, Poli G, Vannini V, Dianzani MU. Free radical metabolism of alcohols by rat liver microsomes. *Free Rad Res Commun* 1987;3:243–249.
225. Albano E, Tomasi A, Goria-Gatti L, Dianzani MU. Spin trapping of free radical species produced during the microsomal metabolism of ethanol. *Chem-Biol Interact* 1988;65:223–234.
226. Albano E, Tomasi A, Persson J, Terelius Y, Goria-Gatti L, Ingelman-Sundberg M, Dianzani MU. Role of ethanol-inducible cytochrome P450 (P450IIE1) in catalysing the free radical activation of aliphatic alcohols. *Biochem Pharmacol* 1991;41:1895–1902.
227. Knecht KT, Bradfort BU, Mason RP, Thurman GR. In vivo formation of a free radical metabolite of ethanol. *Mol Pharmacol* 1990;38:26–30.
228. Albano E, Tomasi A, Parola M, Comoglio A, Ingelman-Sundberg M, Dianzani MU. Mechanisms responsible for free radical formation during ethanol metabolism and their role in causing oxidative injury by alcohol. In: Corongiu F, Banni S, Dessi MA, Rice Evans C, eds. *Free radicals and antioxidants nutrition*. London: Richelieu Press, 1993:77–96.
229. Reinke LA, Kotake Y, McCay PB, Janzen EG. Spin-trapping studies of hepatic free radicals formed following the acute administration of ethanol to rats: in vivo detection of 1-hydroxyethyl radicals with PBN. *Free Rad Biol Med* 1991;11:31–39.
230. Terelius Y, Lindros KO, Albano E, Ingelman-Sundberg M. Isozyme-specificity of cytochrome P450-mediated hepatotoxicity. In: Ruckpaul K, Rein H, eds. *Frontiers in biotransformation*. Berlin: Akademie Verlag, 1993;8:186–232.
231. McCay PB, Reinke LA, Rau JM. Hydroxyl radicals are generated by hepatic microsomes during NADPH oxidation relationship to ethanol metabolism. *Free Rad Res Commun* 1992;15:335–346.

232. Albano E, Parola M, Comoglio A, Dianzani MU. Evidence for the covalent binding of hydroxyethyl radicals to rat microsomal proteins. *Alcohol Alcoholism* 1993;28:453–459.

233. Albano E, Poli G, Tomasi A, Goria-Gatti L, Dianzani MU. Study of the mechanisms responsible for ethanol-induced oxidative damages using isolated rat hepatocytes. In: Hayaishi O, Niki E, Kondo M, Yoshikawa T, eds. *Medical, biochemical and chemical aspects of free radicals.* Amsterdam: Elsevier Biomedical, 1988:1389–1392.

234. Donohur TM, Tuma DJ, Sorrell MF. Acetaldehyde adducts with proteins: binding of ^{14}C-acetaldehyde to serum albumin. *Arch Biochem Biophys* 1983;220:239–246.

235. Moncada C, Torres V, Varghese G, Albano E, Israel Y. Ethanol-derived immunoreactive species formed by free radical mechanisms. *Mol Pharmacol* 1994;46:786–791.

236. Clot P, Bellomo G, Tabone M, Aricòt S, Albano E. Detection of antibodies against proteins modified by hydroxyethyl free radicals in patients with alcoholic cirrhosis. *Gastroenterology* 1995;108:201–207.

237. Grossley IR, Neuberger J, Davis M, Williams R, Eddleston ALWF. Ethanol metabolism in the generation of new antigenic determinants on liver cells. *Gut* 1986;27:186–189.

238. Nanji AA, Khwaja S, Tahan SR, Sadrzaden SMH. Plasma levels of a novel noncyclooxygenase-derived prostanoid (8-isoprostane) correlate with severity of liver injury in experimental alcoholic liver disease. *J Pharmacol Exp Ther* 1994;269:1280–1285.

239. Powell LW, Bassett ML, Halliday JW. Hemochromatosis 1980 update. *Gastroenterology* 1980;78:374–381.

240. Golberg L, Marti LE, Batchelor A. Biochemical changes in the tissues of animals injected with iron. *Biochem J* 1962;83:291–298.

241. Bacon RB, Tavill AS, Brittenham GM, Park CH, Recknagel RO. Hepatic lipid peroxidation in vivo in rats with chronic iron overload. *J Clin Invest* 1983;71:429–439.

242. Dabbagh AJ, Mannion T, Lynch SM, Frei B. The effect of iron overload on rat plasma and liver oxidant status in vivo. *Biochem J* 1994;300:799–803.

243. Comporti M, Signorini C, Ciccoli L, Ferrali M. Phenylhydrazine-induced iron release as a mechanism of membrane and DNA damage. *Free Rad Biol Med* 1993;15:516(A 7:2).

244. Ferrali M, Signorini C, Sugherini L, Pompella A, Lodovici M, Caciotti B, Ciccoli L, Comporti M. Release of free, redox-active iron in the liver and DNA oxidative damage following phenylhydrazine intoxication. *Biochem Pharmacol* 1997;53:1743–1751.

245. Parola M, Leonarduzzi G, Biasi F, Albano E, Biocca ME, Poli G, Dianzani MU. Vitamin E dietary supplementation protects against carbon tetrachloride-induced chronic liver damage and cirrhosis. *Hepatology* 1992;16:1014–1021.

246. Parola M, Muraca R, Dianzani I, Barrera G, Leonarduzzi G, Bendinelli P, Piccoletti R, Poli G. Vitamin E dietary supplementation inhibits transforming growth factor $\beta 1$ gene expression in the rat liver. *FEBS Lett* 1992;308:267–270.

247. Gressner AM. Liver fibrosis: perspectives in pathobiochemical research and clinical outlook. *Eur J Chem Clin Biochem* 1991;29:293–311.

248. Chojkier M, Houglum K, Solis-Herruzo J, Brenner DA. Stimulation of collagen gene expression by ascorbic acid in cultured human fibroblasts: a role for lipid peroxidation? *J Biol Chem* 1989;264:16957–16962.

249. Houglum K, Brenner DA, Chojkier M. D-α-Tocopherol inhibits collagen α_1(I) gene expression in cultured human fibroblasts: modulation of constitutive collagen gene expression by lipid peroxidation. *J Clin Invest* 1991;87:2230–2235.

250. Bedossa P, Houglum K, Trautwein C, Holstage A, Chojkier M. Stimulation of collagen α_1(I) gene expression is associated with lipid peroxidation in hepatocellular injury: a link to tissue fibrosis? *Hepatology* 1994;19:1262–1271.

251. Parola M, Pinzani M, Casini A, et al. Stimulation of lipid peroxidation or 4-hydroxynonenal treatment increases procollagen α_1(I) gene expression in human liver fat-storing cells. *Biochem Biophys Res Commun* 1993;194:1044–1050.

252. Kurose I, Saito H, Suematsu M, et al. Kupffer cell-mediated oxidative stress on colon cancer line visualized by digital imaging fluorescence microscopy. *Cancer Lett* 1991;59:201–1209.

253. Zhu H, Bannenberg GL, Moldéus P, Shertzer HG. Oxidation pathways for the intracellular probe 2′,7′-dichlorofluorescein. *Arch Toxicol* 1994;68:582–587.

254. Babbs CF, Cregor MD, Turek JJ, Badylack SF. Endothelial superoxide production in the isolated rat heart during early reperfusion after ischemia: a histochemical study. *Am J Pathol* 1991;139:1069–1080.

255. Benedetti A, Fulceri R, Ferrali M, Ciccoli L, Esterbauer H, Comporti M. Detection of carbonyl functions in phospholipids of liver microsomes in CCl$_4$- and BrCCl$_3$-poisoned rats. *Biochim Biophys Acta* 1982;712:628–638.

256. Benedetti A, Malvaldi G, Fulceri R, Comporti M. Loss of lipid peroxidation as a histochemical marker for preneoplastic hepatocellular foci of rats. *Cancer Res* 1984;44:5712–5717.

257. Pompella A, Mellaro E, Casini AF, Comporti M. Histochemical detection of lipid peroxidation in the liver of bromobenzene-poisoned mice. *Am J Pathol* 1987;129:295–301.

258. Tanaka M, Sotomatsu A, Kanai H, Hirai S. Combined histochemical and biochemical demonstration of nigral vulnerability to lipid peroxidation induced by dopa and iron. *Neurosci Lett* 1992;140:42–46.

259. Toyokuni S, Okada S, Hamazaki S, Minamiyama Y, Yamada Y, Liang P, Fukunaga Y, Midorikawa O. Combined histochemical and biochemical analysis of sex hormone dependence of ferric nitrilotriacetate-induced renal lipid peroxidation in ddY mice. *Cancer Res* 1990;50:5574–5580.

260. Masuda Y, Yamamori Y. Histologic detection of lipid peroxidation following infusion of tert-butyl hydroperoxide and ADP-iron complex in perfused rat livers. *Jap J Pharmacol* 1991;56:133–142.

261. Pompella A, Comporti M. The use of 3-hydroxy-2-naphthoic acid hydrazide and fast blue B for the histochemical detection of lipid peroxidation in animal tissues: a microphotometrical study. *Histochemistry* 1991;95:255–262.

262. Pompella A, Comporti M. Imaging of oxidative stress at subcellular level by confocal laser scanning microscopy after fluorescent derivativization of cellular carbonyls. *Am J Pathol* 1993;142:1353–1357.

263. Harris ME, Carney JM, Hua DH, Leedle RA. Detection of oxidation products in individual neurons by fluorescence microscopy. *Exp Neurology* 1994;129:95–102.

264. Hedley D, Chow S. Flow cytometric measurement of lipid peroxidation in vital cells using parinaric acid. *Cytometry* 1992;13:686–692.

265. Niemelä O, Parkkila S, Ylä-Herttuala S, Halsted C, Witzum JL, Lanca A, Israel Y. Covalent protein adducts in the liver as a result of ethanol metabolism and lipid peroxidation. *Lab Invest* 1994;70:537–546.

266. Palinski W, Rosenfeld ME, Ylä-Herttuala S, Gurtner GC, Socher SS, Bolter SW, Parthasarathy S, Carew TE, Steinberg D, Witztum JL. Low density lipoprotein undergoes oxidative modification in vivo. *Proc Natl Acad Sci USA* 1989;86:1372–1376.

267. Okamoto K, Toyokuni S, Uchida K, Ogawa O, Takenewa J, Kakehi Y, Kinoshita H, Hattori-Nakakuki Y, Hiai H, Yoshida O. Formation of 8-hydroxy-2′-deoxyguanosine and 4-hydroxy-2-nonenal-modified proteins in human renal-cell carcinoma. *Int J Cancer* 1994;58:825–829.

Toxicology of the Liver, 2nd ed.,
Edited by Gabriel L. Plaa and William R. Hewitt
Copyright © 1998 Taylor & Francis

8

Immunologic Mediation
of Chemical-Induced Hepatotoxicity

Sylvia M. Furst and A. Jay Gandolfi

University of Arizona, Tucson, AZ 85724

Since the end of the 19th century, the metabolic changes effected in foreign substances have been considered to be detoxifying in nature, and for many years the liver has been credited, as the guardian of the body, with the responsibility for detoxification. It is becoming increasingly evident that metabolism of drugs and other foreign chemicals may not always be an innocuous biochemical event leading to detoxification and elimination of the compound. Liver injury induced by chemicals has been recognized as a toxicologic problem for close to 100 years, and because of its strategic situation, the liver is a first-line target for damage (adverse effects) (1).

MECHANISMS OF HEPATOTOXICITY

Toxicities arising in humans through exposure to foreign compounds are traditionally classified into two groups:

Predictable toxicity related to highly hepatotoxic agents is very rarely observed with currently used compounds since direct toxicity occurs as a consequence of the intrinsic properties of the compound and is dose-related. Examples include elemental phosphorus, aflatoxins, carbon tetrachloride, and acetaminophen. With the exception of agents used to treat cancer, most serious adverse chemical reactions are not a result of direct cytotoxicity. This is due to cytotoxic agents' being detected in early toxicity testing and thus discontinued in the early stages of preclinical studies.

Unpredictable or idiosyncratic hepatotoxicity occurs in a very small number of people (1/100–1/100,000). This type of reaction may be host-dependent, dose-independent, and difficult to reproduce in animal models (2). Idiosyncratic reactions are unrelated to the mechanism of action of the compound and cannot be produced in the general population even if the dose is markedly increased. Idiosyncratic hepatotoxicity may be due to direct toxicity of a chemically reactive metabolite, so-called metabolic idiosyncrasy or secondary to an immune reaction. Increased metabolism, though a usually minor route, may arise because of a genetic defect in one of the metabolizing enzymes or an alteration in metabolizing activity associated with one of many factors such as age, sex, concomitant drug ingestion, diet, and preexisting disease. Differences in metabolism could lead to large interindividual and interspecies differences in toxicity, but this does not appear to be the sole basis for the idiosyncratic character of these hepatotoxic reactions. Some reactions may be due to the combined effect of a chemical and some other factor such as an infection. Aspirin hepatotoxicity and other types of idiosyncratic drug reactions appear to be more common in patients with diseases such as lupus (3). Chemical hypersensitivity reactions refer to adverse reactions that involve the immune system. In general, the mechanisms of idiosyncratic chemical reactions are unknown.

It is clear that liver injury can be caused by many different kinds of substances. In addition, a variety of pathologic processes are involved. The question that continually arises is whether the lesion is a manifestation of the hepatotoxic property of the substance in question or whether it is a manifestation of the host's response to the agent. Host response can involve both hypersensitivity reactions and exaggerated responses to minor alterations in hepatic function. The evidence for possible involvement of the immune system in the pathogenesis of some instances of chemical hepatotoxicity is the subject of this chapter.

IMMUNOSUPPRESSION AND HYPERSENSITIVITY REACTIONS

A great variety of chemicals have the potential to influence the functional activity of the immune system. Alteration of the integrity of the immune system can have a profound effect on the ability of the organs within the body, such as the liver, to tolerate toxic insults. Induced changes in immunologic status can be broadly divided into those in which immunosuppression or alteration in immune tolerance results and those that initiate tissue-damaging idiosyncratic immunostimulation. In order to understand the immunologic etiology of these reactions, it is important to grasp the basis of an immune response.

THE BASIS OF AN IMMUNE RESPONSE

The immune system consists of nonspecific and specific components. The nonspecific or innate component is composed of an intact epidermal barrier, phagocytes, and complement. This is a first line of defense against "nonself" invaders. For the host to activate nonspecific immune system components, no prior exposure to the antigen target is required. The specific or adaptive components include T lymphocytes and antibodies that amplify their response after repeated exposure. These seek out specific targets and only interact with a limited subset of closely related nonself invader molecules (antigens), and prior exposure is required for optimal function. Although the immune system is essential for the survival of organisms, perturbations in the function of the immune system can produce profound effects. Congenital or acquired deficiencies of portions of the immune system place the patient at an increased risk for infections. In addition, the loss of the ability to distinguish between self and nonself may lead to problems with autoimmune disease. In the case of drug treatment or chemical exposure, recognition of a compound as foreign or nonself could result in development of an adverse reaction.

Antigen-presenting cells are cells that have a special function in the initial processing and presentation of antigens. These cells are predominantly macrophages, B lymphocytes, dendritic cells, and Langerhans cells (4). Kupffer cells are resident macrophages of the liver and represent the largest population of macrophages in the body (5). Endowed with highly efficient phagocytic and degradative properties, macrophages fulfill major responsibilities in maintaining host defense. They also play a central immunoregulatory role in presenting ingested antigen to immunocompetent lymphocytes to initiate the cascade of specific cell-mediated immunity (6). As antigen uptake, processing, and presentation occur, activated macrophages secrete several potent immunologic mediators known to upregulate or downregulate immunoreactivity, both locally and systemically (7). Antigen-presenting cells internalize antigens, which involves fluid-phase pinocytosis, receptor-mediated endocytosis, or phagocytosis (8). Antigens require some form of internal processing before they can be presented to the T cells in an immunogenic form. Ingested antigen is proteolytically degraded to peptides in an endosomal compartment (9). The cells then express some of the antigenic peptide fragments on the cell surface in association with the major histocompatibility complex (MHC I or MHC II). T cell receptors will recognize only fragments of protein in the context of MHC molecules, rather than the intact antigen from which these fragments are derived (10, 11). The complexes of foreign peptides and host MHC molecules form the antigens that can be recognized by antigen receptors on cytotoxic (killer) T lymphocytes. MHC–peptide complexes are also important in the regulation of immune responses. Recognition of the immunogen in association with MHC II results in production of lymphokines by the helper T cell and leads to proliferation and differentiation of clones of B cells that also recognize the immunogen (10). Antibodies against the immunogen are produced by plasma cells (differentiated B cells) and cross-react with other antigenic determinants (epitopes) on tissue macromolecules. B cells recognize intact immunogen, and this may involve an epitope different from that recognized by T cells. The ability of an antibody to recognize immunogen and cross-react with antigens that share the same or similar epitopes but are otherwise very different may be key to the mechanism of lupus and hypersensitivity reactions.

Since antigen presentation is an important controlling feature of the immune response, and since this phase of the response is determined by class II MHC glycoproteins (coded for by over 50 alleles, making this a highly polymorphic system), the polymorphic nature of this system may be a major contributor to the unpredictable nature of chemical hypersensitivity reactions.

IMMUNOSUPPRESSION AND HEPATOTOXICITY

There now exists substantial literature that reveals a variety of chemicals are able to impair the functional integrity of the immune system of rodents (12). Although the list of chemicals that alter the immune system function is quite large, the mechanisms for only a small group have been investigated. Polychlorinated biphenyls (PCBs), polybrominated biphenyls (PBBs) and 2,3,7,8-tetrachlorodibenzo-p-dioxin (TCDD) are all associated with immunotoxicity in experimental animals (13, 14). The long-chain dialkyltin compounds, in particular di-n-butyl (DBTC) up to di-n-octylin dichloride, have been shown to exert a direct antiproliferative effect on lymphocytes (15). Heavy metals have also been implicated to be immunotoxic and accumulate in human peripheral T and B lymphocytes and monocytes (16).

The epidemic of tumors observed in association with acquired immunodeficiency syndrome has emphasized the role of immunosuppression as a cause. It is apparent from clinical data and experimental studies that impairment of particular components of the immune system is characteristically associated with increased susceptibility to different types of infectious disease and chemical insults, leading to liver damage.

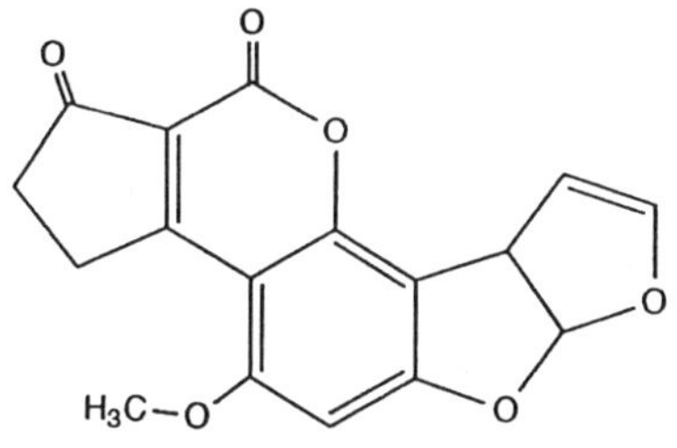

FIG. 1. Aflatoxin B1.

Aflatoxins, particularly aflatoxin B1 (AFB1) (Fig. 1), is an example of a compound associated with liver damage that may be mediated via impairment of the immune system and subsequent susceptibility to infectious disease.

Aflatoxins and Hepatitis

Aflatoxins are mycotoxins that belong to a group of difuranocoumarin metabolites of *Aspergillus flavus* and are the most commonly found mycotoxin in agricultural commodities (17). The incidence of primary liver cancer has been shown to be elevated in certain areas of the world where hepatitis B virus (HBV) is endemic and levels of dietary aflatoxins are high (18). The marked geographic differences in the prevalence of primary liver cancer suggest that the most important risk factors in developing HBV-associated primary liver cancer is dietary exposure to aflatoxin (19–21). A study of HBV status, aflatoxin exposure, and primary liver cancer incidence in southern China found a 10-fold difference in primary liver cancer mortality rates between HBV-infected individuals in two different areas in the region (22). This appeared to be due to a 10-fold difference in aflatoxin food contamination. Several studies have found AFB1 to cause immunosuppression in several animals, resulting in decreased lymphoblastogenesis, delayed type hypersensitivity responses, natural killer cell activity and macrophage phagocytosis (23–29). AFB1 inhibits the proliferation and development of cells of the immune system by inhibiting protein synthesis through chromosomal aberrations (30). Recently AFB1 has been reported to impair the function of Kupffer cells, which are known to be important macrophages involved in the immune response (31). One postulate suggests that aflatoxin causes mutations that complement other mutations induced by the viral infection leading to an accelerated expression of the fully transformed phenotype. Alterations in gene loci were observed such as mutations in the p53 tumor suppressor gene; however, much of the work was done on experimental animals with AFB1-induced liver tumors and human primary liver cancer with no indication of etiology of the primary liver cancer (no HBV antigen detected) (32). Thus, definitive proof of the cocarcinogenic mechanism does not exist as yet. It has been proposed that an AFB1-impaired immune system may not be able to detect/prevent an HBV infection or eradicate small foci of malignancy caused by HBV chronic infection. The known effects of immunosuppression include increases in the incidence of infection and cancer. Mechanisms include decreased immune cell numbers and function, biochemical alterations, and interference in cell–cell cooperation. Although many studies have demonstrated immune impairment via these mechanism, more studies are required to investigate the effects of AFB1 on host resistance to hepatotoxicity and tumor development. This is an example of immunologic mediation of chemical-induced hepatotoxicity via immunosuppression.

IDIOSYNCRATIC IMMUNOSTIMULATION REACTIONS

Apart from the intentional immunosuppression caused by immunomodulatory drugs, at present there is little clear evidence that xenobiotics cause unintended functional immunosuppression. In contrast, immunostimulatory reactions are frequent and often a serious repercussion of human exposure to chemicals. Reactions that are known or suspected to result from an immunostimulatory mechanism are termed hypersensitivity reactions and account for approximately 10–20% of all adverse drug reactions (33). In the case of idiosyncratic reactions, some of these involve the development of untoward effects in susceptible subsets of the population, which may occur on a genetic basis. Although rare, many of these reactions are life-threatening and have resulted in removal of potentially useful drugs from the market. The most common reactions of idiosyncratic nature occur in the skin, the blood, and the liver. In addition, the primary chemical-induced lesion may be accompanied by general manifestations such as lymphadenopathy, fever, arthralgia, and eosinophilia. The mechanism by which these reactions occur is poorly understood or unknown and is generally believed to include the involvement of the immune system (34). Common characteristics that lead investigators to suggest an immunological etiology include the following:

1. A requirement for either a delay of more than a week between starting the drug and the development of toxicity or prior exposure to the drug. This delay can vary between types of reactions, ranging from an almost immediate occurrence up to more than a year for the reaction to manifest itself.
2. Almost immediate recurrence of symptoms on reexposure of a patient who has had an idiosyncratic reaction to the compound; however, with some drugs, such as clozapine, symptoms will reoccur in almost the same amount of time, often requiring months.
3. Insufficient correlation between dose and the risk of toxicity. Although these reactions must be dose-dependent, in some cases the dose-toxicity curve is far to the left of that for the dose-response curve of the desired pharmacologic property.
4. The presence of a skin rash and peripheral blood eosinophilia. In some cases this may be missed because of the brief occurrence of the reaction.
5. An unpredictable nature that cannot be detected by preclinical toxicology testing nor be reproduced in animal models; however, animals have been found that react to some drugs in an idiosyncratic manner. Idiosyncratic hypersensitivity reactions to the sulfonamides, for example, have been reported in dogs (35). The

syndrome is very similar to that seen in humans, with a delayed onset, fever, skin rash, and hepatitis. Another model involves cats and propylthiouracil. About 50% of mongrel cats develop a lupus-like serum sickness reaction when treated with propylthiouracil (36).

Availability of an animal model resembling human idiosyncratic drug reactions permits detailed study of the pathogenesis at both a pharmacologic and an immunologic level as well as examination of potential therapeutic interventions for such reactions. Although animal models do exist, the rarity of these reactions in humans makes it difficult to test all species, and these reactions generally do not occur in the experimental conditions used in pharmaceutical development. For therapeutic agents, it is clear that inbred animals in controlled environments, eating defined diets and remaining disease-free, are unlikely to reflect the heterogeneity of the human population in all of these variables. It is the genetic and environmental heterogeneity of the human population that is, for the most part, responsible for idiosyncratic chemical reactions.

Mechanisms of Hypersensitivity Reactions

The classical description of hypersensitivity reactions was made by Gell and Coombs (37, 38) and includes four possible pathologic processes referred to as types I to IV (Table 1). This classification system serves as a suitable framework for providing avenues for improved understanding of pathogenesis and for facilitating clinical assessment. It must be understood that clinical chemical allergy may not be manifested as a "pure" type I–IV response but that numerous chemicals may produce type I–IV reactions in different persons or occasionally even in the same persons.

Type I–IV Hypersensitivity Reactions

Type I hypersensitivity is used to refer to reactions that are initiated by interactions between an antigen and antigen-specific IgE on the Fc receptors present on mast cells, leading to release of mediators such as histamine, leukotrienes, and platelet-activating factor (37, 38). To most clinicians, the term *allergy* is synonymous with processes mediated by type I hypersensitivity. Most penicillin-induced hypersensitivity reactions are type I reactions, and this is most likely the best understood of the drug hypersensitivity reactions.

TABLE 1. *Mechanisms of systemic hypersensitivity*

Gell and Coombs Classification	
Type I	IgE-mediated anaphylaxis, urticaria, angioedema
Type II	antibody-mediated, complement-dependent, hemolytic anemia, agranulocytosis, thrombocytopenia
Type III	immune-complex–mediated, serum-sickness, vasculitis, glomerulonephritis
Type IV	cell-mediated, delayed fever, exanthema, lymphadenopathy

Type II hypersensitivity is used to describe processes in which antigen-specific antibodies, usually IgG but on occasion IgM, are directed against antigens presented on the cell surface (37, 38). Antibody-antigen interactions then lead to cell damage, either via activated effector cells such as killer lymphocytes, neutrophils, and monocytes, or via activation of complement-induced lysis. The most common example of drug-induced type II hypersensitivity is hemolytic anemia. The mechanism appears to involve binding of the drug to the red blood cell membrane leading to the production of antibodies against the drug followed by antibody coating of the red blood cell, complement activation, and red blood cell lysis. Drugs commonly associated with hemolytic anemia are quinine and penicillin (especially high-dose penicillin).

Type III hypersensitivity is used to describe processes mediated by immune complexes, formed when antigens interact with antibodies. Normally, these immune complexes are rapidly and completely cleared by the reticuloendothelial system; however, in the case of persistent infection (endocarditis), autoimmune disease (systemic lupus erythematosus), or repeated contact with antigens (occupational lung disease), chronic antigen–antibody interactions can lead to tissue deposition of immune complexes. The resulting immune complexes fix and activate the complement cascade, generating chemotactic factors such as C5a, which stimulates immigration of polymorphonuclear leukocytes into the area (39). Release of lysosomal enzymes and reactive oxygen intermediates from infiltrating cells results in tissue destruction and vasculitis. The classical example of type III hypersensitivity is serum sickness, which may present clinically with lymphadenopathy, arthralgia, fever, and rash. Penicillins, cephalosporins, barbiturates, isoniazid, phenytoin, captopril, hydralazine, and sulfonamides produce a serum sickness–like syndrome; however, the antigens involved have never been characterized and the determinants of which patients are at risk remains unknown.

Type IV hypersensitivity refers to reactions that are mediated by T cells. These reactions do not involve immunoglobulins but instead are produced by the cell-mediated immune response. They are also referred to as delayed-type hypersensitivity reactions since the peak response is observed 24–48 hr after antigen challenge. They occur when specific T lymphocytes recognize antigen presented on an antigen-presenting cell and respond by releasing a host of soluble mediators (39).

The classification scheme of Gell and Coombs provides mechanistic explanations for immune responses to chemicals; however, not enough is known about the mechanism of many chemical hypersensitivity reactions to place them into the scheme of Gell and Coombs. It is likely that many chemicals cannot be classified into this scheme, although they could still involve the immune system by some, yet unknown, mechanism. There are a number of drugs and drug-protein conjugates to which antibodies have been detected, but involvement in the pathogenesis of idiosyncratic reactions has not been clearly demonstrated and they do not fit well into the Gell-and-Coombs scheme.

While this scheme aids in understanding the mechanism of certain chemical-induced idiosyncratic reactions, they do not help in predictive capacity. A major problem that confronts clinicians and drug developers alike is the prediction of potential immune reactors to certain chemicals. Elucidating the mechanisms by which these reactions occur is the only means by which we can begin to solve this problem.

Hapten Hypothesis

Immune mechanisms involved in many chemical-induced idiosyncratic reactions and that do not fit the Gell-and-Coombs classification of hypersensitivity may be approached by considering the hapten hypothesis. This hypothesis considers the importance of the metabolic activation of chemicals to reactive intermediates, which can in turn interact with protein molecules and elicit an immune response (40).

In general, in order for an organic molecule to be recognized as nonself and to induce an immune response, it must have a minimum molecular weight of approximately 1000 daltons (41). Many drugs are of small molecular weight, are not very reactive, and therefore cannot be recognized or processed by antigen-processing cells. It is assumed that they must become covalently bound to an endogenous carrier macromolecule to form a drug–protein conjugate before they can interact with the immune system. Hapten formation of a small molecule involves irreversible covalent binding to a macromolecule. The processing of a hapten then permits antigenic determinants in the drug molecule to be expressed in association with the MHC on the cell surface, leading to the induction of an immune response.

REACTIVE METABOLITES INVOLVED IN IDIOSYNCRATIC REACTIONS

Some drugs are chemically reactive and can react directly with tissue macromolecules by direct conjugation. Examples are penicillin and cephalosporin (34, 42). Many idiosyncratic reactions, such as hepatic or bone marrow toxicity, appear to be mediated by metabolites of xenobiotics rather than by the parent compounds (43).

Drugs and other chemicals that do not normally occur in the body are metabolized by a wide variety of enzymes. Most chemicals are metabolized to more polar compounds that are rapidly removed from the body, while some are transformed to therapeutically active metabolites; however, the enzymes that catalyze these processes also catalyze the formation of reactive, toxic metabolites from some chemicals. The differing structural features of the compound and its metabolites determine whether or not the metabolic reaction produces a detoxification product or a potentially toxic metabolite. The biotransformation of relatively inert chemicals to highly reactive metabolites is commonly referred to as *metabolic activation*, (Fig. 2), and it is now recognized to be an obligatory initial event in several kinds of chemical-induced toxicities (44).

Reactive metabolites can be formed by most of the enzymes that are involved in drug metabolism. The liver is the major metabolizing organ and cytochrome P450 the major enzyme; however, the bone marrow is involved just as frequently as the liver in idiosyncratic reactions but has much less cytochrome P450. Epitope density, the number of haptens conjugated to an individual carrier, is an important determinant of immunogenicity and is more relevant than the total amount of covalent binding. The degree of conjugation for individual protein molecules is dependent both on the rate of reaction of metabolite or drug with protein and on the rate of drug distribution (45).

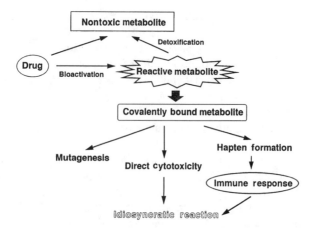

FIG. 2. The biotransformation of chemicals to reactive metabolites ("metabolic acitivation") as an initial event in chemical-induced hepatotoxicity.

HALOGENATED ANESTHETICS

Halothane

Patients anesthetized with halothane may develop mild hepatic damage with elevations in serum transaminase levels; however, a very small fraction of patients (estimated incidence of 1 in 30,000) develops severe hepatic necrosis leading to fatal liver failure (46, 47). Halothane represents one of the best models for an immunologically mediated mechanism of chemical hepatotoxicity based on the hapten hypothesis. The routes of metabolism are well described, and the immune phenomena have been investigated widely.

Bioactivation of halothane occurs in the liver by cytochrome P450 to several reactive metabolites (Fig. 3). The predominant route of halothane metabolism in humans involves hydroxylation followed by spontaneous debromination to a trifluoroacetyl halide (48). This reactive metabolite binds covalently to hepatic proteins via amino groups (49). Immunoblotting studies revealed that the halothane-induced antigens consist of a group of modified hepatic polypeptides that range in molecular mass from 100 kDa to 54 kDa, are concentrated in the liver microsomal fraction, and are expressed in livers from halothane-exposed rabbits, rats, guinea pigs, and humans (50–52). Several of the trifluoroacetylated (TFA)-protein antigens have been purified and have been shown to correspond to trifluoroacetylated forms of proteins believed to be resident normally within the lumen of the endoplasmic reticulum (53).

Direct cytotoxicity as a result of TFA-adduct formation has been demonstrated as a mechanism for hepatic injury, and this would explain the mild hepatic damage observed in up to 20% of halothane-exposed patients (54); however, a variety of clinical characteristics indicate an immune mechanism is most likely involved. Briefly, these

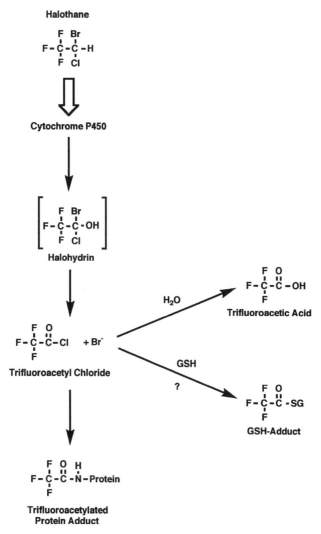

FIG. 3. Halothane biotransformation and interaction with macromolecules.

are a variable delay in onset of liver damage, association of liver damage with postoperative rash, arthralgia, eosinophilia and elevated immune-complexes, autoantibodies to normal liver proteins, and antibodies to TFA-bound proteins.

A role for antibody-mediated injury or humoral immunity in halothane has been explored in both laboratory animals as well as patients with halothane-induced liver injury. Sera from patients with severe hepatic necrosis caused by halothane contain antibodies that recognize distinct neoantigens containing the trifluoroacetyl group, whereas sera from patients exposed to halothane who do not develop hepatitis, or who have viral hepatitis, do not contain these antibodies (47, 55, 56). In addition, the halothane-induced antigens were detected on the hepatocyte surface membrane, and the cytotoxicity studies established that isolated hepatocytes that expressed the antigens were susceptible to cytotoxic killing when cultured in vitro in the presence of the patients' antibodies and normal lymphocytes (57, 58). Controls did not show any cytotoxicity, nor did antibodies react with hepatocytes from control rabbits (55). Overall, the results constitute the first example wherein a specific covalent interaction of drug metabolite-protein neoantigens is implicated in lethal cell injury associated with a drug-induced idiosyncratic reaction and that the immune response to halothane-induced antigens plays an important role in development of halothane hepatitis in patients in vivo.

Analysis of liver samples obtained from a large number of halothane-exposed animals, and from humans anesthetized with halothane, has indicated that all individuals exposed to halothane produce TFA-protein adducts that potentially act as modified-self molecules (59). Why the very small proportion of the population who develop halothane hepatitis mount immune responses to the antigens, but normal, nonsusceptible individuals do not, is unknown. One contributory factor may be variability in the presentation of the antigens to the immune system. Another possibility might be due to the promotion of preexisting immune tolerance against self-epitopes that bear a strong structural resemblance to epitopes on TFA-protein adducts. Breakdown or absence of tolerance toward TFA-protein adducts would then be one factor rendering individuals at an increased risk for the development of halothane hepatitis. The concept of natural tolerance toward TFA-protein adducts has been supported by a series of experiments. Anti-TFA antibody recognized cross-reactive proteins of liver homogenates of rats and humans not exposed to halothane before. These proteins confer molecular mimicry of epitopes present on TFA-protein adducts (60).

So far little is known about the initial steps, such as uptake, processing, and presentation, by which endogenously generated TFA-protein adducts or fragments come into contact with competent cells of the immune system. Macrophages are required for the induction of specific immune responses, where they function to take up and present antigen to responding populations of lymphocytes (4). Studies defining the role of the macrophage in antigen presentation, and in the induction, expression, and regulation of other immune responses, generally have made use of blood monocytes or inflammatory macrophages, such as peritoneal exudate macrophages (61). Resident macrophages of the liver, the Kupffer cells are among the cells lining hepatic sinusoids, where they function to clear antigen and other foreign materials from the bloodstream (5, 62). The development of improved techniques for the isolation of Kupffer cells has provided the opportunity to study the function of this macrophage as an antigen-presenting cell and accessory cell for the induction of an immune response.

Kupffer cells have been shown to both carry and partially process TFA-protein adducts from rats after 18 hr of exposure to a single dose of halothane. Studies have demonstrated Kupffer cells to express TFA antigens similar to those detected in hepatocytes (63); however, similar experiments using an elutriation method to isolate and purify the Kupffer cells from rats was not able to show the presence of TFA-adduct formation (64). Several animal models of halothane-induced hepatic necrosis have been developed. The rat models for anesthetic hepatotoxicity have been under scrutiny as to their accuracy in representing the human situation. In the rat models of halothane-induced liver injury, multiple pretreatments are required to produce a lesion that appears within hours, quickly resolves, does not progress, and is limited to males (65). Obviously, this is in marked contrast to the time course of events in the clinical situation. On the other hand, the guinea pig has also been developed as an animal model to investigate halothane hepatotoxicity. Liver damage is observed within 48 hr after halothane exposure with presence of TFA-covalent binding and recognition by anti-TFA antibodies (54, 66). This is achieved with no pretreatments and similar exposure conditions to human exposure. In the guinea pig, halothane produces centrilobular necrosis or scattered foci throughout the lobules of both sexes. Neither phenobarbital pretreatment nor exposures in hypoxic atmospheres are required for the production of the hepatotoxicity (65, 67). Since the injury is similar to the human situation based on several susceptibility factors such as heritability, sex, obesity, and age, this animal model is a better representation of the clinical situation.

Recently, TFA-adduct formation in Kupffer cells isolated from halothane-exposed guinea pigs has been shown (68). Western blots performed on the various cell fractions collected all demonstrated recognition of TFA-protein adducts by the rabbit anti-TFA antibody. Liver endothelial cells isolated from halothane-exposed animals also demonstrated the presence of TFA-protein adduct formation. Differences in the formation of TFA adducts in Kupffer cells from the rat and guinea pigs may account for the differences in tolerance to halothane hepatotoxicity between these contrasting animal models.

Because of the difficulty of performing assays and equivocal results from cell-mediated immune studies with halothane, the majority of previous investigations have been limited to evaluating the humoral immune response. Although a humoral response could mediate the hepatic hypersensitivity to halothane, a cell-mediated or Tlymphocyte–dependent response should not be discounted and may be paramount in developing hepatotoxicity by the immune system. In previous studies it has been shown that splenic lymphocytes isolated from rabbits, guinea pigs, and mice repeatedly exposed to halothane were stimulated by the presence of TFA-albumin (69). Unfortunately, splenic lymphocytes from animals not exposed to halothane were also stimulated by TFA-albumin. Quite possibly TFA-albumin may not be the proper antigen since it is well established with cell-mediated studies that a positive response in the sensitization assay is dependent on the appropriate choice of antigen. Very low levels of circulating antigen are associated with an immune response, and antigens located on cell membranes are more potent immunologic stimuli than drug albumin conjugates. Recent observations in the guinea pig demonstrated that Kupffer cells are capable of acting as whole-cell antigens by supporting the triggering of mitogen-induced T lymphocyte proliferation (70, 71). In addition, another study investigating the antigen-presenting role of guinea pig Kupffer cells, demonstrated these cells have the capacity to take up and present antigen to primed T lymphocytes for the induction of secondary in vitro antigen-specific proliferative responses (72).

To investigate a cell-mediated immune response as a mechanism for halothane hepatitis, studies used splenocytes and Kupffer cells from guinea pigs receiving multiple exposure to halothane. Splenocytes were incubated with various TFA-albumins as well as Kupffer cells in a lymphocyte transformation test. Stimulation of lymphocyte proliferation in response to TFA-guinea pig albumin occurred only in exposed animals. No response to the carrier protein or other TFA-albumins occurred. In addition, a large increase in splenocyte proliferation in response to Kupffer cells from halothane-exposed animals was demonstrated. Autologous splenocytes demonstrated more of a response from treated versus control animals, indicating the involvement of MHC II antigens (73, 74). These studies demonstrated the involvement of a cellular immune response in a model of halothane hepatitis. These studies also demonstrated that Kupffer cells were capable of functioning as antigen-presenting cells in halothane-induced hepatitis and that the induction of T lymphocyte responsiveness by these cells was restricted by determinants encoded by the MHC antigen (Fig. 4).

Lymphocyte transformation testing has been used to evaluate patients for drug-induced hypersensitivity reactions. Although it is presently being debated as a method for the evaluation of drug allergic hepatic injury (75), researchers are improving its sensitivity with the use of drug metabolites and prostaglandins (76). This assay may be valuable for further identification of susceptible persons and responsible drugs in cases of drug-induced hepatitis.

A role for a cell-mediated mechanism in contributing to liver damage has also been investigated in halothane hepatitis patients. Based on the concept that the antigenic moiety was a metabolic intermediate and not the parent compound halothane, liver homogenates containing metabolite-altered proteins from rabbits exposed to halothane were used (58). These liver homogenates were then incubated with leukocytes from halothane hepatitis patients, and lymphocytes were sensitized as measured by the release of a cytokine. These extensive studies provide good evidence for involvement of a cell-mediated immune response in the induction of halothane hepatotoxicity.

Enflurane and Isoflurane

Of the newer volatile anesthetics, reports concerning enflurane-induced hepatitis had a pattern of hepatocellular damage with striking similarities to halothane-induced hepatitis (77, 78). The incidence of hepatotoxicity seen in patients exposed to enflurane and isoflurane is much rarer than the incidence of halothane hepatitis; however, the clinical studies have indicated that the characteristics of enflurane-induced hepatitis are very similar to the clinical features of halothane hepatitis, and several patients who apparently are cross-sensitized to both halothane and enflurane have been described (79, 80). Studies in humans reveal that 2% of enflurane and 0.2% of isoflurane administered undergoes metabolism and these compounds yield oxidative reactive intermediates analogous to those of halothane; thus, the potential for

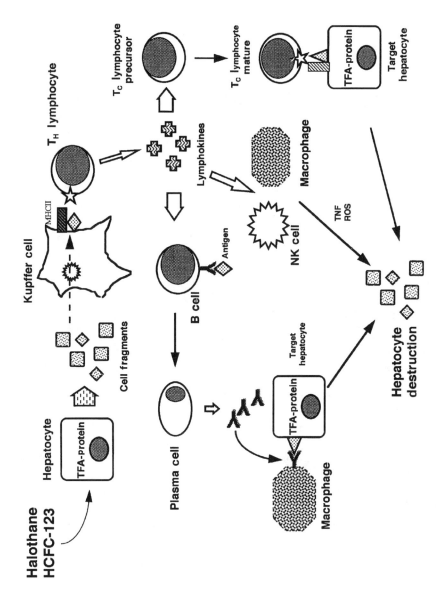

FIG. 4. Proposed mechanism of immune-mediated hepatotoxicity induced by halothane or HCFC analogues as a result of TFA-protein adduct formation.

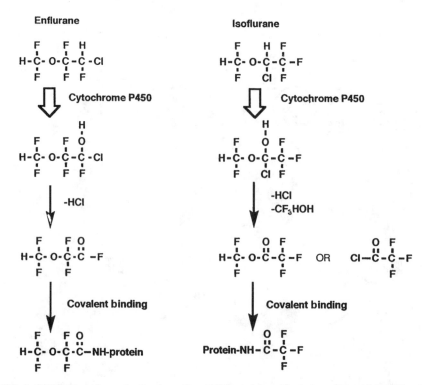

FIG. 5. Metabolic pathway for the formation of TFA-protein adducts from the oxidation of enflurane and isoflurane.

cross-sensitization between anesthetics exists (81, 82) (Fig. 5). Enflurane produced liver microsomal adducts that were detectable on immunoblots with anti-TFA antiserum in rats and serum from halothane hepatitis patients (83). In addition, enflurane and isoflurane are known to form liver adducts and antigens that cross-react with halothane-induced antibodies in the guinea pig (66). This raises the possibility that both anesthetics may cause liver damage via immune processes that are very similar to those that are thought to induce halothane hepatitis.

HYDROCHLOROFLUOROCARBONS

Chlorofluorocarbons (CFCs) (Fig. 6) are widely used throughout industry as industrial refrigerants, foam-blowing agents in the manufacture of plastics, aerosol propellants, food preservatives, and cleaning and sterilizing agents. The venting of automobile and truck air conditioning units is the major source of CFC environmental contamination. 2,2-Dichloro-1,1,1-trifluoroethane (HCFC-123) is a compound currently under investigation as a potential CFC replacement. The addition of hydrogen atoms into CFC

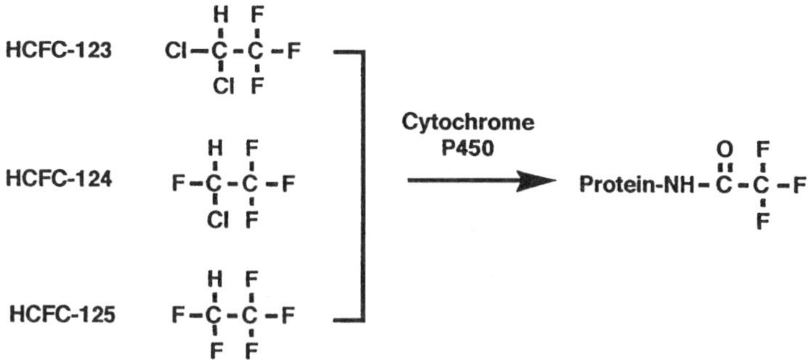

FIG. 6. HCFC analogues metabolized to TFA-protein adducts.

molecules allows degradation of these compounds in the lower atmosphere with little effect on stratospheric ozone. Due to the evident structural similarity between HCFC-123 and halothane and the problem of halothane hepatotoxicity, the metabolism of HCFC-123 was investigated. In a recent report, rat liver microsomes from animals exposed to air, 1% halothane, or 1% or 0.5% HCFC-123 for 2 hr were probed with hapten-specific anti-TFA serum. Immunoblotting demonstrated that HCFC-123 and halothane are metabolized to trifluoroacetylated adducts with identical patterns of TFA labeling (84). More recently, studies done in the guinea pig, a sensitive animal model to hepatotoxic actions of halogenated hydrocarbons, demonstrated inhalation of HCFC-123 can cause acute hepatic injury in the guinea pig that is worsened by low hepatic glutathione concentrations (85). In order to compare these results with those obtained in previous studies with halothane, the same concentrations and length of exposure of HCFC-123 were utilized during the experiments. Since the potentiation of covalent binding by glutathione depletion of HCFC-123-reactive intermediates was similar to that of halothane, this raises the possibility that susceptible individuals repeatedly exposed to this agent might become sensitized and develop hepatitis. It is also possible that individuals sensitized to HCFC-123 without hepatic injury might be at increased risk for hepatic damage following anesthesia with halothane, enflurane, or isoflurane due to possible cross sensitization.

CARDIOVASCULAR AGENTS

Tienilic Acid

Tienilic acid (Fig. 7) is an example of a drug withdrawn from the market due to an unacceptably high incidence of idiosyncratic reactions, namely hepatotoxicity (86). It was used as a uricosuric diuretic for treatment of hypertension. Clinical characteristics such as a delay between initiation of therapy and the development of hepatotoxicity, immediate recurrence of symptoms upon reexposure to drug, and lack of an animal

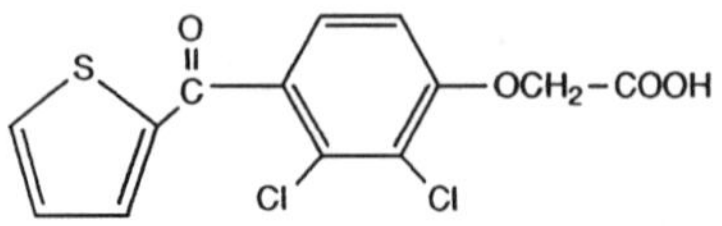

FIG. 7. Tienilic acid.

model all suggest involvement of the immune system (87). Hepatotoxicity by ti-enilic acid has also been associated with a metabolic idiosyncrasy. Tienilic acid is metabolized by a genetically variable cytochrome P450 2C. This cytochrome P450 oxidizes the thiophene ring of the drug to a reactive metabolite, possibly a thiophene S-oxide derivative. This reactive metabolite may be responsible for adduct formation by covalently binding to microsomal proteins (88). Tienilic acid-reactive metabolites, specifically bound to cytochrome P450 2C9, as determined by immunoblotting studies using antitienilic acid antibodies and yeast expressing active enzyme (89). Immunoblots with antitienilic acid antibodies confirmed this evidence since these recognized tienilic acid adducts bound to cytochrome P450 2C9, and covalent binding using ^{14}C-tienilic acid determined binding specificity higher than with any other cytochrome P450 tested, namely 2C8 and 2C18 (90).

Patients with tienilic acidinduced hepatitis have autoantibodies (antiliver/kidney microsomal antibody, anti-LKM2) that specifically recognize cytochrome P450 2C9 (90, 91). These autoantibodies have been found in several drug-induced liver diseases. Anti-LKM2 autoantibodies present in sera of patients with tienilic acid hepatitis strongly recognized native cytochrome P450 2C9 and weakly recognized other 2C cytochrome P450s. Other studies have demonstrated inhibition of covalent binding of tienilic acid by anti-LKM2 and antihuman cytochrome P450 2C, indicating tienilic acid is metabolized to a reactive intermediate by cytochrome P450 2C (92).

Covalent binding of tienilic acid metabolites was confined to one microsomal protein in contrast to covalent binding of chloroform, which was nonspecific (93). Chloroform is well documented as a direct hepatotoxicant. Results from these studies have led investigators to propose that a relationship might exist between specificity of covalent binding of drug metabolites to liver proteins and the type of hepatotoxicity, namely direct or immunostimulatory. It is possible that reactive metabolites are stable enough to leave the site of biotransformation and diffuse throughout the cell, thus leading to direct hepatotoxicity by alkylating many vital target macromolecules. In contrast, a highly reactive metabolite could alkylate an available nucleophile of the protein that generated it. Therefore, large quantities of one particular alkylated protein or even a small peptide that becomes a neoantigen could reach and stimulate the immune system, leading to immune-mediated hepatitis.

Interestingly, the cytochrome P450 apoprotein represents a neoantigen in many cases of drug-induced hepatitis (94). One reason may be that specific cytochrome P450 isoforms both represent the catalytic site for drug bioactivation and are alkylated by the reactive intermediates, eventually leading to the formation of anti-P450 antibodies. Most of these cytochrome P450 isoforms are expressed in the plasma membrane of hepatocytes and could therefore be targets for an immune attack.

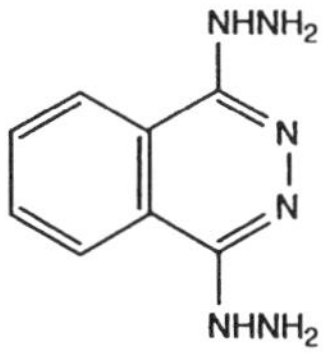

FIG. 8. Dihydralazine.

Dihydralazine

Dihydralazine (Fig. 8) is an antihypertensive drug that is associated with a rare incidence of immunostimulatory hepatitis. Cytochrome P450 1A is responsible for the production of dihydralazine-reactive metabolites (95). Interaction of the reactive intermediates was essentially restricted to cytochrome P450 1A2 that generates the reactive metabolite. Covalent binding of dihydralazine metabolites was observed that reacted with heme and covalently bound to microsomal protein (96). Effects could be increased with pretreatment of animals with B-naphthoflavone, a classical inducer of the cytochrome P450 1A family in rats. Dihydralazine could competitively inhibit catalytic activity characteristic of cytochrome P450 1A2 in human liver microsomes, suggesting this enzyme is involved in the metabolism of the drug (96). Antiliver microsomal autoantibodies (anti-LM) were found only in sera of patients with dihydralazine hepatotoxicity and did not appear in other patients receiving dihydralazine without a toxic response (97). These were clearly distinct from anti-LKM and antiliver antibodies observed in patients with tienilic acid-induced and autoimmune hepatitis. These antibodies specifically recognized cytochrome P450 1A2, responsible for dihydralazine metabolism and not cytochrome P450 1A1. Anti-LM were shown to be specific to the disease. In three cases, these autoantibodies were present at high titers during disease, whereas the titers decreased upon recovery and became undetectable a few months after recovery. Anti-LM could be both a marker of disease and a cause of it and dihydralazine was a specific inducer of the cytochrome P450 A subfamily. This induction might increase the risk of hepatotoxicity by causing formation of reactive metabolites and enhancing the target antigen level of autoantibodies and T cells (98–100). Dihydralazine-induced hepatitis occurs mainly in slow acetylators, and covalent binding to the proteins of a whole homogenate decreased 70% when N-acetyltransferase was activated by the addition of its cofactor, acetyl-CoA. Hence, higher covalent binding in slow acetylators may explain their unique susceptibility; however, 50% of Caucasians are slow acetylators. The rare incidence of this reaction implies that other factors such as HLA phenotype may also be required (101).

One explanation for the presence of autoantibodies may be that the metabolites produced by cytochrome P450s from dihydralazine and tienilic acid are so unstable that they react with, and antigenically alter, the cytochrome P450 proteins that produced the metabolites. These proteins would be convenient targets for the metabolites because they are the nearest to them as they are produced. Reactive metabolites can cause hepatotoxicity by binding to, or reacting with, proteins whose functions are

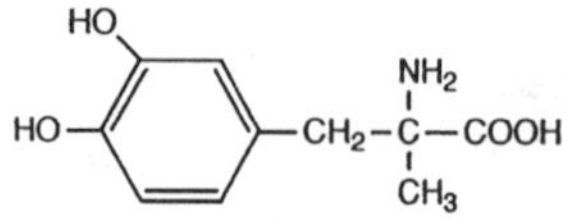

FIG. 9. Methyldopa.

vital to the hepatocyte. The reaction of metabolites with the cytochrome P450 1A family should not directly cause toxicity because these enzymes are unlikely to be of critical importance to the hepatocytes. Antimicrosomal antibodies may directly contribute to the pathogenesis of some forms of chemical-induced liver disease.

Methyldopa

Methyldopa (Fig. 9) is a widely used antihypertensive agent that may cause both reversible liver damage as well as active chronic hepatitis in approximately 6% of the patients (102–104). This is an idiosyncratic reaction, and studies have shown involvement of the immune system. Methyldopa is oxidized by cytochrome P450–generated superoxide anion into a semiquinone or quinone, both reactive metabolites (105, 106). While both may form haptens with liver proteins, methyldopa is not haptenic but appears instead to modify erythrocyte surface antigens (107). Immunoglobulin G against modified erythrocyte surface antigens can be demonstrated in the blood of these patients. Sera from patients with methyldopa-induced severe liver damage were reported to have cytotoxic serum antibodies that reacted with hepatocytes from rabbits pretreated with methyldopa as well as liver sections from patients with methyldopa hepatitis (108). Other indications of immune reactivity have been reported, in particular, the development of positive macrophage migration inhibition tests and the indirect rat mast cell degranulation test. These two in vitro tests indicate the existence of a drug-specific immunologic memory toward methyldopa in the patient (109). A report of circulating lymphocytes from patients with methyldopa hepatitis, sensitized to proliferate in the presence of methyldopa, strongly supports immune reactivity to the drug (110).

ISONIAZID

Isoniazid (Fig. 10) is a tuberculostatic agent implicated in drug-induced lupus and is associated with antinuclear antibodies in about 20% of patients. Isoniazid is also

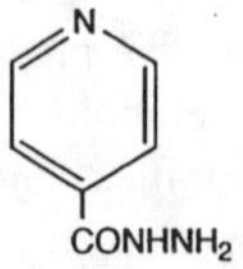

FIG. 10. Isoniazid.

associated with a relatively high incidence of severe hepatic necrosis (111). Isoniazid is a hydrazide chemically similar to hydrazine derivatives that are readily oxidized to reactive intermediates. It has been shown that acetyl-isoniazid hydrolysis produces acetylhydrazine and is further metabolized to an acylating agent, capable of covalently binding to liver protein in the rat. This acylating agent is thought to be the species responsible for liver toxicity (112). Acetyl radicals were produced when isoniazid was incubated with hepatocytes and when acetyl-isoniazid was incubated with hepatocytes, liver microsomes, and NADPH or oxidized chemically. Antibodies have been detected in some patients against isoniazid–albumin conjugate, and the isonicotinic acid portion of the molecule has been implicated to be involved in mediation of the immune reaction. An animal model for isoniazid hepatotoxicity indicates that the toxicity is associated with metabolism to the toxic metabolite acetyl-hydrazine. Acetylation of isoniazid can lead to formation of N-acetylhydrazine, which can be oxidized to a reactive species. Incidence of reactions have been reported higher in slow acetylators. Isoniazid is polymorphically acetylated; however, the correlation with liver toxicity has yet to be explored. Isoniazid was demonstrated to induce drug-specific immune responses in guinea pigs, detected by antibody responses and delayed-type hypersensitivity reactions when injected with complete Freund's adjuvant (113). Antibodies detected in sera from immunized animals had an affinity for isoniazid assessed by the hapten concentration-dependent inhibition of ELISA by the drug. Delayed-type hypersensitivity reactions were induced by isoniazid–albumin and isoniazid–ovalbumin.

It has been demonstrated that persons exposed to isoniazid occupationally or therapeutically can develop antibodies to isoniazid–albumin. In addition, isoniazid was used in the popliteal lymph node assay as a preclinical prediction of xenobiotic-induced autoimmune reaction in humans. The popliteal lymph node assay response was positive to isoniazid only if preincubation and coinjection with S9-mix was performed, indicating that the metabolite rather than the parent drug is involved in an immune-mediated hypersensitivity reaction (114).

IPRONIAZID

Iproniazid (Fig. 11) is a monoamine oxidase inhibitor used as an antidepressive agent and is associated with liver damage. Besides microsomal proteins, a liver mitochondrial protein has been identified as a specific target for covalent interactions in iproniazid-induced hepatotoxicity. In patients suffering from iproniazid hepatitis, anti-M6 (mitochondrial) antibodies directed against liver mitochondria were detected

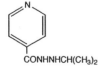

CONHNHCH(CH₃)₂   **FIG. 11.** Iproniazid.

(115). By selective immunoprecipitation, monoamine oxidase (MAO)-B was identified as the specific target protein. In analogy to cytochrome P450, MAO-B itself is probably alkylated during the oxidative bioactivation of iproniazid that occurs via MAO-B. As with tienilic acid, recognition of MAO-B by the immune system and the appearance of anti–MAO-B antibodies could result in the secondary immunologically mediated hepatotoxic effects of iproniazid.

AMODIAQUINE

In the early 1980s amodiaquine was a 4-aminoquinoline antimalarial that was introduced as effective against chloroquine-resistant strains of *Plasmodium falciparum*. Later its prophylactic clinical use was severely restricted due to a high risk of developing hepatotoxicity and agranulocytosis (116). Although neither the precise mechanism nor the causative agent has been identified, studies indicate that these adverse reactions are of an immunologic nature and are a consequence of the oxidation of the drug to chemically reactive metabolites that function as haptens in vivo and initiate an immune response. It has been demonstrated that amodiaquine is readily oxidized to a protein-reactive metabolite, amodiaquine quinone imine (Fig. 12). This process can be catalyzed by several biologic oxidizing systems, including activated white cells and cytochrome P450 enzymes. Electrochemical studies show that the 4-hydroxyaniline side-chain in amodiaquine is readily oxidized to a quinone imine that can conjugate directly with sulfhydryl groups in glutathione and proteins (117). These findings were confirmed by the identification of a 5′-glutathione conjugate as the major biliary metabolite in the rat, and the identification of drug-related antigen in liver.

The quinone imine was found to be more toxic to peripheral blood mononuclear leukocytes than the pharmacologically active desethylamodioquine, a major metabolite of amodiaquine (118). Both direct cytotoxicity and inhibition of cell function and immunologic mechanisms have been implicated. Amodiaquine, amodiaquine quinone imine, and desethylamodiaquine were found to be toxic in vitro toward granulocyte/monocyte colony-forming units and mononuclear leukocytes (119). Although it has been demonstrated that amodiaquine administration in high doses results in direct toxicity, amodiaquine is immunogenic at much lower doses than those required for either direct hepatotoxicity or leukopenia. With lower doses of the drug, it was possible to obtain an antibody response in the absence of any detectable perturbation of liver function.

There has been evidence of circulating amodiaquine-dependent IgG antineutrophil antibodies. Amodiaquine is immunogenic in the rat when given by the oral, intraperitoneal or intramuscular routes, without the requirement for co-administration of immunologic adjuvant (120). The drug is also immunogenic in humans when given in repeated prophylactic doses. Antiamodiaquine antibodies have also been detected in patients with serious adverse reactions (121). Antibodies from patients have been demonstrated to recognize a synthetic drug antigen amodiaquine-metallothionein (121).

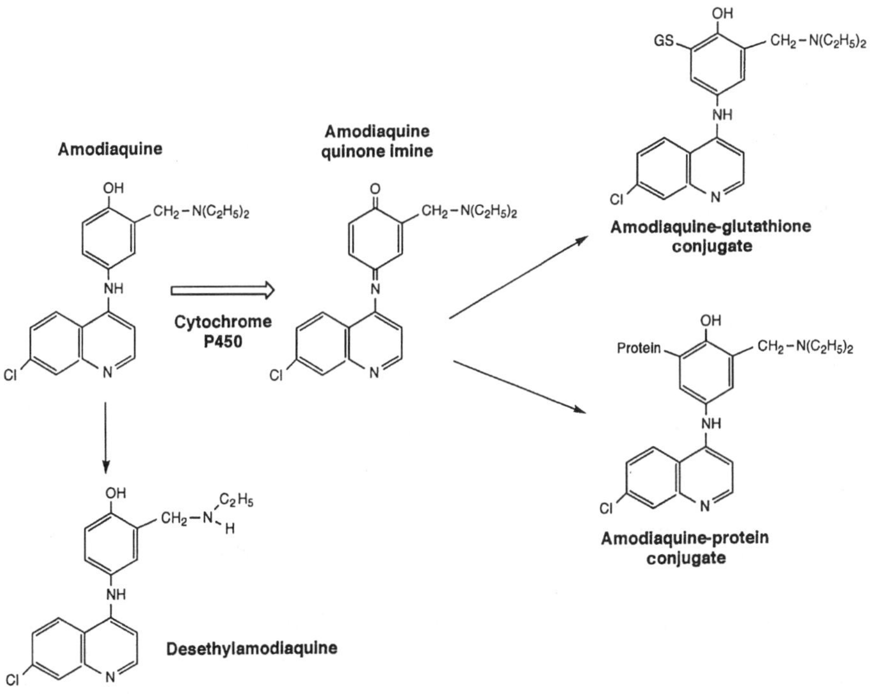

FIG. 12. Metabolic pathway proposed for the formation of amodiaquine-protein adducts by way of the unstable quinone imine intermediate.

Two separate mechanisms of bioactivation may explain the toxicity mediated by amodiaquine. First, the intracellular generation of the quinone imine may result in direct toxicity by interfering with vital cell function; second, the formation of cell-surface antigen may lead to a secondary immune reaction. In vitro studies indicate that rates of glutathione conjugation and also reduction of the quinone imine by microsomal enzymes are host factors that may be important determinants of toxicity. It is unlikely that it will be possible to predict individual susceptibility to amodiaquine toxicity on the basis of the measurement of a single factor; however, based on assays with either malaria parasites or human polymorphonuclear lymphocytes, studies indicate that it is possible to modify amodiaquine chemically and thereby prevent bioactivation without necessarily losing pharmacologic activity (122).

ETHANOL

Ethanol has been demonstrated to be directly cytotoxic in several studies; however, there is great individual variability in susceptibility to the hepatotoxic effects of alcohol. Specific target proteins have recently been identified for acetaldehyde, the major metabolite of ethanol biotransformation. It has been hypothesized that acetaldehyde may covalently bind to lysine residues of hepatic proteins, resulting in structural modification or functional impairment, ultimately leading to tissue injury. Special attention was given to cytoskeletal proteins, acetaldehyde being found to selectively bind to purified tubulin and actin (123). Although the adduct formation was deleterious to the function of these cytoskeletal proteins, and although covalent modification of proteins by acetaldehyde has been demonstrated both in vivo and in vitro, these findings do not, by themselves, establish a mechanism of ethanol-induced hepatocyte injury.

In vivo, acetaldehyde forms stable N-ethyllysine with intracellular proteins such as hemoglobin, cytochrome P450 2E1, and a 37-kDa liver protein (124). Although these various protein adducts have been found, the significance of the acetaldehyde–protein interactions for the development of alcohol-induced hepatic injury and the clinical implications remain largely unknown. As with halothane, studies using both immunofluorescence and antibody-dependent cell-mediated cytotoxicity have shown that about one-half of the patients with alcoholic liver disease have antibodies reacting with alcohol-altered liver cell components (125). Measurement of hemoglobin-acetaldehyde adducts indicated that these adducts are frequently elevated in the erythrocytes of human alcohol consumers (126). Alcoholics have been found to exhibit a significantly higher IgA response than other alcohol groups. This may be a specific marker of alcohol abuse (127). It has also been suggested that those with HLA B8 are more prone to the development of alcoholic cirrhosis (128). Mice treated with alcohol chronically can generate antibodies that recognize acetaldehyde-modified proteins. This directed response is dependent on the formation of stable acetaldehydeprotein surface adducts (129). It also has been suggested that these antibodies may initiate antibody-mediated hepatotoxicity by binding to the surface of hepatocytes. Neutrophils or complement would recognize the antibodies and lyse the cells.

It has been shown that, in an in vitro incubation with rat liver microsomes, acetaldehyde forms a Schiff base with phosphatidylethanolamine, and this adduct is reduced to the corresponding N-ethylphosphatidylethanolamine. Antibodies raised against acetaldehyde adducts of protein, cross-reacted with acetaldehyde adducts of phospholipids, indicating these can serve as haptenic binding sites on the surface of hepatocytes (130, 131). Acetaldehyde adducts and autoantibodies were also detected against VLDL and LDL in alcoholics (132).

Experimental hepatitis could be produced in guinea pigs by immunization with acetaldehyde adducts and ethanol treatment. Peripheral blood lymphocytes obtained from the animals with hepatitis were shown to be stimulated by the adducts to a significantly greater degree than those from control animals who received nothing, ethanol alone, or ethanol and unmodified hemoglobin (133). In vitro, lymphocytes from patients with alcoholic hepatitis are directly cytotoxic to hepatocytes from rabbits and to autologous hepatocytes (134). Intracelluar acetaldehyde adducts occur in the centrilobular region of the liver of individuals consuming excessive amounts of alcohol (135, 136). This cytotoxicity could be blocked by lipoprotein and alcoholic hyaline, suggesting that these agents may have epitopes to which the lymphocytes are sensitized. Acetaldehyde adduct on plasma membranes has also been shown to stimulate complement activation and lead to the appearance of alcoholic hepatitis (137).

These studies investigating alcoholic hepatitis give evidence for the involvement of a humoral and cell-mediated response as well as complement in mediating the liver injury of alcoholic patients.

ANTICONVULSANTS

Carbamazepine

Carbamazepine is an iminostilbene derivative developed in the 1950s for the treatment of complex–partial, generalized tonic–clonic, and other mixed or partial seizures (138). It is now quite commonly used in the treatment of trigeminal neuralgia with less toxic side effects when compared to other anticonvulsants such as phenytoin and primidone (139, 140). Despite the therapeutic value of carbamazepine, adverse effects have been reported in as many as one-third to one-half of all patients treated with this drug (139, 141, 142). About 5% of adverse reactions associated with carbamazepine can be classified as idiosyncratic reactions due to an unknown reactivity of the patient (141). A Swedish survey of 505 reports on 713 idiosyncratic reactions to carbamazepine from 1965 to 1987 reported skin reactions (48%), hematologic disorders (12%), and hepatic disorders (10%) to be the most frequent. Virtually all hepatic disorders and severe skin reactions, as well as the majority (60%) of the hematologic reactions, occurred within the first two months of therapy (143, 144).

Carbamazepine metabolism by cytochrome P450 in the liver has been well studied. The most important pathway of carbamazepine metabolism in the liver is the formation of carbamazepine-10,11-epoxide and its conversion to trans-10,11-dihydro-10,11-dihydroxycarbamazepine (epoxide-diol pathway) (Fig. 13) (145). Direct N-glucurondiation on the carbamoyl side-chain of carbamazepine and hydroxylation of the aromatic rings are also major pathways (146, 147).

The reactive metabolite postulated to be responsible for carbamazepine-induced toxicity is an arene oxide (148, 149). It was suggested that predisposition to idiosyncratic toxicity with carbamazepine is due to a deficiency of the detoxification enzyme, epoxide hydrolase. This is based on the observation that carbamazepine metabolites generated by microsomes in vitro resulted in toxicity to lymphocytes from patients with a history of an idiosyncratic reaction to carbamazepine, which was greater than the toxicity to lymphocytes from normal controls (150, 151). This toxicity was enhanced by 1,1,1-trichloropropene-2,3-oxide (TCPO), an inhibitor of epoxide hydrolase, which suggests that an arene oxide was responsible for the toxicity (152–154). Addition of microsomal epoxide hydrolase caused a 60% reduction in covalent binding and cytotoxicity. Clinical studies suggest that concurrent administration of enzyme inducers is a risk factor. They may operate by altering the critical balance between bioactivation and detoxification. Deduction of the possible nature

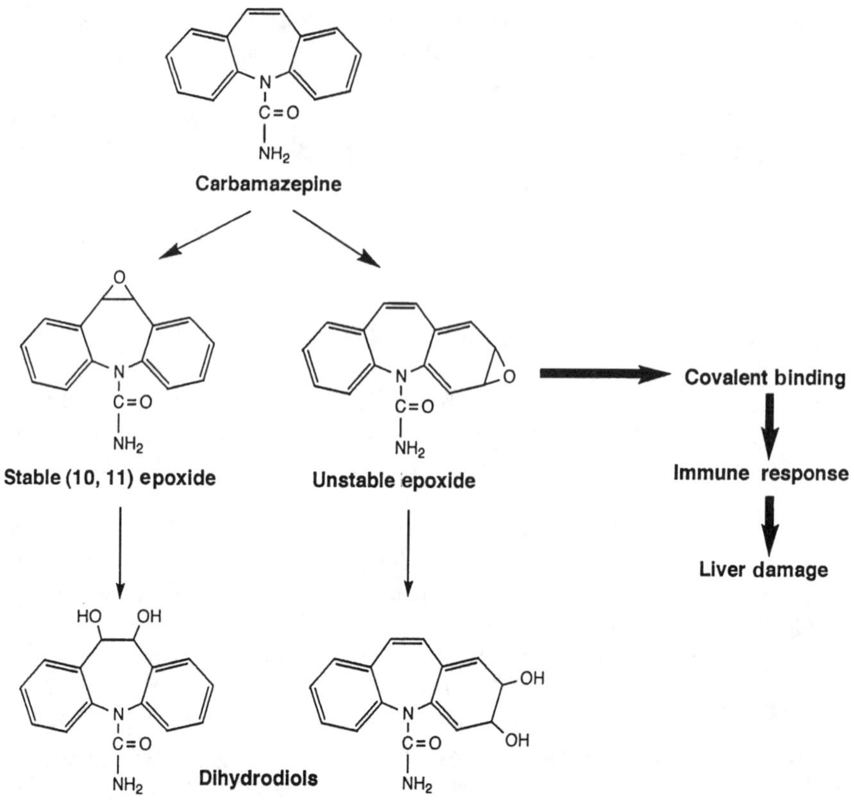

FIG. 13. Carbamazepine activation to a chemically reactive epoxide and its possible involvement in idiosyncratic toxicity.

of the toxic binding metabolite from this evidence is complicated by the fact that TCPO is also known to deplete glutathione and inhibit cytochrome P450 (155). In addition, more than one form of epoxide hydrolase exists. A recent study undertook an evaluation of epoxide hydrolase in large-scale population studies. Outliers indicating enzyme-deficient phenotypes were not observed, and the frequency distribution was unimodal normal (156). Characterization of the microsomal epoxide hydrolase gene in patients with anticonvulsant adverse drug reactions concluded that a genetic defect altering the structure and function of the mEH protein was unlikely to be responsible for predisposing patients to the reactions (157). Further studies are required to prove an enzyme deficiency is associated with carbamazepine-induced idiosyncratic reactions.

Studies have investigated the possible involvement of an antibody-mediated mechanism in carbamazepine-induced adverse reactions (158, 159). Anti-carbamazepine antibodies as well as a specific autoantibody against a human liver microsomal protein in serum of patients were reported (160). Reports of T cell impairment of PHA-induced

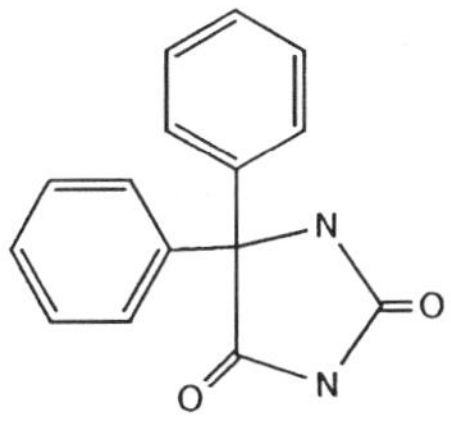

FIG. 14. Phenytoin.

proliferation have been made in patients with serum sickness associated with carbamazepine therapy (161). In addition, carbamazepine treatment of mice resulted in a significant increase in natural killer cell activity, and phagocytosis and killing properties of macrophages (162). Studies were also done using lymphocyte transformation tests to investigate the effect of carbamazepine in patients with severe hypersensitivity to carbamazepine in comparison to controls. In all cases of carbamazepine-induced adverse reactions, lymphocyte transformation tests were positive and all controls gave negative results (163, 164).

These studies provide evidence for immunologic mediation of carbamazepine-induced hepatotoxicity possibly involving immunomodulatory effects and a genetic predispostion in drug metabolism as a susceptibility factor.

Phenytoin

Phenytoin (Fig. 14) is an important anticonvulsant, but it is also associated with a large number of serious adverse effects including drug-induced lupus (165). The pathogenesis of phenytoin hepatotoxicity is proposed to be a result of a defect in arene oxide detoxification leading to covalent binding to macromolecules with resultant cell death and secondary immunologic reactions similar to carbamazepine. Lymphocytes from patients showed a dose-dependent increase in death in comparison to no toxicity in cells from control subjects. Toxicity was dependent on microsomes and NADPH. Inhibition of epoxide hydrolase by TCPO did not alleviate toxicity. Results suggested that predisposition to phenytoin hepatotoxicity derives from an inherited defect in phenytoin arene oxide detoxification (166). Oxidation of phenytoin by activated neutrophils was also determined, and results found that it is chlorinated by the myeloperoxidase system to N,N'-dichlorophenytoin (167). This is the reactive metabolite that appears to be responsible for covalent binding to the neutrophils.

Phenytoin has been shown to cause a variety of alterations in lymphocyte populations and functions. In an early study, 63 patients on long-term phenytoin therapy were screened for abnormalities in immunologic function. It was found that 21% had decreased IgA levels, 9% had a failure of antibody response to *Salmonella typhi* antigen, 22% had an absence of delayed hypersensitivity to three common skin test antigens, and 27% had a depression of in vitro lymphocyte transformation by phytohemagglutinin (168–171). Impairment of polymorphonuclear cell chemotaxis and superoxide generation in phenytoin-treated patients was also reported when compared to controls

(172). A decrease in B lymphocyte number and circulating immunoglobulin was also detected and did not resolve until three years after withdrawal of the drug (173). These studies suggest phenytoin may mediate idiosyncratic reactions such as hepatotoxicity by involving changes in leukocyte function and by genetic predisposition.

NONSTEROIDAL ANTIINFLAMMATORY DRUGS (NSAIDs)

As a class, NSAIDs are associated with a high incidence of idiosyncratic drug reactions, and many of the drugs that have recently been removed from the market for reasons of toxicity belong to this class. Some have functional groups, such as the secondary arylamine of diclofenac, that could be oxidized to a reactive intermediate. In addition, most NSAIDs are carboxylic acids and are metabolized to varying degrees to acyl glucuronides. Acyl glucuronides are chemically reactive and have been demonstrated to covalently bind to protein. Many drugs have been removed from the market shortly after they were introduced because of what was considered to be an unacceptable risk of idiosyncratic reactions. These drugs belong to the class of compounds known as aryl alkanoic nonsteroidal antiinflammatory drugs. Zomepirac and benoxaprofen are examples of NSAIDs withdrawn from use because of an unexplained high incidence of immunologic reactions (174). This group of compounds also includes drugs such as tolmetin, diflunisal, fenoprofen, and diclofenac, which are still on the market but remain under scrutiny because of their potential to form acyl glucuronides (174, 175). This metabolite is unstable in mild alkaline solutions and undergoes rearrangement to positional isomers (176). In the presence of serum albumin these reactions are accompanied by covalent binding of the parent carboxylic acid to the protein. Covalent binding in vitro and in vivo has been demonstrated for bilirubin and for several NSAIDs and is thought to play a role in the adverse reactions associated with these drugs (177). This covalent binding could lead to an immunogen and an immune response. Acyl glucuronides are relatively stable and circulate freely; therefore, adverse reactions are unlikely to be limited to the site of glucuronide formation and could easily be responsible for generalized idiosyncratic reactions as well.

Diclofenac

Diclofenac is an NSAID commonly used against rheumatoid arthritis, osteoarthritis, or ankylosing spondylitis and is associated with the development of hepatic necrosis (178, 179). Both direct toxic effects as well as hypersensitivity reactions have been suggested as possible mechanisms for liver injury, and covalent protein adducts may be involved in either of these mechanisms. Recently, covalent adduct formation of diclofenac to rat and mouse liver proteins in vivo and in cultured hepatocytes was characterized (180). The mechanism of covalent binding of diclofenac to liver proteins has been suggested to involve three different pathways (Fig. 15). The first mechanism involves the conjugation of the carboxylic acid group of diclofenac to glucuronic acid, catalyzed by the microsomal UGTs, forming diclofenac acyl glucuronide. The next

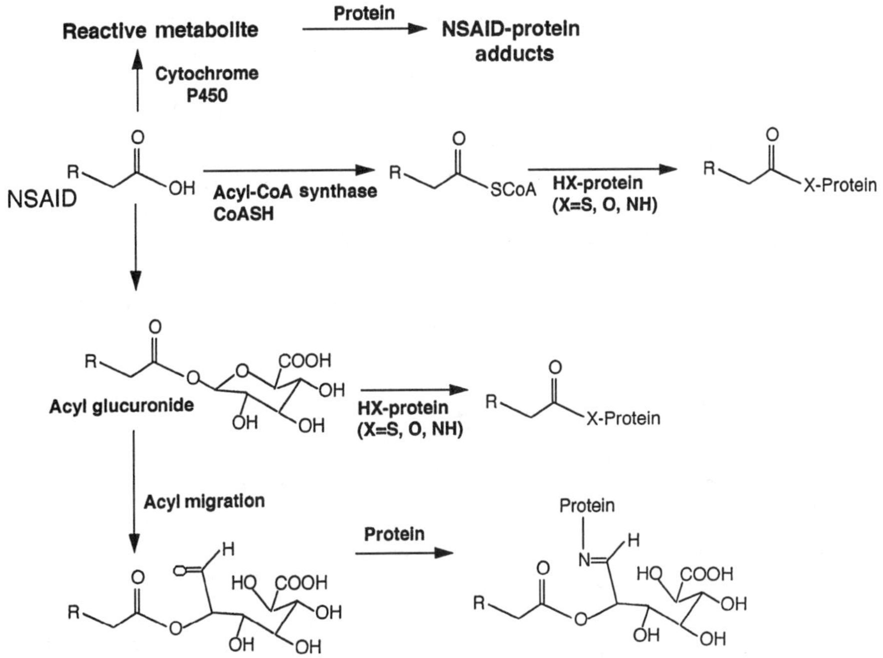

FIG. 15. Mechanisms proposed for the covalent binding of NSAIDs to proteins via their glucuronides.

step in the mechanism was proposed to be a nucleophilic displacement of the glucuronic acid moiety (transacylation) by free cysteine thiols, tyrosine, or lysine residues of the target protein. The other possible mechanism involves direct participation of the glucuronic acid moiety in the adduct formation through a multistep isomerization and rearrangement of the acyl glucuronide. Specifically, an imine would be formed between the free aldehyde of the open sugar chain and a nucleophilic site of a target protein (Schiff base formation), following acyl migration along the ring carbons of the glucuronide. Reduction of the unstable imine would lead to the formation of a more stable 1-amine-2-keto product. A recent study has determined that diclofenac acyl glucuronide covalently binds to hepatic microsomal proteins by these two mechanisms (181, 182). Evidence for acyl migration and imine formation indicates that this may be a general pathway involved in protein adduct formation of carboxylic drugs undergoing conjugation to a reactive acyl glucuronide. It is possible that the glucuronic acid moiety is part of a hapten and is thus involved in the sensitization of the immune system. Epitope density in hepatic proteins would be high since the liver is the major site of glucuroconjugation and levels of glucuronide are high. In conjunction with other factors governing the degree of immunogenicity of drug–protein adducts, formation of reactive acyl glucuronides could then lead to the eliciting of an immune response. Most recently, a second proposed pathway for the formation of diclofenac–protein adducts involved a cytochrome P450 dependent mechanism. The reactive metabolites formed by cytochrome P450 appeared to be very reactive because only one protein was covalently modified. A third pathway that also was proposed for the bioactivation of diclofenac is the formation of diclofenac acyl-CoA, which then binds to proteins by transacylation (183, 184).

Autoantibodies and diclofenac or metabolite-dependent IgG antibodies have been detected in patients with diclofenac-induced immune hemolysis (185). The liver is a key target of the rare NSAID-induced immunostimulatory reactions. It has been suggested that an identical constituent as a common part of the adduct of different drugs may be responsible for the immunologic cross-reactivities observed with several NSAIDs.

CONCLUSIONS

The basis for immunologic mediation of the chemical-induced hepatotoxicity discussed in this chapter remains circumstantial. A major problem is lack of animal models of immune-mediated liver damage for testing and investigative studies of these kind of reactions. Many compounds also generate a direct toxic effect to the liver. It is possible that direct toxicity leading to recognition by the immune system of the drug-generated neoantigens is necessary for the occurrence of immune-mediated hepatotoxicity in humans. The low incidence at which idiosyncratic drug reactions occur suggests that our current approach to preclinical toxicology assessment and evaluation in early human trials is generally quite efficient at screening out compounds with unacceptably high toxicity potential for the population at large; however, many of these reactions are severe, hence there is a great need to develop a means of drug toxicity evaluation to prevent such idiosyncratic drug reactions.

A major problem in evaluating idiosyncratic drug reactions is the difficulty of confirming the diagnosis. Most of the reactions have nonspecific symptoms, and the lack of diagnostic tests limits the ability of clinical pharmacologists to make a definitive diagnosis of an idiosyncratic drug reaction. This inability to diagnose and predict idiosyncratic drug reactions currently creates a risk of morbidity or even mortality for patients. During the process of new drug development, unexpected and unpredictable adverse drug reactions can lead to discontinuation of drug development or post-marketing removal of otherwise useful therapeutic agents with associated adverse publicity, litigation, and immense increases in the cost of drug development. Therefore, we need new approaches to understanding the pathogenesis and pharmacogenetics of such reactions, and hence turn basic knowledge into novel approaches to aid in the diagnosis, prediction, and prevention of idiosyncratic drug reactions.

REFERENCES

1. Zimmerman HL. *Hepatotoxicity*. New York: Appleton-Century-Crofts, 1978.
2. Goldstein R, Patterson R. Summary. *J Allergy Clin Immunol* 1984;74:558–566.

3. Seaman W, Ishak K, Plotz P. Aspirin-induced hepatotoxicity in patients with systemic lupus erythematosus. *Ann Intern Med* 1974;80:1–8.
4. Siljelid R, Eskeland T. The biology of macrophages. I. General principles and properties. *Eur J Haematol* 1993;51:267–275.
5. Shiratori Y, Tananka M, Kawase T, Shiina S, Komatsu Y, Omata M. Quantification of sinusoidal cell function in vivo. *Sem Liver Dis* 1993;13:39–49.
6. Kalish RS. Antigen processing: the gateway to the immune response. *J Am Acad Dermatol* 1995;32:640–652.
7. Nathan C. Secretory products of macrophages. *J Clin Invest* 1987;79:319–326.
8. Rook G. Cell-mediated immune responses. In: Roitt IM, Brostoff J, Male DK, eds. *Immunology*. St Louis: CV Mosby Company, 1989:9.2–9.12.
9. Pierce SK. Molecular chaperones in the processing and presentation of antigen to helper T cells. *Experientia* 1994;50:1026–1030.
10. Paul W, Seder R. Lymphocyte responses and cytokines. *Cell* 1994;76:241–251.
11. Germain R. MHC-dependent antigen presentation and peptide presentation: providing ligands for T lymphocyte activation. *Cell* 1994;76:287–299.
12. Gleichmann E, Kimber I, Purchase I. Immunotoxicology: suppressive and stimulatory effects of drugs and environmental chemicals on the immune system. *Arch Toxicol* 1989;63:257–273.
13. Silkworth JB, Vecchi A. Role of the Ah receptor in halogenated aromatic hydrocarbon immunotoxicity. In: Dean JH, Luster MI, Munson AE, Amos H, eds. *Immunotoxicology and immunopharmacology*. New York: Raven Press, 1985:263–275.
14. Vos J, Moore J. Suppression of cellular immunity in rats and mice by maternal treatment with 2,3,7,8-tetrachlorodibenzo-p-dioxin. *Int Arch Allergy* 1974;47:777–794.
15. Seinen W, Vos J, Brands R, Hooykaas H. Lymphocytotoxicity and immunosuppression by organotin compounds: suppression of GVH activity, blast transformation and E-rosette formation by di-n-butyltin dichloride and di-n-octyltin dichloride. *Immunopharmacology* 1979;1:343–355.
16. Steffensen I, Mesna O, Andruchow E, Namork E, Hylland K, Anderson R. Cytotoxicity and accumulation of Hg, Cd, Cu, Pb and Zn in human peripheral T and B lymphocytes and monocytes in vitro. *Gen Pharmacol* 1995;25:1621–1633.
17. Busby W, Wogan G. In: Riemann H, Bryan F, eds. *Food-borne infections and intoxications*. New York: Academic Press, 1979:519.
18. Rensburg SV, Cook-Mozaffari P, Schakkwyk DV, Watt JVD, Vincent T, Purchase I. Hepatocellular carcinoma and dietary aflatoxin in Mozambique and Transkei. *Br J Cancer* 1985;51:713–726.
19. Peers F, Linsell C. Dietary aflatoxins and liver cancer: a population-based study in Kenya. *Br J Cancer* 1973;27:473–484.
20. Peers F, Bosch K, Kaldor J, Linsell A, Pluijmen M. Aflatoxin exposure, hepatitis B virus infection and liver cancer in Swaziland. *Int J Cancer* 1987;39:545–553.
21. Shank R, Bhamarapravati N, Gordon J, Wogan G. Dietary aflatoxins and human liver cancer. IV. Incidence of primary liver cancer in two municipal populations in Thailand. *Food Cosmet Toxicol* 1972;10:171–179.
22. Yeh F, Yu M, Mo C, Luo S, Tong M, Henderson B. Hepatitis B virus, aflatoxins, and hepatocellular carcinoma in Southern Guangxi, China. *Cancer Res* 1989;49:2506–2509.
23. Giambrone J, Diener U, Davis N, Panangala V, Hoerr F. Effects of aflatoxin on young turkeys and broiler chickens. *Poult Sci* 1985;64:1678–1684.
24. Michael G, Thaxton P, Hamilton R. Impairment of the reticuloendothelial system of chickens during aflatoxicosis. *Poult Sci* 1973;52:1206.
25. Reddy R, Taylor M, Sharma R. Studies of immune function of CD-1 mice exposed to aflatoxin B1. *Toxicology* 1987;43:123–132.
26. Reddy R, Sharma R. Effects of aflatoxin B1 on murine lymphocytic functions. *Toxicology* 1989;54:31–44.
27. Cusumano V, Costa G, Seminara S. Effect of aflatoxins on rat peritoneal macrophages. *Appl Environ Microbiol* 1990;56:3482–3484.
28. Mohapatra N, Roberts J. Effects of aflatoxin B1 on rat peritoneal macrophages and mouse fibroblasts (L-M cells). *Gen Pharmacol* 1979;10:471–474.
29. Richard J, Thurston J. Effect of aflatoxin on phagocytosis of Aspergillus fumigatus spores by rabbit alveolar macrophages. *Appl Microbiol* 1975;30:44–47.
30. Cukrova V, Langrova E, Akao M. Effects of aflatoxin B1 on myelopoiesis in vitro. *Toxicology* 1991;70:203–211.

31. Cusumano V, Costa G, Trifiletti R, Merendino R, Mancuso G. Functional impairment of rat Kupffer cells induced by aflatoxin B1 and its metabolites. *FEMS Immunol Med Microbiol* 1995;10:151–155.

32. Hsia C, Kleiner D, Axiotis C, Di Bisceglie A, Nomura A, Stemmermann G, Tabor E. Mutations of p53 gene in hepatocellular carcinoma: roles of hepatitis-B virus and aflatoxin contamination in the diet. *J Nat Cancer Inst* 1992;84:1638–1641.

33. Park BK, Kitteringham NR. Drug-protein conjugation and its immunological consequences. *Drug Met Rev* 1990;22:87–144.

34. Uetrecht J. Drug metabolism by leukocytes and its role in drug-induced lupus and other idiosyncratic drug reactions. *Crit Rev Toxicol* 1990;20:213–235.

35. Cribb AE, Miller M, Tesoro A, Spielberg SP. Peroxidase-dependent oxidation of sulfonamides by monocytes and neutrophils from man and dog. *Mol Pharmacol* 1990;38:744–751.

36. Aucoin DP. Propylthiouracil-induced immune-mediated disease syndrome in the cat: a novel animal model for a drug-induced lupus disease. *Autoimm Toxicol* 1989:309–322.

37. Coombs RRA, Gell PGH. The classification of allergic reactions underlying disease. In: Gell PGH, Coombs RRA, eds. *Clinical aspects of immunology.* Oxford: Blackwell Scientific Publications, 1963:317–337.

38. Coombs R, Gell P. Classification of allergic reactions responsible for clinical hypersensitivity and disease. In: Coombs R, Gell P, eds. *Clinical aspects of immunology.* New York: FA Davis Co., 1968:575–596.

39. Sanner M, Higgins T. Chemical basis for immune mediated idiosyncratic drug hypersensitivity. In: Michne W, ed. *Annual reports in medicinal chemistry.* New York: Academic Press, Inc., 1991:181–190.

40. Pessayre D. Role of reactive metabolites in drug-induced hepatitis. *J Hepatol* 1995;23:16–24.

41. de Weck AL, Bundgaard H. *Allergic reactions to drugs.* Berlin: Springer, 1983.

42. Ahlstedt S, Kristofferson A. Immune mechanisms for induction of penicillin allergy. *Prog Allergy* 1982;30:67–134.

43. Nelson SD, Pearson PG. Covalent and noncovalent interactions in acute lethal cell injury caused by chemicals. *Annu Rev Pharmacol Toxicol* 1990;30:169–95.

44. Nelson SD. Metabolic activation and drug toxicity. *J Med Chem* 1982;25:753–765.

45. Park BK, Kitteringham N. Drug-protein conjugation and its immunological consequences. *Drug Met Rev* 1990;22:87–144.

46. Kenna JG, Satoh H, Christ DD, Pohl LR. Metabolic basis for a drug hypersensitivity: antibodies in sera from patients with halothane hepatitis recognize liver neoantigens that contain the trifluoroacetyl group derived from halothane. *J Pharmacol Exp Ther* 1988;245:1103–1109.

47. Kenna JG, Neuberger J, Williams R. Identification by immunoblotting of three halothane-induced liver microsomal polypeptide antigens recognized by antibodies in sera from patients with halothane-associated hepatitis. *J Pharmacol Exp Ther* 1987;242:733–740.

48. Sipes I, Gandolfi AJ, Pohl LR, Krishna G, Brown B. Comparison of the biotransformation and hepatotoxicity of halothane and deuterated halothane. *J Pharmacol Exp Ther* 1980;214:716–720.

49. Van Dyke RA, Gandolfi AJ. Studies on irreversible binding of radioactivity from [^{14}C]halothane to rat hepatic microsomal lipids and protein. *Drug Metab Dispos* 1974;2:469–476.

50. Satoh H, Gillette J, Davies H, Schulick R, Pohl L. Immunochemical evidence of trifluoroacetylated cytochrome P-450 in the liver of halothane treated rats. *Mol Pharmacol* 1985;28:568–474.

51. Brown A, Hastings K, Gandolfi AJ. Generation and detection of neoantigens in guinea pig liver slices incubated with halothane. *Int J Immunopharmacol* 1991;13:429–435.

52. Kenna J, Neuberger J, Williams R. Evidence for expression in human liver of halothane-induced neoantigens recognized by antibodies in sera from patients with halothane hepatitis. *Hepatology* 1988;8:1635–1641.

53. Kenna J, Martin J, Pohl L. The topography of trifluoroacetylated protein antigens in liver microsomal fractions from halothane treated rats. *Biochem Pharmacol* 1992;44:621–629.

54. Lind RC, Gandolfi AJ, Hall PDLM. A model for fatal halothane hepatitis in the guinea pig. *Anesthesiology* 1994;81:478–487.

55. Vergani D, Mieli-Vergani G, Alberti A. Antibodies to the surface of halothane-altered rabbit hepatocytes in patients with severe halothane-associated hepatitis. *N Engl J Med* 1980;303:66–71.

56. Kenna JG, Neuberger J, Williams R. Identification by immunoblotting of three halothane-induced liver microsomal polypeptide antigens recognized by antibodies in sera from patients with halothane-associated hepatitis. *J Pharmacol Exp Ther* 1987;242:733–740.

57. Kenna JG, Knight TL, van Pelt FNAM. Immunity to halothane metabolite-modified proteins in halothane hepatitis. *Ann NY Acad Sci* 1993;685:646–661.

58. Vergani D, Tsantoulas D, Eddleston A. Sensitisation to halothane-altered liver components in severe hepatic necrosis after halothane anaesthesia. *Lancet* 1978;ii:801–803.
59. Christen U, Jeno P, Gut J. Halothane metabolism: the dihydrolipoamide acetyltransferase subunit of the pyruvate dehydrogenase complex molecularly mimics trifluoroacetyl-protein adducts. *Biochemistry* 1993;32:1492–1499.
60. Gut J, Christen U, Frey N, Koch V, Stoffler D. Molecular mimicry in halothane hepatitis: biochemical and structural characterization of lipoylated autoantigens. *Toxicology* 1995;97:199–224.
61. Alter BJ, Bach FH. Lymphocyte reactivity in vitro. I. Cellular reconstitution of purified lymphocyte response. *Cell Immunol* 1970;1:207–212.
62. Bjornboe M, Prytz W. The mononuclear phagocytic function of the liver. In: Ferguson A, McSween RWM, eds. *Immunological aspects of the liver and gastrointestinal tract*. Lancaster, England: MTP Press, 1976:251.
63. Christen U, Burgin M, Gut J. Halothane metabolism: Kupffer cells carry and partially process trifluoroacetylated protein adducts. *Biochem Biophys Res Comm* 1991;175:256–262.
64. Amouzadeh H, Pohl LR. Processing of neoantigens associated with halothane hepatitis by hepatic parenchymal cells. *The Toxicologist* 1994;14:425.
65. Clarke JB, Lind RC, Gandolfi AJ. Mechanisms of anesthetic hepatotoxicity. In: Stoelting RK, Barasch PG, Gallagher TJ, eds. *Advances in anesthesia*. New York: Mosby-Year Book, Inc., 1993:219–793.
66. Clarke J, Thomas C, Chen M, Hastings K, Gandolfi A. Halogenated anesthetics form liver adducts and antigens that cross-react with halothane-induced antibodies. *Int Arch Allergy Immunol* 1995;108:24–32.
67. Lind RC, Gandolfi AJ. The role of oxidative biotransformation of halothane in the guinea pig model of halothane-associated hepatotoxicity. *Anesthesiology* 1989;70:649–653.
68. Furst SM, Luedke D, Gandolfi AJ. Kupffer cells from halothane-exposed guinea pigs carry trifluoroacetylated adducts. *Toxicology* 1997;120:119–132.
69. Hubbard AK, Roth TP, Gandolfi AJ. Elicitation of a cell mediated immune response to a reactive intermediate of halothane. *The Toxicologist* 1988;8:12.
70. Squiers ES, Brunson ME, Salomon DR. Kupffer cells can present alloantigen in vitro: an effect abrogated by gadolinium. *J Surg Res* 1993;55:571–574.
71. Waldron JA, Horn RG, Rosenberg AS. Antigen-induced proliferation of guinea pig lymphocytes in vitro: obligatory role of macrophages in the recognition of antigen by immune T lymphocytes. *J Immunol* 1973;111:58–63.
72. Rogoff TM, Lipsky PE. Antigen presentation by isolated guinea pig Kupffer cells. *J Immunol* 1980;124:1740–1744.
73. Furst SM, Luedke D, Gaw HH, Reich RF, Gandolfi AJ. Demonstration of a cellular immune response in halothane-exposed guinea pigs. *Toxicol Appl Pharmacol* 1997;143:245–255.
74. Furst SM, Gandolfi AJ. Interaction of cellular adhesion molecules in a model of halothane hepatotoxicity. *Int Arch Allergy Immunol* 1997 (In press).
75. Berg P, Becker E. The LTT-A debated method for the evaluation of drug allergic hepatic injury. *J Hepatol* 1995;22:115–118.
76. Maria V, Pinto L, Victorino R. Lymphocyte reactivity to ex-vivo drug antigens in drug-induced hepatitis. *J Hepatol* 1994;21:151–158.
77. Ona F, Patanella H, Ayub A. Hepatitis associated with enflurane anesthesia. *Anesth Analg* 1980;59:146–149.
78. van der Reis L, Askin S, Frecker G, Fitzgerald W. Hepatic necrosis after enflurane anesthesia. *JAMA* 1974;227:76.
79. Zimmerman H. Even isoflurane. *Hepatology* 1991;13:1251–1253.
80. Christ D, Satoh H, Kenna J, Pohl L. Potential metabolic basis for enflurane hepatitis and the apparent cross sensitization between enflurane and halothane. *Drug Metab Dispos* 1988;16:135–140.
81. Chase R, Holaday D, Fiserova-Bergerova V, Saidman L, Mack F. The biotransformation of ethrane in man. *Anesthesiology* 1971;35:262–267.
82. Carrigan T, Straughen W. A report of hepatic necrosis and death following isoflurane anesthesia. *Anesthesiology* 1987;67:581–583.
83. Christ D, Kenna J, Kammerer W, Satoh H, Pohl L. Enflurane metabolism produces covalently-bound liver adducts recognized by antibodies from patients with halothane hepatitis. *Anesthesiology* 1988;69:833–838.
84. Urban G, Speerschneider P, Dekant W. Metabolism of the chlorofluorocarbon substitute 1,1-dichloro-2,2,2-trifluoroethane by rat and human liver microsomes: the role of cytochrome P450 2E1. *Chem Res Toxicol* 1994;7:170–176.

85. Lind RC, Gandolfi AJ, Hall PDLM. Biotransformation and hepatotoxicity of HCFC-123 in the guinea pig: potentiation of hepatic injury by prior glutathione depletion. *Toxicol Appl Pharmacol* 1995;134:175–181.

86. Neuberger J, Williams R. Immune mechanisms in tienilic acid associated hepatotoxicity. *Gut* 1989;30:515–519.

87. Zimmerman H, Lewis J, Ishak K, Maddrey W. Ticrynafen-associated hepatic injury: analysis of 340 cases. *Hepatology* 1984;4:315–323.

88. Dansette P, Amar C, Valadon P, Pons C, Beaune P, Mansuy D. Hydroxylation and formation of electrophilic metabolites of tienilic acid and its isomer by human liver microsomes: catalysis by a cytochrome P450 IIC different from that responsible for mephenytoin hydroxylation. *Biochem Pharmacol* 1991;41:553–560.

89. Lopez MG, Dansette P, Valadon P, Amar C, Beaune P, Guengerich F, Mansuy D. Human liver cytochromes P-450 expressed in yeast as tools for reactive-metabolite formation studies: oxidative activation of tienilic acid by P-450 2C9 and P-450 2C10. *Eur J Biochem* 1993;213:223–232.

90. Lecoeur S, Bonierbale E, Challine D, Gautier J, Valadon P, Dansette P, Catinot R, Ballet F, Mansuy D, Beaune P. Specificity of in vitro covalent binding of tienilic acid metabolites to human liver microsomes in relationship to the type of hepatotoxicity: comparison with two directly hepatotoxic drugs. *Chem Res Toxicol* 1994;7:434–442.

91. Lecoeur S, Andre C, Beaune PH. Tienilic acid-induced autoimmune hepatitis: anti-liver and -kidney microsomal type 2 autoantibodies recognize a three-site conformational epitope on cytochrome P450 2C9. *Mol Pharmacol* 1996;50:326–333.

92. Beaune P, Dansette P, Mansuy D, Kiffel L, Finck M, Amar C, Leroux J, Homberg J. Human antiendoplasmic reticulum autoantibodies appearing in a drug induced hepatitis are directed against a human liver cytochrome that hydroxylates the drug. *Proc Natl Acad Sci USA* 1987;84:551–555.

93. Gomez MD, Castro J. Covalent binding of chloroform metabolites to nuclear proteins: no evidence for binding to nucleic acids. *Cancer Letters* 1980;9:213–218.

94. Loeper J, Descatoire V, Maurice M, Beaune P, Belghiti J, Houssin D, Ballet F, Feldmann G, Guengerich F, Pessayre D. Cytochromes P-450 in human hepatocyte plasma membrane: recognition by several autoantibodies. *Gastroenterology* 1993;104:203–216.

95. Pariente E, Pessayre J, Bernuau J, Degott C, Benhamou J-P. Dihydralazine hepatitis: report of a case and review of the literature. *Digestion* 1983;27:47–52.

96. Bourdi M, Tinel M, Beaune P, Pessayre D. Interactions of dihydralazine with cytochromes P450 1A: a possible explanation for the appearance of anti-cytochrome P450 1A2 autoantibodies. *Mol Pharmacol* 1994;45:1287–1295.

97. Nataf J, Bernuau J, Larrey D, Guillin M, Rueff B, Benhamou J-P. A new anti-liver microsome antibody: a specific marker of dihydralazine-induced hepatitis. *Gastroenterology* 1986;90:1751.

98. Bourdi M, Larrey D, Nataf J, Bernuau J, Pessayre D, Iwasaki M, Guengerich F, Beaune P. Anti-liver endoplasmic reticulum autoantibodies are directed against human cytochrome P-450 1A2. *J Clin Invest* 1990;85:1967–1973.

99. Bourdi M, Larrey D, Nataf J, Bernuau J, Pessayre D, Iwasaki M, Guengerich F. Antimicrosomal antibodies: what are they telling us? *Hepatology* 1991;13:385–387.

100. Bourdi M, Gautier J, Mircheva J, Larrey D, Guillouzo A, Andre C, Belloc C, Beaune P. Anti-liver microsomes autoantibodies and dihydralazine-induced hepatitis: specificity of autoantibodies and inductive capacity of the drug. *Mol Pharmacol* 1992;42:280–285.

101. Berson A, Freneaux E, Larrey D, Lepage V, Douay C, Mallet C, Fromenty B, Benhamou J, Pessayre D. Possible role of HLA in hepatotoxicity: an exploratory study in 71 patients with drug-induced idiosyncratic hepatitis. *J Hepatol* 1994;20:336–362.

102. Canals A, Jimenez M, Villa J. Methyldopa-induced granulomatous hepatitis. *Ann Pharmacother* 1991;25:1269–1270.

103. Rodman J, Deutsch D, Gutman S. Methyldopa hepatitis: a report of six cases and a review of the literature. *Am J Med* 1976;60:941–955.

104. Smith G, Piercy W. Methyldopa hepatotoxicity in pregnancy: a case report. *Am J Obstetrics Gynecology* 1995;172:222–224.

105. Hubbard A, Lohr C, Hastings K, Clarke J, Gandolfi A. Immunogenicity studies of a synthetic antigen of alpha methyl dopa. *Immunopharmacol Immunotoxicol* 1993;15:621–637.

106. Dybing E, Nelson S, Mitchell J, Sasame H, Gillette J. Oxidation of methldopa and other catechols by cytochrome P-450 generates superoxide anion: possible mechanism of methyldopa hepatitis. *Mol Pharmacol* 1976;12:911.

107. Cirstea M, Suhaciu G, Cirje M. Spontaneous formation of conjugates of alpha methyldopa and dopa with serum proteins and experimental production of specific antibodies against these haptens. *Physiologie* 1983;20:3–6.
108. Neuberger J, Kenna J, Aria KN. Antibody mediated hepatocyte injury in methyldopa induced hepatotoxicity. *Gut* 1985;26:1233–1239.
109. Wolf R, Tamir A, Werbin N, Brenner S. Methyldopa hypersensitivity syndrome. *Ann Allergy* 1993;71:166–168.
110. Vittorino R, Maria V, Pinto D. Evidence for prostaglandin-producing suppressor cells in drug-induced liver injury and implications in the diagnosis of drug sensitization. *Clin Exp Immunol* 1992;87:132–140.
111. Bickers J, Buechner H, Hood B, Alvarez-Chiesa G. Hypersensitivity reaction to antituberculosis drugs with hepatitis, lupus phenomenon and myocardial infarction. *N Engl J Med* 1961;265:131–133.
112. Timbrell J, Mitchell J, Snodgrass W, Nelson S. Isoniazid hepatotoxicity: the relationship between covalent binding and metabolism in vivo. *J Pharmacol Exp Ther* 1980;213:364–369.
113. Katsutani N, Shionoya H. Drug-specific immune responses induced by procainamide, hydralazine and isoniazid in guinea-pigs. *Int J Immunopharmacol* 1992;14:673–679.
114. Patriarca C, Verdier F, Brouland J, Descotes J. Popliteal lymph node response to procainamide and isoniazid. Role of B-naphthoflavone, phenobarbitone and S9-mix pretreatment. *Toxicology Let* 1993;66:21–28.
115. Homberg J, Abuaf N, Helmy-Khalil S, Biour M. Drug induced hepatitis with anti-intracytoplasmic organelle autoantibodies. *Hepatology* 1985;5:722–727.
116. Neftel K, Woodtly W, Schmid M, Frick P, Fehr J. Amodiaquine induced agranulocytosis and liver damage. *Br Med J* 1986;292:721–723.
117. Jewell H, Maggs JL, Harrison AC, O'Neill PM, Ruscoe JE, Park BK. Role of hepatic metabolism in the bioactivation and detoxification of amodiaquine. *Xenobiotica* 1995;25:199–217.
118. Clarke J, Maggs J, Kitteringham N, Park B. Immunogenicity of amodiaquine in the rat. *Int Arch Allergy Appl Immunol* 1990;91:335–342.
119. Winstanley P, Coleman J, Maggs J, Breckenridge A, Park BK. The toxicity of amodiaquine and its principal metabolites towards mononuclear leucocytes and granulocyte/monocyte colony forming units. *Br J Clin Pharmacol* 1990;29:479–485.
120. Christie G, Breckenridge A, Park BK. Drug-protein conjugates XVIII: detection of antibodies towards the antimalarial amodiaquine and its quinone immine metabolite in man and the rat. *Biochem Pharmacol* 1989;38:1451–1458.
121. Clarke JB, Neftel K, Kitteringham N, Park BK. Detection of antidrug IgG antibodies in patients with adverse drug reactions to amodiaquine. *Int Arch Allergy Appl Immunol* 1991;95:369–375.
122. Ruscoe JE, Jewell H, Maggs JL, O'Neill PM, Storr RC, Ward SA, Park BK. The effect of chemical substitution on the metabolic activation, metabolic detoxification, and pharmacological activity of amodiaquine in the mouse. *J Pharmacol Exp Ther* 1995;273:393–404.
123. Tuma D, Jennett R, Sorrell M. The interaction of acetaldehyde with tubulin. *Ann New York Acad Sci* 1987;492:277–286.
124. Koskinas J, Kenna J, Bird G, Alexander G, Williams R. Immunoglobulin A antibody to a 200-kilodalton cytosolic acetaldehyde adduct in alcoholic hepatitis. *Gastroenterology* 1992;103:1860–1867.
125. Neuberger J, Crossley I, Saunders J. Antibodies to alcohol altered liver cell determinants in patient with alcoholic liver disease. *Gut* 1984;27:300–304.
126. Worrall S, Jersey JD, Nicholls R, Wilce P. Acetaldehyde/protein interactions: are they involved in the pathogenesis of alcoholic liver disease. *Dig Dis* 1993;11:265–277.
127. Worrall S, Jersey Jd, Shanley B, Wilce P. Antibodies against acetaldehyde-modified epitopes: an eleveted IgA response in alcoholics. *Eur J Clin Invest* 1991;21:90–95.
128. Saunders J, Wodak A, Haines A. Accelerated development of alcoholic cirrhosis in patients with HLA B8. *Lancet* 1984;i:1381–1384.
129. Terabayashi H, Kolber M. The generation of cytotoxic T lymphocytes against acetaldehyde-modified syngeneic cells. *Alcoholism: Clin Exp Res* 1990;14:893–899.
130. Trudell J, Ardies C, Green C, Allen K. Binding of anti-acetaldehyde IgG antibodies to hepatocytes with an acetaldehyde-phosphatidylethanolamine adduct on their surface. *Alcoholism: Clin Exp Res* 1991;15:295–299.
131. Trudell J, Ardies C, Anderson W. Cross-reactivity of antibodies raised against acetaldehyde adducts of protein with acetaldehyde adducts of phosphatidylethanolamine: possible role in alcoholic cirrhosis. *Mol Pharmacol* 1990;38:587–593.

132. Wehr H, Rodo M, Lieber C, Baraona E. Acetaldehyde adducts and autoantibodies against VLDL and LDL in alcoholics. *J Lipid Res* 1993;34:1237–1244.
133. Yokoyama H, Nagata S, Moriya S, Kato S, Ito T, Kamegaya K, Ishii H. Hepatic fibrosis produced in guinea pigs by chronic ethanol administration and immunization with acetaldehyde adducts. *Hepatology* 1995;21:1438–1442.
134. Poralla T, Hutteroth T, Meyer Z. Cellular cytotoxicity against autologous hepatocytes in alcoholic liver disease. *Liver* 1984;4:117–121.
135. Niemela O, Juvonen T, Parkkila S. Immunohistochemical demonstration of acetaldehyde-modified epitopes in human liver after alcohol consumption. *J Clin Invest* 1990;87:1367–1374.
136. Niemela O, Israel Y. Hemoglobin-acetaldehyde adducts in human alcohol abusers. *Lab Invest* 1992;67:246–252.
137. Barry R, McGivan J. Acetaldehyde alone may initiate hepatocellular damage in acute alcoholic liver disease. *Gut* 1985;26:1065–1069.
138. Schindler W, Haflinger F. Ueber derivate des imino-debenzyls. *Helv Chim Acta* 1954;37:472–483.
139. Gram L, Jensen P. Carbamazepine toxicity. In: Levy R, Mattson R, Meldrum B, Penry J, Dreifuss F, eds. *Antiepileptic drugs*. New York: Raven Press, 1989:555–565.
140. Smith DB, Mattson RH, Cramer JA, Collins JF, Novelly RA, Craft B. Results of a Nationwide Veterans Administration Cooperative study comparing the efficacy and toxicity of carbamazepine, phenobarbital, phenytoin and primidone. *Epilepsia* 1987;28:S50–S58.
141. Durelli L, Massazza U, Cavallo R. Carbamazepine toxicity and poisoning: incidence, clinical features and management. *Med Tox Adv Drug Exp* 1989;4:95–107.
142. Pellock JM. Carbamazepine side effects in children and adults. *Epilepsia* 1987;28:S64–S70.
143. Askmark H, Wiholm BE. Epidemiology of adverse reactions to carbamazepine as seen in a spontaneous reporting system. *Acta Neurol Scand* 1990;81:131–140.
144. Horowitz S, Patwardhan R, Marcus E. Hepatotoxic reactions associated with carbamazepine therapy. *Epilepsia* 1988;29:149–154.
145. Eichelbaum M, Tomson T, Tybring G, Bertilsson L. Carbamazepine metabolism in man: induction and pharmacogenetic aspects. *Clin Pharm* 1985;10:80–90.
146. Baker KM, Frigerio A, Morselli PL, Pifferi G. Identification of a rearranged degradation product from carbamazepine-10,11-epoxide. *J Pharm Sci* 1973;62:475–476.
147. Frigerio A, Fanelli R, Biandrate P, Passerini G, Morselli PL, Garattini S. Mass spectrometric characterization of carbamazepine-10,11-epoxide, a carbamazepine metabolite isolated from human urine. *J Pharm Sci* 1972;61:1144–1147.
148. Gerson WT, Fine DG, Spielberg SP, Sensenbrenner LL. Anticonvulsant-induced aplastic anemia: increased susceptibility to toxic drug metabolites in vivo. *Blood* 1983;61:889–893.
149. Riley RJ, Kitteringham NR, Park BK. Structural requirements for bioactivation of anticonvulsants to cytotoxic metabolites in vitro. *Br J Clin Pharmacol* 1989;28:482–487.
150. Shear NH, Spielberg SP. In vitro evaluation of a toxic metabolite of sulfadiazine. *Can J Physiol Pharmacol* 1985;63:1370–1372.
151. Shear NH, Spielberg SP. Anticonvulsant hypersensitivity syndrome. *J Clin Invest* 1988;82:1826–1832.
152. Pirmohamed M, Kitteringham N, Guenthner T, Breckenridge A, Park B. An investigation of the formation of cytotoxic, protein-reactive and stable metabolites from carbamazepine in vitro. *Biochem Pharmacol* 1992;43:1675–1682.
153. Pirmohamed M, Kitteringham NR, Breckenridge AM, Park BK. Detection of an autoantibody directed against human liver microsomal protein in a patient with carbamazepine hypersensitivity. *Br J Clin Pharmacol* 1992;33:183–186.
154. Spielberg SP, Gordon GB, Blake DA, Mellits ED, Bross DS. Anticonvulsant toxicity in vitro: possible role of arene oxides. *J Pharmacol Exp Ther* 1981;217:386–389.
155. Ivanetich K, Ziman MR, Bradshaw JJ. 1,1,1-Trichloropropene-2,3-oxide: an alternate mechanism for its inhibition of cytochrome P-450. *Res Commun Chem Path Pharmacol* 1982;35:111–119.
156. Kroetz D, Kerr B, McFarland L, Loiseau P, Wilensky A, Levy R. Measurement of in vivo microsomal epoxide hydrolase activity in white subjects. *Clin Pharmacol Ther* 1993;53:306–315.
157. Gaedigk A, Spielberg S, Grant D. Characterization of the microsomal epoxide hydrolase gene in patients with anticonvulsant adverse drug reactions. *Pharmacogenetics* 1994;4:142–153.
158. Gilhus N, Lea T. Carbamazepine: effect on IgG subclasses in epileptic patients. *Epilepsia* 1988;29:317–320.

159. Sinnige HA, Boender CA, Kyupers EW, Ruitenberg HM. Carbamazepine-induced pseudolymphoma and immune dysregulation. *J Int Med* 1990;227:355–358.
160. Alarcon-Segovia D, Fishbein E, Reyes PA, Dies H, Shwadsky S. Antinuclear antibodies in patients on anticonvulsant therapy. *Clin Exp Immunol* 1972;12:39–47.
161. Virolainen M. Blast transformation in vivo and in vitro in carbamazepine hypersensitivity. *Clin Exp Immunol* 1971;9:429–435.
162. Pacifici R, Carlo SD, Bacosi A, Pichini S, Zuccaro P. Immunomodulating properties of carbamazepine in mice. *Int J Immunopharmacol* 1992;14:605–611.
163. Virolainen M. Blast transformation in vivo and in vitro in carbamazepine hypersensitivity. *Clin Exp Immunol* 1971;9:429–435.
164. Houwerzijl J, Gast GD, Nater J, Esselink M, Nieweg H. Lymphocyte-stimulation tests and patch tests in carbamazepine hypersensitivity. *Clin Exp Immunol* 1977;29:272–277.
165. Powers N, Carson S. Idiosyncratic reactions to phenytoin. *Clin Pediatr* 1987;26:120–124.
166. Spielberg S, Gordon G, Blake D, Goldstein D. Predisposition to phenytoin hepatotoxicity assessed in vitro. *N Engl J Med* 1981;305:722–727.
167. Uetrecht JP, Zahid N. N-Chlorination of phenytoin by myeloperoxidase to a reactive metabolite. *Chem Res Toxicol* 1988;1:148–151.
168. Sorrell T, Forbes I, Burness F, Rischbieth R. Depression of immunological function in patients treated with phenytoin sodium (sodium diphenylhydantoin). *Lancet* 1971;2:1233–1235.
169. Seager J, Jamison D, Wilson J, Hayward A, Soothill J. IgA deficiency, epilepsy and phenytoin treatment. *Lancet* 1975;2 (7936):632–635.
170. Gilhus N, Matre R, Aarli J. Lymphocyte subpopulations and lymphocyte function in phenytoin-treated patients with epilepsy. *Int J Immunopharmacol* 1982;4:43–48.
171. Aarli J, Tonder O. Effect of antiepileptic drugs on serum and salivary IgA. *Scand J Immunol* 1975;4:391–396.
172. Ricevuti G, Marcoli M, Gatti G, Mazzone A, Lecchini S, Frigo G. Assessment of polymorphonucleate leukocyte functions in adult epileptic patients undergoing long-term phenytoin treatment. *Hum Toxicol* 1986;5:237–241.
173. Guerra I, Fawcett W, Redmon A, Lawrence E, Rosenblatt H, Shearer W. Permanent intrinsic B cell immunodeficiency caused by phenytoin hypersensitivity. *J Allergy Clin Immunol* 1986;77:603–607.
174. Samuel SA. Apparent anaphylactic reaction to zomepirac (Zomax). *N Engl J Med* 1981;304:978.
175. Ojingwa J, Spahn-Langguth H, Benet L. Irreversible binding of tolmetin to macromolecules via its glucuronide: binding to blood constituents, tissue homogenates and subcellular fractions in vitro. *Xenobiotica* 1994;24:495–506.
176. Hasegawa J, Smith PC, Benet LZ. Apparent intramolecular acyl migration of zomepirac glucuronide. *Drug Metab Dispos* 1982;10:469–473.
177. Ding A, Ojingwa JC, McDonagh AF, Burlingame AL, Benet LZ. Evidence for covalent binding of acyl glucuronides to serum albumin via an imine mechanism as revealed by tandem mass spectrometry. *Pharmacology* 1993;90:3797–3801.
178. Purcell P, Henry D, Melville G. Diclofenac hepatitis. *Gut* 1991;32:1381–1385.
179. Zimmerman HJ. Update of hepatotoxicity due to classes of drugs in common clinical use: non-steroidal drugs, anti-inflammatory drugs, antibiotics, antihypertensives, and cardiac and psychotropic agents. *Semin Liver Dis* 1990;10:322–338.
180. Pumford N, Myers T, Davila J, Highet R, Pohl L. Immunochemical detection of liver protein adducts of the nonsteroidal antiinflammatory drug diclofenac. *Chem Res Toxicol* 1993;6:147–150.
181. Kretz-Rommel A, Boelsterli UA. Mechanism of covalent adduct formation of diclofenac to rat hepatic microsomal proteins. *Drug Metab Dispos* 1994;22:956–961.
182. Kretz-Rommel A, Boelsterli UA. Selective protein adducts to membrane proteins in cultured rat hepatocytes exposed to diclofenac: radiochemical and immunochemical analysis. *Mol Pharmacol* 1993;45:237–244.
183. Hargus SJ, Amouzedeh HR, Pumford NR, Myers TG, McCoy SC, Pohl LR. Metabolic activation and immunochemical localization of liver protein adducts of the nonsteroidal anti-inflammatory drug diclofenac. *Chem Res Toxicol* 1994;7:575–582.
184. Boelsterli UA, Zimmerman HJ, Kretz-Rommel A. Idiosyncratic liver toxicity of nonsteroidal antiinflammatory drugs: molecular mechanisms and pathology. *Crit Rev Toxicol* 1995;25:207–235.
185. Salama A, Gottsche B, Mueller-Eckhardt C. Autoantibodies and drug- or metabolite-dependent antibodies in patients with diclofenac-induced immune haemolysis. *Br J Haematol* 1991;77:546–549.

Toxicology of the Liver, 2nd ed.,
Edited by Gabriel L. Plaa and William R. Hewitt
Copyright © 1998 Taylor & Francis

9

The Role of Nonparenchymal Cells and Inflammatory Macrophages in Hepatotoxicity

Debra L. Laskin and Carol R. Gardner

*Environmental and Occupational Health Sciences Institute,
Rutgers University
and UMDNJ-Robert Wood Johnson Medical School,
Piscataway, NJ 08855-1179*

Nonparenchymal cells, in particular macrophages, endothelial cells, and stellate cells, have been implicated in the pathogenesis of hepatotoxicity induced by a number of different xenobiotics. Following exposure of experimental animals to hepatotoxicants, these cells, together with newly recruited inflammatory macrophages, are "activated" to release a wide array of proinflammatory and cytotoxic mediators that have the capacity to promote liver damage. These findings, together with the discovery that hepatotoxicity can be modified by agents that modulate inflammatory cell and nonparenchymal cell functioning, provide direct evidence that these cells contribute to tissue injury. The cytotoxic process most likely involves mediators such as reactive

active oxygen intermediates, reactive nitrogen intermediates, cytokines, hydrolytic enzymes, eicosanoids, and lipid mediators released at the site of tissue injury. Whereas some of the mediators are directly cytotoxic (i.e., hydrogen peroxide, nitric oxide, peroxynitrite), others degrade the extracellular matrix (i.e., collagenase, elastase) or promote inflammatory cell infiltration and adhesion and nonparenchymal cell pro-liferation and activation (i.e., chemokines, colony-stimulating factors, interleukin-1 [IL-1], interleukin-6 [IL-6], tumor necrosis factor-α [TNF-α], and platelet-activating factor). There is also evidence that activated nonparenchymal cells produce medi-ators that can modify hepatocyte protein and nucleic acid biosynthesis as well as cytochrome P450–mediated xenobiotic metabolism. This may also contribute to hep-atotoxicity. This chapter reviews experimental data implicating nonparenchymal cells and inflammatory macrophages in hepatotoxicity.

HEPATIC NONPARENCHYMAL CELLS

The majority of the nonparenchymal cells of the liver reside within the hepatic sinu-soids, positioned between the arterial vasculature and the parenchyma. These cells consist predominantly of Kupffer cells, endothelial cells, and stellate cells. Approx-imately 30% of the hepatic sinusoidal cells are Kupffer cells. These cells constitute approximately 80–90% of all the macrophages in the body. Kupffer cells are mainly localized in periportal and central regions of the liver lobule and are anchored to the lumen of the endothelium by long cytoplasmic processes (1). The major function of Kupffer cells is to clear particulate and foreign materials from the portal circulation, primarily through phagocytosis. Kupffer cells possess both Fc and C3 receptors and are known to phagocytize a wide variety of both opsonized and nonopsonized parti-cles as well as tumor cells (2–5). Kupffer cells play a central role in the uptake and detoxification of endotoxin from the portal circulation (6, 7). Like other mononu-clear phagocytes, Kupffer cells respond to chemotactic and inflammatory signals and display both oxidant-dependent and oxidant-independent killing of pathogens and tumor cells (2, 4, 8–18). Kupffer cells also express MHC class II antigens, suggest-ing that they also have the capacity to act as antigen-presenting cells for the induc-tion of specific T-lymphocyte responses (19–21). When activated by xenobiotics or inflammatory stimuli, Kupffer cells release superoxide anion, hydrogen peroxide, nitric oxide, peroxynitrite, hydrolytic enzymes, and eicosanoids that aid in antigen destruction (2, 11, 12, 14, 22–38). Kupffer cells also release a number of different cytokines with immunoregulatory and inflammatory activity including TNF-α, IL-1, IL-6, interleukin-8 (IL-8), transforming growth factor-β (TGF-β), platelet activating factor, and interferons (28, 37–62).

Endothelial cells, which form the walls of the sinusoids, represent a major frac-tion of hepatic sinusoidal cells (approximately 48%). Endothelial cells function as a selective barrier between the blood and the liver parenchyma. They possess pores or fenestrae that allow direct contact between the plasma and the hepatocytes. Unlike endothelial cells in other vascular beds, hepatic sinusoidal endothelial cells are devoid of basement membrane (63). They also possess unique "bristle-coated" membrane invaginations and vesicles, and lysosome-like vacuoles (64). Moreover, they can endocytose a variety of particles including glycoproteins, lipoproteins, albumin, lactoferrin, and hyaluronic acid. Endocytosis is accomplished through pinocytotic vesicles and lysosomes as well as Fc receptors (65, 66). Of particular interest is the observation that endothelial cells display greater levels of phagocytosis than Kupffer cells toward certain types of particles (67–71). In addition, their phagocytic capacity is enhanced when Kupffer cell function is impaired (72, 73). Recent studies have demonstrated that hepatic endothelial cells can be "activated" by inflammatory cytokines to release a variety of mediators that regulate the function of other sinusoidal cells as well as of hepatocytes. These include IL-1, IL-6, fibroblast growth factor, interferon, eicosanoids, lysosomal enzymes, and nitric oxide and its oxidation products as well as reactive oxygen intermediates (11, 23, 39, 74–86). In addition, cell adhesion molecule expression is readily upregulated on these cells in response to inflammatory mediators (87–94). Thus, endothelial cells, like Kupffer cells, appear to be important in immunologic, inflammatory, and regulatory activities in the liver.

Hepatic stellate cells, also referred to as Ito cells, fat-storing cells, perisinusoidal cells, and lipocytes, constitute approximately 20% of the hepatic sinusoidal cells. Stellate cells are located between the endothelial cells and hepatocytes or between the hepatocytes. Morphologically, they resemble fibroblasts in that they possess numerous extensions as well as dilated rough endoplasmic reticulum. The major function of hepatic stellate cells is to store vitamin A, which is localized in intracellular lipid droplets in the form of retinyl esters (95–97). In addition, they have the capacity to synthesize large quantities of extracellular matrix proteins, including types I, III, and IV collagen, and there is evidence that they play a major role in collagen synthesis in both normal and fibrotic liver (98–105). Recent studies have suggested that stellate cells may also contribute to inflammatory and immunologic responses in the liver. These cells express cell adhesion molecules and release a variety of proteins and mediators that have been implicated in tissue injury, including nitric oxide, hydrogen peroxide, prostaglandins, gelatinase, fibronectin, transforming growth factor-β, and macrophage chemotactic protein-1 (100, 106–115).

ROLE OF MACROPHAGES IN HEPATOTOXICITY

A characteristic histologic feature observed after treatment of experimental animals with hepatotoxicants such as acetaminophen, endotoxin, carbon tetrachloride, phenobarbital, allyl alcohol, or galactosamine is an increase in the number macrophages in the liver (2, 26, 28, 116–125). These cells are typically observed in the liver prior to histologic evidence of frank necrosis. Of particular interest is the observation that the specific location of the macrophages within the liver lobule varies with the chemical agent and is directly correlated with areas of the liver that subsequently exhibit signs of injury (126–128). Thus, whereas treatment of rats with acetaminophen or carbon tetrachloride results in an accumulation of macrophages in centrilobular regions of the liver, macrophages that localize in the liver following lipopolysaccharide, phenobarbital, *Corynebacterium parvum* or galactosamine treatment of rats are scattered in clusters throughout the liver lobule (2, 26–28, 117, 124, 127, 129). It has been hypothesized that these macrophages become activated and release mediators that contribute to tissue injury (28, 128, 130). In this regard, several studies demonstrate that macrophages isolated from livers of hepatotoxicant-treated animals display morphologic and functional properties of activated mononuclear phagocytes (2, 12, 13, 24, 26, 27). Thus these cells, which consist of resident Kupffer cells and inflammatory macrophages, appear larger and more stellate than cells from untreated rats, are highly vacuolated, and display an increased cytoplasmic:nuclear ratio (2, 11, 12, 26, 131). In addition, macrophages from animals treated with hepatotoxicants such as phenobarbital, acetaminophen, or endotoxin adhere to and spread on culture dishes more rapidly than resident Kupffer cells (2, 12, 26). These properties are characteristic of morphologically activated macrophages. Liver macrophages from animals treated with hepatotoxicants also exhibit varying degrees of functional activation including enhanced phagocytic, chemotactic, cytotoxic, and metabolic activity as well as increased release of superoxide anion, hydrogen peroxide, nitric oxide, proteolytic enzymes, IL-1, IL-6, and TNF-α (2, 4, 8–13, 15, 39, 43). It is thought that activated Kupffer cells and infiltrating macrophages promote hepatic damage through the release of toxic secretory products (10, 28, 116, 118, 124, 130, 132–134).

Probably the best evidence generated in support of the hypothesis that inflammatory macrophages and Kupffer cells play a role in the pathogenesis of liver injury comes from experiments using agents known to modify the functioning of these cells. Data from these studies clearly demonstrate that the degree of hepatic injury induced by a number of different chemicals is directly correlated with macrophage functioning. Thus, agents that depress macrophage functioning reduce toxicity, while compounds that augment macrophage activity enhance tissue injury. For example, drugs such as hydrocortisone, certain synthetic steroids and natural substances that block inflammatory responses, have been reported to protect against liver injury induced by carbon tetrachloride and acetaminophen (135). Similarly, the accumulation of macrophages in the liver and subsequent toxicity of acetaminophen or carbon tetrachloride is inhibited by pretreatment of rats with gadolinium chloride, carbon particles or dextran sulfate, compounds known to depress macrophage activity (120, 127, 136). Hepatoprotective effects of gadolinium chloride against 1,2-dichlorobenzene, diethyldicarbamate, galactosamine, endotoxin, and alcohol-induced injury have also been described (22, 124, 137–139). A number of studies also demonstrate that activation of hepatic macrophages augments hepatic injury induced by toxic xenobiotics. Thus, pretreatment of rats with macrophage activators such as lipopolysaccharide, glucan, vitamin A, or latex beads has been reported to aggravate liver injury induced by carbon tetrachloride, galactosamine, allyl alcohol, and *C. parvum* (10, 22, 27, 30, 132, 140–146). Taken together, these observations support the hypothesis that macrophages contribute to hepatotoxicity. The specific mediators released by these cells that are involved in the pathogenic process most likely vary with the hepatotoxicant.

ROLE OF ENDOTHELIAL CELLS AND STELLATE CELLS IN HEPATOTOXICITY

Recent studies suggest that endothelial cells and stellate cells also increase in number and become activated following exposure of experimental animals to hepatotoxicants (9, 11, 39, 44, 76, 80, 84, 90, 114, 115, 147–151). Like activated hepatic macrophages, these cells are larger and more granular than cells from untreated rats and produce increased amounts of reactive oxygen and nitrogen intermediates, IL-1 and IL-6 (11, 22, 80, 86, 114, 115, 152–154). The capacity of endothelial cells and stellate cells to produce these mediators may represent an important mechanism by which they partic-ipate in inflammatory and immune reactions associated with hepatotoxicity. Vascular endothelial cells have been reported to produce increased amounts of IL-1, IL-6, IL-8, TGF-α, and endothelin-1, as well as reactive oxygen and nitrogen intermediates in response to macrophage-derived cytokines (79, 153, 155–172). Similarly, it is possi-ble that cytokines released by nonparenchymal cells and inflammatory macrophages in the liver induce the production of mediators from hepatic endothelial cells and stellate cells. These may act in a paracrine or autocrine manner to promote cellular proliferation and activation and to induce cytotoxicity.

INFLAMMATORY MEDIATORS IMPLICATED IN HEPATOTOXICITY

Over the past 10 years evidence has accumulated that clearly demonstrates that tissue damage induced by a number of different hepatotoxicants is due not only to a direct action of the chemical on hepatocytes but also to the actions of inflammatory media-tors produced at the injured site by nonparenchymal cells and infiltrating leukocytes. Whereas some of these mediators exert cytotoxic activity directly, others promote the inflammatory response. Among the more prominent proinflammatory and cyto-toxic mediators that have been implicated in hepatotoxicity are TNF-α, IL-1, reactive oxygen intermediates, nitric oxide, bioactive lipids, and hydrolytic enzymes. These mediators are likely to act in concert to promote hepatotoxicity.

Inflammatory Cytokines

Cytokines consist of a family of proteins that act in an autocrine and paracrine man-ner to regulate immune and inflammatory responses. Hepatic nonparenchymal cells and inflammatory macrophages are known to release a number of different cytokines that may contribute to tissue injury (28, 128, 130). Of particular interest in terms of liver injury are IL-1 and TNF-α, which can act directly on hepatocytes to induce injury or alter function or, indirectly, on other nonparenchymal cells or infiltrating leukocytes that accumulate in the liver, thus amplifying the inflammatory response (60, 173–182). IL-1 and TNF-α are low-molecular-weight multifunctional proteins that mediate a wide variety of diverse and overlapping biologic effects (183–187). Considered "early response cytokines," they are rapidly produced by macrophages in response to inflammatory stimuli. Among their prominent proinflammatory actions is their ability to upregulate cell adhesion molecule expression on endothelial cells (87, 89, 90, 93), thus facilitating phagocyte margination and emigration to sites of injury. IL-1 also induces proliferation and activation of macrophages and endothelial cells as well as T- and B-lymphocytes and epithelial cells (24, 183, 187–194). Both IL-1 and TNF-α augment macrophage-mediated cytotoxicity and nitric oxide production (195–204). TNF-α also sensitizes neutrophils and monocytes to release reactive oxygen intermediates (60, 205–212) and stimulates the release of other inflammatory mediators including IL-1, IL-6, colony-stimulating factor, platelet-activating factor, and eicosanoids from parenchymal and nonparenchymal liver cells (37, 40, 47, 56, 60, 62, 204, 213). In conjunction with IL-6, IL-1 and TNF-α also regulate hepatocyte acute-phase protein and gene expression (40, 47, 51, 179, 180) and cytochrome P450 activity (173, 177, 214). TNF-α is unique among inflammatory cytokines in that it has the capacity to induce cytotoxicity directly (198, 215–217). In hepatocytes TNF-α stimulates nitric oxide production and induces both necrosis and apoptosis (178, 218, 219).

Both IL-1 and TNF-α have been directly implicated in chemical-induced hepatotoxicity. Thus, many of the observed clinical features of liver disease and injury, including fever, inflammation, cirrhosis, and acute phase protein production, can be induced by administration of these inflammatory cytokines (60, 181, 183, 220, 221). Conversely, administration of neutralizing antibodies to IL-1 or TNF-α, soluble cytokine receptors, or cytokine receptor antagonists prevents inflammatory cell accumulation and tissue injury induced by toxicants such as acetaminophen, endotoxin, cadmium, and carbon tetrachloride (222–231). These data, together with the findings that macrophage or nonparenchymal cell production of IL-1 and TNF-α is increased following exposure of animals to various hepatotoxicants (24, 25, 39, 44, 107, 114, 115, 140, 160–162, 164, 224–227, 229, 232–235), suggest that these cytokines play a role in tissue injury. The specific mechanism underlying their actions is unknown and may be due to production of cytotoxic mediators such as nitric oxide, superoxide anion, and hydroxyl radicals by inflammatory cells or by hepatic parenchymal and nonparenchymal cells.

Reactive Oxygen Intermediates

Reactive oxygen intermediates are generated enzymatically by macrophages via a membrane-bound NADPH oxidase. Activated by inflammatory and phagocytic stimuli, this enzyme adds one electron to molecular oxygen, resulting in the formation of superoxide anion. Two molecules of superoxide anion subsequently react spontaneously or enzymatically as a consequence of the actions of superoxide dismutase to form oxygen and hydrogen peroxide. In the presence of transition metals such as ferrous iron or cuprous ion, hydrogen peroxide is reduced to hydroxyl radical, an even more potent oxidizing species. Under physiologic conditions, the abundant antioxidant defenses of most cells prevent reactive oxygen intermediates from causing cytotoxicity. However, when the rate of formation of reactive oxygen intermediates is increased or intracellular antioxidant defense systems are compromised, oxidative cell injury can occur. This can lead to cell membrane, protein, and DNA damage; lipid peroxidation; and cytotoxicity (10, 236–241). Peroxidation of membrane lipids by reactive oxygen intermediates can also induce the formation and release of a number of other vasoactive agents, including prostaglandins, thromboxanes, and leukotrienes. Recent studies have demonstrated that macrophages, as well as endothelial cells and stellate cells isolated from the livers of hepatotoxicant-treated rats, are activated to release reactive oxygen intermediates (2, 11, 80). Moreover, stimulation of hepatic macrophages to produce additional reactive oxygen intermediates by administration of agents such as retinol, glucan, or latex beads augments liver injury induced by agents such as *C. parvum*, carbon tetrachloride, 1,2-dichlorobenzene, and galactosamine. In contrast, administration of antioxidants like superoxide dismutase, catalase, allopurinol, methyl palmitate, endotoxin, or quinone derivatives is hepatoprotective (10, 29, 30, 121, 122, 132, 137, 141, 145, 242–250). These studies support the hypothesis that oxygen-derived free radicals contribute to the pathogenesis of chemical-induced hepatotoxicity (28, 30, 122, 132, 242).

Reactive Nitrogen Intermediates

Recent studies have also implicated reactive nitrogen intermediates, in particular nitric oxide and peroxynitrite, in the pathogenesis of hepatotoxicity. Nitric oxide is produced by the NADPH-dependent oxidation of L-arginine by the enzyme nitric oxide synthase. At least three major isoforms of nitric oxide synthase have been cloned and characterized (251). Two forms (types I and III) are produced in cells constitutively and are calcium- and calmodulin-dependent. The type I form is localized in neuronal tissue (252–254), while the type III form is found in vascular endothelium (255). In contrast, the type II or macrophage form of nitric oxide synthase is induced only after activation of these cells by bacterially derived pathogens or cytokines (256, 257). Type II or inducible nitric oxide synthase activity has been identified in both resident and inflammatory liver macrophages as well as hepatocytes, endothelial cells, stellate cells, smooth muscle cells, fibroblasts, and certain epithelial cells (9, 23, 60, 114, 115, 152, 153, 155, 170, 195, 258–261).

Nitric oxide is a small, relatively stable free radical gas that readily diffuses into cells and cell membranes, where it reacts with molecular targets such as heme- and thiol-containing proteins and amines (251, 262). This can result in decreased cellular proliferation and nucleic acid biosynthesis as well as altered enzyme activity, cytotoxicity, and apoptosis (219, 262–265). It has been established that nitric oxide produced by macrophages is involved in the destruction of certain intracellular pathogens and tumor cells and in cytostasis (201, 202, 265–268). In the liver, macrophages, as well as endothelial cells, stellate cells, and hepatocytes, have been reported to produce excess quantities of nitric oxide and to express inducible nitric oxide synthase following treatment of animals with hepatotoxicants such as acetaminophen, carbon tetrachloride, and endotoxin (114, 115, 140, 258, 268). These findings, together with the observation that administration of inhibitors of inducible nitric oxide synthase, such as aminoguanidine, block toxicity in some of these models, demonstrate that this reactive nitrogen intermediate contributes to inflammation and injury in the liver (227, 269–274). Nitric oxide may also modulate drug-induced hepatotoxicity by altering cytochrome P450 mixed-function oxidase activity. Nitric oxide binds to heme-containing proteins, and this may result in either inhibition or activation of enzymes involved in hepatic drug metabolism (258, 262–264, 272).

Nitric oxide is also known to react with superoxide anion forming peroxynitrite, a relatively long-lived cytotoxic oxidant that has been implicated in stroke, heart disease, and immune complex–mediated pulmonary edema (275–280). Peroxynitrite may also initiate lipid peroxidation and can react directly with sulfhydryl groups in cell membranes (281–283). Recent studies have also demonstrated that peroxynitrite can induce apoptosis (284–286). It has also been suggested that the reaction of superoxide and nitric oxide may function as a defense against oxidant stress by reducing intracellular levels of these reactive intermediates (275–277). In this regard, inhibition of nitric oxide synthesis has been reported to augment oxidant-dependent tissue injury induced by *C. parvum* and endotoxin, and it has been proposed to play a protective role in the hepatotoxicity of endotoxin (287, 288). Thus, nitric oxide or secondary oxidants generated from nitric oxide may be cytotoxic or hepatoprotective, depending on levels of superoxide anion present and the extent to which tissue injury is mediated by reactive oxygen intermediates (275–277).

Bioactive Lipids

Eicosanoids consist of a family of biologically active lipid mediators derived from 20-carbon essential fatty acids and include prostaglandins, thromboxanes, and leukotrienes. The most abundant precursor of the eicosanoids is arachidonic acid, which is found esterified to cell membrane phospholipids. Metabolism of arachidonic acid via cyclooxygenase leads to the generation of various prostaglandins (PG) and thromboxanes (Tx), while lipoxygenase oxidation initiates leukotriene (LT) biosynthesis. Activated liver macrophages, as well as endothelial cells and stellate cells, have been reported to synthesize a number of different eicosanoids including LTB_4, TxA_2, PGE_2, PGD_2, $PGF_{2\alpha}$ and PGI_2 (31, 32, 35–37, 50, 60, 74–76, 82, 83, 106). The precise role of these reactive species in hepatotoxicity is unknown. Prostaglandins such as PGE_2 and PGD_2 play a key role in regulating inflammatory and immune reactions and also have the capacity to modify hepatocyte carbohydrate metabolism and calcium homeostasis as well as protein synthesis and phosphorylation (35, 289, 290). Enhanced release of prostaglandins has been described following exposure of animals to toxins such as acetaminophen and endotoxin (35, 37, 50, 76, 83, 290–292). Moreover, administration of cyclooxygenase inhibitors to animals prevents tissue injury induced by these toxicants (36, 146, 230, 292–294). Similarly, TxB_2 synthase inhibition protects against endotoxic shock and liver injury (295, 296).

Several of the leukotrienes exhibit proinflammatory activity and are thought to play a role in chemical-induced tissue injury (36, 123, 297). For example, LTB_4 is known to be a potent polymorphonuclear leukocyte chemoattractant and to induce monocyte IL-1, TNF-α and hydrogen peroxide production (34, 35, 298). Thus, release of LTB_4 by macrophages in the liver following hepatotoxicant exposure may constitute a local control mechanism for the recruitment and activation of inflammatory cells. In this regard, recent studies have demonstrated that administration of lipoxygenase inhibitors or antagonists to mice protected against galactosamine-induced hepatitis (117, 293). These data suggest that leukotrienes contribute to inflammatory liver disease and injury.

Another biologically active lipid that has been implicated in tissue injury is platelet-activating factor (PAF) (185, 299–301). This phospholipid mediator of anaphylaxis was originally named for its ability to induce platelets to change shape, aggregate, and release their granule contents. PAF is released by a variety of cell types including macrophages, neutrophils and endothelial cells and is thought to act in an autocrine and paracrine manner to amplify and propagate early stages of the inflammatory response. Thus, PAF released from inflammatory phagocytes stimulates macrophage chemotaxis and oxidative metabolism (32, 79, 302). Following exposure of animals to endotoxin, liver macrophages and endothelial cells produce increased quantities of PAF (303, 304). Interestingly, these cells also express increased numbers of functionally active receptors for this bioactive lipid (305). Upregulation of PAF receptors may represent an important mechanism underlying macrophage and endothelial cell activation following hepatotoxicant exposure. In support of this possibility is the finding that administration of a PAF receptor antagonist reduces tissue injury induced by endotoxin (306).

Hydrolytic Enzymes

Macrophages and endothelial cells activated by inflammatory stimuli are known to produce proteolytic and lysosomal enzymes. These include various proteases, lipases, plasminogen activator, collagenase, elastase, gelatinase, acid phosphatase, and cathepsin D (14, 60, 307–321). These can act directly on hepatocyte membranes, inducing damage. Some of these proteases have been shown to play a role in macrophage-mediated target cell destruction as well as in altered hepatocyte functioning (14, 60, 308, 310), and similar effects may occur in vivo after hepatotoxicant exposure.

MODEL OF HEPATOTOXICITY

A schematic model for the role of nonparenchymal cells and inflammatory macrophages in chemical-induced hepatotoxicity is shown in Fig. 1. According to this model, macrophages, endotheliai cells, and stellate cells increase in number and become activated following hepatotoxicant exposure. These cells release mediators such as reactive oxygen intermediates, reactive nitrogen intermediates, cytokines,

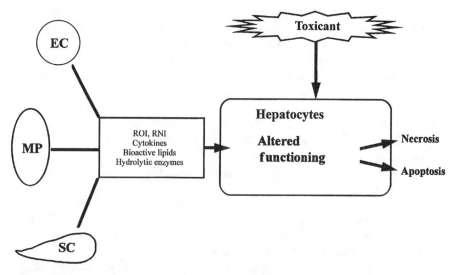

FIG. 1. Model for the role of nonparenchymal cells and inflammatory macrophages in chemical-induced hepatotoxicity. Macrophages (MP), endothelial cells (EC), and stellate cells (SC) become "activated" following hepatotoxicant treatment of animals. These cells release reactive oxygen intermediates (ROI) and reactive nitrogen intermediates (RNI), as well as cytokines, bioactive lipids, and hydrolytic enzymes, which contribute to toxicant-induced alterations in hepatocyte functioning, necrosis, or apoptosis.

bioactive lipids, and hydrolytic enzymes that contribute to hepatotoxicant-induced alterations in liver functioning, necrosis or apoptosis. Data from our laboratory and those of other investigators support this model of hepatotoxicity.

CONCLUSION

It is becoming increasingly apparent that chemical-induced hepatotoxicity is a multi-factor process involving a variety of soluble and lipid mediators derived from different cell types in the liver. These include not only resident cells (hepatocytes, Kupffer cells, stellate cells and endothelial cells) but also infiltrating leukocytes. While toxicity may be a direct result of chemical-induced injury to hepatocytes leading to apoptosis or necrosis, it may also be due to proliferation and activation of nonparenchymal cells and inflammatory phagocytes. Reactive mediators including nitric oxide, peroxynitrite, superoxide anion, hydrogen peroxide, and hydroxyl radicals produced by activated nonparenchymal cells and infiltrating leukocytes may be cytotoxic, proinflammatory, and can compromise normal liver functioning. Defining the precise role of each of these mediators in tissue injury is essential in our understanding of the mechanism of action of hepatotoxic chemicals and for devising steps to prevent or reverse toxicity.

ACKNOWLEDGMENTS

Dr. Laskin is a Burroughs Wellcome Toxicology Scholar. This work was supported by an award from the Burroughs Wellcome Fund and by USPHS National Institutes of Health grants GM34310, ES05022, and ES04738.

REFERENCES

1. Bouwens L, Baekeland M, De Zanger R, Wisse E. Quantitation, tissue distribution and proliferation kinetics of Kupffer cells in normal rat liver. *Hepatology* 1986;6:718–722.
2. Pilaro AM, Laskin DL. Accumulation of activated mononuclear phagocytes in the liver following lipopolysaccharide treatment of rats. *J Leukoc Biol* 1986;40:29–41.
3. Gardner CR, Wasserman AJ, Laskin DL. Differential sensitivity of tumor targets to liver macrophage-mediated cytotoxicity. *Cancer Res* 1987;47:6686–6691.
4. Gardner CR, Wasserman AJ, Laskin DL. Liver macrophage mediated cytotoxicity involves phagocytosis of tumor targets. *Hepatology* 1991;14:318–324.
5. Reske SN, Vyska K, Feinendegen LE. *In vivo* assessment of phagocytic properties of Kupffer cells. *J Nucl Med* 1981;22:405–410.
6. Mathison JC, Ulevitch RJ. The clearance, tissue distribution, and cellular localization of intravenously injected lipopolysaccharide in rabbits. *J Immunol* 1979;123:2133–2143.
7. Nolan J. Endotoxin, reticuloendothelial function and liver injury. *Hepatology* 1981;1:458–465.
8. Abril ER, Simm WE, Earnest DL. Kupffer cell secretion of cytotoxin cytokines is enhanced by hypervitaminosis A. In: Wisse E, Knook DL, Decker K, eds. *Cells of the Hepatic Sinusoid* Vol. 2. Rijswijk: Kupffer Cell Foundation, 1989;73–75.
9. Laskin DL, Heck DE, Gardner CR, Feder LS, Laskin JD. Distinct patterns of nitric oxide production in hepatic macrophages and endothelial cells following acute exposure of rats to endotoxin. *J Leukoc Biol* 1994;56:751–758.
10. Arthur MJP, Bentley IS, Tanner A, Saunders PK, Millward-Sadler GH, Wright R. Oxygen-derived free radicals promote hepatic injury in the rat. *Gastroenterology* 1985;89:1114–1122.
11. Mc Closkey TW, Todaro JA, Laskin DL. Lipopolysaccharide treatment of rats alters antigen expression and oxidative metabolism in hepatic macrophages and endothelial cells. *Hepatology* 1992;16:191–203.
12. Laskin DL, Pilaro AM. Potential role of activated macrophages in acetaminophen hepatotoxicity. I. Isolation and characterization of activated macrophages from rat liver. *Toxicol Appl Pharmacol* 1986;86:204–215.
13. Shiratori Y, Takikawa H, Kawase T, Sugimoto T. Superoxide anion generating capacity and lysosomal enzyme activities of Kupffer cells in galactosamine-induced hepatitis. *Gastroenterol Jpn* 1986;21:135–144.
14. Tanner A, Keyhani A, Reiner R, Holdstock G, Wright R. Proteolytic enzymes released by liver macrophages may promote injury in a rat model of hepatic damage. *Gastroenterology* 1980;80:647–654.
15. Mochia S, Ogata I, Ohta Y, Yamada S, Fujiwara K. *In situ* evaluation of the stimulatory state of hepatic macrophages based on their ability to produce superoxide anions in rats. *J Pathol* 1989;158:67–71.
16. Bautista AP, Meszaros K, Bojta J, Spitzer JJ. Superoxide anion generation in the liver during the early stages of endotoxemia in rats. *J Leukoc Biol* 1990;48:123–128.
17. Bautista AP, Spitzer JJ. Superoxide anion generation by *in situ* perfused rat liver: effect of *in vivo* endotoxin. *Am J Physiol* 1990;259:G907–G912.
18. Mayer A, Spitzer J. Continuous infusion of *Escherichia coli* endotoxin *in vivo* primes *in vitro* superoxide anion release in rat polymorphonuclear leukocytes and Kupffer cells in a time-dependent manner. *Am Soc Microbiol* 1991;12:4590.
19. Rogoff TM, Lipsky PE. Antigen presentation by isolated guinea pig Kupffer cells. *J Immunol* 1980;124:1740–1744.

20. Itoh Y, Okanoue T, Morimoto M, Nagao Y, Mori T, Hori N, Kagawa K, Kashima K. Functional heterogeneity of rat liver macrophages: interleukin-1 secretion and Ia antigen expression in contrast with phagocytic activity. *Liver* 1992;12:26–33.
21. Lohse AW, Knolle PA, Bilo K, Uhrig A, Waldmann C, Ibe M, Schmitt E, Gerken G, Meyer Zum Buschenfelde KH. Antigen-presenting function and B7 expression of murine sinusoidal endothelial cells and Kupffer cells. *Gastroenterology* 1996;110:1175–1181.
22. Liu P, McGuire GM, Fisher MA, Farhood A, Smith CW, Jaeschke H. Activation of Kupffer cells and neutrophils for reactive oxygen formation is responsible for endotoxin-enhanced liver injury after hepatic ischemia. *Shock* 1995;3:56–62.
23. Feder LS, Laskin DL. Regulation of hepatic endothelial cell and macrophage proliferation and nitric oxide production by GM-CSF, M-CSF and IL-1β following acute endotoxemia. *J Leukoc Biol* 1994;55:507–513.
24. Kamimura S, Tsukamoto H. Cytokine gene expression by Kupffer cells in experimental alcoholic liver disease. *Hepatology* 1995;22:1304–1309.
25. Furutani M, Arii S, Monden K, Adachi Y, Funaki H, Higashitsuji H, Fujita S, Mise M, Ishiguro S, Kitao T, Nakamura T, Imamura M, Tainatani T, Miyasaka M, Nakayama H, Fujita J. Immunological activation of hepatic macrophages in septic rats: a possible mechanism of sepsis-associated liver injury. *J Lab Clin Med* 1994;123:430–436.
26. Laskin DL, Robertson FM, Pilaro AM, Laskin JD. Activation of liver macrophages following phenobarbital treatment of rats. *Hepatology* 1988;8:1051–1055.
27. Arthur MJP, Kowalski-Sanders P, Wright R. *Corynebacterium parvum*-elicited hepatic macrophages demonstrate enhanced respiratory burst activity compared with resident Kupffer cells in the rat. *Gastroenterology* 1986;91:174–181.
28. Laskin DL. Potential role of activated macrophages in chemical and drug induced liver injury. In: Wisse E, Knook DL, Decker K, eds. *Cells of the Hepatic Sinusoid* Vol. 2. Rijswijk: Kupffer Cell Foundation, 1989:284–287.
29. Arai M, Mochida S, Ohno A, Ogata I, Fujiwara K. Sinusoidal endothelial cell damage by activated macrophages in rat liver necrosis. *Gastroenterology* 1993;104:466–471.
30. Shiratori Y, Kawase T, Shiina S, Okano K, Sugimoto T, Teraoka H, Matano S, Matsumoto K, Kamii K. Modulation of hepatotoxicity by macrophages in the liver. *Hepatology* 1988;8:815–821.
31. Kuiper J, De Rijke YB, Zijlstra FJ, Van Waas MP, van Berkel TJ. The induction of glucogenolysis in the perfused liver by platelet activating factor is mediated by prostaglandin D_2 from Kupffer cells. *Biochem Biophys Res Commun* 1988;157:1288–1295.
32. Dieter P, Schulze-Specking A, Decker K. Differential inhibition of prostaglandin and superoxide production by dexamethasone in primary cultures of rat Kupffer cells. *Eur J Biochem* 1986;159:451–457.
33. Keppler D, Hagmann W, Rapp S. Role of leukotrienes in endotoxin action *in vivo*. *Rev Infect Dis* 1987;9:S580–S584.
34. Henderson WR. The role of leukotrienes in inflammation. *Ann Intern Med* 1994;121:684–697.
35. Decker K. Eicosanoids, signal molecules of liver cells. *Semin Liver Dis* 1985;5:175–190.
36. Keppler D, Hagmann W, Rapp S, Denzlinger C, Koch HK. The relation of leukotrienes to liver injury. *Hepatology* 1985;5:883–891.
37. Peters T, Karck U, Decker K. Interdependence of tumor necrosis factor, prostaglandin E_2 and protein synthesis in lipopolysaccharide-exposed rat Kupffer cells. *Eur J Biochem* 1990;191:583–589.
38. Goss JA, Mangino MJ, Flye MW. Kupffer cell autoregulation of IL-1 production by PGE_2 during hepatic regeneration. *J Surg Res* 1992;52:422–428.
39. Feder LS, Todaro JA, Laskin DL. Characterization of interleukin-1 and interleukin-6 production by hepatic endothelial cells and macrophages. *J Leukoc Biol* 1993;53:126–132.
40. Wu J-Z, Ogle CK, Mao J-X, Szczur K, Fischer JE, Ogle JD. The increased potential for the production of inflammatory cytokines by Kupffer cells and splenic macrophages eight days after thermal injury. *Inflammation* 1995;19:529–541.
41. Karck U, Peters T, Decker K. The release of tumor necrosis factor from endotoxin-stimulated rat Kupffer cells is regulated by prostaglandin E_2 and dexamethasone. *J Hepatol* 1988;7:352–361.
42. Callery MP, Mangino MJ, Kamei T, Flye MW. Interleukin-6 production by endotoxin-stimulated Kupffer cells is regulated by prostaglandin E_2. *J Surg Res* 1990;48:523–527.
43. Armendariz-Borunda J, Seyer JM, Postlethwaite AE, Kang AH. Kupffer cells from carbon tetrachloride-injured rat livers produce chemotactic factors for fibroblasts and monocytes: the role of tumor necrosis factor-alpha. *Hepatology* 1991;14:895–900.

44. Tsukamoto H, Rippe RA, Niemela O, Lin M. Roles of oxidative stress in activation of Kupffer and Ito cells in liver fibrogenesis. *J Gastroenterol Hepatol* 1995;10:S50–S53.

45. Gressner AM. Liver fibrosis: Perspectives in pathobiological research and clinical outlook. *Eur J Clin Chem Biochem* 1991;29:293–311.

46. Meyer DH, Bachem MG, Gressner AM. Bidirectional effects of Kupffer cells on hepatocyte proliferation *in vitro*. *FEBS Lett* 1991;283:150–154.

47. Ayala A, Perrin MM, Wang P, Chaudry IH. Sepsis induces an early increased spontaneous release of hepatocellular stimulatory factor (interleukin-6) by Kupffer cells in both endotoxin tolerant and intolerant mice. *J Surg Res* 1992;52:635–641.

48. Bautista AP. Chronic alcohol intoxication enhances the expression of CD18 adhesion molecules on rat neutrophils and release of a chemotactic factor by Kupffer cells. *Alcohol Clin Exp Res* 1995;19:285–290.

49. Chensue SW, Terebuh PD, Remick DG, Scales WE, Kunkel SL. *In vivo* biologic and immunohistochemical analysis of interleukin-1α, β and tumor necrosis factor during experimental endotoxemia: kinetics, Kupffer cell expression, and glucocorticoid effects. *Am J Pathol* 1991;138:395–402.

50. Decker T, Lohmann-Matthes ML, Karck U, Peters T, Decker K. Comparative study of cytotoxicity, tumor necrosis factor, and prostaglandin release after stimulation of rat Kupffer cells, murine Kupffer cells, and murine inflammatory liver macrophages. *J Leukoc Biol* 1989;45:139–146.

51. Grewe M, Gausling R, Gyufko K, Hoffmann R, Decker K. Regulation of mRNA expression for tumor necrosis factor-alpha in rat liver macrophages. *J Hepatol* 1994;20:811–818.

52. Hoffmann R, Henninger H, Schulze-Specking A, Decker K. Regulation of interleukin-6 receptor expression in rat Kupffer cells: modulation by cytokines, dexamethasone and prostaglandin E_2. *J Hepatol* 1994;21:543–550.

53. Kawada N, Mizoguchi Y, Kobayashi K, Morisawa S, Monna T, Yamamoto S. Interferon-gamma modulates production of interleukin-1 and tumor necrosis factor by murine Kupffer cells. *Liver* 1991;11:42–47.

54. Hisama N, Yamaguchi Y, Miyanari N, Ichiguchi O, Goto M, Mori K, Ogawa M. Ischemia-reperfusion injury: the role of Kupffer cells in the production of cytokine-induced neutrophil chemoattractant, a member of the interleukin-8 family. *Transplant Proc* 1995;27:1604–1606.

55. Maher JJ. Rat hepatocytes and Kupffer cells interact to produce interleukin-8 (CINC) in the setting of ethanol. *Am J Physiol* 1995;269:G518–G523.

56. Ogle CK, Wu JZ, Mao X, Szczur K, Alexander JW, Ogle JD. Heterogeneity of Kupffer cells and splenic, alveolar, and peritoneal macrophages for the production of TNF, IL-1, and IL-6. *Inflammation* 1994;18:511–523.

57. Shirahama M, Ishibashi H, Tsuchiya Y, Kurokawa S, Okumura Y, Niho Y. Kinetics and parameters of the induction of interleukin-1 secretion by rat Kupffer cells. *J Clin Lab Immunol* 1988;27:127–132.

58. Tran-Thi TA, Weinhold L, Weinstock C, Hoffmann R, Schulze-Specking A, Northoff H, Decker K. Production of tumor necrosis factor-alpha, interleukin-1 and interleukin-6 in perfused rat liver. *Eur Cytokine Netw* 1993;4:363–370.

59. Tzung SP, Cohen SA. Endogenous interferon α/β produced by Kupffer cells inhibits interleukin-1, tumor necrosis factor alpha production and interleukin-2-induced activation of nonparenchymal cells. *Cancer Immunol Immunother* 1991;34:150–156.

60. Decker K. Biologically active products of stimulated liver macrophages (Kupffer cells). *Eur J Biochem* 1990;192:245–261.

61. Callery MP, Kamei T, Flye MW. Endotoxin stimulates interleukin-6 production by human Kupffer cells. *Circ Shock* 1992;37:185–188.

62. Busam KJ, Bauer TM, Bauer J, Gerok W, Decker K. Interleukin-6 release by rat liver macrophages. *J Hepatol* 1990;11:367–373.

63. Wisse E, Knook DL. The investigation of sinusoidal cells: a new approach to the study of liver function. *Prog Liver Dis* 1979;6:153–171.

64. Hahn E, Wick G, Pencev D, Timpl R. Distribution of basement membrane protein in normal and fibrotic human liver: collagen type IV, laminin, and fibronectin. *Gut* 1980;21:63–71.

65. Dini L, Lentini A, Diez GD, Rocha M, Falasca L, Serafino L, Vidal-Vanaclocha F. Phagocytosis of apoptotic bodies by liver endothelial cells. *J Cell Sci* 1995;108:967–973.

66. De Leeuw AM, Praaning-Van Dalen DP, Brouwer A, Knook DL. Endocytosis in liver sinusoidal endothelial cells. In: Wisse E, Knook DL, Decker K, eds. *Cells of the Hepatic Sinusoid* Vol. 2, Rijswijk: Kupffer Cell Foundation, 1989:94–98.

67. Smedstod B, Pertoft H, Eggertsen G, Sundstrom C. Functional and morphological characterization of cultures of Kupffer cells and liver endothelial cells prepared by means of density separation in Percoll, and selective substrate adherence. *Cell Tissue Res* 1985;241:639–649.
68. Kosugi I, Muro H, Shirasawa H, Ito I. Endocytosis of soluble IgG immune complex and its transport to lysosomes in hepatic sinusoidal endothelial cells. *J Hepatol* 1992;16:106–114.
69. Praaning-Van Dalen DP, De Leeuw AM, Brower A, Knook DL. Rat liver endothelial cells have a greater capacity that Kupffer cells to endocytose N-acetylglucosamine- and mannose-terminated glycoproteins. *Hepatology* 1987;7:672–679.
70. Smedsrod B, Pertoft H, Gustanfson S, Laurent TC. Scavenger functions of the liver endothelial cell. *Biochem J* 1990;266:313–327.
71. Steffan A-M, Gendrault J-L, McCuskey RS, McCuskey PA, Kirn A. Phagocytosis, an unrecognized property of murine endothelial liver cells. *Hepatology* 1986;6:830–836.
72. Shiratori Y, Jiñnai H, Teraoka H, Matano S, Matsumoto K, Kamii K, Tanaka M, Okano K. Phagocytic properties of hepatic endothelial cells and splenic macrophages compensating for a decreased phagocytic function of Kupffer cells in the chronically ethanol-fed rats. *Exp Cell Biol* 1989;57:300–309.
73. Bogers WMJM, Stad RK, Janssen DJ, Prins FA, Van Rooijen N, Vanes LA, Daha MR. Kupffer cell depletion *in vivo* results in clearance of large-sized IgA aggregates in rats by liver endothelial cells. *Clin Exp Immunol* 1991;85:128-136.
74. Hashimoto N, Watanabe T, Shiratori Y, Ikeda Y, Kato H, Han K, Yamada H, Toda G, Kurokawa K. Prostanoid secretion by rat hepatic sinusoidal endothelial cells and its regulation by exogenous adenosine triphosphate. *Hepatology* 1995;21:1713–1718.
75. Kuiper J, Zijlstra FJ, Kamps JA, van Berkel TJ. Identification of prostaglandin D_2 as the major eicosanoid from liver endothelial and Kupffer cells. *Biochim Biophys Acta* 1988;959:143–152.
76. Rieder H, Ramadori G, Allmann KH, Meyer zum Buschenfelde KH. Prostanoid release of cultured liver sinusoidal endothelial cells in response to endotoxin and tumor necrosis factor: comparison with umbilical vein endothelial cells. *J Hepatol* 1990;11:359–366.
77. Rosenbaum J, Mavier P, Preaux AM, Dhumeaux D. Demonstration of a basic fibroblast growth factor-like molecule in mouse hepatic endothelial cells. *Biochem Biophys Res Commun* 1989;164:1099–1104.
78. Feng Q, Hedner T. Endothelium-derived relaxing factor (EDRF) and nitric oxide (NO). I. Physiology, pharmacology and pathophysiology implications. *Clin Pharmacol* 1990;10:407–426.
79. Gardner CR, Laskin JD, Laskin DL. Platelet-activating factor-induced calcium mobilization and oxidative metabolism in hepatic macrophages and endothelial cells. *J Leukoc Biol* 1993;53:190–196.
80. Mc Closkey TW, Todaro JA, Feder LS, Gardner CR, Laskin DL. Activation of liver macrophages and endothelial cells following lipopolysaccharide treatment of rats. In: Wisse E, Knook DL, McCuskey R, eds. *Cells of the Hepatic Sinusoid* Vol. 3. Leiden: Kupffer Cell Foundation, 1991:112–114.
81. Misquith S, Wattiaux-De Coninck S, Wattiaux R. Intracellular degradation by liver endothelial cells. *Molec Cell Biochem* 1989;91:63–74.
82. Nolan KD, Keagy BA, Ramadan FM, Johnson G, Jr. Endothelial cells can synthesize leukotriene B_4. *J Vascular Surg* 1990;12:298–304.
83. Rodriguez de Turco EB, Spitzer JA. Eicosanoid production in nonparenchymal liver cells isolated from rats infused with *E. coli* endotoxin. *J Leukoc Biol* 1990;48:488–494.
84. Salvemini D, Korbut R, Anggard E, Vane JR. Lipopolysaccharide increases release of a nitric oxide-like factor from endothelial cells. *Eur J Pharmacol* 1989;171:135–136.
85. Sironi M, Breviario F, Proserpio P, Biondi A, Vecchi A, Van Damme J, Dejana E, Mantovani A. IL-1 stimulates IL-6 production in endothelial cells. *J Immunol* 1989;142:549–553.
86. Spolarics Z. Endotoxin stimulates gene expression of ROS-eliminating pathways in rat hepatic endothelial and Kupffer cells. *Am J Physiol* 1996;270:G660–G666.
87. Gorczynski RM, Cohen Z, Fu XM, Levy G, Plapler H, Sullivan B. Hepatic regulation of lymphocyte adhesion to, and activation on, syngeneic endothelial monolayers. *Immunology* 1994;83:58–64.
88. Komatsu Y, Shiratori Y, Kawase T, Hashimoto N, Han K, Shiina S, Matsumura M, Niwa Y, Kato H, Tada M, Ikeda Y, Tanaka M, Omata M. Role of polymorphonuclear leukocytes in galactosamine hepatitis: mechanism of adherence to hepatic endothelial cells. *Hepatology* 1994;20:1548–1556.
89. Ohira H, Ueno T, Shakado S, Sakamoto M, Torimura J, Inuzuka S, Sata M, Tanikawa K. Cultured rat hepatic endothelial cells express intercellular adhesion molecule-1 (ICAM-1) by tumor necrosis factor-alpha or interleukin-1alpha stimulation. *J Hepatol* 1994;20:729–734.

90. Schlayer HJ, Karck U, Ganter U, Hermann R, Decker K. Enhancement of neutrophil adherence to isolated rat liver sinusoidal endothelial cells by supernatants of lipopolysaccharide-activated monocytes: role of tumor necrosis factor. *J Hepatol* 1987;5:311–321.

91. Aronson FR, Libby P, Brandon EP, Janicka MW, Mier JW. IL-2 rapidly induces natural killer cell adhesion to human endothelial cells: a potential mechanism for endothelial injury. *J Immunol* 1988;141:158–163.

92. Dejana E, Breviario F, Caveda L. Leukocyte-endothelial cell adhesive receptors. *Clin Exp Rheumatol* 1994;12:S25–S28.

93. Doherty DE, Zagarella L, Henson PM, Worthen GS. Lipopolysaccharide stimulates monocyte adherence by effects on both the monocyte and the endothelial cell. *J Immunol* 1989;143:3673–3679.

94. Scoazec JY, Feldmann G. The cell adhesion molecules of hepatic sinusoidal endothelial cells. *J Hepatol* 1994;20:296–300.

95. Blomhoff R, Wake K. Perisinusoidal stellate cells of the liver: important roles in retinol metabolism and fibrosis. *FASEB J* 1991;5:271–277.

96. Matsuura T, Nagamori S, Fijise K, Hasumura S, Homma S, Sujino H, Shimizu H, Niiya M, Kameda H. Retinol transport in cultured fat-storing cells of rat liver. *Lab Invest* 1989;61:107–115.

97. Hendriks HF, Verhoofstad WA, Brouwer A, De Leeuw AM, Knook DL. Perisinusoidal fat-storing cells are the main vitamin A storage cells in rat liver. *Exp Cell Res* 1985;160:138–149.

98. Ogata I, Mochida S, Tomiya T, Fujiwara W. Minor contribution of hepatocytes to collagen production in normal and early fibrotic rat livers. *Hepatology* 1991;14:361–367.

99. Shiratori Y, Ichida T, Geerts A, Wisse E. Modulation of collagen synthesis by fat-storing cells, isolated from CCl₄- or vitamin A-treated rats. *Digestive Dis Sci* 1987;32:1281–1289.

100. Arthur MJ, Stanley A, Iredale JP, Rafferty JA, Hembry RM, Friedman SL. Secretion of 72 kDa type IV collagenase/gelatinase by cultured human lipocytes: analysis of gene expression, protein synthesis and proteinase activity. *Biochem J* 1992;287:701–707.

101. Friedman SL. Cellular sources of collagen and regulation of collagen production in liver. *Semin Liver Dis* 1990;10:20–29.

102. Friedman SL, Roll FJ, Boyles JK, Bissell DM. Hepatic lipocytes: the principle collagen-producing cells of normal rat liver. *Proc Natl Acad Sci USA* 1985;82:8681–8685.

103. Geerts A, Vrijsen R, Rauterberg J, Burt A, Schellinck P, Wisse E. *In vitro* differentiation of fat-storing cells parallels marked increase of collagen synthesis and secretion. *J Hepatol* 1989;9:59–68.

104. Loreal O, Levavasseur F, Fromaget C, Gros D, Guillouzo A, Clement B. Cooperation of Ito cells and hepatocytes in the deposition of an extracellular matrix *in vitro. Am J Pathol* 1993;143:538–544.

105. Weiner FR, Giambrone MA, Czaja MJ, Shah A, Annoni G, Takahashi S, Eghbali M, Zern MA. Ito-cell expression and collagen regulation. *Hepatology* 1990;11:111–117.

106. Athari A, Hanecke K, Jungermann K. Prostaglandin F₂ alpha and D₂ release from primary Ito cell cultures after stimulation with noradrenaline and ATP but not adenosine. *Hepatology* 1994;20:142–148.

107. Xu Y, Rojkind M, Czaja MJ. Regulation of monocyte chemoattractant protein 1 by cytokines and oxygen free radicals in rat hepatic fat-storing cells. *Gastroenterology* 1996;110:1870–1877.

108. Marra F, Grandaliano G, Valente AJ, Abboud HE. Thrombin stimulates proliferation of liver fat-storing cells and expression of monocyte chemotactic protein-1: potential role in liver injury. *Hepatology* 1995;22:780–787.

109. Marra F, Valente AJ, Pinzani M, Abboud HE. Cultured human liver fat-storing cells produce monocyte chemotactic protein-1. Regulation by proinflammatory cytokines. *J Clin Invest* 1993;92:1674–1680.

110. Bachem MG, Sell KM, Melchior R, Kropf J, Eller T, Gressner AM. Tumor necrosis factor α (TNF α) and transforming growth factor β1 (TGF β1) stimulate fibronectin synthesis and the transdifferentiation of fat-storing cells in the rat liver into myofibroblasts. *Virchows Arch B Cell Pathol Incl Mol Pathol* 1993;63:123–130.

111. Knittel T, Janneck T, Muller L, Fellmer P, Ramadori G. Transforming growth factor β 1-regulated gene expression of Ito cells. *Hepatology* 1996;24:352–360.

112. Ramadori G, Knittel T, Odenthal M, Schwogler S, Neubauer K, Meyer zum Buschenfelde K. Synthesis of cellular fibronectin by rat liver fat-storing (Ito) cells: regulation by cytokines. *Gastroenterology* 1992;103:1313–1321.

113. Davis BH, Kramer RT, Davidson NO. Retinoic acid modulates rat Ito cell proliferation, collagen, and transforming growth factor β production. *J Clin Invest* 1990;86:2062–2070.

114. Helyar L, Bundschuh DS, Laskin JD, Laskin DL. Hepatic fat storing cells produce nitric oxide and hydrogen peroxide in response to bacterially-derived lipopolysaccharide. In: Knook DL, Decker K, eds. *Cells of the Hepatic Sinusoid* Vol. 4. Leiden: Kupffer Cell Foundation, 1993;394–396.
115. Helyar L, Bundschuh DS, Laskin JD, Laskin DL. Induction of hepatic Ito cell nitric oxide production by acute endotoxemia. *Hepatology* 1994;12:1509–1515.
116. Laskin DL, Pilaro AM, Ji S. Potential role of macrophages in acetaminophen hepatotoxicity. II. Mechanisms of macrophage accumulation and activation. *Toxicol Appl Pharmacol* 1986;86:216–226.
117. Shiratori Y, Hai K, Takada H, Kiriyama H, Nagura T, Matsumoto K, Kamii K, Okano T, Tanaka M. Mechanism of accumulation of macrophages in galactosamine-induced liver injury: effect of lipoxygenase inhibitors on chemotaxis of spleen cells. *Pathobiology* 1992;60:316–321.
118. Thompson WD, Jack AS, Patrick RS. Possible role of macrophages in transient hepatic fibrogenesis induced by acute carbon tetrachloride injury. *J Pathol* 1980;130:65–73.
119. Lloyd RS, Triger DR. Studies on hepatic uptake of antigen. III. Studies of liver macrophage function in normal rats and following carbon tetrachloride administration. *Immunology* 1975;29:253–263.
120. Edwards MJ, Keller BJ, Kauffman FC, Thurman RG. The involvement of Kupffer cells in carbon tetrachloride toxicity. *Toxicol Appl Pharmacol* 1993;119:275–279.
121. Towner RA, Reinke LA, Janzen EG, Yamashiro S. *In vivo* magnetic resonance imaging study of Kupffer cell involvement in CCl_4-induced hepatotoxicity in rats. *Can J Physiol Pharmacol* 1994;72:441–446.
122. Shiratori Y, Tanaka M, Hai K, Kawase T, Shirna S, Sugimoto T. Role of endotoxin-responsive macrophages in hepatic injury. *Hepatology* 1990;11:183–192.
123. Jonker AM, Kijkhuis FW, Kroese FG, Hardonk MJ, Grond J. Immunopathology of acute galactosamine hepatitis in rats. *Hepatology* 1990;11:622–627.
124. Przybocki JM, Reuhl KR, Thurman RG, Kauffman FC. Involvement of nonparenchymal cells in oxygen-dependent hepatic injury by allyl alcohol. *Toxicol Appl Pharmacol* 1992;115:57–63.
125. Belinsky SA, Popp JA, Kauffman FC, Thurman RG. Trypan blue uptake as a new method to investigate hepatotoxicity in periportal and pericentral regions of the liver lobule: studies with allyl alcohol in the perfused liver. *J Pharmacol Exp Ther* 1984;230:755–760.
126. James R, Desmond P, Kupfer A, Schenker S, Branch RA. The differential localization of various drug metabolizing systems within the rat liver lobule as determined by the hepatotoxins ally alcohol, carbon tetrachloride and bromobenzene. *J Pharmacol Exp Ther* 1981;217:127–132.
127. Laskin DL, Gardner CR, Price VF, Jollow DJ. Modulation of macrophage functioning abrogates the acute hepatotoxicity of acetaminophen. *Hepatology* 1995;21:1045–1050.
128. Laskin DL. Sinusoidal lining cells and hepatotoxicity. *Toxicol Pathol* 1996;24:112–118.
129. MacDonald JR, Beckstead JH, Smuckler EA. An ultrastructural and histochemical study of the prominent inflammatory response in D(+)-galactosamine hepatotoxicity. *Br J Exp Pathol* 1987;68:189–199.
130. Laskin DL. Nonparenchymal cells and hepatotoxicity. *Semin Liver Dis* 1990;10:293–304.
131. Earnst DL, Brouwer A, Sim W, Horan MA, Hendriks HF, De Leeuw AM, Knook DL. Hypervitaminosis A activates Kupffer cells and lowers the threshold for endotoxin liver injury. In: Kirn A, Knook DL, Wisse E, eds. *Cells of the Hepatic Sinusoid* Vol. 1. Rijswijk: Kupffer Cell Foundation, 1986;277–283.
132. elSisi AE, Earnest DL, Sipes IG. Vitamin A potentiation of carbon tetrachloride hepatotoxicity: role of liver macrophages and active oxygen species. *Toxicol Appl Pharmacol* 1993;119:295–301.
133. Ferluga J, Allison AC. Role of mononuclear infiltrating cells in the pathogenesis of hepatitis. *Lancet* 1978;2:610–611.
134. Freudenberg MA, Keppler D, Galanos C. Requirement for lipopolysaccharide-responsive macrophages in galactosamine-induced sensitization to endotoxin. *Infect Immun* 1986;51:891–895.
135. Sudhir S, Budhiraja RD. Comparison of the protective effect of Withaferin-A and hydrocortisone against CCl_4 induced hepatotoxicity in rats. *Indian J Physiol Pharmacol* 1992;36:127–129.
136. Stenger RJ, Petrelli M, McPath DCP, Segel A. Modification of carbon tetrachloride hepatotoxicity by prior loading of the reticuloendothelial system with carbon particles. *Am J Pathol* 1969;57:689–697.
137. Ishiyama H, Ogino K, Hobara T. Kupffer cells in rat liver injury induced by diethyldithiocarbamate. *Eur J Pharmacol* 1995;292:135–141.
138. Iimuro Y, Yamamoto M, Kohno H, Itakura J, Fujii H, Matsumoto Y. Blockade of liver macrophages by gadolinium chloride reduces lethality in endotoxemic rats: analysis of mechanisms of lethality in endotoxemia. *J Leukoc Biol* 1994;55:723–728.

139. Knecht KT, Adachi Y, Bradford BU, Iimuro Y, Kadiiska M, Xuang QH, Thurman RG. Free radicals adducts in the bile of rats treated chronically with intragastric alcohol: inhibition by destruction of Kupffer cells. *Mol Pharmacol* 1995;47:1028–1034.
140. Chamulitrat W, Blazaka ME, Jordan SJ, Luster MI, Mason RP. Tumor necrosis factor-α and nitric oxide production in endotoxin-primed rats administered carbon tetrachloride. *Life Sci* 1995;57:2273–2280.
141. Al-Tuwaijri A, Akdamar K, Di Luzio NR. Modification of galactosamine-induced liver injury in rats by reticuloendothelial system stimulation or depression. *Hepatology* 1981;1:107–113.
142. Chojkier M, Fierer J. D-Galactosamine hepatotoxicity is associated with endotoxin sensitivity and mediated by lymphoreticular cells in mice. *Gastroenterology* 1985;88:115–121.
143. Galanos C, Freudenberg MA, Reuter W. Galactosamine-induced sensitization to the lethal effects of endotoxin. *Proc Natl Acad Sci USA* 1979;76:5939–5943.
144. Nolan JP, Leibowitz AI. Endotoxin and the liver. III. Modification of acute carbon tetrachloride injury by polymyxin B—an antiendotoxin. *Gastroenterology* 1978;75:445–449.
145. Sauer JM, Hooser SB, Badger DA, Baines A, Sipes IG. Alterations in chemically induced tissue injury related to all-*trans*-retinol pretreatment in rodents. *Drug Metabol Rev* 1995;27:299–323.
146. Tiegs G, Wolter M, Wendel A. Tumor necrosis factor is a terminal mediator in galactosamine/endotoxin-induced hepatitis in mice. *Biochem Pharmacol* 1989;38:627–631.
147. Vajta G, Kovacs L, Lapis K. Light, fluorescence and electron microscopic observations on vitamin A storing cells in allyl-alcohol induced liver damage. *Acta Morphol Acad Sci Hung* 1982;30:309–317.
148. Rockey DC, Housset CN, Friedman SL. Activation-dependent contractility of rat hepatic lipocytes in culture and *in vivo*. *J Clin Invest* 1993;92:1795–1804.
149. Rockey DC, Maher JJ, Jarnagin WR, Gabbiani G, Friedman SL. Inhibition of rat hepatic lipocyte activation in culture by interferon-gamma. *Hepatology* 1992;16:776–784.
150. Friedman SL, Arthur MJ. Activation of cultured rat hepatic lipocytes by Kupffer cell conditioned medium. Direct enhancement of matrix synthesis and stimulation of cell proliferation via induction of platelet-derived growth factor receptors. *J Clin Invest* 1989;84:1780–1785.
151. Gressner AM. Cytokines and cellular crosstalk involved in the activation of fat-storing cells. *J Hepatol* 1995;22:28–36.
152. Kilbourn RG, Belloni P. Endothelial cell production of nitrogen oxides in response to interferon gamma in combination with tumor necrosis factor, interleukin-1, or endotoxin. *J Natl Cancer Inst* 1990;82:772–776.
153. Laskin DL, Gardner CR, Feder LS, Heck DE, Laskin JD. Nitric oxide derived from nonparenchymal liver cells (NPC) as a mediator of hepatotoxicity: (abstr.) *The Toxicologist* 1991;11:170.
154. Pober JS, Cotran RS. The role of endothelial cells in inflammation. *Transplantation* 1990;50:537–544.
155. Spolarics Z, Spitzer JJ, Wang JF, Xie J, Kolls J, Greenberg S. Alcohol administration attenuates LPS-induced expression of inducible nitric oxide synthase in Kupffer and hepatic endothelial cells. *Biochem Biophys Res Commun* 1993;197:606–611.
156. Arditi M, Zhou J, Huang SH, Luckett PM, Marra MN, Kim KS. Bactericidal/permeability-increasing protein protects vascular endothelial cells from lipopolysacchride-induced activation and injury. *Infect Immun* 1994;62:3930–3936.
157. Doukas J, Cutler AH, Mordes JP. Polyinosinic:polycytidylic acid is a potent activator of endothelial cells. *Am J Pathol* 1994;145:137–147.
158. Fibbe WE, Daha MR, Hiemstra PS, DuinKerKen N, Lurvink E, Ralph P, Altrock BW, Kaushansky K, Willemze R, Falkeuburg JHF. Interleukin 1 and poly (rI).poly(rC) induce production of granulocyte CSF, macrophage CSF, and granulocyte-macrophage CSF by human endothelial cells. *Exp Hematol* 1989;17:229–234.
159. Herbert CA, Luscinskas FW, Kiely J-M, Luis EA, Darbonne WC, Bennett GL, Liu CC, Obin MS, Gimbroue MA, Jr., Baker JB. Endothelial and leukocyte forms of IL-8: conversion by thrombin and interactions with neutrophils. *J Immunol* 1990;145:3033–3040.
160. Jirik FR, Podor TJ, Hirano T, Kishimoto T, Loskutoff DJ, Carson DA, Lotz M. Bacterial lipopolysaccharide and inflammatory mediators augment IL-6 secretion by human endothelial cells. *J Immunol* 1989;142:144–147.
161. Libby P, Ordovas J, Auger K, Robbins A, Birinyl L, Dinarello C. Endotoxin and tumor necrosis factor induce interleukin-1 gene expression in adult human vascular endothelial cells. *Am J Pathol* 1986;124:179–185.
162. Loppnow H, Libby P. Adult human vascular endothelial cells express the IL-6 gene differently in response to LPS or IL-1. *Cell Immunol* 1989;122:493–503.

163. Loppnow H, Libby P. Comparative analysis of cytokine induction in human vascular endothelial and smooth muscle cells. *Lymphokine Res* 1989;8:293–299.
164. Miossec P, Cavender D, Ziff M. Production of interleukin-1 by human endothelial cells. *J Immunol* 1986;136:2486–2491.
165. Modat G, Dornand J, Bernad N, Junguero D, Mary A, Muller A, Bonne C. LPS-stimulated bovine aortic endothelial cells produce IL-1 and IL-6 like activities. *Agents Actions* 1990;30:403–411.
166. Norioka K, Hara M, Harigai M, Kitani, Hirose T, Suzuki K, Kawakumi M, Tabata H, Kawagoe M, Nakamura H. Production of B cell stimulatory factor-2/interleukin-6 activity by human endothelial cells. *Biochem Biophys Res Commun* 1988;153:1045–1050.
167. Phan SH, Gharaee-Kermani M, McGarry B, Kunkel SL, Wolber FW. Regulation of rat pulmonary artery endothelial cell transforming growth factor-α production by IL-1α and tumor necrosis factor-α. *J Immunol* 1992;149:103–106.
168. Sica A, Wang JM, Colotta F, Dejana E, Mantovani A, Oppenheim JJ, Larsen CG, Zachariae COC, Matsushima K. Monocyte chemotactic and activating factor gene expression induced in endothelial cells by IL-1 and tumor necrosis factor. *J Immunol* 1990;144:3034–3038.
169. Strieter R, Kunkel SL, Showell H, Remick D, Phan SH, Ward P, Marks R. Endothelial cell gene expression of neutrophil chemotactic factor by TNF-α, LPS and IL-1 β. *Science* 1989;17:1467–1469.
170. Suschek C, Rothe H, Fehsel K, Enczmann J, Kolb-Bachofen V. Induction of a macrophage-like nitric oxide synthase in cultured rat aortic endothelial cells: IL-1 α-mediated induction regulated by tumor necrosis factor-α and IFN-γ. *J Immunol* 1993;151:3283–3291.
171. Warner SJC, Auger KR, Libby P. Interleukin-1 induces interleukin-1: recombinant human interleukin-1 production by adult human vascular endothelial cells. *J Immunol* 1987;139:1911–1917.
172. Yoshizumi M, Kurihara H, Morita T, Yamashita J, Oh-hashi MI, Sugiyama J, Takaku F, Yanagisawa M, Masaki T, Yazaki Y. Interleukin-1 increases the production of endothelin-1 by cultured endothelial cells. *Biochem Biophys Res Commun* 1990;166:324–329.
173. Bertini R, Bianchi M, Erroi A, Villa P, Ghezzi P. Dexamethasone modulation of in vivo effects of endotoxin, tumor necrosis factor, and interleukin-1 on liver cytochrome P-450, plasma fibrinogen, and serum iron. *J Leukoc Biol* 1989;46:254–262.
174. Hagiwara T, Suzuki H, Kono I, Kashiwagi H, Akiyama Y, Onozaki K. Regulation of fibronectin synthesis by interleukin-1 and interleukin-6 in rat hepatocytes. *Am J Pathol* 1990;136:39–47.
175. Tsutsumi Y, Kakumu S, Yoshioka K, Arao M, Inoue M, Wakita T. Effects of various cytokines on collagen synthesis by normal rat hepatocytes in primary cultures and fibroblasts. *Digestion* 1989;44:191–199.
176. Lin B-F, Ku N-O, Zahedi K, Whitehead AS, Mortensen RF. IL-1 and IL-6 mediate increased production and synthesis by hepatocytes of acute-phase reactant mouse serum amyloid p-component (SAP). *Inflammation* 1990;14:297–313.
177. Pous C, Giroud J-P, Damais C, Raichvarg D, Chauvelot-Moachon L. Effect of recombinant human interleukin-1β and tumor necrosis factor α on liver cytochrome P-450 and serum α-1-acid glycoprotein concentrations in the rat. *Drug Metabol Disposit* 1990;18:467–470.
178. Curran RD, Billiar TR, Stuehr DJ, Ochoa JB, Harbrecht BG, Flint SG, Simmons RL. Multiple cytokines are required to induce hepatocyte nitric oxide production and inhibit total protein synthesis. *Ann Surg* 1990;212:462–469.
179. Tilg H, Wilmer A, Vogel W, Herold M, Nolchen B, Judmaier G, Huber C. Serum levels of cytokines in chronic liver diseases. *Gastroenterology* 1992;103:264–274.
180. Fey GH, Hocke GM, Wilson DR, Ripperger JA, Juan TS-C, Cui M-Z, Darlington GJ. Cytokines and the acute phase response of the liver. In: Arias IM, Boyer JL, Fausto N, Jakoby WB, Schachter DA, Shafritz DA, eds. *The Liver: Biology and Pathology,* 3rd ed. New York: Raven Press, 1994:113–143.
181. Shedlofsky SI, McClain CJ. Hepatic dysfunction due to cytokines. In: Kimball ES, ed. *Cytokines and inflammation.* Boca Raton: CRC Press, 1991:235–273.
182. Volpes R, van den Oord JJ, Desmet VJ. Can hepatocytes serve as "activated" immunomodulating cells in the immune response? *J Hepatol* 1992;16:228–240.
183. Larrick JW, Kunkel SL. The role of tumor necrosis factor and interleukin 1 in the immunoinflammatory response. *Pharmaceut Res* 1988;5:129–139.
184. Sherry B, Cerami A. Cachectin/tumor necrosis factor exerts endocrine, paracrine, and autocrine control of inflammatory responses. *J Cell Biol* 1988;107:1269–1277.
185. Whicher JT, Evans SW. Cytokines in disease. *Clin Chem* 1990;36/7:1269–1281.
186. Dinarello CA. Biology of interleukin 1. *FASEB J* 1988;2:108–115.

187. Cerami A. Inflammatory cytokines. *Clin Immunol Immunopathol* 1992;62:S3–S10.
188. Detmar M, Tenorio S, Hettmannsperger U, Ruszczak Z, Orfanos CE. Cytokine regulation of proliferation and ICAM-1 expression of human dermal microvascular endothelial cells *in vitro. J Invest Dermatol* 1992;98:147–153.
189. Helle M, Boeije L, Aarden LA. IL-6 is an intermediate in IL-1 induced thymocyte proliferation. *J Immunol* 1989;12:4335–4338.
190. Sztein M, Vogel S, Sipe J, Murphy P, Mizel S, Oppenheim J, Rosenstreich D. The role of macrophages in the acute-phase response: SAA inducer is closely related to lymphocyte activating factor and endogenous pyrogen. *Cell Immunol* 1981;63:164–176.
191. Bollag W, Peck R, Frey JR. Inhibition of proliferation by retinoids, cytokines and their combination in four human transformed epithelial cell lines. *Cancer Lett* 1992;62:167–172.
192. Sherwood ER, Williams DL, McNamee RB, Jones EL, Browder IW, Di Luzio NR. Enhancement of interleukin-1 and interleukin-2 production by soluble glucan. *Br J Immunopharmacol* 1987;9:261–267.
193. Saklatvala J, Sarsfield SJ, Townsend Y. Pig interleukin. 1. Purification of two immunologically different leukocyte proteins that cause cartilage resorption, lymphocyte activation, and fever. *J Exp Med* 1985;162:1208–1222.
194. Punjabi CJ, Laskin JD, Hwang S-M, MacEachern L, Laskin DL. Enhanced production of nitric oxide by bone marrow cells and increased sensitivity to macrophage colony-stimulating factor (CSF) and granulocyte-macrophage CSF after benzene treatment of mice. *Blood* 1994;83:3255–3262.
195. Lavnikova N, Drapier J-C, Laskin DL. A single exogenous stimulus activates rat macrophages for nitric oxide production and cytotoxicity. *J Leukoc Biol* 1993;54:322–328.
196. Hibbs JB Jr, Taintor RR, Vavrin Z, Rachlin EM. Nitric oxide: a cytotoxic activated macrophage effector molecule. *Biochem Biophys Res Commun* 1988;157:87–94.
197. Hori K, Ehrke MJ, Mace K, Maccubbin D, Doyle MJ, Otsuka Y, Mihich E. Effect of recombinant human tumor necrosis factor on the induction of murine macrophage tumoricidal activity. *Cancer Res* 1987;47:2793–2798.
198. Mace KF, Ehrke MJ, Hori K, Maccubbin DL, Mihich E. Role of tumor necrosis factor in macrophage activation and tumoricidal activity. *Cancer Res* 1988;48:5427–5432.
199. Kos FJ. Augmentation of recombinant interleukin-2-dependent murine macrophage-mediated tumor cytotoxicity by recombinant tumor necrosis factor-α. *Immunol Cell Biol* 1989;67:433–436.
200. Reif DW, Simmons RD. Nitric oxide mediates iron release from ferritin. *Arch Biochem Biophys* 1990;283:537–541.
201. Keller R, Keist R, Wechsler A, Leist TP, van der Meide PH. Mechanisms of macrophage-mediated tumor cell killing: a comparative analysis of the roles of reactive nitrogen intermediates and tumor necrosis factor. *Int J Cancer* 1990;46:682–686.
202. Denis M. Tumor necrosis factor and granulocyte macrophage-colony stimulating factor stimulate human macrophages to restrict growth of virulent Mycobacterium avium and to kill avirulent *M. avium*: Killing effector mechanism depends on the generation of reactive nitrogen intermediates. *J Leukoc Biol* 1991;49:380–387.
203. Woods KM, Chapes SK. Three distinct cell phenotypes of induced-TNF cytotoxicity and their relationship to apoptosis. *J Leukoc Biol* 1993;53:37–45.
204. Bonta IL, Ben-Efraim S. Involvement of inflammatory mediators in macrophage antitumor activity. *J Leukoc Biol* 1993;54:613–626.
205. Hoffman M, Weinberg JB. Tumor necrosis factor-α induces increased hydrogen peroxide production and Fc receptor expression, but not increased Ia antigen expression by peritoneal macrophages. *J Leukoc Biol* 1987;42:704–707.
206. Kharazmi A, Nielsen H, Bendtzen K. Modulation of human neutrophil and monocyte chemotaxis and superoxide responses by recombinant TNF-α and GM-CSF. *Immunobiol* 1988;177:363–370.
207. Kownatzki E, Kapp A, Uhrich S. Modulation of human neutrophilic granulocyte functions by recombinant human tumor necrosis factor and recombinant human lymphotoxin. Promotion of adherence, inhibition of chemotactic migration and superoxide anion release from adherent cells. *Clin Exp Immunol* 1988;74:143–148.
208. Paubert-Braquet M, Hosford D, Klotz P, Guibaud J, Braquet P. Tumor necrosis factor-α "primes" the platelet-activating factor-induced superoxide production by human neutrophils: possible involvement of G proteins. *J Lipid Mediators* 1990;2:S1–S14.
209. McColl SR, Beauseigle D, Gilbert C, Naccache PH. Priming of the human neutrophil respiratory burst by granulocyte-macrophage colony-stimulating factor and tumor necrosis factor-α involves regulation at a post-cell surface receptor level. *J Immunol* 1990;145:3047–3053.

210. Humbert JR, Winsor EL. Tumor necrosis factor primes neutrophils by shortening the lag period of the respiratory burst. *Am J Med Sci* 1990;299:209–213.
211. Ferrante A, Hauptmann B, Seckinger P, Dayer J-M. Inhibition of tumour necrosis factor alpha (TNF-α)-induced neutrophil respiratory burst by a TNF inhibitor. *Immunology* 1991;72:440–442.
212. Nathan CF. Neutrophil activation on biological surfaces: massive secretion of hydrogen peroxide in response to products of macrophages and lymphocytes. *J Clin Invest* 1987;80:1550–1560.
213. Waga I, Nakamura M, Honda Z-i, Ferbij I, Toyoshima S, Ishiguro S, Shimizu T. Two distinct signal transduction pathways for the activation of guinea-pig macrophages and neutrophils by endotoxin. *Biochem Biophys Res Commun* 1993;197:465–472.
214. Sujita K, Okuno F, Tanaka Y, Hirano Y, Inamoto Y, Eto S, Arai M. Effect of interleukin 1 (IL-1) on the level of cytochrome P-450 involving IL-1 receptor on the isolated hepatocytes of rat. *Biochem Biophys Res Commun* 1990;168:1217–1222.
215. Kriegler M, Perez C, DeFay K, Albert I, Lu SD. A novel form of TNF/cachectin is a cell surface cytotoxic transmembrane protein: ramifications for the complex physiology of TNF. *Cell* 1988;53:45–53.
216. Suffys P, Beyaert R, Van Roy F, Fiers W. Reduced tumour necrosis factor-induced cytotoxicity by inhibitors of the arachidonic acid metabolism. *Biochem Biophys Res Comm* 1987;149:735–743.
217. Hepburn A, Boeynaems J-M, Fiers W, Dumont JE. Modulation of tumor necrosis factor-α cytotoxicity in L929 cells by bacterial toxins, hydrocortisone and inhibitors of arachidonic acid metabolism. *Biochem Biophys Res Comm* 1987;149:815–822.
218. Spitzer JA. Cytokine stimulation of nitric oxide formation and differential regulation in hepatocytes and nonparenchymal cells of endotoxemic rats. *Hepatology* 1994;19:217–228.
219. Nussler AK, Beger H-G, Liu ZZ, Billiar TR. Nitric oxide, hepatocytes and inflammation. *Res Immunol* 1995;146:671–677.
220. Fey GH, Gauldie J. The acute phase response of the liver in inflammation. *Prog Liver Dis* 1990;9:89–116.
221. Dinarello CA. Interleukin-1 and its biologically related cytokines. *Adv Immunol* 1989;44:153–205.
222. Fiedler VB, Loof I, Sander E, Voehringer V, Galanos C, Fournel MA. Monoclonal antibody to tumor necrosis factor-α prevents lethal endotoxin sepsis in adult rhesus monkeys. *J Lab Clin Med* 1992;120:574–588.
223. Russell DA, Tucker KK, Chinookoswong N, Thompson RC, Koho T. Combined inhibition of interleukin-1 and tumor necrosis factor in rodent endotoxemia: improved survival and organ function. *J Infect Dis* 1995;171:1528–1538.
224. Hishinuma I, Nagakawa J, Hirota K, Miyamoto K, Tsukidate K, Yamanaka T, Katayama K, Yamatsu I. Involvement of tumor necrosis factor-α in development of hepatic injury in galactosamine-sensitized mice. *Hepatology* 1990;12:1187–1191.
225. Kayama F, Yoshida T, Elwell MR, Luster MI. Role of tumor necrosis factor-α in cadmium-induced hepatotoxicity. *Toxicol Appl Pharmacol* 1995;131:224–234.
226. Czaja MJ, Xu J, Alt E. Prevention of carbon tetrachloride-induced rat liver injury by soluble tumor necrosis factor receptor. *Gastroenterology* 1995;108:1849–1854.
227. Gardner CR, Barton D, Goller N, Durham S, Laskin DL. Role of tumor necrosis factor-α and nitric oxide in acetaminophen hepatotoxicity (abstr.). *The Toxicologist* 1995;15:136.
228. Silva AT, Bayston KF, Cohen J. Prophylatic and therapeutic effects of a monoclonal antibody to tumor necrosis factor-α in experimental gram-negative shock. *J Infect Dis* 1990;162:421–427.
229. Blazaka ME, Wilmer JL, Holladay SD, Wilson RE, Luster MI. Role of proinflammatory cytokines in acetaminophen hepatotoxicity. *Toxicol Appl Pharmacol* 1995;133:43–52.
230. Mancuso G, Cusumano V, Cook JA, Smith E, Squadlrito F, Blandino G, Teti G. Efficacy of tumor necrosis factor alpha and eicosanoid inhibitors in experimental models of neonatal sepsis. *FEMS Immunol Med Microbiol* 1994;9:49–54.
231. Dinarello CA. Interleukin-1 and interleukin-1 antagonism. *Blood* 1991;77:1627–1652.
232. Zerbe O, Gressner AM. Proliferation of fat-storing cells is stimulated by secretions of Kupffer cells from normal and injured liver. *Exp Mol Pathol* 1988;49:87–101.
233. Tsukamoto H, Cheng S, Blaner WS. Effects of dietary polyunsaturated fat on ethanol-induced Ito cell activation. *Am J Physiol* 1996;270:G581–G586.
234. Kakumu S, Fukatsu A, Shinagawa T, Kurokawa S, Kusakabe A. Localisation of intrahepatic inter-leukin 6 in patients with acute and chronic liver disease. *J Clin Pathol* 1992;45:408–411.

235. Czaja MJ, Flanders KC, Biempica L, Klein C, Zern MA, Weiner FR. Expression of tumor necrosis factor-α and transforming growth factor-β1 in acute liver injury. *Growth Factors* 1989;1:219–226.
236. Babior BM. Oxidants from phagocytes: agents of defense and destruction. *Blood* 1984;64:959–966.
237. Del Maestro RF, Thaw H, Bjork J, Planker M, Arfors KE. Free radicals as mediators of tissue injury. *Acta Physiol Scand* 1980;492(suppl):43–57.
238. Fantone JC, Ward PA. Role of oxygen-derived free radicals and metabolites in leukocyte-dependent inflammatory reactions. *Am J Pathol* 1982;107:397–418.
239. Halliwell B, Gutteridge JMC. Oxygen toxicity, oxygen radicals, transition metals and disease. *Biochem J* 1984;219:1-14.
240. Rubin R, Farber JL. Mechanisms of the killing of cultured hepatocytes with hydrogen peroxide. *Arch Biochem Biophys* 1984;228:450–459.
241. Sevanian A, Hochstein P. Mechanisms and consequences of lipid peroxidation in biological systems. *Annu Rev Nutr* 1985;5:365–390.
242. Guanawardhana L, Mobley SA, Sipes IG. Modulation of 1,2-dichlorobenzene hepatotoxicity in the Fischer-344 rat by a scavenger of superoxide anions and an inhibitor of Kupffer cells. *Toxicol Appl Pharmacol* 1993;119:205–213.
243. Nakae D, Yamamoto K, Yoshiji H, Kinugawa T, Maruyama H, Farber JL, Konishi Y. Liposome-encapsulated superoxide dismutase prevents liver necrosis induced by acetaminophen. *Am J Pathol* 1990;136:787–795.
244. Kyle ME, Miccadei S, Nakae D, Farber JL. Superoxide dismutase and catalase protect cultured hepatocytes from the cytotoxicity of acetaminophen. *Biochem Biophys Res Comm* 1987;149:889–896.
245. Kyle ME, Nakae D, Sakaida I, Miccadei S, Farber JL. Endocytosis of superoxide dismutase is required in order for the enzyme to protect hepatocytes from the cytotoxicity of hydrogen peroxide. *J Biol Chem* 1988;263:3784–3789.
246. Fujita S, Arai S, Monden K, Adachi Y, Funaki N, Higashitsuji H. Participation of hepatic macrophages and plasma factors in endotoxin-induced liver injury. *J Surg Res* 1995;59:263–270.
247. Ma TT, Ischiropoulos H, Brass CA. Endotoxin-stimulated nitric oxide production increases injury and reduces rat liver chemiluminescence during reperfusion. *Gastroenterology* 1995;108:463–469.
248. Amimoto T, Matsura T, Koyama SY, Nakanishi T, Yamada K, Kajiyama G. Acetaminophen-induced hepatic injury in mice: the role of lipid peroxidation and effects of pretreatment with coenzyme Q10 and alpha-tocopherol. *Free Radical Biol Med* 1995;19:169–176.
249. Nagabubu E, Sesikeran B, Lakshmaiah L. The protective effects of eugeol on carbon tetrachloride induced hepatotoxicity in rats. *Free Radical Res* 1995;23:617–627.
250. Sugino K, Dohi K, Yamada K, Kawaski T. Changes in the levels of endogenous antioxidants in the liver of mice with experimental endotoxemia and the protective effects of antioxidants. *Surgery* 1989;105:200–206.
251. Gross SS, Wolin MS. Nitric oxide: pathophysiological mechanisms. *Annu Rev Physiol* 1995;57:737–769.
252. Bredt DS, Snyder SH. Nitric oxide mediates glutamate-linked enhancement of cGMP levels in the cerebellum. *Proc Natl Acad Sci USA* 1989;86:9030–9033.
253. Schmidt HH, Warner TD, Ishii K, Scheng H, Murad F. Insulin secretion from α-pancreatic cells caused by l-arginine-derived nitrogen oxides. *Science* 1992;258:1376–1378.
254. Kobzik L, Bredt DS, Lowenstein CJ, Drazen J, Gaston B, Sugarbaker D, Stamler JS. Nitric oxide synthase in human and rat lung: immunocytochemical and immunohistochemical localization. *Am J Respir Cell Mol Biol* 1993;9:371–377.
255. Palmer RMJ, Ashton DS, Moncada S. Vascular endothelial cells synthesize nitric oxide from L-arginine. *Nature* 1988;333:664–666.
256. Stuehr DJ, Marletta MA. Induction of nitrite/nitrate synthesis in murine macrophages by BCG infection, lymphokines or interferon-γ. *J Immunol* 1987;139:518–525.
257. Nathan CF, Hibbs JB. Role of nitric oxide synthesis in macrophage antimicrobial activity. *Curr Opin Immunol* 1991;3:65–70.
258. Laskin DL, Rodriguez del Valle M, Heck DE, Hwang S-M, Ohnishi ST, Durham S, Goller N, Laskin JD. Hepatic nitric oxide production following acute endotoxemia in rats is mediated by increased nitric oxide synthase gene expression. *Hepatology* 1995;22:223–234.
259. Lavnikova N, Lakhotia A, Patel N, Prokhorova S, Laskin DL. Cytostasis is required for IL-1 induced nitric oxide production in transformed hamster fibroblasts. *J Cell Physiol* 1996;169:532–537.

260. Curran RD, Ferrari FK, Kispert PH, Stadler J, Stuehr DJ. Nitric oxide and nitric-oxide-generating compounds inhibit hepatocyte protein synthesis. *FASEB J* 1991;5:2085–2092.
261. Weisbrodt NW, Pressley TA, Li YF, Zembowicz MJ, Higham SC, Zembowicz A, Lodato RF, Moody FG. Decreased ileal muscle contractility and increased NOS II expression induced by lipopolysaccharide. *Am J Physiol* 1996;271:G454–G460.
262. Stadler J, Schmalix WA, Doehmer J. Inhibition of biotransformation by nitric oxide (NO) overproduction and toxic consequences. *Toxicol Lett* 1995;82/83:215–219.
263. Hodgson PD, Renton KW. The role of nitric oxide generation in interferon-evoked cytochrome P450 down-regulation. *Int J Immunopharmacol* 1995;17:995–1000.
264. Muller CM, Scierka A, Stiller RL, Kim Y-M, Cook DR, Lancaster JR, Buffington CW. Nitric oxide mediates hepatic cytochrome P450 dysfunction induced by endotoxin. *Anesthesiology* 1996;84:35–42.
265. Green SJ, Meltzer MS, Hibbs JB Jr, Nacy CA. Activated macrophages destroy intracellular *Leishmania major* amastigotes by an L-arginine-dependent killing mechanism. *J Immunol* 1990;144:278–283.
266. Keller R, Gehri R, Keist R, Huf E, Kayser F. The interaction of macrophages and bacteria: a comparative study of the induction of tumoricidal activity and of reactive nitrogen intermediates. *Cell Immunol* 1991;134:249–256.
267. Kilbourn R, Lopez-Berestein G. Protease inhibitors block the macrophage-mediated inhibition of tumor cell mitochondrial respiration. *J Immunol* 1990;144:1042–1045.
268. Takema M, Inaba K, Okazaki K-I, Uno K, Tawara K, Muramatsu S. Effect of L-arginine on the retention of macrophage tumoricidal activity. *J Immunol* 1991;146:1928–1933.
269. Gardner CR, Laskin JD, Heck DE, Thomas PE, Yang CS, Laskin DL. The role of nitric oxide in acetaminophen-induced hepatotoxicity (abstr). *Hepatology* 1996;24(4, pt. 2):335A.
270. Kilbourn RG, Jubran A, Gross SS, Griffith OW, Levi R, Adams J, Lodato RF. Reversal of endotoxin-mediated shock by N'-methyl-L-arginine, an inhibitor of nitric oxide synthesis. *Biochem Biophys Res Commun* 1990;172:1132–1138.
271. Wu C-C, Chen S-J, Szabo C, Thiemermann C, Vane JR. Aminoguanidine attenuates the delayed circulatory failure and improves survival in rodent models of endotoxic shock. *Br J Pharmacol* 1995;114:1666–1672.
272. Milbourne EA, Bygrave FL. Does nitric oxide play a role in liver function? *Cell Signal* 1995;7:313–318.
273. Wright CE, Rees DD, Moncada S. Protective and pathological roles of nitric oxide in endotoxin shock. *Cardiovasc Res* 1992;26:48–57.
274. Ialenti A, Ianaro A, Moncada S, Di Rosa M. Modulation of acute inflammation by endogenous nitric oxide. *Eur J Pharmacol* 1992;211:177–182.
275. Beckman J. The double-edged role of nitric oxide in brain function and superoxide-mediated injury. *J Dev Physiol* 1991;15:53–59.
276. Beckman J, Crow JP. Pathological implications of nitric, superoxide and peroxynitrite formation. *Biochem Soc Trans* 1993;21:330–334.
277. Freeman B. Free radical chemistry of nitric oxide: looking at the dark side. *Chest* 1994;105:79S–84S.
278. Buttery LD, Springall DR, Chester AH, Evans TJ, Stanfield EN, Parums DV, Yacoub MH, Polak JM. Inducible nitric oxide synthase is present within human atherosclerotic lesions and promotes the formation and activity of peroxynitrite. *Lab Invest* 1996;75:77–85.
279. Kooy NW, Royall JA, Ye YZ, Kelly DR, Beckman JS. Evidence for *in vivo* peroxynitrite production in human acute lung injury. *Am J Respir Crit Care Med* 1995;151:1250–1254.
280. Beckman JS, Koppenol WH. Nitric oxide, superoxide, and peroxynitrite: the good, the bad, and ugly. *Am J Physiol* 1996;271:C1424–C1437.
281. Radi R, Beckman JS, Bush KM, Freeman B. Peroxynitrite oxidation of sulfhydrols: the cytotoxic potential of superoxide and nitric oxide. *J Biol Chem* 1991;266:4244–4250.
282. Radi R, Beckman JS, Bush KM, Freeman B. Peroxynitrite-induced membrane lipid peroxidation: the cytotoxic potential of superoxide and nitric oxide. *Arch Biochem Biophys* 1991;288:481–487.
283. Rubbo H, Radi R, Trujillo M, Telleri R, Kalyanaraman B, Barnes S, Kirk M, Freeman BA. Nitric oxide regulation of superoxide and peroxynitrite-dependent lipid peroxidation. Formation of novel nitrogen-containing oxidized lipid derivatives. *J Biol Chem* 1994;269:26066–26075.
284. Lin KT, Xue JY, Nomen M, Spur B, Wong PY. Peroxynitrite-induced apoptosis in HL-60 cells. *J Biol Chem* 1995;270:16487–16490.
285. Estevez AG, Radi R, Barbeito L, Shin JT, Thompson JA, Beckman JS. Peroxynitrite-induced cytotoxicity in PC12 cells: evidence for an apoptotic mechanism differentially modulated by neurotrophic factors. *J Neurochem* 1995;65:1543–1550.

286. Troy CM, Derossi D, Prochiantz A, Greene LA, Shelanski ML. Downregulation of Cu/Zn superoxide dismutase leads to cell death via the nitric oxide-peroxynitrite pathway. *J Neurosci* 1996;16:253–261.

287. Billiar TR, Curran RD, Harbrecht BG, Stueher DJ, Demetris AJ, Simmons RL. Modulation of nitrogen oxide synthesis *in vivo*: N^G-monomethyl-L-arginine inhibits endotoxin-induced nitrite/nitrate biosynthesis while promoting hepatic damage. *J Leukoc Biol* 1990;48:565–569.

288. Harbrecht BG, Billiar TR, Stadler J, Demetris AJ, Ochoa JB, Curran RD, Simmons RL. Inhibition of nitric oxide synthesis during endotoxemia promotes intrahepatic thrombosis and an oxygen radical-mediated hepatic injury. *J Leukoc Biol* 1992;52:390–394.

289. vom Dahl S, Hallbrucker C, Lang F, Haussinger D. Role of eicosanoids, inositol phosphates and extracellular Ca^{2+} in cell-volume regulation of rat liver. *Eur J Biochem* 1991;198:73–83.

290. Ogle CK, Wu JZ, Alexander JW, Fischer JE, Ogle JD. The effects of *in vivo* administration of endotoxin on the functions and interaction of hepatocytes and Kupffer cells. *Prostaglandins* 1991;41:169–183.

291. Ben-Zvi Z, Weissman-Teitellman B, Katz S, Danon A. Acetaminophen hepatotoxicity: is there a role for prostaglandin synthesis? *Arch Toxicol* 1990;64:299–304.

292. Horton AA, Wood JM. Effects of inhibitors of phospholipase A_2, cyclooxygenase and thromboxane synthase on paracetamol hepatotoxicity in the rat. *Eicosanoids* 1989;2:123–129.

293. Shiratori Y, Tanaka M, Umihara J, Kawase T, Shiina S, Sugimoto T. Leukotriene inhibitors modulate hepatic injury induced by lipopolysaccharide-activated macrophages. *J Hepatol* 1990;10:51–61.

294. Tiegs G, Wendel A. Leukotriene-mediated liver injury. *Biochem Pharmacol* 1988;37:2569–2573.

295. Casey LC, Fletcher JR, Zmudka MI, Ramwell PW. The role of thromboxane in primate endotoxin shock. *J Surg Res* 1985;39:140–149.

296. Smith EF III, Jugus M, Kinter LB. Effect of thromboxane receptor antagonist, BM 13.505, on the sequelae of endotoxemia in the conscious rat. *Eicosanoids* 1998;1:27–33.

297. Hagmann W, Denzlinger C, Keppler D. Role of peptide leukotrienes and their hepatobilliary elimination in endotoxin action. *Circ Shock* 1984;14:223–235.

298. Goetzl EJ, Pickett WC. Novel structural determinants of the human neutrophil chemotactic activity of leukotriene B. *J Exp Med* 1981;153:482–487.

299. Spencer DA. An update on PAF. *Clin Exp Allergy* 1992;22:521–524.

300. Camussi G, Tetta C, Baglioni C. The role of platelet-activating factor in inflammation. *Clin Immunol Immunopathol* 1990;57:331–338.

301. Koltai M, Hosford D, Guinot P, Esanu A, Braquet P. Platelet activating factor (PAF): I. A review of its effects, antagonists and future implications. *Drugs* 1991;42:9–29.

302. Locati M, Zhou D, Luini W, Evanelista V, Mantovani A, Sozzani S. Rapid induction of arachidonic acid release by monocyte chemotactic protein-1 and related chemokines: role of Ca^{2+} influx, synergism with platelet-activating factor and significance for chemotaxis. *J Biol Chem* 1994;269:4746–4753.

303. Anderson BO, Bensard DD, Harken AH. The role of platelet activating factor and its antagonists in shock, sepsis and multiple organ failure. *Surg Gynecol Obstet* 1991;172:415–424.

304. Bussolino F, Arese M, Silvestro L, Soldi R, Benfenati E, Sanavio F, Aglietla M, Bosia A, Camussi G. Involvement of a serine protease in the synthesis of platelet-activating factor by endothelial cells stimulated by tumor necrosis factor-α or interleukin-1 α. *Eur J Immunol* 1994;24:3131–3139.

305. Gardner CR, Laskin JD, Laskin DL. Distinct biochemical responses of hepatic macrophages and endothelial cells to platelet-activating factor during endotoxemia. *J Leukoc Biol* 1995;57:269–274.

306. Yue TL, Farhat M, Rabinovici R, Perera PY, Vogel SN, Feuerstein G. Protective effect of BN 50739, a new platelet-activating factor antagonist, in endotoxin-treated rabbits. *J Pharmacol Exp Ther* 1990;254:976–981.

307. Tanner A, Keyhani A, Wright R. The influence of endotoxin *in vitro* on hepatic macrophage lysosomal enzyme release in different models of hepatic injury. *Liver* 1983;3:151–160.

308. Hamilton JA. Stimulation of macrophage prostaglandin and neutral protease production by phorbol esters as a model for the induction of vascular changes associated with tumor promotion. *Cancer Res* 1980;40:2273–2280.

309. Magilavy DB, Zhan R, Black DD. Modulation of murine hepatic lipase activity by exogenous and endogenous Kupffer-cell activation. *Biochem J* 1993;292:249–252.

310. Hart PH, Vitti GF, Burgess DR, Whitty GA, Royston K, Hamilton JA. Activation of human monocytes by granulocyte-macrophage colony-stimulating factor: increased urokinase-type plasminogen activator activity. *Blood* 1991;77:841–848.

311. Winwood PJ, Schuppan D, Iredale JP, Kawser CA, Docherty AJ, Arthur MJP. Kupffer cell-derived 95-kd type IV collagenase/gelatinase B: characterization and expression in cultured cells. *Hepatology* 1995;22:304–315.

312. Petty HR, Hermann W, McConnell HM. Cytochemical study of macrophage lysosomal inorganic trimetaphosphatase and acid phosphatase. *J Ultrastruct Res* 1985;90:80–88.

313. Diment S, Leech MS, Stahl PD. Cathepsin D is membrane-associated in macrophage endosomes. *J Biol Chem* 1988;263:6901–6907.

314. Ashworth EM, Herring MB, Hoagland WP, Arnold M, Glover JL, Dalsing MC. Endothelial linings: the effect of serine protease inhibition. *J Surg Res* 1987;43:10–13.

315. Peinado-Onsurbe J, Soler C, Galan X, Proveda B, Soley M, Llobera M, Ramirez I. Involvement of catecholamines in the effect of fasting on hepatic endothelial lipase activity in the rat. *Endocrinology* 1991;129:2599–2606.

316. Sobel MI, Winkel CA, Macy LB, Liao P, Bjornsson TD. The regulation of plasminogen activators and plasminogen activator inhibitor type 1 in endothelial cells by sex hormones. *Am J Obstet Gynecol* 1995;173:801–808.

317. Moscatelli D, Jaffe E, Rifkin DB. Tetradecanoyl phorbol acetate stimulates latent collagenase production by cultured human endothelial cells. *Cell* 1980;20:343–351.

318. Toborek M, Hennig B. Vitamin E attenuates induction of elastase-like activity by tumor necrosis factor-α, cholestan-3β, 5α, 6β-triol and linoleic acid in cultured endothelial cells. *Clin Chim Acta* 1993;215:201–211.

319. Foda HD, George S, Conner C, Drews M, Tompkins DC, Zucker S. Activation of human umbilical vein endothelial cell progelatinase A by phorbol myristate acetate: a protein kinase C-dependent mechanism involving a membrane-type matrix metalloproteinase. *Lab Invest* 1996;74:538–545.

320. deBruyn PP, Cho Y, Michelson S. *In vivo* endocytosis by bristle coated pits of protein tracers and their intracellular transport in endothelial cells lining the sinuses of the liver. I. The endosomal disposition. *J Ultrastruct Res* 1983;85:272–289.

321. Sawmura T, Kimura S, Shinmi O, Sugita Y, Kobayashi M, Mitsui Y, Yanagisawa M, Goto K, Masaki T. Characterization of endothelin converting enzyme activities in soluble fraction of bovine cultured endothelial cells. *Biochem Biophys Res Commun* 1990;169:1138–1144.

PART III

Cholestasis

Toxicology of the Liver, 2nd ed.,
Edited by Gabriel L. Plaa and William R. Hewitt
Copyright © 1998 Taylor & Francis

10

Cholestatic Properties
of Steroid Glucuronides

Mary Vore

University of Kentucky, Lexington, KY 40536-0035

Kim L. R. Brouwer

University of North Carolina, Chapel Hill, NC 27599-7360

The physiologic and clinical significance of the cholestatic activity of the glucuronide conjugates of the steroid D-ring of the estrogens is apparent primarily in light of the ability of the parent estrogens to induce cholestasis and decrease hepatic excretory function in animals and humans. Recognition of the ability of estrogens to induce cholestasis began with the description of intrahepatic cholestasis of pregnancy (ICP) in 1954 (1). ICP is characterized by symptoms of generalized pruritus, mild anorexia, nausea, occasional vomiting, and, in the more severe cases, jaundice that may be accompanied by a slightly enlarged and tender liver. Liver function tests show elevated levels of 5′-mononucleotidase, alkaline phosphatase, and conjugated bilirubin and retention of bromosulfophthalein (BSP) (2). Soon after the introduction of the oral contraceptives in 1960, intrahepatic cholestasis was observed in a few subjects taking these drugs (3). It was quickly recognized that 50% of women with intrahepatic cholestasis attributable to the oral contraceptives also had ICP (4, 5). Kreek et al. (6) carried out key rechallenge studies showing that administration of ethinylestradiol to women who had a history of pruritus or jaundice in pregnancy precipitated symptoms similar to those experienced in pregnancy, suggesting that the estrogens were the active agents. Mueller and Kappas (7) had already shown that administration of high doses of estradiol or estriol for a week or more in humans increased BSP retention and decreased its transport maximum (T_m). Taken together, these studies confirmed the suggestion of Combes et al. (8) that the decreased T_m for BSP observed in normal gravid compared to nongravid women was due to the elevated hormone levels in pregnancy, and further identified the estrogens as the relevant hormones.

Subsequent animal studies demonstrated that pregnancy and both synthetic and natural estrogens were effective in decreasing the biliary excretion of several organic anions, including BSP (9), dibromosulfophthalein, and the glucuronide conjugate metabolites of phenytoin and morphine (10–15). Ethinylestradiol, at dosages of 0.5–1 mg/day for 5–10 days, also decreased basal bile flow and the maximal taurocholate secretory capacity (16–19). Both pregnancy and treatment of rats with estradiol or ethinylestradiol decrease the uptake of taurocholate and several steroid glucuronides in isolated hepatocytes (20, 21), indicating inhibition of basolateral as well as canalicular transport processes. Indeed, ethinylestradiol treatment decreases both Na^+/taurocholate cotransport in basolateral membrane vesicles and ATP-dependent taurocholate transport in canalicular membrane vesicles (22). The decrease in Na^+/taurocholate cotransport is accompanied by a decrease in steady-state mRNA levels for Na^+/taurocholate cotransporter (23, 24). The effects of pregnancy, however, are less pronounced. While the V_{max} for Na^+/taurocholate cotransport is decreased in isolated hepatocytes from pregnant rats (25), this value is not different in hepatic basolateral membrane vesicles isolated from pregnant versus nonpregnant rats (26, 27), consistent with the lack of effect of pregnancy on the expression of mRNA (26, 28) and protein (27) for the Na^+/taurocholate cotransporter.

These data indicate clear differences in the effects of estrogen treatment versus pregnancy, possibly due to differences in the amount of estrogens to which the animal is exposed as well as differences in transport measured in whole cells versus membrane vesicles in pregnant versus nonpregnant rats. Nevertheless, it is clear that estrogens and pregnancy decrease the transhepatic transport of bile acids and the ability of the liver to excrete glucuronide conjugates into the bile under physiologic conditions. An important question that remains is whether these effects are mediated by estrogen metabolites, specifically the glucuronide conjugates of the steroid D-ring. These are naturally occurring metabolites, several of which are formed in significant quantities in pregnancy, and that have been shown in many laboratories to be potent cholestatic agents. The purpose of this chapter is to review our present knowledge about the cholestatic properties of these glucuronides, with a view toward understanding the mechanism by which they inhibit bile flow and the likelihood that they are responsible for the decreased bile secretory function in pregnancy.

BILE SECRETION AND HEPATIC TRANSPORT

Bile serves diverse and essential functions. Biliary excretion is the only route of elimination for cholesterol; many endogenous waste products such as the glucuronide conjugates of bilirubin and steroids and the glucuronide and glutathione conjugates of many xenobiotics are also excreted in bile. Furthermore, the secretion of bile salts is essential for the emulsification of fats and fat-soluble vitamins in the intestinal tract (29, 30). Secretion of bile consumes significant energy and metabolic resources in order to maintain the vectorial transport of solutes directed from the sinusoidal or basolateral domain of the cell to the canalicular or apical domain (Fig. 1). The hepatocyte is a polarized secretory epithelial cell with specific transporters localized to the basolateral and canalicular domains of the plasma membrane. The active vectorial transport of osmotically active solutes into a confined space, the canaliculus, followed by the passive movement of water until osmotic equilibrium is reached, is the basis for the formation of bile flow. Bile salts are the most concentrated organic solutes in bile and are considered to be the major determinant of bile secretion (29). Bile flow is proportional to the concentration of bile salts (or the accompanying counterions) when their concentration in bile exceeds the critical micellar concentration for each bile salt. This portion of bile flow is defined as *bile acid–dependent bile flow*. Bile flow is not completely abolished in the absence of bile salts but remains at 40–50% of total bile flow. This fraction of bile flow is referred to as *bile acid–independent flow*, and the proportion varies somewhat among species (31). While it is likely that other factors also contribute, the secretion of glutathione into bile contributes significantly to the bile acid–independent component of bile flow (32).

The hepatocyte must continuously transport bile salts from the portal blood into bile to maintain their efficient enterohepatic circulation (30). Several active transport systems provide this essential vectorial transport. Taurocholate, a major conjugated bile salt, is taken up across the basolateral domain by a Na^+-dependent transporter, the Na^+/taurocholate-cotransporting polypeptide (Ntcp) (30). The driving force for the concentrative uptake of taurocholate is derived from the electrochemical sodium gradient, generated by Na^+, K^+-activated adenosine triphosphatase (Na^+, K^+-ATPase), localized to the basolateral domain of the hepatocyte. Ntcp is a glycoprotein with an apparent molecular mass of 51 kDa, is localized exclusively in basolateral rat liver plasma membranes, and appears to account for all of the Na^+-dependent taurocholate uptake of the hepatocyte (30, 33). A less clearly defined Na^+-independent bile salt uptake system, the *organic anion transporting polypeptide*, or Oatp1, is also localized to the basolateral membrane of the hepatocyte (34). Oatp1, a glycoprotein with an apparent molecular weight of 80 kDa, is responsible for the uptake of BSP by the hepatocyte as well as much of the Na^+-independent uptake of taurocholate and cholate

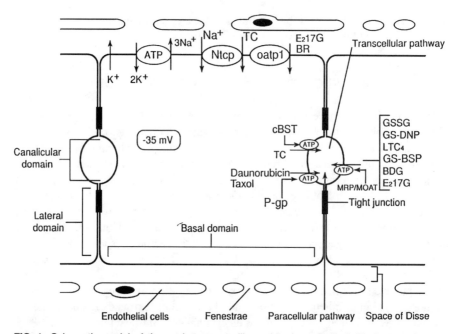

FIG. 1. Schematic model of the rat hepatocyte illustrating the polarized distribution of transporters in the plasma membrane. Two organic anion transporters in the basolateral plasma membrane have been identified: a Na^+/taurocholate-cotransporting polypeptide (Ntcp) and a Na^+-independent organic anion transorter (oatp1). Ntcp transports taurocholate (TC) in a Na^+-dependent manner, while oatp1 transports bile acids and other organic anions, such as $E_2 17G$, BSP, and perhaps bilirubin (BR), in a Na^+-independent manner. The intracellular membrane potential of –35 mV is derived from Na^+, K^+-activated ATPase and a K^+ conductance channel localized to the basolateral membrane. Three ATP-dependent transporters are shown in the canalicular domain. The "canalicular bile salt transporter," cBST, mediates the secretion of monovalent bile salts, while the "multispecific organic anion transporter" or "multidrug resistance protein" (MRP/MOAT) mediates secretion of monovalent and divalent anions including glutathione disulfide (GSSG), glutathione conjugates of BSP (GS-BSP), and dinitrophenyl (GS-DNP) as well as bilirubin diglucuronide (BDG), leukotriene C_4 (LTC_4), and $E_2 17G$. The multidrug-resistant gene product, P-glycoprotein (P-gp), transports hydrophobic drugs, including daunorubicin and taxol. (Reprinted from [66], with permission.)

(30, 34). Oatp1 transports several anionic steroid conjugates, including estrone-3-sulfate and estradiol-17β(β-D-glucuronide) ($E_2 17G$), a prototype cholestatic estrogen glucuronide; neutral steroids, such as ouabain and aldosterone; and even some cations (35, 36).

Secretion of taurocholate into the canaliculus is the rate-limiting step in its transhepatic transport (29, 30). While taurocholate transport across the canalicular membrane was initially thought to be dependent on the intracellular negative membrane potential, recent studies have identified a canalicular primary active, ATP-dependent taurocholate transporter, which is able to generate the 10–100:1 bile acid concentration gradient observed between bile and the hepatocyte (37–40). This transporter has not been conclusively identified but is likely to be a member of the ATP-Binding

Cassette (ABC) superfamily of membrane transporters, as are other ATP-dependent transporters present in the canalicular membrane discussed below.

Two additional ATP-dependent transporters, P-glycoprotein and the *multispecific organic anion transporter* (cMOAT), are localized to the canalicular membrane and are important for understanding the cholestatic action of the steroid glucuronides. P-glycoprotein, the product of the multidrug resistance gene, *MDR1* in humans and *mdr1a/1b* in rodents, is a 170-kDa glycoprotein and a member of the ABC superfamily of membrane transporters. P-glycoprotein mediates the ATP-dependent efflux of hydrophobic polycyclic compounds such as the Vinca alkaloids, the anthracyclines, colchicine, and the epipodophyllotoxins and many other drugs, some of which are widely used in cancer chemotherapy (41). Overexpression of P-glycoprotein increases the efflux of substrates from the cell, resulting in decreased intracellular accumulation, decreased cytotoxicity, and hence resistance to these drugs. P-glycoprotein is constitutively expressed in the canalicular domain of the hepatocyte, where its function resembles that in resistant tumor cells (42). Although P-glycoprotein was the first ATP-dependent transporter identified in canalicular membranes, its physiologic role in liver is not known. It is postulated to protect the cell from toxic insult by eliminating into bile toxic products or metabolites of endogenous or exogenous origin (43).

cMOAT has a broad substrate specificity for the ATP-dependent transport of glutathione and glucuronide conjugates and is believed to be responsible for the biliary clearance of these metabolites (44). Substrates identified include glutathione disulfide (GSSG), cysteinyl leukotrienes, dinitrophenylglutathione (DNP-SG), BSP-glutathione, bilirubin glucuronides, and the 3-OH-sulfated and -glucuronidated bile salts. Monovalent anions such as p-nitrophenyl glucuronide and $E_2 17G$, as discussed below, are also substrates of cMOAT (44). The selective absence of cMOAT expression in TR-mutant rats, a strain of Wistar rats that has an autosomal recessive defect in the biliary excretion of classic cMOAT substrates, has led to the cloning of cMOAT in Wistar rats and its identification as a liver-specific homolog of the Multidrug Resistance Protein (MRP) (45–47). MRP is also a member of the ABC superfamily of transport proteins whose overexpression confers resistance to some cancer chemotherapeutic agents in tumor cells that do not express P-glycoprotein. Human leukemia cells that overexpress MRP, and HeLa cells transfected with MRP, demonstrate ATP-dependent transport of classic cMOAT substrates such as cysteinyl leukotrienes, GS-DNP, GSSG, $E_2 17G$, glucuronosyletoposide, glucuronosylhyodeoxycholate and sulfotaurolithocholate (48–50).

CHOLESTATIC EFFECTS OF STEROID GLUCURONIDES

Effects Following Bolus Administration

Appreciation of the decreased biliary excretion of drug metabolites in pregnancy suggested the possibility that this "defect" might serve a useful purpose, i.e., retention of estrogens in the body during pregnancy. We therefore investigated the biliary excretion of ^{3}H-E$_2$17G, a natural metabolite of estradiol that was commercially available in the radioactive form, in pregnant and nonpregnant rats. Unexpectedly, we found that intravenous administration of E$_2$17G to female rats caused an immediate, reversible, and dose-dependent inhibition of bile flow (51). In contrast, similar doses of estradiol-3-(β-D-glucuronide) (E$_2$3G) and estriol-3-(β-D-glucuronide) (E$_3$3G) increased bile flow under the same experimental conditions. Maximal inhibition of flow following E$_2$17G administration occurs within 15–30 min and recovery is essentially complete within 2–3 hours, depending on the extent of the initial cholestasis. Essentially the same degree of cholestasis is obtained if E$_2$17G is administered repeatedly after recovery of bile flow, such that there is no evidence for tolerance or sensitization to its cholestatic effects.

Early studies examined the cholestatic response to E$_2$17G in several species. Intravenous administration of E$_2$17G at 11 μmol/kg ($n = 1$) or 22 μmol/kg ($n = 1$) to female New Zealand white rabbits resulted in no observable cholestasis. Female Golden Syrian hamsters were also refractory to the cholestatic effects of E$_2$17G at doses of 11 μmol/kg ($n = 4$) and 44 μmol/kg ($n = 3$) (52). Studies by Roy et al. (53) in the isolated perfused male guinea pig liver have shown that administration of 5 μmol E$_2$17G is not cholestatic. In recent studies we found that 0.33 μmol E$_2$17G decreased bile flow 72% in isolated perfused livers from male FVB Taconic mice (Y Liu, M Vore, unpublished observations). In order to determine if the cholestatic activity of E$_2$17G extended to primates, we investigated the effects of E$_2$17G on the clearance of indocyanine green, a dye excreted almost exclusively in the bile (54). Intravenous administration of E$_2$17G to the rhesus monkey significantly decreased the clearance of indocyanine green in a dose-dependent manner. In contrast, E$_2$3G had no effect on indocyanine green clearance in the rhesus, consistent with its ability to increase bile flow in the rat. The amounts of E$_2$17G that decrease indocyanine green clearance in the rhesus, 5.5 and 11 μmol/kg intravenously, are in the same range as the amounts of another cholestatic estrogen glucuronide (see below), estriol-16α-glucuronide (E$_3$16G), excreted in the urine of women in the third trimester of pregnancy, i.e., 140 μmol/day, or 2–3 μmol/kg/day. While we do not know the cholestatic activity of E$_3$16G in women, its formation and constant presence in the liver during the latter stages of pregnancy could certainly contribute to the observed decrease in bile secretory function in normal pregnancy.

A clear structure-activity relationship for the cholestatic activity of estrogen glucuronides is apparent, with other glucuronide conjugates of the steroid D-ring decreasing bile flow in the same manner. Thus, E$_3$16G, estriol-17-glucuronide (E$_3$17G), testosterone glucuronide, and 17α-ethinylestradiol-17β-glucuronide (EE$_2$17G) also decrease bile flow in an immediate, reversible, and dose-dependent manner following intravenous administration in rats (55, 56). Characterization of the log-dose response curves for the maximal percent inhibition of bile of these conjugates yielded a family of curves that are parallel (Fig. 2) (36). Two additional steroid glucuronides were also cholestatic: 17α-ethinylestradiol-17β(α-D-glucuronide) (EE$_2$17αG) (56) and dihydrotestosterone glucuronide (57). The former is the synthetic anomer of

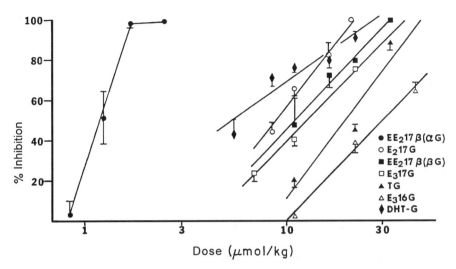

FIG. 2. The relationship between the logarithm of the dose of the cholestatic agents and the maximal percent inhibition of bile flow. Points represent the mean ±SE of the maximal percent inhibition of bile flow following intravenous administration to female rats. (Data are taken from [58], with permission.) Abbreviations: $EE_217\beta(\alpha$-G), 17α-ethinylestradiol-$17\beta(\alpha$-D-glucuronide); E_217G, estradiol-$17\beta(\beta$-D-glucuronide); $EE_217\beta(\beta$G), 17α-ethinylestradiol-$17\beta(\beta$-D-glucuronide); E_317G, estriol-$17\beta(\beta$-D-glucuronide); TG, testosterone $17\beta(\beta$-D-glucuronide); E_316G, estriol-$16\alpha(\beta$-D-glucuronide); DHT-G, dihydrotestosterone $17\beta(\beta$-D-glucuronide).

17α-ethinylestradiol-$17\beta(\beta$-D-glucuronide) ($EE_217\beta$G) and is not formed biologically but is an extremely potent cholestatic agent in the rat (56). The log-dose response curves of these last two agents are not parallel to each other or to the other "family" of cholestatic steroid glucuronides (58). Interestingly, the log-dose response curves for the cholestasis induced by dihydrotestosterone glucuronide, a series of allo bile acids, and lithocholate were all parallel, with dihydrotestosterone glucuronide being almost five times more potent than lithocholate (57). We have postulated that cholestatic glucuronides with parallel log-dose response curves have the same target or mechanism of action, whereas cholestatic glucuronides with log-dose response curves of differing slopes have either different target sites or differing mechanisms of action. We and others have used E_217G, the most potent of the naturally occurring estrogen cholestatic glucuronides, as a prototype to investigate the mechanism of action of this group of cholestatic agents.

Effects Following Continuous Infusion

In preliminary studies we investigated the effects of E_217G on liver function following continuous infusion. Female rats were prepared as described previously (51), and given a 7.5 μmol/kg intravenous bolus loading dose of E_217G, followed by a

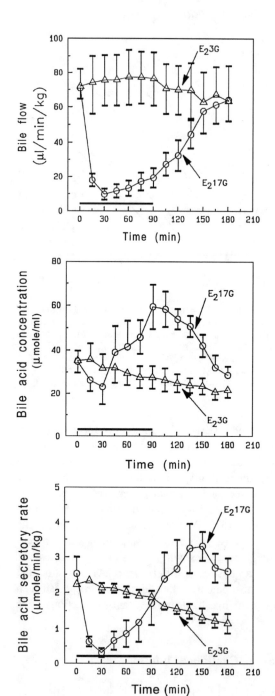

FIG. 3. Bile flow (top panel), bile acid concentration (middle panel), and bile acid secretory rate (bottom panel) in female rats administered a loading dose (7.5 μmol/kg, intravenously) followed by a continuous infusion (12.5 μmol/kg/hr, intravenously) of $E_2 17G$ or $E_2 3G$ (control) for 90 min. The bar indicates the duration of infusion. Cholestasis (20% of initial bile flow) was maintained throughout the infusion of $E_2 17G$. Bile flow recovered within 90 min when the infusion of $E_2 17G$ was replaced with a saline infusion.

12.5 μmol/kg/hr continuous infusion (1 ml/hr) of $E_2$17G for 90 min. Doses were calculated based on the pharmacokinetic disposition of $E_2$17G previously reported (54) to achieve a steady-state plasma concentration of 25 μmol/ml. In the control group, rats were given the same loading dose and maintenance infusion of $E_2$3G, the noncholestatic steroid A-ring glucuronide. At the end of the 90-min period, the $E_2$17G infusion was stopped and saline (1 ml/hr) was infused for an additional 90 min. Bile flow, bile acid concentration, and bile acid secretory rates were determined as described (51) and are shown in Fig. 3. These data demonstrate that constant infusion of $E_2$17G maintains cholestasis (20% of initial bile flow) for at least 90 min and that the effect is reversible so that bile flow quickly recovers upon discontinuation of the infusion. These data indicate that the ability of $E_2$17G to decrease bile flow is directly proportional to its concentration in liver or bile at any point in time.

Kossor et al. (59) examined the effect of repetitive administration of $E_2$17G for 48 hr on biliary epithelial cell hyperplasia in male rats. In these studies, $E_2$17G was administered hourly (21 μmol/kg/hr, intravenously) for 48 hr to produce nonobstructive cholestasis (23% of initial bile flow). At the end of the 48-hr period of cholestasis, microscopic evaluation of the liver showed biliary epithelial cell hyperplasia accompanied by hypertrophy of the epithelium of bile ducts and ductules that regressed upon discontinuation of $E_2$17G. While bile duct ligation and treatment with α-naphthylisothiocyanate, which cause bile duct obstruction, are known to cause biliary epithelial cell hyperplasia, these studies demonstrate that the relatively short-term (i.e., 48 hr) inhibition of bile flow by $E_2$17G in the absence of obstruction also can induce hyperplasia.

PROPOSED MECHANISMS OF CHOLESTASIS

Inhibition of Bile Salt Transport

The structure–activity relationship observed and the series of parallel dose-response curves obtained for the cholestatic steroid D-ring β-glucuronides suggested the possibility that these agents could induce cholestasis by interacting with a specific "receptor" site in the hepatocyte. The structural similarity between the bile salts and the steroid D-ring glucuronides further suggested that such a receptor site might serve as a bile salt transporter. Indeed, receptor binding studies with ^{3}H-$E_2$17G in canalicular membranes had shown that the cholestatic steroid glucuronides and taurocholate, but not the non-cholestatic estrogen glucuronides or BSP, competed with ^{3}H-$E_2$17G for binding to a high-affinity site, suggesting that competition between taurocholate and the cholestatic glucuronides at this site could mediate cholestasis (60). The interactions between bile salts, with differing detergent and micelle-forming properties, and the cholestatic steroid D-ring glucuronides, have been examined systematically. Adinolfi et al. (61) used the isolated perfused male rat liver to demonstrate that infusion of increasing concentrations of taurocholate prevented $E_2$17G-induced cholestasis, with infusion of 0.75 μmol/min taurocholate offering complete protection against

17.5 μM $E_2$17G. In contrast, infusion of 0.75 μmol/min dehydrocholate, a nonmicelle-forming bile salt, did not protect against the cholestasis. Taurocholate did not affect the hepatic uptake of $E_2$17G but markedly stimulated its biliary excretion, consistent with prevention of the inhibition of bile flow. $E_2$17G also increased the bile:plasma concentration ratio of ^{14}C-sucrose (from 0.27 to 0.87), and this increase was prevented by infusion of 0.75 μmol/min taurocholate, but not dehydrocholate. These authors suggested that $E_2$17G induced cholestasis by increasing the permeability of the tight junction, consistent with the increased bile:plasma sucrose concentration; the protective effect of taurocholate was attributed to incorporation of $E_2$17G into biliary micelles and enhanced excretion into bile. In further studies, Utili et al. (62) demonstrated that tauroursodeoxycholate and taurocholate reversed the cholestasis induced by $E_2$17G, whereas dehydrocholate was less effective. Tauroursodeoxycholate, which is less hydrophobic than taurocholate, was not as potent as taurocholate in reversing the cholestasis but was less toxic than taurocholate.

We also investigated the protective effects of taurocholate on $E_2$17G cholestasis in the female rat perfused liver (63). Consistent with the protective effect shown by Adinolfi et al. (61), infusion of taurocholate protected against $E_2$17G cholestasis. Characterization of the $E_2$17G dose-response curve showed that taurocholate shifted the curve to the right but increased the slope of the line five- to sixfold. These data indicate that the protective effect of taurocholate is not competitive in nature. Taurocholate clearly increases the biliary excretion of $E_2$17G; however, it is not clear if this is the cause or the result of its ability to prevent cholestasis. Surprisingly, these experiments also showed that both $E_2$17G and the noncholestatic $E_2$3G increased the biliary secretion of taurocholate, with $E_2$17G being more effective, and protected against the cholestasis induced by high doses of taurocholate. These data indicate that there is an interaction between taurocholate and $E_2$17G transport into bile, but the nature of this interaction is not clear. Numerous studies have shown that infusion of taurocholate stimulates the biliary secretion of non–bile acid organic anions; however, these data indicate that the converse is also possible.

Studies in basolateral and canalicular membrane vesicles have provided some additional insights into potential interactions between taurocholate and $E_2$17G transport. $E_2$17G is taken up by liver basolateral membrane vesicles as an anion by facilitated diffusion (64) and has been shown to be a high-affinity substrate of Oatp1 in transfected HeLa cells (35). $E_2$17G does not alter Na^+/taurocholate cotransport, which is responsible for about 80% of taurocholate uptake by the hepatocyte. While $E_2$17G could inhibit Na^+-independent Oatp1-mediated uptake of taurocholate, it seems unlikely that inhibition of this minor pathway could contribute to $E_2$17G-mediated cholestasis. Similarly, studies in canalicular membrane vesicles have demonstrated that taurocholate does not inhibit ATP-dependent $E_2$17G transport and, conversely, that $E_2$17G does not inhibit ATP-dependent taurocholate transport (65, 66). Thus, in vitro, $E_2$17G has no detectable effects on taurocholate transport. It is difficult to understand how an agent that can inhibit bile flow completely without causing obstruction of the biliary tree is able to do so without affecting the transport of bile acids, the major determinant of bile flow.

Increased Permeability of Tight Junctions

While Adinolfi et al. (61) had noted an increase in the bile:perfusate concentration ratio of sucrose following administration of $E_2 17G$, suggestive of increased permeability of the tight junctions, the reliability of this technique as a measure of tight junction permeability has been questioned. Under basal conditions, greater that 80% of sucrose is transported from plasma (or perfusate) to bile by a transcellular route, with the remainder reaching bile via the paracellular pathway (67). Furthermore, under cholestatic conditions, decreased bile flow increases the opportunity for sucrose to diffuse from perfusate to bile, thus artificially increasing the bile:perfusate concentration ratio. In order to investigate the effect of $E_2 17G$ on tight junction permeability under conditions that avoided these limitations, Kan et al. (68) determined the effect of $E_2 17G$ on the biliary excretion of horseradish peroxidase (HRP) administered as a single pulse in the single-pass isolated perfused rat liver. HRP is excreted into bile via two pathways; an early peak represents penetration of HRP through tight junctions, whereas a later peak represents a transcellular pathway. In a second study, taurodehydrocholate was infused to increase basal bile flow and control for the decreased bile flow following $E_2 17G$. Thus, bile flow in the presence of taurodehydrocholate and $E_2 17G$ was equal to control bile flow in the absence of $E_2 17G$ and taurodehydrocholate. In both the presence and the absence of taurodehydrocholate, administration of $E_2 17G$ increased the biliary excretion of HRP in the early peak more than twofold. While these data indicate that $E_2 17G$ increases permeability of the tight junction, Kan et al. (68) are careful to point out that it is not possible to determine if this permeability change is causally related to the cholestatic effects of $E_2 17G$. Whether a cause or an effect, these data indicate that increased permeability of the tight junctions is a part of the cholestasis induced by $E_2 17G$.

Effects of $E_2 17G$ on Membrane Fluidity

Several studies have indicated that treatment with ethinylestradiol decreases the fluidity of liver plasma membranes as well as bile flow and that the cholestasis can be countered by increasing membrane fluidity (69). Thus, Triton WR 1339, S-adenosyl-L-methionine, and various dietary regimens were shown to increase membrane fluidity and to reverse, at least in part, the cholestasis induced by ethinylestradiol treatment. Alvaro et al. (70) have pursued the hypothesis that $E_2 17G$-induced cholestasis is due to decreased membrane fluidity by characterizing the effect of treatment of rats with dimethylethanolamine (DME) on cholestasis induced by $E_2 17G$. Intravenous infusion of DME, the polar head group of phosphatidylethanolamine, enhances the synthesis of phosphatidyldimethylethanolamine, which replaces phosphatidylethanolamine as the substrate for microsomal N-methyltransferase. The net effect is an increase in the synthesis of polyunsaturated phosphatidylcholine and an increase in membrane fluidity. In the studies by Alvaro et al. (70), three groups of rats were drained of endogenous bile salts, then infused with taurocholate in the presence (group 1) or absence (groups

2 and 3) of 0.3 mg/kg/min DME for 15 hr. Subsequently, rats in groups 1 and 2 were treated with a cholestatic dose (10.4 mg/kg) of $E_2$17G, and bile flow as well as the biliary secretion of cholesterol, phosphatidylcholine, and bile salts was monitored for 3 hr. Portions of liver were also taken for electron microscopy and fluorescence polarization studies of microsomes and sinusoidal and canalicular liver plasma membranes. Pretreatment with DME antagonized the cholestatic effect of $E_2$17G such that bile flow was decreased 74% in controls but only 28% in DME-pretreated rats. The $E_2$17G-induced decreases in biliary secretion of bile salts, phosphatidylcholine, and cholesterol were blunted to a similar extent by DME treatment. Microscopic examination of the liver showed no ultrastructural alterations at the time of maximum cholestasis; however cholestatic features were evident in non–DME-treated rats 3 hr after $E_2$17G administration. These cholestatic features included dilated canaliculi with a decreased number of microvilli, an increased number of pericanalicular vesicles, and a thickened pericanalicular ectoplasm. Mitochondria with curled cristae were apparent, as were free ribosomes and degranulated rough endoplasmic reticulum cisternae. These classic features of cholestasis were not present in DME-treated rats given $E_2$17G. Finally, fluidity of endoplasmic reticulum and sinusoidal and canalicular plasma membranes was decreased by $E_2$17G treatment and was associated with an enrichment of cholesterol and a higher cholesterol/phospholipid ratio. All of these effects were antagonized by DME pretreatment. These authors suggest that the increased incorporation of the sn-1 stearoyl phosphatidylcholine in DME-treated rats influences the interaction between $E_2$17G and the membranes to blunt the cholestatic response. Questions that remain relate to the precise site of the interactions between $E_2$17G and the membrane and how such an interaction can profoundly inhibit bile flow.

Roles of P-Glycoprotein and cMOAT in $E_2$17G Cholestasis

Studies characterizing $E_2$17G transport in canalicular membrane vesicles demonstrated ATP-dependent transport via both cMOAT and P-glycoprotein (65). ATP-dependent $E_2$17G transport in canalicular membranes is temperature-dependent, occurs into an osmotically sensitive space, and is saturable, with an apparent K_m of 75 μM and V_{max} of about 600 pmol/min/mg protein (65). This ATP-dependent transport is inhibited by the classic cMOAT substrates GSSG, GS-DNP, BSP, BSP-glutathione, and several glucuronide conjugates such as estradiol-3-glucuronide, estriol-16α-glucuronide and morphine glucuronide (see Table 2). Studies in membrane vesicles from MRP-transfected HeLa cells recently demonstrated that $E_2$17G is a high-affinity substrate (K_m, 1.5–2.5 μM) of human MRP (50, 71). Taken together, these studies provide very strong evidence that $E_2$17G is a substrate of cMOAT in rat liver.

Additional evidence for cMOAT-mediated biliary excretion of $E_2$17G, and its importance in the cholestatic response is derived from studies in Eisai hyperbilirubinemic rats (EHBRs). EHBRs, a strain of the Sprague-Dawley rat, are deficient in cMOAT and therefore do not excrete a variety of organic anions into bile (72). This trait exhibits autosomal recessive inheritance and is due to a mutation that introduces a premature stop codon, preventing expression of cMOAT (73). The biliary excretion of $E_2 17G$ in EHBR is markedly decreased (74, 75), i.e., 12% and 90% of a tracer dose of $E_2 17G$ are excreted in bile in EHBR and Sprague-Dawley rats, respectively. Infusion of $E_2 17G$ (0.075 μmol/100 g/min for 20 min) to EHBR rats did not inhibit bile flow, while this dose induced a profound cholestasis in Sprague-Dawley rats. These authors concluded that biliary excretion of $E_2 17G$ is essential for the cholestatic response and that the cholestasis is not an intrahepatic event but rather occurs in the canalicular membrane or within the canalicular lumen.

Studies in two well-characterized cell lines, a human sarcoma cell line, MES-SA, and a leukemia cell line, K562, and their doxorubicin-selected MDR variants, Dx5 and K562/MDR, respectively, provided initial evidence that $E_2 17G$ is also a substrate of P-glycoprotein (76). Dx5 cells are 35-fold resistant to doxorubicin compared to the parental cell line MES-SA and are 35- to 40-fold cross-resistant to both etoposide and vinblastine and 60-fold cross-resistant to taxol. However, addition of 100 μM $E_2 17G$ to the MDR-positive cell lines restored their sensitivity to doxorubicin, vinblastine, etoposide, and taxol, whereas 100 μM $E_3 3G$ was without effect. Accordingly, Dx5 cells accumulated only about 25% as much of the MDR substrates vinblastine and taxol as did the parental MESSA cells, and addition of 100 μM $E_2 17G$ to Dx5 cells reversed this accumulation defect; again, $E_3 3G$ was without effect. As shown in Table 1, the MDR-positive cell lines were also two- to fivefold resistant to the cytotoxicity induced by the cholestatic estrogen D-ring glucuronides, relative to the parental cell lines. In contrast, there was no difference in the cytotoxic effects of the noncholestatic

TABLE 1. Cytotoxicity of steroid glucuronides in parental (MES-SA, K562) and MDR (Dx5, K562MDR) cells

Compound	Cell line	IC_{50} (μM)[1]	Resistance
$E_2 17G$	MES-SA	72.0 ± 3.0	
	Dx5	336 ± 40	4.7
	K562	76.0 ± 6.0	
	K562MDR	393 ± 15	5.2
$E_3 16G$	MES-SA	92.0 ± 7.0	
	Dx5	350 ± 70	3.8
$EE_2 17\alpha G$	MES-SA	94.0 ± 5.0	
	Dx5	520 ± 27	5.5
$EE_2 17\beta G$	MES-SA	185 ± 30	
	Dx5	360 ± 52	1.9
$E_3 3G$	MES-SA	172 ± 30	
	Dx5	165 ± 20	1.0
	K562	176 ± 60	
	K562MDR	193 ± 15	1.1

[1] Mean $\pm$ SD of three to six determinations; the IC_{50} represent the concentration that decreased cell survival 50% determined from semilogarithmic dose-response curves as described by Gosland et al. (76).

estriol 3-glucuronide ($E_3$3G) in these cell lines. Dx5 cells accumulated about 30% as much ^{3}H-$E_2$17G (10 μM) as MES-SA, and this accumulation defect was reversed by etoposide (20 μM), vinblastine (10 μM), taxol (10 μM), verapamil (10 μM), PSC-833 (1.0 μM), and cyclosporine (2.5 μM), all classic substrates or modulators of P-glycoprotein. Cisplatin (20 μM), which is not a substrate or modulator of P-glycoprotein, was without effect. These data strongly suggested that $E_2$17G, but not $E_3$3G, is a substrate of P-glycoprotein that could itself be transported from the cell as well as compete with classic P-glycoprotein substrates for efflux.

Recently, Loe et al. (71) have countered this hypothesis, based on data demonstrating minimal ATP-dependent uptake of 50 nM ^{3}H-$E_2$17G in membrane vesicles from cells overexpressing P-glycoprotein. As indicated above, $E_2$17G is a high-affinity substrate of MRP in membrane vesicles from transfected HeLa cells ($K_m = 2.5$ μM). These authors (71) demonstrated that the cysteinyl leukotriene LTC$_4$ is a potent inhibitor of MRP-mediated $E_2$17G transport, in that 1 μM LTC$_4$ inhibited the transport of 50 nM $E_2$17G by 90%. In contrast, the 3-glucuronide conjugates, $E_3$3G and $E_2$3G, were not inhibitory at concentrations of 10 μM. Loe et al. (71) argue that potentially contaminating MRP present in resistant Dx5 and K562/MDR cells, rather than P-glycoprotein, could account for the transport of $E_2$17G and the selective reversal of doxorubicin resistance by $E_2$17G, but not $E_3$3G. However, while MRP does mediate low levels of transport of daunorubicin, etoposide, and vincristine, taxol is not a substrate of MRP (77), and MRP transfection does not confer resistance to taxol (78). Furthermore, cyclosporine and PSC-833 are potent modulators of P-glycoprotein but are much less effective for MRP (49). Thus, while the selectivity of human MRP for $E_2$17G versus the 3-glucuronide conjugates of estradiol and estriol is intriguing, the data of Gosland et al. (76) are highly consistent with the hypothesis that P-glycoprotein is important in $E_2$17G transport.

Takikawa et al. (75) recently compared the biliary excretion of tracer doses of $E_2$17G, vinblastine, and taurocholate transport in EHBR and Sprague-Dawley rats and demonstrated that only the biliary excretion of $E_2$17G is inhibited significantly in EHBR, consistent with the lack of expression of cMOAT. Furthermore, infusion of BSP markedly inhibited the biliary excretion of a tracer dose of $E_2$17G in Sprague-Dawley rats, suggesting that they are transported by the same carrier, i.e., cMOAT. Treatment of Sprague-Dawley rats with a phenothiazine (5 mg/100 g for 3 days; the specific drug is not indicated), a treatment regimen proposed to increase expression of P-glycoprotein, increased the biliary excretion of a tracer dose of vinblastine, but did not increase the biliary excretion of a tracer dose of $E_2$17G. However, phenothiazine treatment increased the biliary excretion of a cholestatic dose of $E_2$17G and offered some protection against the cholestasis. Takikawa et al. (75) conclude that cMOAT is a high-affinity transporter for $E_2$17G whereas P-glycoprotein has a relatively low affinity for $E_2$17G, participating only in the biliary excretion of cholestatic concentrations of $E_2$17G. These results are consistent with the relatively high-affinity (1–2 μM K_m) of $E_2$17G determined for MRP and could explain why P-glycoprotein–mediated transport was not detectable at the low $E_2$17G concentrations (50 nM) examined by Loe et al. (71).

TABLE 2. *Effect of inhibitors on ATP-dependent transport of $E_2 17G$ in canalicular membrane vesicles from rat liver*

Inhibitor	Activity (% of control)
Control	100 ± 9.2
+TC (50 μM)	96.7 ± 3.3
+E$_2$3G (100 μM)	46.5 ± 8.9[1]
+E$_3$3G (100 μM)	59.0 ± 13[1]
+TG (100 μM)	56.7 ± 17[1]
+E$_3$16G (100 μM)	18.2 ± 6.8[1]
+E$_2$3SO$_4$17G (100 μM)	29.1 ± 9.4[1]
+BSP (50 μM)	43.2 ± 7.0[1]
+GSSG (100 μM)	63.8 ± 14[1]
+GS-DNP (10 μM)	34.4 ± 21[1]
+MG (100 μM)	34.9 ± 15[1]
+Vinblastine (100 μM)	40.6 ± 1.9[1]
+Etoposide (100 μM)	66.0 ± 42[1]
+Daunorubicin (100 μM)	12.9 ± 6.5[1]
+Daunorubicin (50 μM)	40.6 ± 16[1]
+Cyclosporine (10 μM)	17.2 ± 14[1]
+Cyclosporine (1 μM)	72.3 ± 2.8[1]
+PSC-833 (10 μM)	3.9 ± 9.9[1]
+Taxol (50 μM)	19.5 ± 7.9[1]
+Taxol (10 μM)	52.9 ± 11[1]
+Verapamil (100 μM)	92.5 ± 7.8

ATP-dependent uptake was determined in the absence and presence of inhibitors. Data represent the mean $\pm$ SE of three to five determinations and are modified from (65, 76, 79).
[1]$P < .05$, significantly different from control.
Abbreviations: TC, taurocholate; E$_2$3G, estradiol-3-glucuronide; E$_3$3G, estriol-3-glucuronide; TG, testosterone glucuronide; E$_3$16G, estriol-16α-glucuronide; E$_2$3SO$_4$17G, estradiol-3-sulfate-17-glucuronide; BSP, bromosulfophthalein; GSSG, glutathione dissulfide; GS-DNP, S-(2,4-dinitrophenyl) glutathione; MG, morphine glucuronide.

Subsequent studies in canalicular membrane vesicles have confirmed the initial observations that $E_2 17G$ is a substrate of P-glycoprotein (65). As shown in Table 1, etoposide, vinblastine, daunorubicin, taxol, cyclosporine, and PSC-833 all inhibited the ATP-dependent transport of $E_2 17G$ in canalicular vesicles (65, 79). Verapamil, however, had no effect on $E_2 17G$ transport in these vesicles. $E_2 17G$ competitively inhibited the ATP-dependent transport of daunorubicin, whereas $E_2 3G$ had no effect on daunorubicin transport. In contrast, both $E_2 17G$ and $E_2 3G$ inhibited the ATP-dependent transport of GS-DNP, a classic cMOAT substrate. Finally, C219, a monoclonal antibody against an internal epitope of P-glycoprotein, inhibited ATP-dependent $E_2 17G$ and daunorubicin transport but had no effect on the ATP-dependent transport of taurocholate or GS-DNP. These data are consistent with the hypothesis that while the noncholestatic $E_2 3G$ is a substrate of cMOAT, $E_2 17G$ is transported by both cMOAT and P-glycoprotein in canalicular membrane vesicles. These data suggest that the substrate specificities for human MRP and rat liver cMOAT differ in that while the 3-glucuronide conjugates of estradiol and estriol do not inhibit MRP-mediated transport of $E_2$17G or LTC4, they are very effective inhibitors of cMOAT-mediated transport of GS-DNP. Similarly, the substrate specificities of human MDR and rat liver mdr1a/1b differ with respect to verapamil-mediated inhibition of $E_2$17G transport.

The observation that the cholestatic estrogen glucuronides, but not the noncholestatic 3-glucuronide conjugates of estradiol and estriol, are substrates of P-glycoprotein suggested that P-glycoprotein could be involved in $E_2$17G cholestasis. The localization of P-glycoprotein in secretory epithelial cells (e.g., liver, kidney, and intestine) has led to the suggestion that P-glycoprotein may function physiologically to excrete toxic metabolites of endogenous or exogenous origin (43). We therefore postulated that P-glycoprotein, like cMOAT, could also excrete the toxic $E_2$17G into bile and that biliary excretion would serve as a detoxification process. To test this hypothesis, we used the isolated perfused rat liver to monitor the cholestatic response to $E_2$17G in the presence or absence of alternative P-glycoprotein substrates, such as daunorubicin, taxol or the modulator, cyclosporine (79). We postulated that if P-glycoprotein serves a protective role and excretes $E_2$17G into bile, then infusion of alternative substrates should compete with $E_2$17G for excretion, leading to accumulation of $E_2$17G in the hepatocyte and potentiation of cholestasis. Similarly, we postulated that infusion of BSP, a cMOAT substrate, would block cMOAT-mediated biliary excretion of $E_2$17G and potentiate cholestasis. $E_2$17G was administered as a bolus dose into the portal vein cannula, and taxol, daunorubicin, BSP, or cyclosporine were given as a constant infusion into the portal vein in the single-pass isolated perfused rat liver. As shown in Fig. 4 (top panel), a bolus dose (2 μmol) of $E_2$17G alone decreased bile flow by 70% within 10 min, and bile flow remained significantly depressed throughout the remainder of the experiment. A constant infusion of 1.5 μM daunorubicin (final concentration) in the perfusate had no effect on basal bile flow but markedly attenuated the cholestatic response to subsequent administration of 2 μmol $E_2$17G. Similarly, a constant infusion of 1 μM taxol (final concentration) significantly inhibited the cholestatic response to 2 μmol $E_2$17G. Infusion of cyclosporine (Fig. 4, bottom panel) alone (6 μM, final concentration, for 20 min) decreased bile flow by 10–15%, but administration of 2 μmol $E_2$17G had no further inhibitory effect on bile flow. In contrast, in the presence of an infusion of 3.6 μM BSP (final concentration), 2 μmol $E_2$17G decreased bile flow by 72%, such that BSP had no effect on the cholestatic response to $E_2$17G (Fig. 4, top panel). Thus, rather than the anticipated potentiation of cholestasis, the presence of alternative P-glycoprotein substrates/modulators dramatically protected against the cholestatic response to $E_2$17G.

The nature of the protective effects of daunorubicin, taxol, and cyclosporine against $E_2$17G-induced cholestasis were further characterized by examining the log-dose response relationships between the maximal percent inhibition of bile flow and the dose of $E_2$17G in the presence and absence of these agents. $E_2$17G-induced cholestasis showed a linear relationship between the logarithm of the dose as shown in Fig. 5,

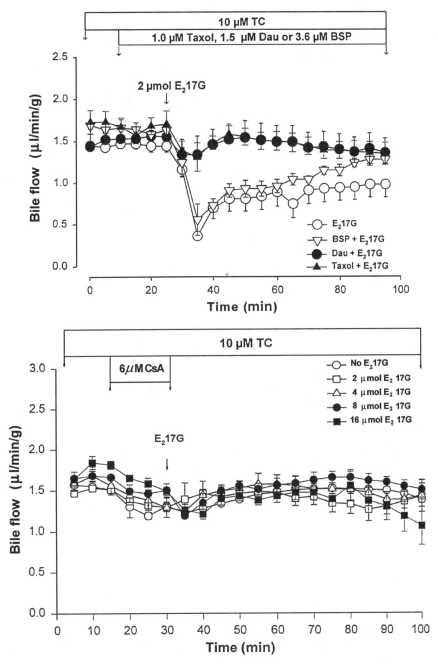

FIG. 4. *Top panel.* Daunorubicin (Dau) or Taxol, but not BSP, protects against $E_2 17G$-mediated cholestasis in the isolated perfused male rat liver. Taurocholate (TC, 10 μM final concentration) was infused to maintain stable bile flow; Taxol, Dau, or BSP were infused for 15 min before administration of 2 μmol $E_2 17G$, and infusion was continued for the remainder of the experiment. *Bottom panel.* Cyclosporine (CsA) protects against $E_2 17G$-mediated cholestasis. CsA was infused for 15 min before and 5 min after administration of the indicated doses of $E_2 17G$. Data represent the mean $\pm$SE of three to four rat livers. (Taken from [79], with permission.)

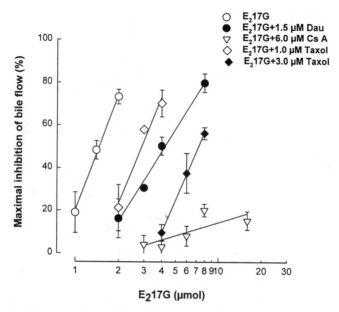

FIG. 5. The maximum percent inhibition of bile flow versus the logarithm of the dose of $E_2 17G$ alone and in the presence of daunorubicin (Dau), Taxol, or cyclosporine (CsA). Data represent the mean $\pm$SE of three to four replications for each group. (Taken from [79], with permission.)

consistent with earlier studies (63). In the presence of daunorubicin (1.5 μM) the log-dose response curve for $E_2 17G$ cholestasis was shifted to the right about fourfold, in a near parallel manner. In the presence of 1 and 3 μM taxol, the dose-response curves for $E_2 17G$ cholestasis were shifted to the right two- and fivefold, respectively, in a parallel manner. These data clearly indicate that taxol competitively inhibits the cholestatic action of $E_2 17G$. In contrast, in the presence of cyclosporine, the dose-response curve was shifted markedly to the right and the slope was decreased significantly, such that doses as high as 16 μmol $E_2 17G$ had only a slight cholestatic effect.

We also characterized the biliary excretion of ^{3}H-$E_2 17G$ to determine if these agents had altered its elimination, as postulated (79). Neither BSP nor daunorubicin had any effect on the overall concentration of $E_2 17G$ equivalents in bile, whereas taxol (1 μM) and cyclosporine significantly decreased these measures. Because of the protection against cholestasis, the biliary secretory rate (the product of bile flow and bile concentration) of $E_2 17G$ equivalents was not decreased by taxol or daunorubicin relative to $E_2 17G$ given alone. Cyclosporine, however, significantly inhibited the biliary excretion of $E_2 17G$. Studies in basolateral membrane vesicles showed that cyclosporine did not inhibit $E_2 17G$ uptake, thus ruling out decreased hepatic uptake of $E_2 17G$ as the basis for cyclosporine protection against cholestasis. Analysis of the bile by high-pressure liquid chromatography demonstrated that the proportion of

$E_2 17G$ metabolized to the noncholestatic 3-sulfate-$E_2 17G$ was not altered by any of the treatment conditions (79).

These results clearly do not support our initial hypothesis that infusion of alternative P-glycoprotein or cMOAT substrates would inhibit biliary excretion and potentiate cholestasis. Rather, cyclosporine, a potent inhibitor of both P-glycoprotein and cMOAT (80), decreased the biliary concentration and excretion of $E_2 17G$ and essentially abolished the cholestatic response. The ability of the P-glycoprotein substrates daunorubicin and taxol to protect against $E_2 17G$ cholestasis supports the hypothesis that P-glycoprotein plays an essential role in the cholestatic response, whereas the lack of effect of BSP argues against a key role for cMOAT. However, the ability of cyclosporine to inhibit the biliary excretion of $E_2 17G$ and to essentially abolish the cholestatic response suggests a role for both transporters in the cholestatic response. As discussed above, Sano et al. (74) have postulated that accumulation of $E_2 17G$ in the canaliculus is essential for its cholestasis. While the concomitant inhibition of biliary excretion and protection against cholestasis mediated by cyclosporine support this hypothesis, the ability of daunorubicin to protect against $E_2 17G$ cholestasis without altering its concentration in bile indicates that although accumulation of $E_2 17G$ in bile may be an important variable, access to P-glycoprotein is an essential component of the cholestatic response. The highly effective protection conveyed by cyclosporine may therefore by due to a synergism between its ability to inhibit both cMOAT- and P-glycoprotein-mediated $E_2 17G$ transport, resulting in a decreased concentration in bile coupled to a blockade of P-glycoprotein.

Collectively, these data support a model in which both cMOAT and P-glycoprotein contribute to $E_2 17G$-induced cholestasis. In this model (Fig. 6) cMOAT functions under most physiologic conditions to excrete the normally low levels of $E_2 17G$ into bile. This usually serves as a detoxification mechanism, preventing its intracellular accumulation and access to P-glycoprotein from the intracellular domain. However, when high cholestatic concentrations of $E_2 17G$ are present, cMOAT delivers such high concentrations (up to 2–3 mM) (79) to the canaliculus that $E_2 17G$ is able to partition into the canalicular membrane and gain access to P-glycoprotein from the extracellular domain and induce cholestasis. Theoretically, high intracellular concentrations of $E_2 17G$ could also gain direct access to P-glycoprotein and induce cholestasis. According to the "hydrophobic vacuum cleaner" model of P-glycoprotein–mediated transport, P-glycoprotein can remove substrates directly from the plasma membrane (81); recent studies suggest that removal of substrate from the inner and the outer leaflet of the plasma membrane may occur by different mechanisms (82).

Much more work is needed to identify the relative roles of cMOAT and P-glycoprotein in $E_2 17G$ cholestasis. Conclusive evidence of P-glycoprotein-mediated transport of $E_2 17G$ in transfected cell lines lacking MRP/cMOAT is also needed, along with a measure of its affinity for P-glycoprotein. We also do not know why P-glycoprotein-mediated transport of $E_2 17G$ is essential to the cholestatic response. The data suggest that either the mechanism by which P-glycoprotein transports $E_2 17G$ or the

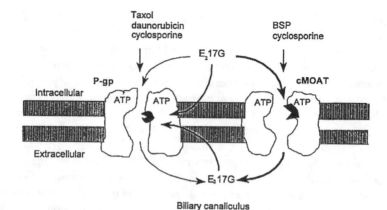

FIG. 6. A schematic model of the roles of P-glycoprotein (P-gp) and cMOAT in the transport of $E_2 17G$ and the resulting cholestasis. According to this model, $E_2 17G$ may access P-glycoprotein from either the intracellular compartment or the canaliculus. cMOAT is postulated to deliver high concentrations of $E_2 17G$ to the canaliculus, from which it can access P-glycoprotein via the canalicular membrane. $E_2 17G$ may also access P-glycoprotein from the intracellular compartment either directly, or most likely, via the canalicular membrane.

site to which it delivers $E_2 17G$ is critical. Potential key delivery sites include the ATP-dependent taurocholate transporter, since it is responsible for the transport of the most prevalent osmotically active solutes into bile. It is not known if $E_2 17G$ directly inhibits the canalicular taurocholate transporter or, as suggested by the data of Alvaro et al. (70), it alters canalicular membrane fluidity and thus inhibits taurocholate transport. Alternatively, P-glycoprotein may regulate a chloride channel in a manner analogous to that of CFTR, the cystic fibrosis transmembrane conductance regulator, as proposed by Higgins (83). While chloride channels have been identified in the canalicular membrane, they have been thought to be most important in the regulation of the volume of the hepatocyte in response to altered osmotic conditions, rather than to bile flow per se (84).

In summary, identification of the endogenously formed glucuronide conjugates of the estrogen D-ring as cholestatic agents has provided an important set of tools for investigating mechanisms of cholestasis associated with pregnancy and the cholestatic response to estrogens. Investigation of the mechanism of cholestatic action of the prototypic agent, $E_2 17G$, has identified taurocholate, the fluidity of the membrane, and the transporters cMOAT and P-glycoprotein as key pieces of this puzzle. The challenge of the next several years will be to identify how these pieces fit together. It seems likely that the emerging picture will demonstrate that cMOAT, P-glycoprotein, and the ATP-dependent bile salt transporter all work together in a coordinated manner, requiring a relatively fluid membrane for these postulated interactions, to deliver high concentrations of bile salts, followed by the movement of water, i.e., bile flow, which then permits the excretion of endogenous and exogenous waste products.

ACKNOWLEDGMENTS

This work was supported by HD13250 (GM55343) and by DK46923. We thank the many individuals in our laboratory who have contributed significantly over the years with their insights and experiments. We are particularly grateful to Dr. Yong Liu, Liyue Huang, and Tim Hoffman, who helped significantly in the preparation of this manuscript.

REFERENCES

1. Svanborg A. A study of recurrent jaundice in pregnancy. *Acta Gynecol* 1954;33:434–44.
2. Vore M. Estrogen cholestasis: membranes, metabolites, or receptors? *Gastroenterology* 1987;93: 643–649.
3. Kreek MJ. Female sex steroids and cholestasis. *Semin Liver Dis* 1987;7:8–23.
4. Furhoff AK, Hellstrom K. Jaundice in pregnancy: a follow-up study of the series of women originally reported by L. Thorling. I. The pregnancies. *Acta Med Scand* 1973;193:259–266.
5. Furhoff AK, Hellstrom K. Jaundice in pregnancy: a follow-up study of the series of women originally reported by L. Thorling. II Present health of the women. *Acta Med Scand* 1974;196:181–189.
6. Kreek MJ, Weser E, Sleisenger MH, Jeffries GH. Idiopathic cholestasis of pregnancy. *N Engl J Med* 1967;277:1391–1395.
7. Mueller MN, Kappas A. Estrogen pharmacology. I. The influence of estradiol and estriol on hepatic disposal of sulfobromophthalein (BSP) in man. *J Clin Invest* 1964;43:1905–1914.
8. Combes B, Shibata H, Adams R, Mitchell BD, Trammel V. Alterations in sulfobromophthalein sodium-removal mechanisms from blood during normal pregnancy. *J Clin Invest* 1963;42:1431–1442.
9. Gallagher TF, Mueller MN, Kappas A. Estrogen pharmacology. IV. Studies of the structural basis for estrogen-induced impairment of liver function. *Medicine* 1966;45:471–479.
10. Vore M, Bauer J, Pascucci V. The effect of pregnancy on the metabolism of ^{14}C-phenytoin in the isolated perfused rat liver. *J Pharmacol Exp Ther* 1978;206:439–447.
11. Vore M, Soliven E, Blunden M. The effect of pregnancy on the biliary excretion of ^{14}C-phenytoin in the rat. *J Pharmacol Exp Ther* 1979;208:257–262.
12. Vore M, Montgomery C. The effect of estradiol-17β treatment on the metabolism and biliary excretion of phenytoin in the isolated perfused rat liver and in vivo. *J Pharmacol Exp Ther* 1980;214:71–76.
13. Montgomery C, Vore M. The effect of diethylstilbestrol treatment on the metabolism and biliary excretion of ^{14}C-phenytoin in the isolated perfused rat liver. *Toxicol Appl Pharmacol* 1981;58:510–519.
14. Auansakul A, Vore M. The effect of pregnancy and estradiol-17β treatment on the biliary transport maximum of dibromosulfophthalein and the glucuronide conjugates of 5-phenyl-5-hydroxyphenyl-^{14}C-hydantoin and ^{14}C-morphine in the isolated perfused rat liver. *Drug Metab Dispos* 1982;10:344–349.
15. Durham S, Mack R, Vore M. Effects of taurocholate infusion on biliary excretion in isolated perfused rat livers. Decreased biliary excretion of dibromosulfophthalein in pregnancy. *Drug Metab Dispos* 1985;13:695–699.
16. Kreek MJ, Peterson RE, Sleisenger MH, Jeffries GH. Effects of ethinylestradiol-induced cholestasis on bile flow and biliary excretion of estradiol and estradiol glucuronide by the rat. *Proc Soc Exp Biol Med* 1969;131:646–650.
17. Forker EL. The effect of estrogen on bile formation in the rat. *J Clin Invest* 1969;48:654–663.
18. Gumucio J, Valdivieso V. Studies on the mechanisms of ethinylestradiol impairment of bile flow and bile salt excretion in the rat. *Gastroenterology* 1971;61:339–344.
19. Kern F, Eriksson H, Curstedt T, Sjövall J. Effect of ethinylestradiol on biliary excretion of bile acids, phosphatidylcholines and cholesterol in the bile fistula rat. *J Lipid Res* 1977;18:623–634.
20. Brock WJ, Vore M. The effect of pregnancy and treatment with estradiol-17β on the transport of organic anions into isolated rat hepatocytes. *Drug Metab Dispos* 1984;12:712–716.
21. Berr F, Simon FR, Reichen J. Ethynylestradiol impairs bile salt uptake and Na-K pump function of rat hepatocytes. *Am J Physiol* 1984;247:G437–G443.

22. Bossard R, Stieger B, O'Neill B, Fricker G, Meier PJ. Ethinylestradiol treatment induces multiple canalicular membrane transport alterations in rat liver. *J Clin Invest* 1993;91:2714–2720.
23. Kupferschmidt H, Hagenbuch B, Stieger B, Kraehenbühl, Meier PJ. Ethinylestradiol induces differential effects on various transporter mRNA and protein levels in rat liver. *Hepatology* 1994;20:175A.
24. Bowman SB, Fortune J, Sutherland E, Wolkoff A, Simon FR. Sex differences and hormonal regulation of hepatic organic anion transporters. *Hepatology* 1995;22:312A.
25. Ganguly T, Hyde JF, Vore M. Prolactin increases Na$^+$/taurocholate cotransport in isolated hepatocytes from postpartum rats and ovariectomized rats. *J Pharmacol Exp Therap* 1993;267:82–87.
26. Ganguly TC, Liu Y, Hyde JF, Hagenbuch B, Meier PJ, Vore M. Prolactin increases hepatic Na$^+$/taurocholate co-transport activity and messenger RNA *post partum*. *Biochem J* 1994;303:33–36.
27. Liu Y, Stieger B, Meier P, Vore M. Increased Na$^+$/taurocholate (TC) cotransport in basolateral liver plasma membrane vesicles post partum is due to overexpression of Na$^+$/TC cotransport polypeptide. *Hepatology* 1995;22:319A.
28. Vore M, Liu Y, Ganguly T. Prolactin and bile secretory function. In: Reyes HB, Leuschner U, Arias IM, eds. *Pregnancy, sex hormones and the liver*. Falk Symposium 89. London: Kluwer Academic Publishers, 1995.
29. Nathanson MH, Boyer JL. Mechanisms and regulation of bile formation. *Hepatology* 1991;14:551–566.
30. Meier PJ. Molecular mechanisms of hepatic bile salt transport from sinusoidal blood into bile. *Am J Physiol* 1995;269:G801–G812.
31. Lenzen R, Tarsetti F, Salvi R, Ekkehard S, Dembitzer R, Tavoloni N. Physiology of canalicular bile formation. In: Tavoloni N, Berk PD, eds. *Hepatic transport and bile secretion: physiology and pathophysiology*. New York: Raven Press, 1993:539–551.
32. Ballatori N, Truong AT. Relation between biliary glutathione excretion and bile acid-independent bile flow. *Am J Physiol* 1989;256:G22–G30.
33. Hagenbuch B, Stieger B, Foguet M, Lübbert H, Meier PJ. Functional expression cloning and characterization of the hepatocyte Na$^+$/bile acid cotransport system. *Proc Natl Acad Sci USA* 1991;88:10629–10633.
34. Jacquemin E, Hagenbuch B, Stieger B, Wolkoff AW, Meier PJ. Expression cloning of a rat liver Na$^+$-independent organic anion transporter. *Proc Natl Acad Sci USA* 1994;91:133–137.
35. Kanai N, Lu R, Bao Y, Wolkoff AW, Vore M, Schuster VL. Estradiol 17β-D-glucuronide is a high-affinity substrate for oatp organic anion transporter. *Am J Physiol* 1996;270:F326–F331.
36. Bossuyt X, Müller M, Hagenbuch B, Meier PJ. Polyspecific drug and steroid clearance by an organic anion transporter of mammalian liver. *J Pharmacol Exp Ther* 1996;276:891–896.
37. Nishida T, Gatmaitan Z, Che NM, Arias IM. Rat liver canalicular membrane vesicles contain an ATP-dependent bile acid transport system. *Proc Natl Acad Sci USA* 1991;88:6590–6594.
38. Adachi Y, Kobayashi H, Jurumi Y, Shouji M, Kitano M, Yamamoto T. ATP-dependent taurocholate transport by rat liver canalicular membrane vesicles. *Hepatology* 1991;14:655–659.
39. Müller M, Ishikawa T, Berger U, Klünemann C, Lucka L, Schreyer A, Kannicht C, Reutter W, Kurz G, Keppler D. ATP-dependent transport of taurocholate across the hepatocyte canalicular membrane mediated by a 110-kDa glycoprotein binding ATP and bile salt. *J Biol Chem* 1991;266:18920–18926.
40. Stieger B, O'Neill B, Meier PJ. ATP-dependent bile salt transport in canalicular rat liver plasma-membrane vesicles. *Biochem J* 1992;284:67–74.
41. Endicott JA, Ling V. The biochemistry of P-glycoprotein-mediated multidrug resistance. *Annu Rev Biochem* 1989;58:137–171.
42. Kamimoto Y, Gatmaitan Z, Hsu J, Arias IM. The function of Gp-170, the multidrug resistance gene product in rat liver canalicular membrane vesicles. *J Biol Chem* 1989;264:11693–11698.
43. Schrenk D, Gant TW, Preisegger J-H, Silverman JA, Marino PA, Thorgeirsson SS. Induction of multidrug resistance gene expression during cholestasis in rats and nonhuman primates. *Hepatology* 1993;17:854–860.
44. Vore M. Canalicular transport: discovery of ATP-dependent mechanisms. *Toxicol Appl Pharmacol* 1993;118:2–7.
45. Mayer R, Kartenbeck J, Büchler M, Jedlitschky G, Leier I, Keppler D. Expression of the *MRP* Gene-encoded conjugate export pump in liver and its selective absence from the canalicular membrane in transport-deficient mutant hepatocytes. *J Cell Biol* 1995;131:137–150.
46. Paulusma CC, Bosma PJ, Zaman GJR, Bakker CTM, Otter M, Scheffer GL, Scheper RJ, Borst P, Oude Elferink RPJ. Congenital jaundice in rats with a mutation in a multidrug resistance-associated protein gene. *Science* 1996;271:1126–1128.

47. Büchler M, König J, Brom M, Kartenbeck J, Spring J, Horie T, Keppler D. cDNA cloning of the hepatocyte canalicular isoform of the multidrug resistance protein, cMrp, reveals a novel conjugate export pump deficient in hyperbilirubinemic mutant rats. *J Biol Chem* 1996;271:15091–15098.

48. Jedlitschky G, Leier I, Buchholz U, Center M, Keppler D. ATP-dependent transport of glutathione S-conjugates by the multidrug resistance-associated protein. *Cancer Res* 1994;54:4833–4836.

49. Leier I, Jedlitschky G, Buchholz U, Cole SPC, Deeley RG, Keppler D. The *MRP* gene encodes an ATP-dependent export pump for leukotriene C$_4$ and structurally related conjugates. *J Biol Chem* 1994;269:27807–27810.

50. Jedlitschky G, Leir I, Buchholz U, Barnouin K, Kurz G, Keppler D. Transport of glutathione, glucuronate, and sulfate conjugates by the *MRP* gene-encoded conjugate export pump. *Cancer Res* 1996;56:988–994.

51. Meyers M, Slikker W, Pascoe G, Vore M. Characterization of cholestasis induced by estradiol-17β-D-glucuronide in the rat. *J Pharmacol Exp Ther* 1980;214:87–93.

52. Meyers MB. Characterization of steroid D-ring glucuronide-induced cholestasis in the rat. *Dissertation.* University of Kentucky, 1981.

53. Roy AB, Curtis CG, Powell GM. The metabolism of oestrone and some other steroids in isolated perfused rat and guinea pig livers. *Xenobiotica* 1987;17:1299–1313.

54. Slikker W, Vore M, Bailey J, Meyers M, Montgomery C. Hepatotoxic effects of estradiol-17β-D-glucuronide in the rat and monkey. *J Pharmacol Exp Ther* 1983;225:138–143.

55. Meyers M, Slikker W, Vore M. Steroid D-ring glucuronides: characterization of a new class of cholestatic agents in the rat. *J Pharmacol Exp Ther* 1981;218:63–73.

56. Vore M, Hadd H, Slikker W. Ethynylestradiol-17β D-ring glucuronide conjugates are potent cholestatic agents in the rat. *Life Sci* 1983;32:2989–2993.

57. Vore M, Montgomery C, Durham S, Schlarman D, Elliott, WH. Structure-activity relationship of the cholestatic activity of dihydrotestosterone glucuronide, allo bile acids and lithocholate. *Life Sci* 1989;44:2033–2040.

58. Vore M, Slikker W. Steroid D-ring glucuronides: a new class of cholestatic agents. *Trends Pharmacol Sci* 1985;6:256–259.

59. Kossor DC, Goldstein RS, Dulik DM, Meunier PC. Bile duct obstruction is not a prerequisite for biliary epithelial cell hyperplasia. *Toxicologist* 1993;13:394.

60. Changchit A, Durham S, Vore M. Characterization of ^{3}H-estradiol-17β-(β-D-glucuronide) binding sites in basolateral and canalicular liver plasma membranes. *Biochem Pharmacol* 1990;40:1219–1225.

61. Adinolfi LE, Utili R, Gaeta GB, Abernathy CO, Zimmerman HJ. Cholestasis induced by estradiol-17β-D-glucuronide: mechanisms and prevention by sodium taurocholate. *Hepatology* 1984;4:30–37.

62. Utili R, Tripodi MF, Adinolfi LE, Gaeta GB, Abernathy CO, Zimmerman, HJ. Estradiol-17β-D-glucuronide (E-17G) cholestasis in perfused rat liver: fate of E-17G and choleretic responses to bile salts. *Hepatology* 1990;11:735–742.

63. Durham S, Vore M. Taurocholate and steroid glucuronides: mutual protection against cholestasis in the isolated perfused rat liver. *J Pharmacol Exp Ther* 1986;237:490–495.

64. Vore M, Hoffman T. Carrier-mediated electrogenic transport of estradiol-17β-glucuronide in rat liver BMV. *Am J Physiol* 1994;267:G546–G551.

65. Vore M, Hoffman T, Gosland M. ATP-dependent transport of β-estradiol 17-(β-D-glucuronide) in rat canalicular membrane vesicles. *Am J Physiol* 1996;271:G791–G798.

66. Vore M, Liu Y, Huang L. Cholestatic properties and hepatic transport of steroid glucuronides. *Drug Metab Rev* 1997;29:183–203.

67. Jaeschke J, Krell H, Pfaff E. Quantitative estimation of transcellular and paracellular pathways of biliary sucrose in isolated perfused rat liver. *Biochem J* 1987;241:635–640.

68. Kan KS, Monte MJ, Parslow RA, Coleman R. Oestradiol 17β-glucuronide increases tight-junctional permeability in rat liver. *Biochem J* 1989;261:297–300.

69. Simon FR. Role of membrane lipids and fluidity in hepatic plasma membrane transport processes. In: Tavoloni N, Berk PD, eds. *Hepatic transport and bile secretion: physiology and pathophysiology.* New York: Raven Press,1993:297–312.

70. Alvaro D, Angelico M, Cantafora A, Gaudio E, Gandin C, Santini MT, Masella R, Capocaccia L. Improvement of estradiol 17β-D-glucuronide cholestasis by intravenous administration of dimethylethanolamine in the rat. *Hepatology* 1991;13:1158–1172.

71. Loe DW, Almquist KC, Cole SPC, Deeley RG. ATP-dependent 17β-estradiol 17-(β-D-glucuronide)

transport by multidrug resistance protein (MRP). Inhibition by cholestatic steroids. *J Biol Chem* 1996;271:9683–9689.

72. Takikawa H, Sano N, Narita T, Uchida Y, Yamanaka M, Horie T, Mikami T, Tagaya O. Biliary excretion of bile acid conjugates in hyperbilirubinemic mutant Sprague-Dawley rat. *Hepatology* 1991;14:352–360.

73. Ito K, Suzuki H, Hirohashi T, Kume K, Shimizu T, Sugiyama Y. Molecular cloning of canalicular multispecific organic anion transporter defective in EHBR. *Am J Physiol* 1997;272:G16–G22.

74. Sano N, Takikawa H, Yamanaka M. Estradiol-17β-glucuronide-induced cholestasis: effects of ursodeoxycholate-3-O-glucuronide and 3,7-disulfate. *J Hepatol* 1993;17:241–246.

75. Takikawa J, Yamazaki R, Sano N, Yamanaka M. Biliary excretion of estradiol-17β-glucuronide in the rat. *Hepatology* 1996;23:607–613.

76. Gosland M, Tsuboi C, Hoffman T, Goodin S, Vore M. 17β-estradiol glucuronide: an inducer of cholestasis and a physiological substrate for the multidrug resistance transporter. *Cancer Res* 1993;53:5382–5385.

77. Paul S, Breuninger LM, Tew KD, Shen H, Kruh GD. ATP-dependent uptake of natural product cytotoxic drugs by membrane vesicles establishes *MRP* as a broad specificity transporter. *Proc Natl Acad Sci USA* 1996;93:6929–6934.

78. Breuninger LM, Paul S, Gaughan K, Miki T, Chan A, Aaronson SA, Kruh GD. Expression of multidrug resistance-associated protein in NIH/3T3 cells confers multidrug resistance associated with increased drug efflux and altered intracellular drug distribution. *Cancer Res* 195;55:5342–5347.

79. Liu Y, Huang L, Hoffman T, Gosland M, Vore M. MDR1 substrates/modulators protect against β-estradiol-17β-D-glucuronide cholestasis in rat liver. *Cancer Res* 1996;56:4992–4997.

80. Bohme M, Jedlitschky G, Leier I, Buchler M, Keppler D. ATP-dependent export pumps and their inhibition by cyclosporins. *Adv Enzyme Regul* 1994;34:371–380.

81. Gottesman MM. How cancer cells evade chemotherapy: sixteenth Richard and Hinda Rosenthal foundation award lecture. *Cancer Res* 1993;53:747–754.

82. Stein WD, Cardarelli C, Pastan I, Gottesman MM. Kinetic evidence suggesting that the multidrug transporter differentially handles infux and efflux of its substrates. *Mol Pharmacol* 1994;45:763–772.

83. Higgins CF. P-glycoprotein and cell volume-activated chloride channels. *J Bioenerg Biomembr* 1995;27:63–70.

84. Boyer JL, Graf J, Meier PJ. Hepatic transport systems regulating pH$_i$, cell volume and bile secretion. *Annu Rev Physiol* 1992;54:415–438.

Toxicology of the Liver, 2nd ed.,
Edited by Gabriel L. Plaa and William R. Hewitt
Copyright © 1998 Taylor & Francis

11

Mechanisms Involved in Bile Acid–Induced Cholestasis

Ibrahim M. Yousef, Guylaine Bouchard, Beatriz Tuchweber, and Gabriel L. Plaa

Université de Montréal, Montréal, Québec, Canada H3C 3J7

Cholestasis has been defined by many hepatologists, including clinicans, toxicologists, and basic scientists. All agree that the term means bile stagnation resulting in failure of bile formation. Since most bile acids (BA) can be hepatotoxic, their role becomes an important factor in the development or maintenance of the cholestatic process. The purpose of this chapter is to review the experimental models used in BA-induced cholestasis and the possible cellular events and mechanisms underlying cholestasis.

BILE ACID BIOSYNTHESIS

BA biosynthesis and secretion are major pathways of cholesterol elimination from the body. They are also important for global lipid homeostasis. Cholesterol biotransformation to BA is a complex process. Its regulation has still not been fully elucidated. The process involves modification of the steroid nucleus, followed by side-chain transformation. Side-chain modification, however, can also initiate the biotransformation process. At least 15 enzymes are involved in the biosynthesis of BA. They are distributed in various hepatic cellular subfractions: microsomes, mitochondria, cytosol, and peroxysomes. Some are even present in extrahepatic cells. Many of these enzymes have been identified and isolated and their cDNA characterized. Recent reviews have been published (1–4).

Neosynthetized BA, mostly in their aminated form, join the preexisting BA pool and undergo enterohepatic circulation. BA secreted in the intestine are efficiently (95–97%) reabsorbed by an active Na-dependent ileal transporter (mainly the conjugated form) and by passive diffusion (mostly free BA) through the gastrointestinal tract (5). Through various reactions, which include deconjugation, dehydroxylation, desulfation, reduction, desaturation, and oxidation, the intestinal flora and enzymes generate a large number of metabolites, theoretically exceeding 1000 compounds, of which at least 20 have been definitely identified. BA metabolites formed in the intestine are partially reabsorbed by passive diffusion into the enterohepatic and systemic circulations (6, 7). The BA returning to the liver, particularly BA that have been deconjugated and metabolized in the intestine, undergo additional metabolism. Besides the hydroxylation process, there are numerous phase II metabolism processes such as conjugation, sulfation, glucuronidation, glycosylation, and N-acetylglucosamination (3, 7, 8).

BILE ACID METABOLISM IN CHOLESTASIS

As pointed out above, the composition of the BA pool is dependent on a large number of enzymes that regulate BA formation and biotransformation. Although the global regulation of these pathways remains to be clarified, relatively constant BA profiles are usually observed under normal conditions in plasma, feces, bile, and urine as well as in the BA pool, suggesting a high level of integration. Cholestasis, on the other hand, results in some deregulation of BA homeostasis. An excellent review on changes in BA composition and distribution in cholestasis was published by Ostrow

(9). The three classic features associated with virtually all cholestatic syndromes are increased BA concentrations, increased levels of sulfation and glucuronidation, and the presence of atypical BA, including polyhydroxylated BA and BA precursors (3, 9–13). Atypical BA contribute to changes in the conjugation profile (3, 14). The number of hydroxyl groups is an important factor in sulfation and glucuronidation of BA, since monohydroxylated BA are exclusively found in sulfate form in human cholestasis while only a small proportion of chenodeoxycholic (CDCA) and cholic acid (CA) forms ester sulfate (8). Furthermore, cholestasis is associated with impaired biliary secretion of BA, decreased availability in the enterohepatic circulation, hepatic retention and elevated systemic levels (3, 9, 11, 12, 15), producing major changes in the distribution and compartmentalization of the BA pool.

Serum and Plasma

In cholestasis, decreased biliary secretion increases BA reflux into plasma, which can reach up to 100 times the level in controls (9). In general, serum BA appears to be in good correlation with the severity of hepatobiliary diseases (9, 12). Primary BA are classically increased. The increase, however, appears to be greater for CA than CDCA in the early stages or in mild cholestasis, and the adverse phenomenon occurs in severe cholestasis (9). The percent contributions of the secondary BA deoxycholic acid (DCA) and lithocholic acid (LCA, the dehydroxylated product of the primary BA) are decreased. Another constant finding is the elevated plasma level of BA precursors such as 7-α-hydroxy-cholesterol and 3-β-hydroxy-5-cholenoic acid, as well as polyhydroxylated BA (3, 16, 17). The presence of 3-β-hydroxy-5-cholenoic acid, which is 90% sulfated or glucuronidated, is a characteristic feature of cholestasis, as this compound is absent or present in trace amounts under normal conditions (18). Taurine-conjugated BA are increased in cholestasis. Indeed, the level of the taurine-conjugated form appears to be in good correlation with the pruritus of cholestasis (18). Higher levels of glucuronidated, glucoside, and sulfated BA are also observed, with sulfates usually exceeding glucuronides (8, 9, 19). Ostrow (9) postulated that the increased percent contribution of BA sulfate esters in many subjects with liver disease may be related to disease progression or severity. In neonatal cholestasis, sulfated LCA shows the largest relative increase compared to CA and CDCA sulfates (20). However, CDCA constitutes an important part of the pool of BA glucuronides (7–8% of total BA) (21).

Urine and Renal Clearance

While urinary BA elimination is minor under normal conditions, it becomes a major factor in BA kinetics in cholestasis. Increased plasma BA levels and conjugation appear to be direct mediators of augmented urinary BA content (8, 22). The elimination rate, however, is highly variable for various BA: Sulfated BA are excreted 15–100 times more rapidly than free BA, and glucuronides 7–10 times more rapidly (9, 23). Furthermore, different sulfated BA show different renal clearance rates:

CA>CDCA>DCA>LCA>3-β-hydroxy-δ5-cholenoic acid (9). Compared to 25% of plasma BA in ester form, urinary BA contain 46% sulfated BA, 18% glucuronides, and 22% nonsulfated nonglucuronides (8). However, rates of sulfated BA as high as 80% have been reported (24). They could be related to the severity of the disease. The main urinary BA are sulfated CDCA and CA (22), mainly in monosulfate (3α) and disulfate (3,7 or 3,12) form, but some trisulfate BA are also present (9). The contributions of secondary BA, DCA, and LCA mostly secreted in ester form are largely decreased in cholestasis. Inversely, a much larger proportion of unusual and atypical BA, representing up to one-third of total BA, is observed (8, 9, 24). The major unusual BA are hydroxylated derivatives of primary BA, mostly C6α for CA and CDCA and C1β for CA (8, 24) although C2- and C4-hydroxylated derivatives are also found (25). More than 50 atypical BA have been identified (9). They include nor, oxo, allo, and unsaturated BA and bile alcohols. However, they usually remain relatively minor constituents of urinary BA.

Hepatic Content

Whatever the etiopathology of cholestasis, BA accumulation in the liver can reach about 10 times the normal concentration, and the plasma level can go up by two to 30 times (8, 9, 11) due mainly to impaired BA excretion from the canalicular pathway rather than aberrant hepatic uptake. The liver BA profile is also perturbed throughout cholestasis, with an initial increase of CA and then of CDCA as the disease progresses (9). There is also a gradual decrease of DCA, LCA, and sulfated BA (9). Hepatic BA mainly remains conjugated, with a significant increase in the proportion of taurine conjugates (7, 26). Hepatic BA accumulation is associated with a degenerative profile of cholestatic liver disease. A high correlation between the hepatic concentrations of dihydroxylated BA and feathery liver degeneration in chronic cholestasis suggests that they contribute to hepatic damage (8).

Bile

In cholestatic conditions, BA output has been found to decrease by 50% or more. This decrease is pronounced for the secondary BA, DCA. As in the liver, a proportionate increase of taurine conjugates is observed. The contribution of sulfates and glucuronides also appears to be augmented by up to fourfold but not more than 20% of the total circulation. Similarly, the unusual BA and bile alcohols may increase to about 10% of total BA (versus less than 5% in the controls) mostly as glucuronides of pentols, bile alcohols, or sulfates of 3-β-hydroxy-δ5-cholenoic acid (9).

Altered Bile Acid Kinetics, Turnover, and Metabolism

It is usually suggested that changes in BA kinetics are induced by cholestasis and that kinetic changes do not initiate cholestasis (6, 27). In humans, the kinetics of BA uptake by the liver do not appear to be affected in cholestasis. However, 30 min after the administration of free CA, a large reflux of amidated CA is observed in plasma supposedly mediated by impaired biliary secretion (9). The decreased enterohepatic circulation results in diminished intestinal BA and reduced fecal BA elimination (8). Thus, increased plasma levels culminate in higher urinary clearance. A few studies have focused on BA pool size in cholestasis. Evidence in humans suggests that the primary BA pool remains normal or decreases slightly (9, 22). This may be related to maintenance of balance between fractional turnover and synthesis, which have been reported to stay normal for CDCA but decline a little for CA. A higher turnover rate of CDCA is associated with an elevated level of sulfation, which apparently goes up by 27% (6). DCA pool size is decreased in relation to the severity and duration of cholestasis while the presence of novel BA and bile alcohols is augmented, suggesting higher synthesis than turnover rates of the latter. The synthesis rate appears to be inversely related to the degree of obstruction. The higher concentration of BA found in the liver with increasingly severe cholestasis, particularly of CDCA, which is a potent inhibitor of 7α-hydroxylase (28), could be important for decreasing synthesis. Other factors, however, such as rising bile alcohols or unusual BA derivatives, could have regulatory effects on BA synthesis.

EXPERIMENTAL CHOLESTASIS INDUCED BY BILE ACIDS

BA appear to be important mediators of cholestasis. Indeed, numerous investigators consider BA to be major initiators of this condition (29). The decreased efficiency of the enterohepatic circulation and biliary secretion is associated with increased liver and systemic BA concentrations that produce numerous secondary defects and worsen the pathology (8, 9, 30). Furthermore, altered BA profiles in cholestasis could also be important factors in hepatotoxicity, since the physiologic properties of BA are modulated by their chemical structure. Perturbations in the usual homeostasis of BA may also initiate cholestasis seen with intravenous infusion of stepwise increasing doses of BA (12, 31–35).

Monohydroxy Bile Acids

LCA is the principal monohydroxy BA in many species. It usually represents less than 5% of the BA pool (36, 37). LCA is a potent cholestatic agent (12, 38–50), and its accumulation may initiate or contribute to hepatic toxicity. LCA accumulation is known to occur in various cholestatic conditions in humans as in total parenteral nutrition-induced cholestasis (51), in cholestatic cystic fibrosis patients (12), and in some subjects treated with BA for gallstone or chronic liver diseases (52). Administration of LCA or its amidated conjugates causes rapid, dose-dependent, but reversible cholestasis in many animal species (12, 38–50). Chronic LCA administration can lead to BA retention and cirrhosis (53).

In experimental LCA-induced cholestasis, BA uptake does not appear to be affected while its canalicular secretion is decreased, culminating in global liver accumulation

(54). High-dose pulse administration of LCA, however, evokes a severe cholestatic response associated with an increased bile salt secretion rate (BSSR) (46). Decreased biliary lipid secretion, reduced transport maximum (Tm) of organic anions, and augmented secretion of membrane and cytoplasmic proteins are also associated with cholestasis (55, 56). Many canalicular changes are observed, mostly in periportal areas (57). These include canaliculus dilatation, loss of microvilli, modifications in the ectoplasm, and large increases of cholesterol but not of phospholipid (PL) in canalicular membranes, resulting in decreased fluidity (38, 39, 47, 55). The elevation of canalicular cholesterol is believed to be supplied by de novo synthesis and from the microsomal pool (58, 59). It is noteworthy that LCA does not produce cholestasis by retrograde perfusion (57) and that perivenous hepatocytes do not appear to synthesize cholesterol (60). Changes in membrane contents are linked with the incorporation of LCA in canalicular membranes (38, 39, 46, 47), although LCA seems to be mostly concentrated in cytosol (46), and cytosolic proteins are involved in LCA binding as well as in cholesterol transport to these membranes. Many other localized effects also occur, such as the formation of vacuoles (61, 62) and the secondary decrease of NaK-ATPase activity (38, 39, 63) in liver cell plasma membranes. Proliferation of the smooth endoplasmic reticulum (SER) is also observed with minimal mitochondrial defects (41) but appears to be a late event. The formation of biliary precipitates has also been suggested (44, 64). LCA provokes increased permeability of tight junctions but this change is insufficient to produce cholestasis (42, 47, 65).

A complex structure-effect relationship is evident in the cholestatic potency of monohydroxylated BA. In the guinea pig, sulfation of LCA or glyco-LCA does not protect against the cholestatic effect of the BA, while sulfation of tauro-LCA does (66, 67). Both sulfated-LCA and glyco-LCA are secreted in small amounts in bile. They induce cytoplasmic vacuoles with the lamellated myelin characteristics of phospholipidosis (49). Conjugation of LCA with glucuronides demonstrates cholestatic potency, and, in fact, LCA-glucuronidate is one of the more potent cholestatic agents among monohydroxylated BA (50, 68, 69). These characteristics may prove to be important in LCA cholestasis since LCA appears to be extensively metabolized, and only 6–10% is secreted in free form in bile (57, 69, 70). It is of interest that in LCA cholestasis, the biliary secretion of glucuronides of LCA has been found to be more significant in the cholestatic period, while hydroxylation and amidation increase with recovery from the cholestasis, suggesting that LCA-glucuronide formation contributes to LCA cholestasis (46, 70). Acinar zonation of LCA metabolism has also been implicated (70).

Although monohydroxylated BA–induced cholestasis has mostly been studied using LCA, it is obvious that cholestatic potency is not specific to LCA. Many unusual monohydroxylated BA such as 3-β-hydroxy-5-cholenoic acid (44), 3-β-hydroxy-5-β-cholanic acid (71), and mono-allo BA (48) are cholestatic agents. These monohydroxy derivatives are also amidated, glucuronidated, or sulfated. Their cholestatic potency is modulated by these biotransformations (53, 71, 72).

The total availability of monohydroxylated BA cannot in itself be sufficient to predict cholestasis. Their relative proportion to other noncholestatic or toxic BA appears to be just as important. Administration of less toxic dihydroxy or trihydroxy BA such as CDCA or CA, in appropriate doses, can prevent cholestasis or speed recovery from cholestasis induced by LCA (73), taurolithocholate (74), glucuronidated-LCA (75), or 5-β-hydroxy-5-cholenoic acid (44), which indicates a neutralizing effect of less hydrophobic BA. Protection of LCA cholestasis by tauro-CA or tauroursodeoxycholic acid has been shown to be associated not with decreased uptake but with increased LCA secretion, reduced LCA biotransformation, and heightened percent secretion in free form (56, 73). Cholestasis is inhibited or at least diminished by inhibitors of protein synthesis (cycloheximide) or the hypocholesterolemiant clofibrate (27, 59, 76). Cycloheximide and clofibrate protection is linked with decreased canalicular accumulation of cholesterol, which is suggested to be dependent on cytosolic proteins, since diminished BA binding has been reported in these conditions (59, 76).

Dihydroxy Bile Acids

Administration of CDCA in animals is associated with inhibition of bile flow (BF) and BSSR as well as with increased albumin and lactate dehydrogenase biliary secretion (77). In the isolated perfused female rat liver, infusion of CDCA induces complete cholestasis. Three hours after the addition of CDCA, "light" and "dark" liver cells are seen extensively. Nucleoli and chromatin are clumped, and there are dense granular aggregates within nucleoli. The rough endoplasmic reticulum (RER) is extensively disorganized, and autophagic vacuoles are prominent. Numerous indentations of the plasma membrane are seen along the sinusoidal surface, with clear, single, membrane-bound vacuoles in the cytoplasm, especially near the cell surface. In some light cells, ultrastructural breakdown is complete. These changes are less advanced in dark cells. These morphologic differences between LCA- and CDCA-induced cholestasis suggest that both are mediated through different pathogenic mechanisms (78). It is of interest that a similar dose of CDCA is not cholestatic in the isolated perfused liver obtained from male rats. This was explained by the greater capacity of the male liver to convert toxic CDCA to less hydrophobic β-muricholic acid (79). The lack of correlation between LCA levels and cholestasis in gallstone-bearing patients treated with CDCA may also suggest direct CDCA toxicity (80). The toxicity of CDCA is further supported by the observation that high-dose infusion of CDCA or its conjugates produces cholestasis, which follows their secretory rate maximum (SRm) values in bile duct–canulated rats (81, 82). It is puzzling, however, that high-dose infusion of tauro-CDCA, which is cholestatic in normal rats, does not demonstrate a classical SRm in the Eizai hyperbilirubinemic rat (EHBR) (83, 84). This animal has defective organic anion canalicular secretion but shows normal transport capacity in isolated canalicular membrane vesicles toward bilirubin (83). The other major dihydroxylated BA, DCA, is also a very cholestatic agent (85, 86). It is reported to be more hepatotoxic than LCA after 2 weeks of oral administration at 0.5% in the diet, being the only BA found to accumulate in liver and to induce lipid peroxidation (87). Both tauro-CDCA and tauro-DCA produce severe cholestasis and hepatocellular necrosis within hours (88).

High Bile Acid Concentrations

The relatively more hydrophilic BA such as CA are choleretic at doses that result in cholestasis with mono- or dihydroxylated BA. With infusion of stepwise increasing doses of CA, however, biliary secretion reaches its SRm and subsequently produces a decrease in the BSSR. Bile formation and lipid secretion are reduced, but biliary leakage of such proteins as albumin, LDH, alkaline phosphatase, and 5'-nucleotidase is increased (33, 35, 82, 89, 90). Cholestasis can be produced both in vivo (33, 35, 90) and in the isolated perfused liver (91). Although CA shows a much higher SRm than other BA, the change in subsequently occurring bile formation appears to be quite similar to the cholestasis induced by infusion of stepwise increasing doses of other BA. In one study of CA-induced cholestasis, PL secretion reached its SRm before the BA SRm (35, 92, 93). A change in biliary PL composition is observed at this point, the usual percent phosphatidylcholine decrease being associated with increased sphingomyelin and phosphatidylethanolamine levels. It should be emphasized that the SRm of BA is not stable and can be altered significantly by BA availability. It is greatly increased with an expanded BA pool but appears to be much more limited in BA pool–depleted animals (93–95).

Effect of Conjugation

BA secreted are almost totally conjugated with glycine or taurine in a ratio dependent mainly on taurine availability (96). Experimental studies have revealed that both glyco- and tauroconjugation do not abolish the cholestatic potency of BA (38, 97–99). Despite a decreased pKa and higher resistance to metal precipitation, the minimal effect of conjugation could be related to the lack of influence on relative BA lipophilicity, which usually matches the cholestatic potency of BA (100–102). Taurine-conjugated BA, however, demonstrate a higher SRm than glycoconjugates, and taurine administration in the guinea pig, which conjugates mostly with glycine, results in an increased SRm in relation to the level of conjugation with taurine (103), thus facilitating hepatic secretion. Another major effect of BA conjugation and cholestatic potency is found in further phase II metabolism, particularly sulfation, which generates BA with totally different cholestatic potency. It is worth mentioning, however, that conjugation sometimes appears to modulate the intracellular effect. As an example, glyco-CDCA but not CDCA or tauro-CDCA at a dose level of 250 μM elicits intracellular ATP depletion that could be related to impaired mitochondrial function (104).

Effect of Sulfation

BA sulfation is associated with a decrease in half-life and an increase in solubility, which are equated with reduced hepatotoxicity and cholestatic potency (3, 99). However, sulfation of monohydroxylated BA, particularly LCA, is not necessarily a protective mechanism. In fact, sulfation of LCA carries very little, if any, urinary secretion (7), appearing to be reabsorbed as well as the nonsulfated form (105), thus showing no facilitation of the elimination process. Most important, both sulfated LCA and sulfated glyco-LCA, but not sulfated tauro-LCA, remain highly cholestatic agents (12, 49). Sulfated-LCA, however, appears much less cholestatic than LCA itself in tauroconjugation species since sulfated tauro-LCA is mostly formed (50, 66). This observation, however, cannot be generalized since the sulfate of tauro-3β-hydroxy-5-cholenoate is as cholestatic as the nonsulfate form in rats (71). Cholestasis has been observed without signs of hepatic damage, as evaluated by light and electron microscopy, including normal canalicular morphology, although cytoplasmic vacuole accumulation and phospholipidosis are seen (49, 106). The physicochemical properties of sulfated tauro- and glyco-LCA have been studied, and major variations noted, particularly in regard to precipitation by metals. Sulfated glyco-LCA presents very strong Ca-binding capacity, unlike sulfated tauro-LCA (107, 108). Sulfated glyco-LCA is thought to be precipitated in the bile canaliculus (106–108). In addition, sulfated glyco-LCA does not, while sulfated tauro-LCA does, solubilize PL (109) and shows very low biliary secretion when compared to sulfated tauro-LCA, which suggests that intracellular hepatic accumulation may be related to cholestatic potency. However, the lack of cholestatic action of sulfated glyco-LCA in the GY mutant rat, which does not present significant canalicular secretion of the BA (108), could argue against such an intracellular effect. Thus, it has been proposed that canalicular secretion of the BA is essential for cholestatic action. Another possibility is that the cholestatic action of sulfated glyco-LCA is associated with a defective process already found in these mutants which have decreased basal BF. Pan-sulfation of dihydroxy and trihydroxy BA, on the other hand, prevents the cholestatic effect of high concentrations of non-sulfated analogues (99, 110).

Effect of Glucuronidation

For a long period of time, despite the known presence of glucuronidated BA, information regarding their effect on BF has remained very limited. Infusion of low amounts of ursodeoxycholic acid (UDCA)–glucuronide results in high choleretic potency of the BA, as expected from the presence of highly polar glucuronides (111). However, the best studied BA, LCA-glucuronide, has been demonstrated to be one of the more potent cholestatic BA identified to date (50, 68, 69). In normal rats, LCA-glucuronide is rapidly secreted in bile, mostly without being biotransformed (50, 112). As for LCA, cholestasis is reversible and can be prevented or reduced by more hydrophilic BA. In fact, administration of tauro-CA allows faster recuperation of BF (68). Faster hepatic elimination of LCA-glucuronide, which appears to be secreted by multiorganic anions transporter (MOAT) (113), can be expected since tauro-CA is known to stimulate the biliary secretion rate of components through MOAT transport. It is noteworthy, however, that although uptake of LCA-glucuronide is not affected in GY rats, this BA is not cholestatic in this mutant or in EHBR at doses that reduce BF in normal animals (114), suggesting that the hepatic level of the biliary BA is not associated per se with the development of cholestasis. LCA-glucuronide is known to be precipitated with calcium (Ca), and cholestasis is accompanied by white crystalline precipitates in bile (68). Secretion of this component into the canaliculus has also been proposed to be necessary into cholestasis induction on the basis of mutant studies. It is possible, however, that LCA-glucuronide may mediate cholestasis through a mechanism already defective in mutant rats. Inhibitors of protein synthesis (as in LCA cholestasis) or of vesicular transport (115) decrease or suppress cholestatic potency in normal rats (68), indicating that intracellular binding/transport to or through the canalicular membrane may be a major factor. A better comprehension of the properties of glucuronide-LCA and of other glucuronided-BA, particularly in high doses, would be useful since all usual unconjugated BA have been shown to be glucuronidated to various degrees, depending on the BA, in an apparent dose-related manner (116).

Although not discussed here, many other factors may influence the cholestatic effect of BA. These include prior treatment with ketogenic compounds (117–120), diet (121), and age (122–124). Improved knowledge via the integration of already-observed phenomena and mechanistic processes is needed for a better understanding of BA-induced cholestasis.

MECHANISMS OF BILE ACID–INDUCED CHOLESTASIS

Cholestasis can result from perturbation of any step involved in bile formation. Extensive investigation of abnormalities induced by BA revealed that they can affect numerous cellular functions. BA have been found in many cell compartments, including microsomes, mitochondria, cytosol, and nuclei. They induce anomalies in membrane composition and function, intracellular binding, distribution and metabolism of BA, mitochondrial energy supply, canalicular membrane supply, and microtubule and microfilament functions as well as intracellular second messenger signal lines, all possibly implicated in cholestasis (53, 125, 126). However, the exact mechanism of decreased BF after BA administration remains unclear (125). The following are some of the mechanisms proposed. It must be stressed that these mechanisms are not necessarily separated from each other, and in fact may constitute an integrated process.

Cellular Transport of Bile Acids

Polarized BA transport in hepatocytes is responsible for the high concentration gradient of BA from blood to intrahepatic content to canalicular space. This process is important because BA are a major osmotic driving force of bile formation and of cytotoxic effects via increased concentrations in hepatocytes (127). Perturbation of any steps involved in this process could thus produce cholestasis. Although their respective roles in cholestasis have not been well characterized, the three major steps of BA transport in hepatocytes must be considered (128, 129): basolateral uptake, intracellular transport, and canalicular secretion. Basolateral BA uptake into hepatocytes is mediated by at least two carrier transport systems, one Na-dependent, which appears to transport at least 80% of amidated BA, and the other Na-independent, which is mostly implicated in sulfate and glucuronide conjugate transport. Free hydrophobic BA seem to be transported by non-ionic diffusion (130, 131). Although often affected in cholestasis, basolateral BA uptake does not appear to be an initiating event in BA cholestasis (54) but could contribute to it. Intracellular BA transport remains a less characterized stage even though at least three families of cytosolic binding proteins are known to be involved (132, 133), and coordinated vectorial transport by vesicles involves the Golgi apparatus directly or indirectly (134–136). Cytosolic and vesicular apical proteins may also be an important factor in intracellular BA transport and BA-induced cholestasis. Canalicular BA transport, which is usually considered to be the rate-limiting step in hepatocyte transport, appears to be mediated by at least a BA electrogenic carrier, an ATP-dependent carrier, and the MOAT-dependent carrier (113, 137, 138). The relative capacity of the BA-ATP-dependent carrier, however, is estimated to be limited to 7 nmol/min/g liver (139) while the MOAT transporter is related to sulfated and glucuronidated BA (8). Electrogenic transport, which is probably mediated by a 100-kD transporter, appears to be the major canalicular vehicle for usually amidated BA. The direct contribution of these transporters to cholestasis still remains obscure. Another major factor in canalicular bile secretory capacity could be the structure and contraction of canaliculi, which are at least partly dependent on the microfilaments. In view of the possible importance of these steps in the pathogenesis of BA cholestasis, and because of the limited information available in some areas, we will concentrate only on the role of binding proteins, vesicular transport and microfilaments.

Effect on Cellular Binding

BA binding to intracellular proteins is reported to be directly related to hydrophobicity. The exact repercussions of these different binding ratios need to be characterized because they could significantly modulate the cholestatic potency of BA, which is known to be correlated with hydrophilicity (55). In isolated hepatocytes, derivatives of CA and CDCA are rapidly transferred to the canalicular space while LCA accumulates within the cell and is less concentrated in the canaliculus (140). It is well known that intracellular binding of BA to cytosolic proteins allows BA to concentrate in hepatocytes and limits their reflux to plasma but it also appears to limit their canalicular secretion (33). Thus, there seems to be a relationship between the level of BA binding to cytosolic proteins, possible liver accumulation and the BA-SRm. The level of intracellular binding proteins might thus directly contribute to both the rate of canalicular secretion and the extent of hepatic BA accumulation. Experimental evidence supports the role of binding proteins in cholestasis. Particularly in the LCA cholestasis model, it is known that increased protein synthesis (with methyl isobutyl ketone [MIBK]) is associated with greater cholestatic conditions while reversal with inhibitors of protein synthesis minimizes cholestasis. In the suckling guinea pig, which is resistant to LCA cholestasis, and in adults following pretreatment with cycloheximide, which prevents LCA cholestasis, decreased intracellular binding of BA to the cytosolic fraction has been observed (76, 97, 141–144), lending credance to the view that changes in intracellular binding protein levels may be responsible. In vitro, the presence of cytosol increases LCA binding to plasma membranes and microsomes (40), an effect known to be related to the peak of cholestasis in vivo (45). These findings suggest that cytosolic binding proteins could serve in transport of BA to the intracellular compartments. As an example, BA, by analogy with steroids (145), could utilize cytosolic binding proteins for transport to the nuclei, where they could mediate their known effects on gene regulatory elements. In addition, increased hepatic BA levels could saturate cytosol binding proteins and also lead to greater intracellular distribution, which could be implicated in the development of cholestasis. In this regard, it has been shown that binding to microsomal and plasma membranes is augmented at the cholestatic peak induced by LCA while it is decreased in the recovery phase (46). Although the role of elevated amounts of LCA in plasma membranes and microsomes remains obscure, LCA binding to canalicular membranes has been proposed to alter membrane structure, which, in addition to allowing incorporation of additional cholesterol in membranes, could change membrane transport and permeability capacities. It is possible that binding to plasma membranes follows binding to microsomes since both fractions show similar binding levels in cholestasis and also in recuperation from cholestasis, in which LCA content is decreased by more than 50% (46). Vesicles derived from the endoplasmic reticulum (ER) could thus contribute to changes in plasma membranes.

Effect on Vesicle Transport

The exact role of vesicular transport in normal bile formation and in cholestasis is not quite clear. However, stimulation of BF by many agents including BA (146, 147), or directly through cAMP elevation, cell response to increased hydration or intracellular pH is associated with stimulation of vesicular transport to the apical membrane (148). This stimulation of the vesicular pathway is suggested by the blockade of bile stimulation in many of these processes by colchicine (149–152), an inhibitor of tubulin polymerization that appears to be necessary for apical vesicular transport (153). Note that colchicine only blocks the slow, microtubule-dependent vesicular pathway since the so-called rapid transit vesicular pathway is microtubule-independent (146).

Following high-dose administration, BA have been shown to accumulate in the Golgi and ER (154, 155), which initially suggested BA vesicular transport. An alternative hypothesis, however, may involve the binding of the BA to the canalicular transporters in these organelles (156). Hepatocytes, however, appear to be dependent on transcytosis for the supply of protein to the canalicular membrane to maintain cell polarization (157–159). Such a mechanism has been proposed for the BA transporter, for MOAT (156, 160), and for ecto-ATPase. Experimental evidence supports a direct contribution of vesicular transport to bile formation and cholestasis. First, exposure to isoosmotic stress (150, 156, 161, 162) is known to result in regulatory volume processes that occur rapidly, reestablishing new cell equilibrium. Although cell swelling and the associated regulatory volume decrease have been shown to stimulate vesicular transport (horseradish peroxidase [HRP] biliary secretion), this effect appears to return to normal with the new equilibrium level. BA administration in this last stage, however, elicits a much higher BA secretory rate than in normoosmotic conditions, indicating increased transporter transport through the membrane during the stimulated vesicular transport phase (162). More direct evidence has recently been provided in isolated couplets treated with stimulators or inhibitors of apical vesicular transport, which showed that direct stimulation of this pathway resulted in increased canalicular content of fluorescent BA and to heightened expression of the canalicular membrane protein ecto-ATPase. Inversely, inhibitors of microtubules decrease BA content in canaliculi (148), still indicating some needed supply from vesicular sources. As discussed by Maurice et al. (159), the transcytosis process appears to be affected in experimental cholestasis evidenced, for example, by abnormal basolateral localization of many canalicular proteins or evaluated by HPR biliary secretion (163–165). It might thus be suggested that decreased canalicular insertion of vesicles into membranes, by reduced vesicular availability or decreased insertion of vesicules into membranes, may be a major factor leading to cholestasis. The accumulation of vesicular structures in the pericanalicular region in humans but also in experimental cholestasis, including the BA model (148, 164, 165), points to such a defect.

Vesicular transport to the apical membrane could also play a pivotal role in the observed BA SRm since colchicine, which does not affect BA uptake, potentiates the cholestatic effect of BA occurring at much lower doses and with a decreased SRm and lipid secretion, suggesting that physiologic blockade of directed vesicular transport could mediate cholestasis (166–169).

It is also of major importance that BA themselves are able to modulate their SRm. After depletion of the endogenous pool, a 50% decrease in the secretion of administered TC is observed and associated with fewer membrane binding sites, but reflux is increased. Prefeeding with TC, in the absence of cycloheximide, expands the endogenous pool by 50%, and this effect is abolished by cycloheximide pretreatment (94, 95, 170). These results strongly suggest that BA themselves modulate or induce the modulation of expression of some proteins implicated in their vectorial transport and that such action is needed to reach very high secretory rates. Since canalicular secretion is considered to be the limiting factor, BA may exert effects on their own canalicular transporters. Tauro-LCA and other BA under supraphysiologic conditions are known to inhibit NaK-ATPase activity (139). Although decreased activity is associated with lower intracellular K concentrations in other models, a direct action of BA should be considered since inhibition is observed in isolated membranes. Whatever the mechanism, reduced NaK activity would dissipate the Na gradient and result in diminished BA uptake.

Microfilaments

Microfilaments are concentrated in the hepatocyte pericanalicular zone (171). Evidence has been provided for their role in mechanical canalicular contraction and bile propulsion (172), regulation of tight junction permeability, and canalicular translocation of vesicles (173). Disruption of microfilaments could thus be an important contributing factor in cholestasis. Well-known microfilaments disrupting agents such as phalloidin, which produces irreversible polymerization of actin, and cytochalasin B, which destroys the microfilament network, lead to decreased BF (174, 175) through proposed ileus spastic and ileus paralytic cholestasis, respectively.

Although limited information is available on the role of microfilaments in BA-induced cholestasis, high BA doses in vitro produce bleb formation (176) that may be related to cytoskeleton disruption (55). In fact, in isolated rat couplets, tauro-LCA has been shown, as with many other cholestatic agents, to cause F-actin accumulation, evaluated by fluorescein-isothiocyanate phalloidin staining, although no signs of change could be observed by electron microscopy (177). Accumulation of pericanalicular ectoplasm following chronic tauro-LCA administration is, however, visible by electron microscopy (43). In vitro, a decreased rate of actin polymerization with BA has been observed (178). This suggests changes in the globular and filamentous actin ratio or reduced interactions of actin and myosin filaments, which appears to be necessary for canalicular contraction (179, 180). Such interactions seem to be ATP-dependent, and the contribution of MgATPase has been proposed (181). Decreased activity of this ATPase could thus lead to BA cholestasis. Globally, these observations suggest a loss of functional integrity through the destruction of microfilaments. Such an effect could be related to dilation of the canaliculus (171), which is a feature of BA cholestasis. Intracellular perturbations of other microfilament functions in BA cholestasis support the view that BA evoke their disruption. First, significantly increased permeation of inert solutes by tauro-LCA or high doses of tauro-CA produces disruption of junctional strands with a loss of parallel orientation (139). Second, pericanalicular vesicles are found to accumulate in some BA cholestasis models, suggesting that all usual microfilament functions are affected. However, the initiating role of microfilament disruption remains unproven, and, in fact, the ectoplasm accumulation observed without a defect in BF after tauro-LCA indicates a dissociation (43). Evidence from better characterized models of cytochalasin B and work in our laboratory with phalloidin suggest that the respective changes in microfilaments are insufficient to explain the etiology of cholestasis (182). In fact, cytochalasin B in cultured hepatocytes does not affect secretory function (183), so it has been proposed that the integrity of microfilaments is not necessary if the pericanalicular sheath of intermediate filaments is intact. Intermediate filaments are distributed in all hepatocyte spaces but are concentrated in pericanalicular areas where they form a continuous sheath. An intact peric analicular sheath has been suggested to be necessary for normal secretory capacity (173). Disruption of the intermediate filaments is associated with the formation of Mallory bodies in cholestasis, mostly in the periportal zone (184). As for microfilaments, they are found to be increased by phalloidin (185). However, their exact role in bile formation and cholestasis remains obscure.

Bile Acid Metabolism

The role of BA metabolism in the development of BA cholestasis has not been thoroughly investigated. It has, however, become obvious that BA metabolism plays an important role in the resulting effect on BF. LCA hydroxylation is found to be increased in the recovery phase of acute cholestasis (46), and the absence of a cholestatic action of tauro-LCA by retrograde perfusion has been partially explained by increased tauro-LCA metabolism to more hydrophilic BA (57). In a more chronic model (43), the very low cholestatic potency of LCA has been attributed to the formation of hydroxylated metabolites, suggesting that the relative hydrophobic/hydrophilic balance of BA may be important. It is clear that increased hydrophilicity is not sufficient to predict cholestatic potency since both sulfated- and glucuronidated-LCA are highly cholestatic (49, 50, 68, 69). In fact, in the rat, which does not appear to conjugate usual BA with sulfate, LCA cholestasis correlates with higher levels of glucuronide biliary secretion (46). The reason for LCA-glucuronide formation is not well understood but it has been proposed to be indirectly controlled by liver amidation capacity and saturation of the system results in more glucuronide formation. The reason behind the higher cholestatic potency of LCA-glucuronide remains unclear. LCA-glucuronide, like the very cholestatic agent estradiol-glucuronide, is known to be transported through a more distinct canalicular transporter (113) than in the amidated form, and some direct action on this MOAT transporter has been postulated. Administration of similar amounts of UDCA- or CA-glucuronides, however, has proven to be choleretic (186, 187). It should be pointed out that LCA-glucuronides are significantly less cytotoxic than LCA itself (188): 50% cytotoxicity has been observed at the 150 and 50 μM dose levels, respectively, as measured by lactate dehydrogenase release in isolated rat hepatocytes, pointing to a distinct mechanism of BA action inducing cholestasis and cytotoxicity.

Membrane Effects

BA interactions with membranes are well known to occur. Changes in lipid composition and fluidity as well as permeability have been reported in many types of cell membranes, including erythrocytes and hepatocytes (38, 47, 73, 88, 92, 181, 189–191). In high concentration (critical micellar concentration [CMC]), BA solubilize membrane lipids and proteins (35, 55). All usual BA are known to be potent detergents and have been shown to be incorporated into various membranes, including plasma, inner mitochondria, Golgi, and ER (192), inducing lipid solubilization. Changes in some membrane protein activities, such as of NaK-ATPase, could be related to global membrane perturbations (63). In isolated hepatocytes, BA cause enzyme release and membrane lysis that appear to be directly correlated with the relative lipophilic balance of BA in free or conjugated form (190). Although these studies showed a definite role of BA in cytotoxicity at levels found in cholestasis, it has never been obvious that BA changes are related to the induction of cholestasis. Leuschner et al. (55) proposed, however, that even in concentrations below their CMC, BA can induce membrane damage. BA accumulate in membranes, partitioning the deep layer and modulating the orientation of lipids. Thus, they produce transient holes and leaky membranes. Such an effect, which is supported by observations of membrane fluidity, could induce some intracellular content leakage as lactate dehydrogenase canalicular secretion (55, 125). A similar mechanism was proposed by Kakis and Yousef (38, 73).

In vivo studies have shown that near the initiation of acute cholestasis, although through apparently different mechanisms, BA produce changes in cholesterol and PL ratios of the membrane lipid, including the ER and the canalicular membrane. Mixed plasma membrane (mostly basolateral) composition also appears to be rapidly affected and presents reversible decreases of ATPase activity with increased fluidity (181). A detailed investigation of membrane composition following high-dose administration of CA revealed that major changes were induced (92). In enriched canalicular membrane fractions, a threefold decrease in total PL content was observed without changes in cholesterol content, resulting in a threefold increase in the cholesterol/PL ratio. Enriched microsomal membranes also demonstrated a decrease in PL content (twofold). In terms of total solubilization, about three times more PL appeared to be withdrawn from microsomes. At the SRm level, biliary PL composition was modulated, with increased phosphatidylethanolamine and sphingomyelin contributions, and their global fatty acids showed decreases in C16:0 and C18:2 (usual major constituents) but with elevated fatty acid membrane constituents such as C24:0. These changes could well correlate with depletion of supply of the specific PL pool to the canalicular membrane, which has been postulated to initiate cholestasis (92, 93). Some evidence has been provided that BA are secreted through the canalicular lumen and then solubilize biliary lipids from specific canalicular membrane vesicle microdomains (92, 166, 193) that are resupplied by transport of vesicles to the apical membrane. However, sources of biliary PL appear to include de novo synthesis, as well as microsome, Golgi, and preformed extrahepatic pools (194, 195). Evidence suggests, however, that the microsome and extrahepatic pools are major contributors (195, 196). The specific decrease in PL of both canalicular and microsomal membranes during BA cholestasis indicates microsomal depletion with reduced supply to the canalicular membrane. A recent investigation showed that the total PL secretion in bile produced by micellar BA is similar before reaching the SRm, with more hydrophobic BA inducing higher PL secretion rate per BA (197). DCA and CDCA have been shown to solubilize plasma and microsomal membrane lipids at lower concentrations than CA (191), and possible depletion of the specifically directed PL pool could thus also be implicated in these types of cholestasis. It is noteworthy that BA potency to extract PL from ER membranes is related to their hydrophobicity (198). Such a lack of PL might impair vesicle formation and could thus mediate a decrease in apical vesicular transport or membrane insertion.

Interaction with Calcium

Regulation and oscillation of intracellular Ca levels are associated with various cell functions, including secretion, metabolism, motility, cell division, and structural integrity of the cytoskeleton. However, Ca is also a cofactor for many proteases, phospholipases, and endonucleases. A sustained increase of intracellular Ca has been implicated in cell death (199). The cell blebbing seen in isolated hepatocytes exposed to high BA concentrations indicates that cell death might occur through Ca-dependent mechanisms (189). The observation that LCA elevates intracellular Ca levels led to the proposal of a role for Ca in BA-induced cholestasis. In fact, all usual BA have been shown to produce an increase in intracellular Ca in isolated cells. The rise in intracellular Ca has been found to be dose-dependent and in good correlation to the relative hydrophobicity of BA, both free and conjugated LCA augmenting cytosolic Ca more than CDCA and DCA, which are more efficient than CA (200–202). Increases in cytosolic Ca have been reported to be mediated by various endogenous pools, mostly the ER pool independent of inositol triphosphate, but possibly dependent on protein kinase c, at least for tauro-LCA (203–206), and an extracellular pool through an ionophoric action (139, 207, 208) for most BA. In isolated hepatocytes, most BA investigated, including LCA, CDCA, and DCA; some conjugates; and LCA-sulfate, tauro-LCA-sulfate, and LCA-glucuronide have been shown to induce a biphasic change in cytosolic calcium: a very large increase followed by a gradual decrease that appears to be associated with Ca efflux. Ca efflux is related to hydrophobicity of the steroid nucleus in the isolated perfused liver (IPL) (209, 210). It is thought to be mediated by a plasma membrane Ca pump. Increased intracellular Ca also appears to produce activation of Ca-dependent K and Cl current efflux, as reported for sulfated-tauro-LCA and tauro-DCA (207, 211). In very high amounts, mono- and dihydroxy BA cause a secondary and irreversible rise in intracellular Ca that is associated with toxicity (202).

It is quite clear, however, that the elevation of intracellular Ca produced by BA is in itself insufficient to explain cholestasis. In the LCA cholestasis model, increased intracellular Ca is associated with heightened metabolic activity but shows no sign of toxicity (189). Indirect evaluation of Ca levels in LCA cholestasis as determined by augmented phosphorylase a activity in vivo (45) was not associated with changes in bile flow. A sustained increase of intracellular Ca by depletion of ER stores associated with a loss of response to vasopressin and phenylephrine did not produce changes in BF in IPL (212), suggesting that cholestasis cannot be attributed to prolonged liberation of Ca from ER stores. The increase in intracellular Ca and activation of phosphorylase a observed with the hepatoprotective and noncholestatic BA UDCA (204) further support an indirect relationship, if any. In isolated rat hepatocytes, tauro-UDCA has been shown to produce a sustained rise in intracellular Ca in the presence of extracellular Ca, being even a more potent inducer of intracellular Ca levels than other usually cholestatic BA (203). Tauro-UDCA abolishes further responses to tauro-CA (203), but the fact that tauro-LCA and -UDCA result in a much higher increase than with tauro-LCA alone in hepatocytes (204) but not in couplets (202), although being hepatoprotective against both BA, still points to a dissociation between global intracellular Ca and cholestasis. A role of Ca, however, cannot be excluded, and more precise analysis of Ca movements is needed. As an example, both tauro-LCA and sulfated-tauro-LCA, which are thought to liberate Ca from a common intracellular pool, increase cytosolic Ca but produce very distinct changes in intracellular Ca movement. Tauro-LCA evokes a sustained rise in cytosolic Ca and does not appear to elicit Ca-induced Ca release, while sulfated-tauro-LCA produces repetitive oscillating pulses of intracellular Ca that are significantly blocked by ryanodine, an inhibitor of Ca-induced Ca release (206), suggesting that distinct Ca-induced patterns could exert diverse hepatocellular effects and cholestatic responses.

Other types of interactions between BA and Ca have been investigated. BA binding to Ca is related to their hydrophobic balance, the more hydrophobic BA usually showing greater binding affinity (213). Binding of BA, particularly of hydrophobic BA, to Ca could result in the formation of insoluble aggregates leading to blockade of the canaliculus (44). What is puzzling, however, is that there is no consistency between the presence of precipitates and cholestasis, which strongly argues against solely precipitation-related cholestasis. It should be noted that sulfated-glyco-LCA, but not sulfated-tauro-LCA, which is not cholestatic, binds avidly to Ca. Although other possibilities exist, the lack of cholestatic effect of sulfated-glyco-LCA in mutant GY rats that show normal uptake but limited secretion of this BA is considered to support the precipitation hypothesis (108).

Effect on Bile Salt–Independent Bile Flow (BSIF)

Although BA provide an important driving force for osmotic canaliculus bile formation (138), other factors also contribute to this process. Although still subject to controversy, evaluation of the intercept between BF and BSSR allows estimation of the BSIF, which might not be really independent of BA since they appear to modulate BSIF in relation to their concentration and composition. BSIF evaluation in LCA cholestasis demonstrates a decrease in the Y-intercept (214), suggestive of BSIF inhibition. In fact, both the very significant cholestasis produced by LCA in rats, which is sometimes associated with increased BSSR, and the dissociation between BF and BSSR observed near the development of cholestasis with dihydroxylated BA (46, 99) implicate decreased BSIF. Unpublished results from this laboratory have revealed that, following high-dose infusions of various BA (CA, CDCA, DCA, LCA), diminished bile formation is accompanied by a major drop in the percent BSIF contribution to total BF in rats when compared with periods preceding the SRm. In other cholestatic models, decreased bile formation has been shown to produce specific inhibition of BSIF (215), suggesting that this portion of flow does not solely follow BA as a driving force and is somehow independently regulated. The effect observed after BA administration, however, indicates that they interfere with BSIF generation by an actually uncharacterized, most probably hepatic, process.

It is difficult to identify the precise inhibitory impact of BA on BSIF because the factors implicated in its generation are not fully understood. However, glutathione

(GSH) was demonstrated to be an important osmotic driving force (216). It appears to mediate about 50% of BSIF generation. Hepatic evaluation of GSH levels after LCA cholestasis supports an effect of BA on GSH homeostasis. However, although subsequently decreased, hepatic GSH level was found to be normal at the beginning of cholestasis (45). Although hepatic GSH levels usually correlate with biliary secretion, this relationship has been reported to be disturbed in cholestasis (215). Direct investigation of the effect of LCA on biliary GSH secretion with the progression of cholestasis would be interesting, particularly since glucuronidated-LCA, with its biliary secretion increased at the beginning of cholestasis, has been shown to inhibit biliary GSH secretion (217). Although the extent of its contribution to cholestasis has not been studied, tauro-CA has been demonstrated to decrease biliary GSH content in cholestatic conditions while increasing plasma reflux (218), an effect attributed to greater tight junction permeability produced by BA. Raiford et al. (219), however, provided evidence against a change in tight junction permeability significantly modulating biliary GSH and sinusoidal efflux or content, suggesting that other mechanisms, such as directed GSH transport, may be involved.

In addition to GSH, many other biliary components, particularly electrolytes, have been implicated but, with the exception of bicarbonate, they do not appear efficient enough to constitute a driving force due to their low reflection coefficient which will allow back diffusion to plasma, even if they were actively secreted by hepatocytes (220). More controversially, the electrochemical equilibrium of canalicular pH with extracellular pH, suggestive of hydrogen and bicarbonate diffusion through paracellular pathways (132), supports the view that bicarbonate is not directly involved in the generation of canalicular BF although it probably plays a role in ductular bile formation. As estimated by Alpini et al. (221), ductular bile contributes about 10% of total BF in rats, and the lack of effect of usual BA on HCO_3 biliary concentration (222, 223) does not validate a strong interaction at this level. Finally, fluid phase endocytosis/canalicular exocytosis appears to contribute to BSIF generation. It has been estimated to represent less than 2–6% or as much as 30% of BF (132, 224, 225). The exact contribution of fluid phase endocytosis to BA cholestasis has not yet been determined. Many more studies are needed to clarify the importance of BSIF inhibition in BA cholestasis and its contributing mechanisms.

Effect on Redox Cycling, ATP Levels, and Free Radical Formation (or Lipid Peroxidation)

Although subject to controversy, increased O_2 consumption induced by BA appears to parallel their hydrophobicity under some conditions (189, 226) and thus could participate in the cholestatic process. Evidence has been provided that higher O_2 consumption could be associated with mitochondrial uncoupling observed after high-dose BA administration (227). However, as discussed by Reichen (125), lower BA concentrations, in the order of 10 μM, which are more likely to be obtained in the mitochondrial environment, even in cholestasis, inhibit mitochondrial respiration through direct suppression of complexes I (succinate dehydrogenase) and III (bc complex), without producing uncoupling associated with enhanced O_2 consumption. Another hypothesis linking increased O_2 consumption with augmentation of lipid peroxidation products by hydrophobic BA in microsomal membranes (125, 228) or isolated hepatocytes (229) suggests that elevated amounts of hydrophobic BA could stimulate oxygen radical formation. The BA binder 3-α-hydroxysteroid dehydrogenase has been proposed to be responsible for this initiation since it could mediate cyclical oxidation in hepatocytes and IPL (125, 230, 231), resulting in higher O_2 consumption. In fact, BA may be important contributors to the redox state in hepatocytes. In vitro, BA have been shown to have direct antioxidant properties like scavenging peroxyl radicals on polyunsaturated lipids by BA oxidation, producing keto-7 BA for CA and CDCA (228). However, BA appear to enhance lipid peroxidation at a higher lipid:BA concentration (228). Increased hydroperoxide formation observed in hepatocytes following incubation with high BA doses would thus result in oxidative stress and elevated levels of intracellular oxidized GSH, intracellular Ca, and inositol triphosphate; accelerated K release; and cell shrinkage, probably via activation of K channels sensitive to barium (232) and leading subsequently to cell death. The known effect of BA on the release of oxygen radicals by neutrophils (233) and the increased degranulation of mast cells (234) could also contribute to amplification of toxicity. It could be mentioned that a high concentration of glyco-CDCA (but not LCA) produces mitochondrial membrane permeability transition (235) by a mechanism not yet well defined. This may be associated with a loss of membrane PL, which are known to be necessary for electron chain integrity (190, 236), thus eliciting uncoupling of the respiratory chain, leading to ATP depletion and possible secondary defects of this depletion, such as decreased NaK-ATPase activity and BA uptake or diminished canalicular BA secretion. ATP depletion, however, causes more serious perturbations, including a sustained increase of intracellular Ca and activation of Ca-dependent proteases that result in cell necrosis (237). Although it is obvious that any of these derangements would aggravate cholestasis, their contribution to its initiation remains unclear. In fact, there appears to be no relationship between the BF and O_2 consumption. The best example seems to be the increased O_2 consumption produced by tauro-LCA in both anterograde and retrograde perfusion while backward perfusion is not cholestatic. However, tauro-LCA is hepatotoxic by anterograde perfusion, suggesting that O_2 consumption may be solely related to toxicity (226).

Effect on the Major Histocompatibility Complex (MHC) in Hepatocytes

The aberrant expression of class I MHC antigen in humans has recently been demonstrated in hepatic autoimmune diseases and viral hepatitis as well as in various chronic cholestatic conditions (238–240). In fact, such aberrant expression also appears to be a feature of experimental cholestasis (239, 241). Investigation of the possible role of BA in this process recently revealed that at least some BA, particularly CDCA but not UDCA, induce the aberrant expression of class I MHC antigen on human and rat hepatocytes in primary cultures or in human hepatoma cell lines (242, 243) in association with elevated mRNA levels, possibly through increased transcriptional activity. The effect of CDCA appears to occur at the transcription level, perhaps through protein kinase c and protein kinase a activation. This unexpected effect of BA and cholestasis may obviously increase vulnerability of the liver to immune destruction, allowing the action of cytotoxic lymphocytes on hepatocytes. Thus, such expression of antigens could directly contribute to the initiation of cholestasis.

CONCLUSIONS

It is tempting to classify the effects of bile acid on the reduction of bile flow (cholestasis) into two categories: bile acid–induced cholestatic effects and bile acid–induced cytotoxicity resulting in cholestasis.

The first group of these bile acids is those that induce cholestasis at low concentration, in a dose-dependent fashion, reversible and independent of their hydrophobicity. This group includes mainly the 3α- or 3β-monohydroxy bile acids whether they are saturated or unsaturated, free, conjugated, sulfated, glucuronidated, or in other derivatives described thus far. This suggests that the pathogenesis of the cholestasis induced by these compounds must involve the hydroxyl group in the 3 position, which possibly confers the cholestatic effect on the molecule despite its hydrophobicity. Figure 1 summarizes the pathogenesis of the cholestasis induced by these molecules. After their uptake by the liver, these bile acids bind to cytosolic protein. This binding increases its concentration in the liver cell and causes disturbance in its intracellular distribution and transport to cellular organelles such as plasma membrane, microsome, and possibly the nuclei. Apparently, this disturbance and binding to cellular organelles may be the initial step in the cholestasis. For example, the binding of these bile acids to the canalicular membrane (which has been confirmed for lithocholic acid) disturbs the structural stability of these membranes and may even cause initial choleresis. The binding to the microsome may have a similar effect on the microsome, causing an increase in cholesterol synthesis; or, at least, more newly synthesized cholesterol is released and transported to the canalicular membranes by means involving the cytosolic protein that carries lithocholate in the cytosol. Such an alteration in the canalicular membrane structure may be the final step in the pathogenesis of the cholestasis induced by this molecule. It is interesting that this lithocholic acid–binding protein in lithocholic acid–induced cholestasis is different from the normal "bile acid–binding" proteins, suggesting the possibility that interaction of lithocholic acid in the nuclei may be involved in the synthesis of this protein. This protein is not present in sufficient concentration in newborn animals, which are less sensitive to the cholestatic effect of lithocholic acid, but becomes more prominent in adult and older animals. This suggests that continuous exposure of the liver to lithocholic acid at even low concentrations (noncholestatic), which is produced by the bacterial dehydroxylation of chenodeoxycholic acid in adult animals, may be involved in the gene expression of this binding protein. It may be also suggested that binding of these bile acids to the nuclei may affect vesicle transport of membrane components as well as the transport

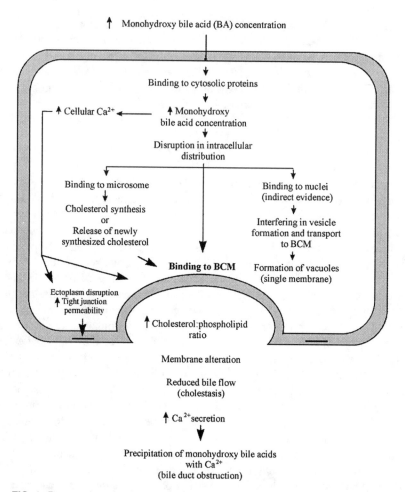

FIG. 1. Proposed mechanisms for monohydroxy bile acid (BA)–induced cholestasis.

of certain bile acids, resulting in the formation of single-membrane vacuoles seen in the cholestasis induced by other monohydroxy bile acids.

Other factors may be involved in the severity and the duration of the cholestatic effect of the monohydroxy bile acids. These factors may include, as previously mentioned, the degree of the structural changes in cellular membranes, alteration in the anatomy of the canalicular membrane such as alteration in the microfilamental structure, alteration of the tight junction permeability due either to stagnation of bile flow or alteration in the cell ectoplasm, and precipitation of the bile acids, either alone or in complex with other ions such as calcium, which can cause an extrahepatic obstruction. It is interesting that this cholestasis can be completely prevented by cycloheximide, supporting the concept that binding to the cytosolic protein is the initial step in the cholestasis. Thus, we need to know the regulation of this protein. What is the role of the 3 hydroxyl group in this process and how may it regulate the binding to the membrane or even the production of the binding protein. This information will be important in understanding the pathogenesis of monohydroxy bile acid–induced cholestasis and in designing an effective prevention strategy.

The second group of bile acids is those that induce cell toxicity resulting in cholestasis, and cholestasis thus appears to be secondary to the toxic effect of these bile acids. These bile acids induce cholestasis only when infused in high concentrations such as those of cholic acid, chenodeoxycholic acid, and deoxycholic acid. In this group the cholestasis appears, with the exception of ursodeoxycholic acid, to be related to their hydrophobicity. To support the concept of cytotoxicity, infusion of these bile acids increases bile flow (choleresis) until it reaches a maximum secretion rate, and then cholestasis occurs; thus, the failure in bile flow occurs without an indication of a direct cholestatic effect of these bile acids such as that seen in monohydroxy bile acid–induced cholestasis. To differentiate between direct cholestatic effect and cholestasis resulting from cellular toxicity of the bile acids, this type of cholestasis will be referred to as cholestasis-induced by toxicity of bile acids. Figure 2 shows the possible mechanism of this cholestasis. It has been shown that infusion of bile acids promotes the secretion of biliary phospholipid and cholesterol. The mechanism of biliary phospholipid and cholesterol secretion is still controversial, as is the origin of these lipids. However, recent studies suggest that bile acids secreted in the canalicular membranes solubilize certain microdomains of the phospholipids in the canalicular membranes, which is replaced by phospholipids mainly of cellular origin to preserve the integrity of the canalicular membranes. The mechanism of the secretion of biliary cholesterol is less well understood, but it may be similar to that of the phospholipids. When bile acids are infused in high concentration, these bile acids are extracted with high efficiency by the liver, increasing their cellular concentrations. These bile acids possess certain detergent properties that may be conferred by the increasing number of the hydroxyl groups and their position. The high secretion of these bile acids through the canalicular membranes promotes the speed of the solubilization of the canalicular domain phospholipids, which are also replaced by the intracellular biliary pool of phospholipids. The biliary pool of phospholipids may be depleted or not replaced at the same rate of the depletion; thus, the bile acid detergent effect may start affecting the intracellular membrane structures, releasing structural lipids in the bile. The detergent effect of bile acids on these intracellular membranes manifest toxicity to cellular organelles such as that seen in the intracellular structure in chenodeoxycholic acid toxicity. These cellular changes either impair cell function by reducing its energy (as for chenodeoxycholic acid) or cellular membrane function in general. The intracellular toxicity is not reversible and often leads to cell death. During this cellular toxicity the bile flow is reduced and the term cholestasis may be used during this period. Two pieces of evidence support the theory of cytotoxicity due to the detergent effect of the bile acids. First, this cholestasis may be reduced by previous feeding of phosphatidylcholine, which presumably increases biliary phospholipid pool in the cell. Second, the infusion of ursodeoxycholic acid also increases bile flow and phospholipid

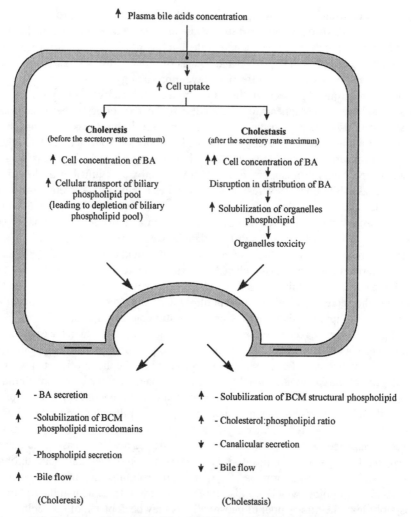

FIG. 2. Mechanisms of high bile acid (BA) concentration–induced cholestasis.

secretion, but in contrast to other bile acids, instead of reaching maximum secretion rates and then proceeding to cholestasis, bile flow plateaus. This can be explained by the fact that solubilization of membrane phospholipid per unit time in the case of ursodeoxycholic acid is smaller than that caused by other bile acids, allowing time for replacement of the biliary bile acid pool. It is also interesting that ursodeoxycholic acid hydrophilicity is higher than that of other toxic bile acids, and it may be that hydrophilicity in multiple hydroxy bile acids is related to its detergent properties. Therefore, many aspects need to be clarified before we have complete understanding of bile acid toxicity resulting in cholestasis, such as the origin and mechanisms of biliary lipid secretion and the role of these lipids in cellular membranes function on bile formation. These have been difficult areas of study because of the involvement of these lipids not only in bile formation but in all cell function.

It is clear that much work is needed to understand the mechanisms of BA-induced cholestasis, including better identification of BA and their precursors. Isolation and characterization of various membranes and cytosolic transport proteins of BA may be critical in elaborating the pathogenesis of BA-induced cholestasis. Better characterization of the so-called BSIF component of BF and its regulation is also important as it is almost always reduced in all models of cholestasis. New experimental models need to be developed to investigate these theories. They may include transgenic or knock-out animals. These developments are currently under way, with recent advances in mass-spectrometry for BA identification, in the molecular biology of some membrane transporters, and in the refinement of certain animal models such as the multiple drug resistance (MDR). The next decade will definitely bring us closer to understanding the role and mechanisms of BA-induced cholestasis.

ACKNOWLEDGMENTS

The research of the authors (I.M.Y., B.T.) cited in this review was supported by the Medical Research Council of Canada. G.B. was supported by a fellowship from the Canadian Liver Foundation.

REFERENCES

1. Bjorkhem I. Mechanism of degradation of the steroid side chain in the formation of the steroid side chain in the formation of bile acids. *J Lipid Res* 1992;33:455–471.
2. Javitt NB. Bile acid synthesis from cholesterol: regulatory and auxiliary pathways. *FASEB J* 1994;8:1308–1311.
3. Radominska A, Treat S, Little J. Bile acid metabolism and the pathophysiology of cholestasis. *Semin Liver Dis* 1993;13:219–234.
4. Russell DW, Setchell KD. Bile acid biosynthesis. *Biochemistry* 1992;31:4737–4749.
5. Galatola G, Jazrawi RP, Bridges C, Joseph AEA, Northfield TC. Direct measurement of first-pass ileal clearance of a bile acid in humans. *Gastroenterology* 1991;100:1100–1105.
6. Carey MC, Duane WC. Enterohepatic circulation. In: Arias IM, Boyer JL, Fausto N, Jakoby WB, Schachter D, Shafritz DA, eds. *The liver: biology and pathobiology*, 3rd ed. New York: Raven Press, 1994, 719–768.
7. Hofmann AF. Bile acids. In: Arias IM, Boyer JL, Fausto N, Jakoby WB, Schachter D, Shafritz DA, eds. *The liver: biology and pathobiology*, 3rd ed. New York: Raven Press, 1994, 769–795.
8. Stiehl A. Pattern of bile acids in cholestasis. In: Gentilini P, Arias IM, McIntyre N, Rodes J, eds. *Cholestasis*. New York: Elsevier Science, 1994, 231–238.
9. Ostrow JD. Metabolism of bile salts in cholestasis in humans. In: Tavaloni N, Berk PD, eds. *Hepatic transport and bile secretion: physiology and pathophysiology*. New York: Raven Press, 1993, 673–712.
10. Back P, Spaczynski K, Gerok W. Bile-salt glucuronides in urine. *Hoppe-Seylers Z Physiol Chem* 1974;355:749–752.
11. Queneau PE, Montet JC. Hepatoprotection by hydrophilic bile salts. *J Hepatol* 1994;21:260–268.
12. Roy CC, Tuchweber B, Weber AM, Yousef IM. Update on bile formation and on mechanism of bile acid-induced cholestasis. In: Shaffer E, Thompson AA, eds. *Advances in gastroenterology*. New York: Plenum Press, 1989, 41–67.

13. Stiehl A, Raedsch R, Rudolph G, Gundert-Remy U, Senn M. Biliary and urinary excretion of sulfated, glucuronidated and tetrahydroxylated bile acids in cirrhotic patients. *Hepatology* 1985;5:492–495.

14. Kirkpatrick RB, Green MD, Hagey LR, Hofmann AF, Tephly TR. Effect of side chain length on bile acid conjugation: glucuronidation, sulfation and coenzyme A formation of nor-bile acids and their natural C24 homologs by human and rat liver fractions. *Hepatology* 1988;8:353–357.

15. Watkins JB. Neonatal cholestasis: developmental aspects and current concepts. *Semin Liver Dis* 1993;13:276–288.

16. Shoda J, Osuga T, Matsuura K, Mahara R, Tohma M, Tanaka N, Matsuzaki Y, Miyazaki H. Concurrent occurrence of 3-beta,12-alpha-dihydroxy-5-cholenoic acid associated with 3-beta-hydroxy-5-cholenoic acid and their preferential urinary excretion in liver diseases. *J Lipid Res* 1989;30:1233–1242.

17. Shoda J, Tanaka N, Osuga T, Matsuura K, Miyazaki H. Altered bile acid metabolism in liver disease: concurrent occurrence of C-1 and C-6 hydroxylated bile acid metabolites and their preferential excretion into urine. *J Lipid Res* 1990;31:249–259.

18. Sugiyama K, Okuyama S, Okumura K, Takagi K, Satake T. Clinical evaluation of serum 3-beta-hydroxy-5-cholenoic acid in hepatobiliary diseases. *Gastroenterol Jpn* 1986;21:608–616.

19. Takikawa H, Otsuka H, Beppu T, Seyama Y. Determination of 3-beta-hydroxy-5-cholenoic acid in serum of hepatobiliary diseases: its glucuronidated and sulfated conjugates. *Biochem Med* 1985;33:393–400.

20. Balisterli WF, Suchy FJ, Farrell MK, Heubi JE. Pathologic versus physiologic cholestasis: elevated serum concentration of a secondary bile acid in the presence of hepatobiliary disease. *J Pediatr* 1981;98:399–402.

21. Takikawa H, Otsuka H, Beppu T, Seyama Y, Yamakawa T. Serum concentrations of bile acid glucuronides in hepatobiliary diseases. *Digestion* 1983;27:189–195.

22. Raedsch R, Lauterburg B, Hofmann AF. Altered bile acid metabolism in primary biliary cirrhosis. *Dig Dis Sci* 1981;26:394–401.

23. Corbett CL, Bartholomew TC, Billing BH, Summerfield JA. Urinary excretion of bile acids in cholestasis: evidence for renal tubular excretion in man. *Clin Sci* 1981;61:773–780.

24. Bremelgaard A, Slovall J. Hydroxylation of cholic, chenodeoxycholic, and deoxycholic acids in patients with intrahepatic cholestasis. *J Lipid Res* 1980;21:1071–1081.

25. Crosignani A, Podda M, Bertolini E, Battezzati PM, Zuin M, Setchell KD. Failure of ursodeoxycholic acid to prevent a cholestatic episode in a patient with benign recurrent intrahepatic cholestasis: a study of bile acid metabolism. *Hepatology* 1991;13:1076–1083.

26. Nakashima T, Shima T, Sakamoto Y, Nakajima T, Seto Y, Sano A, Iwai M, Okanoue T, Kashima K. Effects of bile acids and taurine on the lipid fluidity of hepatic microsomes in normal and bile-duct ligated rats: a spin label study. *J Hepatol* 1993;18:74–79.

27. Dahlstrom-King L, du Souich P, Couture J, Plaa GL. The influence of severity of bile flow reduction, cycloheximide, and methyl isobutyl ketone pretreatment on the kinetics of taurolithocholic acid disposition in the rat. *Toxicol Appl Pharmacol* 1990;104:312–321.

28. Taniguchi T, Chen J, Cooper AD. Regulation of cholesterol 7 alpha-hydroxylase gene expression in Hep-G2 cells. Effect of serum, bile salts, and coordinate and noncoordinate regulation with other sterol-responsive genes. *J Biol Chem* 1994;269:10071–10078.

29. Fromm H. Cholestasis: pathogenetic role and therapeutic action of bile acids. In: Gentilini P, Arias IM, McIntyre N, Rodes J, eds. *Cholestasis*. New York: Elsevier Science, 1994, 239–246.

30. Luketic VA, Sanyal AJ. The current status of ursodeoxycholate in the treatment of chronic cholestatic liver disease. *Gastroenterologist* 1994;2:74–79.

31. Drew R, Priestly BG. Choleretic and cholestatic effects of infused bile salts in the rat. *Experientia* 1979;35:809–811.

32. Hall TJ, Baker AL, Cooper MJ, Moossa AR. Choleresis and cholestasis produced by infusion of taurocholic acid or taurodehydrocholic acid combined with BSP in the rhesus monkey. *Dig Dis Sci* 1979;24:351–357.

33. Hardison WG, Hatoff DE, Miyai K, Weiner RG. Nature of bile acid maximum secretory rate in the rat. *Am J Physiol* 1981;241:G337–G343.

34. Herz R, Paumgartner G, Preisig R. Bile salt metabolism and bile formation in the rat with a portacaval shunt. *Eur J Clin Invest* 1974;4:223–228.

35. Barnwell SG, Yousef IM, Tuchweber B. Biliary secretion in rats during infusion of increasing doses of unconjugated bile acids. *Biochim Biophys Acta* 1987;992:221–233.

36. Yousef IM, Kakis G, Fisher MM. Bile acid metabolism in mammals. III. Sex difference in the bile acid composition of rat bile. *Can J Biochem* 1972;50:402–408.
37. Fisher MM, Kakis G, Yousef IM. Bile acid pool in Wistar rats. *Lipids* 1976;11:93–96.
38. Kakis G, Yousef IM. Pathogenesis of lithocholate and taurolithocholate induced intrahepatic cholestasis in rats. *Gastroenterology* 1978;75:595–607.
39. Kakis G, Phillips MJ, Yousef IM. The respective roles of membrane cholesterol and of sodium potassium adenosine triphosphate in the pathogenesis of lithocholate-induced cholestasis. *Lab Invest* 1980;43:73–81.
40. Yousef IM, Lewittes M, Tuchweber B, Roy CC, Weber A. Lithocholic acid-cholesterol interactions in rat liver plasma membrane fractions. *Biochim Biophys Acta* 1984;796:345–353.
41. Bonvicini F, Gautier A, Gardiol D, Borel GA. Cholesterol in acute cholestasis induced by taurolithocholic acid. a cytochemical study in transmission and scanning electron microscopy. *Lab Invest* 1978;38:487–495.
42. Boyer JL. Tight junctions in normal and cholestatic livers: does the paracellular pathway have functional significance? *Hepatology* 1983;3:614–617.
43. Gratton F, Weber AM, Tuchweber B, Morazain R, Roy CC, Yousef IM. Effect of chronic administration of taurolithocholate on bile formation and liver ultrastructure in the rat. *Liver* 1987;7:130–137.
44. Miyai K, Richardson AL, Mayr W, Javitt NB. Subcellular pathology of rat liver in cholestasis and choleresis induced by bile salts. 1. Effects of lithocholic, 3 beta-hydroxy-5-cholenoic, cholic, and dehydrocholic acids. *Lab Invest* 1977;36:249–258.
45. Vu DD, Tuchweber B, Plaa GL, Yousef IM. Do intracellular Ca^{2+} activity and hepatic glutathione play a role in the pathogenesis of lithocholic acid-induced cholestasis? *Toxicol Lett* 1992;61:255–264.
46. Vu DD, Tuchweber B, Plaa GL, Yousef IM. Pathogenesis of lithocholate-induced intrahepatic cholestasis: role of glucuronidation and hydroxylation of lithocholate. *Biochim Biophys Acta* 1992;1126:53–59.
47. Vu DD, Tuchweber B, Raymond P, Yousef IM. Tight junction permeability and liver plasma membrane fluidity in lithocholate-induced cholestasis. *Exp Mol Pathol* 1992;57:47–61.
48. Vonk RJ, Tuchweber B, Masse D, Perea A, Audet M, Roy CC, Yousef IM. Intrahepatic cholestasis induced by allo monohydroxy bile acid in rats. *Gastroenterology* 1981;80:242–249.
49. Yousef IM, Tuchweber B, Vonk RK, Masse D, Audet M, Roy CC. Lithocholate cholestasis: sulfated glycolithocholate-induced intrahepatic cholestasis in rats. *Gastroenterology* 1981;80:233–241.
50. Takikawa H, Ohki H, Sano N, Kasama T, Yamanaka M. Cholestasis induced by lithocholate and its glucuronide: their biliary excretion and metabolism. *Biochim Biophys Acta* 1991;1081:39–44.
51. Farrell MK, Balistreri WF, Suchy FJ. Serum-sulfated lithocholate as an indicator of cholestasis during parenteral nutrition in infants and children. *JPEN* 1982;6:30–33.
52. Jazrawi RP, de Caestecker JS, Goggin PM, Britten AJ, Joseph AEA, Maxwell JD, Northfield TC. Kinetics of hepatic bile acid handling in cholestatic liver disease: effect of ursodeoxycholic acid. *Gastroenterology* 1994;106:134–142.
53. Feuer G, Di Fonzo CJ. Intrahepatic cholestasis: a review of biochemical-pathological mechanisms. *Drug Metab Drug Interact* 1992;10:1–161.
54. Tuchweber B, Weber A, Roy CC, Yousef IM. Mechanisms of experimentally induced intrahepatic cholestasis. *Prog Liver Dis* 1986;8:161–178.
55. Leuschner U, Guldutuna S, Bhatti S, You T, Sipos P, Zimmer G. Cytotoxicity and membrane protection by bile acids. In: Meyer zum Buschenfelde KH, Paumgartner G, Scholmerich J, eds. *Perspectives in gastroenterology: current facts and future trends*. Baltimore: Urban & Schwarzenberg, 1995, 153–164.
56. Scholmerich J, Baumgartner U, Miyai K, Gerok W. Tauroursodeoxycholate prevents taurolithocholate-induced cholestasis and toxicity in the rat liver. *J Hepatol* 1990;10:280–283.
57. Baumgartner U, Hardison WG, Miyai K. Reduced cholestatic potency of taurolithocholate during backward perfusion of the rat liver. *Lab Invest* 1987;56:576–582.
58. Barnwell SG, Yousef IM, Tuchweber B. The effect of colchicine on the development of lithocholic acid-induced cholestasis: a study of the role of microtubules in intracellular cholesterol transport. *Biochem J* 1986;236:345–350.
59. Yousef IM, Tuchweber B, Morazain R, Kugelmass R, Gauvin M, Roy CC, Weber AM. Cholesterol synthesis in the pathogenesis of lithocholic acid-induced cholestasis. *Lipids* 1988;23:230–233.
60. Groothuis GM, Meijer DK. Hepatocyte heterogeneity in bile formation and hepatobiliary transport of drugs. *Enzyme* 1992;46:94–138.
61. Priestly BG, Côté G, Plaa GL. Biochemical and morphological parameters of taurolithocholate-induced cholestasis. *Can J Physiol Pharmacol* 1971;49:1078–1091.

62. Schaffner F, Javitt NB. Morphological changes in hamster liver during intrahepatic cholestasis induced by taurolithocholate. *Lab Invest* 1966;15:1783–1792.
63. Reichen J, Paumgartner G. Inhibition of hepatic Na⁺,K⁺-adenosinetriphosphate in taurolithocholate-induced cholestasis in the rat. *Experientia* 1979;35:1186–1189.
64. Javitt NB, Emerman S. Effect of sodium taurolithocholate on bile flow and bile acid excretion. *J Clin Invest* 1968;47:1002–1014.
65. Hardison WGM, Dalle-Molle E, Gosink E, Lowe PJ, Steinbach JH, Yamaguchi Y. Function of rat hepatocyte tight junctions: studies with bile acid infusions. *Am J Physiol* 1991;260:G167–G174.
66. Paul-Dorvil N, Yousef IM, Tuchweber B, Roy CC. Effect of dietary taurine on sulfated lithocholate induced cholestasis. *Am J Clin Nutr* 1983;37:221–232.
67. Belli DC, Roy CC, Fournier LA, Tuchweber B, Giguere R, Yousef IM. The effect of taurine on the cholestatic potential of sulfated lithocholate and its conjugates. *Liver* 1991;11:162–169.
68. Oelberg DG, Chari MV, Little JM, Adcock EW, Lester R. Lithocholate glucuronide is a cholestatic agent. *J Clin Invest* 1984;73:1507–1514.
69. Little JM, Zimniak P, Shattuch KE, Lester R, Radominska A. Metabolism of lithocholic acid in rat: formation of lithocholic acid-3-O-glucuronide in vivo. *J Lipid Res* 1990;31:615–622.
70. Dionne S, Tuchweber B, Plaa GL, Yousef IM. Phase I and phase II metabolism of lithocholic acid in hepatic acinar zone 3 necrosis. Evaluation in rats by chromatography-mass spectrometry. *Biochem Pharmacol* 1994;48:1187–1197.
71. Mathis U, Karlaganis G, Preisig R. Monohydroxy bile salt sulfates: tauro-3-beta-hydroxy-5-cholenoate-3-sulfate induces intrahepatic cholestasis in rats. *Gastroenterology* 1983;85:674–681.
72. Kuipers F, Havinga R, Vonk RJ. Cholestasis induced by sulphated glycolithocholic acid in the rat: protection by endogenous bile acids. *Clin Sci* 1985;68:127–134.
73. Kakis G, Yousef IM. Mechanisms of cholic acid protection in lithocholate-induced intrahepatic cholestasis in rats. *Gastroenterology* 1980;78:1402–1411.
74. Layden TJ, Boyer JL. Taurolithocholate-induced cholestasis: taurocholate but not dehydrocholate, reverses cholestasis and bile canalicular membrane injury. *Gastroenterology* 1977;73:120–128.
75. Zimniak P, Radominska A, Lester R. The pathogenesis of cholestasis. *Hosp Pract* 1990;25:107–125.
76. Yousef IM, Tuchweber B, Weber A. Prevention of lithocholate-induced cholestasis by cycloheximide, an inhibitor of protein synthesis. *Life Sci* 1983;33:103–110.
77. Kitani K, Kanai S, Sato Y, Ohta M. Tauro alpha-muricholate is as effective as tauro beta-muricholate and tauroursodeoxycholate in preventing taurochenodeoxycholate-induced liver damage in the rat. *Hepatology* 1994;19:1007–1012.
78. Miyai K, Price VM, Fisher MM. Bile acid metabolism in mammals. Ultrastructural studies on intrahepatic cholestasis induced by lithocholic and chenodeoxycholic acids in rats. *Lab Invest* 1971;24:292–302.
79. Yousef IM, Magnusson R, Price V, Fisher M. Bile acid metabolism in mammals. V. Studies on the sex difference in response of the isolated perfused rat liver to chenodeoxycholic acid. *Can J Physiol Pharmacol* 1973;6:418–423.
80. Fisher RL, Hofmann AF, Converse JL, Rossi SS, Lan SP. The lack of relationship between hepatotoxicity and lithocholate-acid sulfation in biliary bile acids during chenodiol therapy in the National Cooperative Gallstone Study. *Hepatology* 1991;14:454–463.
81. Kanai S, Ohta MM, Kitani K, Sato Y. Tauro beta-muricholate is as effective as tauroursodeoxycholate in preventing taurochenodeoxycholate-induced liver damage in the rat. *Life Sci* 1990;47:2421–2428.
82. Kitani K, Ohta M, Kanai S. Tauroursodeoxycholate prevents biliary protein excretion induced by other bile salts in the rat. *Am J Physiol* 1985;248:G407–G417.
83. Adachi Y, Kobayashi H, Shouji M, Kitano M, Okuyama Y, Yamamoto T. Functional integrity of hepatocytes canalicular membrane transport of taurocholate and bilirubin diglucuronide in Eisai hyperbilirubinuria rats. *Life Sci* 1993;52:777–784.
84. Hoshino M, Hayakawa T, Hirano A, Kamiya Y, Ohiwa T, Tanaka A, Kumai T, Inagaki T, Miyaji M, Takeuchi T. The mutant Eisai hyperbilirubinemic rat is resistant to bile acid-induced cholestasis and cytotoxicity. *Hepatology* 1994;20:932–939.
85. Fisher M, Price VM, Magnusson RJ, Yousef IM. Bile acid metabolism in mammals. VII. Studies on the sex difference in deoxycholic acid metabolism in isolated perfused rat liver. *Lipids* 1974;9:786–794.
86. Fisher MM, Yousef IM. Bile acids, sex and the liver. *Ann Roy Coll Phys Surg Can* 1972;5:132–150.
87. Delzenne NM, Calderon PB, Taper HS, Roberfroid MB. Comparative hepatotoxicity of cholic acid, deoxycholic acid and lithocholic acid in the rat: in vivo and in vitro studies. *Toxicol Lett* 1992;61:291–304.

88. Heuman DM, Mills AS, McCall J, Hylemon PB, Pandak WM, Vlahcevic ZR. Conjugates of ursodeoxycholate protect against cholestasis and hepatocellular necrosis caused by more hydrophobic bile salts: in vivo studies in the rat. *Gastroenterology* 1991;100:203–211.

89. Fukumoto Y, Ando M, Yasunaga M, Okuda M, Okita K. Secretin prevents taurocholate-induced intrahepatic cholestasis in the rat. *J Hepatol* 1994;20:750–754.

90. Kanai S, Kitani K. Glycoursodeoxycholate is as effective as tauroursodeoxycholate in preventing the taurocholate-induced cholestasis in the rat. *Res Com Chem Pathol Pharmacol* 1983;42:423–430.

91. Durham S, Vore M. Taurocholate and steroid glucuronides: mutual protection against cholestasis in the isolated perfused rat liver. *J Pharmacol Exp Ther* 1986;237:490–495.

92. Yousef IM, Barnwell S, Gratton F, Tuchweber B, Weber A, Roy CC. Liver cell membrane solubilization may control maximum secretory rate of cholic acid in the rat. *Am J Physiol* 1987;252:G84–G91.

93. Rioux F, Perea A, Yousef IM, Levy E, Malli L, Carillo MC, Tuchweber B. Short-term feeding of a diet enriched in phospholipids increases bile formation and the bile acid transport maximum in rats. *Biochim Biophys Acta* 1994;1214:193–202.

94. Accatino L, Hono J, Maldonado M, Icarte MA, Persico R. Adaptative regulation of hepatic bile salt transport: effect of prolonged bile salt depletion in the rat. *J Hepatol* 1988;7:215–223.

95. Adler RA, Wannagat FJ, Ockner RK. Bile secretion in selective biliary obstruction. Adaptation of taurocholate transport maximum to increased secretory load in the rat. *Gastroenterology* 1977;73:129–136.

96. Hardison WGM, Proffit JH. Influence of hepatic taurine concentration on bile acid conjugation with taurine. *Am J Physiol* 1977;232:E75–E79.

97. Dahlstrom-King L, Plaa GL. Effect of inhibition of protein synthesis on cholestasis induced by taurolithocholate, lithocholate and a manganese-bilirubin combination in the rat. *Biochem Pharmacol* 1989;38:2543–2549.

98. Yousef IM, Barnwell SG, Tuchweber B, Weber A, Roy CC. Effect of complete sulfation of bile acids on bile formation in rats. *Hepatology* 1987;7:535–542.

99. Yousef I, Mignault D, Tuchweber B. Effect of complete sulfation of bile acids on bile formation: role of conjugation and number of sulfate groups. *Hepatology* 1992;15:438–445.

100. Hofmann AF. Bile acids. In: Arias IM, Jakoby WB, Popper H, Schachter D, Shafritz DA, eds. *The liver: biology and pathobiology*, 2nd ed. New York: Raven Press, 1988, 553–572.

101. Roda A, Hofmann AF, Mysels KJ. The influence of bile salt structure on self-association in aqueous solutions. *J Biol Chem* 1983;258:6362–6370.

102. Strange RC. Hepatic bile flow. *Physiol Rev* 1984;64:1055–1103.

103. Belli DC, Fournier LA, Lepage G, Tremblay P, Yousef IM, Roy CC. The influence of taurine on the bile acid maximum secretory rate in the guinea pig. *Pediatr Res* 1988;24:34–37.

104. Spivey JR, Bronk SF, Gores GL. Glycochenodeoxycholate-induced lethal hepatocellular injury in rat hepatocytes: roles of ATP depletion and cytosolic calcium. *J Clin Invest* 1993;92:17–24.

105. Kuipers F, Heslinga H, Havinga R, Vonk RJ. Intestinal absorption of lithocholic acid sulfates in the rat: inhibitory effect of calcium. *Am J Physiol* 1986;251:G189–G194.

106. Bellentani S, Armocida C, Pecorari M, Saccoccio G, Marchegiano P, Angeloni A, Manenti F, Ricci GL. The role of calcium precipitation in the sulfoglycolithocholate-induced cholestasis of the bile fistula hamster. *J Hepatol* 1990;10:356–363.

107. van der Meer R, Vonk RJ, Kuipers F. Cholestasis and the interaction of sulfated glyco- and taurolithocholate with calcium. *Am J Physiol* 1988;254:G644–G649.

108. Kuipers F, Hardonk MJ, Vonk RJ, van der Meer R. Bile secretion of sulfated glycolithocholic acid is required for its cholestatic action in the rats. *Am J Physiol* 1992;262:G267–G273.

109. Carey MC, Wu SF, Watkins JB. Solution properties of sulfated monohydroxy bile salts. Relative insolubility of the disodium salt of glycolithocholate sulfate. *Biochim Biophys Acta* 1979;575:16–26.

110. Yousef IM, Tuchweber B, Mignault D, Weber A. Effect of co-infusion of cholic acid and sulfated cholic acid on bile formation in rats. *Am J Physiol* 1989;256:G62–G66.

111. Takikawa H, Sano N, Narita T, Yamanaka M. The ursodeoxycholate dose-dependent formation of ursodeoxycholate glucuronide in the rat and choleretic potencies. *Hepatology* 1990;11:743–749.

112. Takikawa H, Sano N, Ohki H, Yamanaka M. Comparison of biliary excretion and metabolism of lithocholic acid and its sulfate and glucuronide conjugates in rats. *Biochim Biophys Acta* 1989;1004:147–150.

113. Oude Elferink RP, Ottenhoff R, Radominska A, Hofmann AF, Kuipers F, Jansen PL. Inhibition of glutathione-conjugate secretion from isolated hepatocytes by dipolar bile acids and other organic anions. *Biochem J* 1991;274:281–286.

114. Takikawa H, Minagawa K, Sano N, Yamanaka M. Lithocholate-3-O-glucuronide-induced cholestasis: a study with congenital hyperbilirubinemic rats and effects of ursodeoxycholate conjugates. *Dig Dis Sci* 1993;38:1543–1548.

115. Takikawa H, Sano N, Yamazaki R, Yamanaka M. Colchicine inhibits lithocholate-3-O-glucuronide-induced cholestasis in rats. *J Hepatol* 1995;22:88–93.

116. Takikawa H, Narita T, Sano N. Glucuronidation of bile acids by their high-dose infusion into rats. *Hepatology* 1991;13:1222–1228.

117. De Lamirande E, Plaa GL. 1,3-Butanediol pretreatment on the cholestasis induced in rats by manganese-bilirubin combination, taurolithocholic acid, or alpha-naphthylisothiocyanate. *Toxicol Appl Pharmacol* 1981;59:467–475.

118. Plaa GL, Ayotte P. Taurolithocholate-induced intrahepatic cholestasis: potentiation by methyl isobutyl ketone and methyl n-butyl ketone in rats. *Toxicol Appl Pharmacol* 1985;80:228–234.

119. Vézina M, Plaa GL. Potentiation by methyl isobutyl ketone of the cholestasis induced in rats by a Mn-Br combination or manganese alone. *Toxicol Appl Pharmacol* 1987;91:477–483.

120. Vézina M, Plaa GL. Methyl isobutyl ketone metabolites and potentiation of the cholestasis induced in rats by a Mn-BR combination or manganese alone. *Toxicol Appl Pharmacol* 1988;92:419–427.

121. Villalon L, Tuchweber B, Yousef IM. Low protein diets potentiate lithocholic acid-induced cholestasis in rats. *J Nutr* 1992;122:1587–1596.

122. Kroger R, Hegner D, Anwer MS. Altered hepatobiliary transport of taurocholic acid in aged rats. *Mech Ageing Dev* 1980;12:367–373.

123. Schmucker JL. Aging and drug disposition. In: Rothstein M, ed. *Review of biological research in aging*, vol. 2. New York: Alan R Liss, 1985, 465–501.

124. Bouchard G, Carrillo MC, Tuchweber B, Perea A, Ledoux M, Poulin D, Yousef IM. Moderate exercise improves the age related decline in bile formation and bile salt secretion in rats. *Proc Soc Exp Biol Med* 1994;206:409–415.

125. Reichen J. Pharmacologic treatment of cholestasis. *Semin Liver Dis* 1993;13:302–315.

126. Strange RC, Chapman BT, Johnston JD, Mimmo IA, Percy-Robb IW. Partitioning of bile acids into subcellular organelles and the in vivo distribution of bile acids in rat liver. *Biochim Biophys Acta* 1979;573:535–545.

127. Schmucker DL, Ohta M, Kanai S, Sato Y, Kitani K. Hepatic injury induced by bile salts: correlation between biochemical and morphological events. *Hepatology* 1990;12:1216–1221.

128. Boyer JL. Perspectives on progress and future developments of the cellular and molecular biology of bile acid transport mechanisms. In: Meyer zum Buschenfelde KH, Paumgartner G, Scholmerich J, eds. *Perspectives in gastroenterology: current facts and future trends*. Baltimore: Urban & Schwarzenberg, 1995, 123–127.

129. Suchy FJ. Hepatocellular transport of bile acids. *Semin Liver Dis* 1993;13:235–247.

130. Bartholomew TC, Billing BH. The effect of 3-sulphation and taurine conjugation on the uptake of chenodeoxycholic acid by rat hepatocytes. *Biochim Biophys Acta* 1983;754:101–109.

131. Boyer JL, Graf J, Meier PJ. Hepatic transport systems regulating pHi, cell volume, and bile secretion. *Ann Rev Physiol* 1992;54:415–438.

132. Stolz A, Takikawa H, Ookhtens M, Kaplowitz N. The role of cytoplasmic proteins in hepatic bile acid transport. *Ann Rev Physiol* 1989;51:161–176.

133. Takikawa H, Sano N, Narita T, Uchida Y, Yamanaka M, Horie T, Mikami T, Tagaya O. Biliary excretion of bile acid conjugates in a hyperbilirubinemic mutant Sprague-Dawley rat. *Hepatology* 1991;14:352–360.

134. Erlinger S. Recent concepts in bile formation and cholestasis. *Recenti Prog Med* 1990;81:387–391.

135. Lin MC, Kramer W, Wilson FA. Identification of cytosolic and microsomal bile acid-binding proteins in rat ileal enterocytes. *J Biol Chem* 1990;265:14986–14995.

136. Meier-Abt PJ. Cellular mechanisms of intrahepatic cholestasis. *Drugs* 1990;40 (suppl 3):084–97.

137. Elferink RPJO, Jansen PLM. The role of the canalicular multispecific organic anion transporter in the disposal of endo- and xenobiotics. *Pharmacol Ther* 1994;64:77–97.

138. Reichen J. Mechanisms of cholestasis. In: Tavaloni N, Berk PD, eds. *Hepatic transport and bile secretion: physiology and pathophysiology*. New York: Raven Press, 1993, 665–672.

139. Stieger B, O'Neill B, Meier PJ. ATP-dependent bile-salt transport in canalicular rat liver plasma-membrane vesicles. *Biochem J* 1992;284:67–84.

140. Wilton JC, Matthews GM, Burgoyne RD, Mills CO, Cipman JK, Coleman R. Fluorescent choleretic and cholestatic bile salts take different paths across the hepatocytes: transcytosis of glycolithocholate leads to an extensive redistribution of annexin II. *J Cell Biology* 1994;127:401–410.

141. Lewittes M, Tuchweber B, Weber A, Roy CC, Yousef IM. Resistance of the suckling guinea pig to lithocholic acid-induced cholestasis. *Hepatology* 1984;4:486–491.
142. Joseph LD, Yousef IM, Plaa GL, Sharkawi M. Potentiation of lithocholic-acid-induced cholestasis by methyl isobutyl ketone. *Toxicol Lett* 1992;61:39–47.
143. Stolz A, Sugiyama Y, Kunlenkamp J, Osadchey B, Yamada T, Belknap W, Balistreri W, Kaplowitz N. Cytosolic bile acid binding protein in rat liver: radioimmunoassay, molecular forms, developmental characteristics and organ distribution. *Hepatology* 1986;6:433–439.
144. Tuchweber B, Perea A, Lee D, Yousef IM. Lithocholic acid-induced cholestasis in newborn rats. *Toxicol Lett* 1983;19:107–112.
145. Svec F. Glucocorticoid receptor regulation. *Life Sci* 1985;36:2359–2366.
146. Hayakawa T, Cheng OI, Ma A, Boyer JL. Taurocholate stimulates transcytotic vesicular pathways labeled by horseradish peroxidase in the isolated perfused rat liver. *Gastroenterology* 1990;99:216–228.
147. Sakisaka S, Ng OC, Boyer JL. Tubulovesicular transcytotic pathway in isolated rat hepatocyte couplets in culture: effect of colchicine and taurocholate. *Gastroenterology* 1988;95:793–804.
148. Boyer JL. The role of vesicle transport and exocytosis in bile formation and cholestasis: influence of cell volume, pHi, hormones and bile acids. In: Gentilini P, Arias IM, McIntyre N, Rodes J, eds. *Cholestasis*. New York: Elsevier Science, 1994, 69–78.
149. Bruck R, Benedetti A, Strazzabosco M, Boyer JL. Intracellular alkalinization stimulates bile flow and vesicular-mediated exocytosis in IPRL. *Am J Physiol* 1993;265:G347–G353.
150. Bruck R, Haddad P, Graf J, Boyer JL. Regulatory volume decrease stimulates bile flow, bile acid excretion, and exocytosis in the isolated perfused rat liver. *Am J Physiol* 1992;262:G806–G812.
151. Hayakawa T, Bruck R, Ng OC, Boyer JL. DBcAMP stimulates vesicle transport and HRP excretion in isolated perfused rat liver. *Am J Physiol* 1990;259:G727–G735.
152. Lenzen R, Hruby VJ, Tavoloni N. Mechanism of glucagon choleresis in guinea pigs. *Am J Physiol* 1990;259:G736–G744.
153. Avila J. Microtubule dynamics. *FASEB J* 1990;4:3284–3290.
154. Erlinger S. Role of intracellular organelles in the hepatic transport of bile acids. *Biomed Pharmacother* 1990;44:409–416.
155. Lamri Y, Roda A, Dumont M, Feldmann G, Erlinger S. Immonuperoxidase localization of bile salts in rat liver cells. Evidence for a role of the Golgi apparatus in bile salt transport. *J Clin Invest* 1988;82:1173–1182.
156. Haussinger D, Saha N, Hallbrucker C, Lang F, Gerok W. Involvement of microtubules in the swelling-induced stimulation of transcellular taurocholate transport in the perfused rat liver. *Biochem J* 1993;291:355–360.
157. Bartles JF, Feracci HM, Stieger B, Hubbard AL. Biogenesis of the rat hepatocyte plasma membrane in vivo: comparison of the pathway taken by apical and basolateral proteins using subcellular fractionation. *J Cell Biol* 1987;105:1241–1251.
158. Larkin JM. Vesicle-mediated transcytosis: insights from the cholestatic rat liver. *Gastroenterology* 1993;105:594–597
159. Maurice M, Schell MJ, Lardeux B, Hubbard AL. Biosynthesis and intracellular transport of a bile canalicular plasma membrane protein: studies in vivo and in the perfused rat liver. *Hepatology* 1994;19:648–655.
160. Oude Elferink RP, Bakker CT, Roelofsen H, Middlekoop E, Ottenhoff R, Heijn M, Jansen PL. Accumulation of organic anion in intracellular vesicles of cultured rat hepatocytes is mediated by the canalicular multispecific organic anion transporter. *Hepatology* 1993;17:434–444.
161. Hallbrucker C, Lang F, Gerok W, Haussinger D. Cell swelling increases bile flow and taurocholate excretion into bile in isolated prefused rat liver. *Biochem J* 1992;281:593–595.
162. Haussinger D, Hallbrucker C, Saha N, Lang F, Gerok W. Cell volume and bile acid excretion. *Biochem J* 1992;288:681–689.
163. Barr VA, Hubbard AL. Newly synthetized hepatocyte plasma membrane proteins are transported in transcytotic vesicles in the bile duct-ligated rat. *Gastroenterology* 1993;105:554–571.
164. Okanoue T, Kondo I, Ihrig T, French SW. Effect of ethanol and chlorpromazine on transhepatic transport and biliary secretion of horseradish peroxidase. *Hepatology* 1984;4:253–260.
165. Roman ID, Monte MJ, Gonzalez-Buitrago JM, Esteller A, Jimenez R. Inhibition of hepatocytary vesicular transport by cyclosporine A in the rat: relationship with cholestasis and hyperbilirubinemia. *Hepatology* 1990;12:83–91.
166. Barnwell SG, Lowe PJ, Coleman R. The effects of colchicine on secretion into bile of bile salts,

phospholipids, cholesterol and plasma membrane enzymes: bile salts are secreted unaccompanied by phospholipids and cholesterol. *Biochem J* 1984;220:723–731.

167. Crawford JN, Berken CA, Gollan JL. Role of the hepatocyte microtubular system in the excretion of bile salts and biliary lipids: implications for intracellular vesicular transport. *J Lipid Res* 1988;29:144–156.

168. Dubin M, Maurice M, Feldmann G, Erlinger S. Influence of colchicine and phalloidin on bile secretion and hepatic ultrastructure in the rat. Possible interaction between microtubules and microfilaments. *Gastroenterology* 1980;79:646–654.

169. Gregory DH, Vlahcevic ZR, Prugh MF, Swell L. Mechanism of secretion of biliary lipids: role of a microtubular system in hepatocellular transport of biliary lipids in the rat. *Gastroenterology* 1978;74:93–100.

170. Baumgartner U, Scholmerich J, Karsch J, Gerok W, Farthmann EH. Loss of zonal heterogeneity and cell polarity in rat liver with respect to bile acid secretion after bile drainage. *Gastroenterology* 1991;100:1054–1061.

171. Phillips MJ, Oda M, Mak E, Fisher MM, Jeejeebhoy KN. Microfilament dysfunction as a possible cause of intrahepatic cholestasis. *Gastroenterology* 1975;69:48–58.

172. Watanabe S, Smith CR, Phillips MJ. Coordination of the contractile activity of bile canaliculus: evidence from calcium microinjection of triplet hepatocytes. *Lab Invest* 1985;53:275–280.

173. Desmet VJ. The bile secretory apparatus. In: Gentilini P, Arias IM, McIntyre N, Rodes J, eds. *Cholestasis*. New York: Elsevier Science, 1994, 19–30.

174. Vonk RJ, Yousef IM, Corriveau JP, Tuchweber B. Phalloidin-induced morphological and functional changes of rat liver. *Liver* 1982;2:133–140.

175. Phillips MJ, Satir P. The cytoskeleton of the hepatocyte: organization, relationships, and pathology. In: Arias IM, Jakoby WB, Popper H, Schachter D, Shafritz DA, eds. *The liver: biology and pathobiology*, 2nd ed. New York: Raven Press, 1988, 11–28.

176. Lemasters JJ, DiGuiseppi J, Nieminen AL, Herman B. Blebbing, free Ca^{2+} and mitochondrial membrane potential preceding cell death in hepatocytes. *Nature* 1987;325:78–81.

177. Thibault N, Maurice M, Maratrat M, Cordier A, Feldmann G, Ballet F. Effect of tauroursodeoxycholate on actin filament alteration induced by cholestatic agents: a study in isolated rat hepatocyte couplets. *J Hepatol* 1993;19:367–376.

178. Tuchweber B, Roy S, Desroches S, Yousef IM, Gicquaud C, Weber AM, Loranger A. Effects of bile acids on actin polymerization in vitro. *Life Sci* 1990;47:1299–1307.

179. Oshio C, Phillips MJ. Contractility of bile canaliculi: implications for liver function. *Science* 1981;212:1041–1042.

180. Watanabe S, Miyazaki A, Hirose M, Takeuchi M, Ohide H, Kitamura T, Ueno T, Kominami E, Sato N. Myosin in hepatocytes is essential for bile canalicular contraction. *Liver* 1991;11:185–189.

181. Scharschmidt BF, Keeffe EB, Vessey DA, Blankenship NM, Ockner RK. In vitro effect of bile salts on rat liver plasma membrane, lipid fluidity, and ATPase activity. *Hepatology* 1981;1:137–145.

182. Loranger A, Barriault C, Yousef IM, Tuchweber B. Structural and functional alterations of hepato cytes during transient phalloidin-induced cholestasis in rats. *Toxicol Appl Pharmacol* 1966;137;100–111.

183. Kawahara H, Marceau N, French SW. Effect of agents which rearrange the cytoskeleton in vitro on the structure and function of hepatocytic canaliculi. *Lab Invest* 1989;60:692–704.

184. Kunze D, Rustow B. Pathobiochemical aspects of cytoskeleton components. *Eur J Clin Chem Clin Biochem* 1993;31:477–489.

185. Ohta M, Marceau N, French SW. Pathologic changes in the cytokeratin pericanalicular sheath in experimental cholestasis and alcoholic fatty liver. *Lab Invest* 1988;59:60–74.

186. Little JM, Chari MV, Lester R. Excretion of cholate glucuronide. *J Lip Res* 1985;26:583–592.

187. Takikawa H, Sano N, Minagawa K, Yamanaka M. Effects of ursodeoxycholate, its glucuronide and disulfate and beta-muricholate on biliary bicarbonate concentration and biliary lipid secretion. *J Hepatol* 1992;15:77–84.

188. Takikawa H, Tomita J, Takemura T, Yamanaka M. Cytotoxic effect and uptake mechanism by isolated rat hepatocytes of lithocholate and its glucuronide and sulfate. *Biochim Biophys Acta* 1991;1091:173–178.

189. Reichen J, Krahenbuhl S, Zimmermann H. Impact of cholestasis on hepatic function: retention of cholephiles and their potential targets. In: Gentilini P, Arias IM, McIntyre N, Rodes J, eds. *Cholestasis*. New York: Elsevier Science, 1994, 167–176.

190. Scholmerich J, Becher MS, Schmidt K, Schubert R, Kremer B, Feldhaus S, Gerok W. Influence of hydroxylation and conjugation of bile salts on their membrane-damaging properties: studies on isolated hepatocytes and lipid membrane vesicles. *Hepatology* 1984;4:661–666.
191. Yousef IM, Fisher MM. In vitro effect of free bile acids on the bile canalicular membrane phospholipids in the rat. *Can J Biochem* 1976;54:1040–1046.
192. Crawford JM, Barnes S, Stearns RC, Hastings CL, Godleski JJ. Ultrastructural localization of a fluorinated bile salt in hepatocytes. *Lab Invest* 1994;71:42–51.
193. Lowe PJ, Barnwell SG, Coleman R. Rapid kinetic analysis of the bile-salt-dependent secretion of phospholipid, cholesterol and a plasma-membrane enzyme into bile. *Biochem J* 1984;222:631–637.
194. Chanussot F, Lafont H, Hauton J, Tuchweber B, Yousef I. Studies on the origin of biliary phospholipid: effect of dehydrocholic acid and cholic acid infusion on hepatic and biliary phospholipids. *Biochem J* 1990;270:691–695.
195. Portal I, Clerc T, Sbarra V, Portugal H, Pauli AM, Lafont H, Tuchweber B, Yousef I, Chanussot F. Importance of high-density lipoprotein-phosphatidylcholine in secretion of phospholipid and cholesterol in bile. *Am J Physiol* 1993;264:G1052–G1056.
196. el-Hariri LM, Marriott C, Martin GP. The mitigating effects of phosphatidylcholines on bile salt- and lysophosphatidylcholine-induced membrane damage. *J Pharm Pharmacol* 1992;44:651–654.
197. Baumgartner U, Scholmerich J, Leible P, Farthmann EH. Cholestasis, metabolism and biliary lipid secretion during perfusion of rat liver with different bile salts. *Biochim Biophys Acta* 1992;1125:142–149.
198. Cohen DE, Leonard R, Carey MC. In vitro evidence that phospholipid secretion into bile may be coordinated intracellularly by the combined action of bile salts and the specific phosphatidylcholine transfer protein of liver. *Biochemistry* 1994;33:9975–9980.
199. Farber JL. The role of calcium in lethal cell injury. *Chem Res Toxicol* 1990;3:503–508.
200. Anwer MS, Emgelking LR, Nolan K, Sullivan D, Zimniak P, Lester R. Hepatotoxic bile acids increase cytosolic Ca^{++} activity of isolated rat hepatocytes. *Hepatology* 1988;8:887–891.
201. Combettes L, Berthon B, Doucet E, Erlinger S, Claret M. Characteristics of bile acid-mediated Ca^{2+} release from permeabilized liver cells and liver microsomes. *J Biol Chem* 1989;264:157–167.
202. Thibault N, Ballet F. Effects of bile acids on intracellular calcium in isolated rat hepatocyte couplets. *Biochem Pharmacol* 1993;45:289–293.
203. Beuers U, Nathanson MH, Boyer JL. Effects of tauroursodeoxycholic acid on cytosolic Ca^{2+} signals in isolated rat hepatocytes. *Gastroenterology* 1993;104:604–612.
204. Bouscarel B, Fromm H, Nussbaum R. Ursodeoxycholate mobilizes intracellular Ca^{2+} and activates phosphorylase a in isolated hepatocytes. *Am J Physiol* 1993;264:G243–G251.
205. Combettes L, Berthon B, Claret M. Taurolithocholate-induced Ca^{2+} release is inhibited by phorbol esters in isolated hepatocytes. *Biochem J* 1992;287:891–896.
206. Marrero I, Sanchez-Bueno A, Cobbold P, Dixon CJ. Taurolithocholate and taurolithocholate-3-sulphate exert different effects on cytosolic free Ca^{2+} concentration in rat hepatocytes. *Biochem J* 1994;300:383–386.
207. Devor DC, Sekar MC, Frizzeli RA, Duffey ME. Taurodeoxycholate activates potassium and chloride conductance via an IP3-mediated release of calcium from intracellular stores in a colonic cell line (T84). *J Clin Invest* 1993;92:2173–2181.
208. Zimniak P, Little JM, Radominska A, Oelberg DG, Anwer MS, Lester R. Taurine-conjugated bile acids act as Ca^{2+} ionophores. *Biochemistry* 1991;30:8598–8604.
209. Anwer MS, Little JM, Oelberg DG, Zimniak P, Lester R. Effect of bile acids on calcium efflux from isolated rat hepatocytes and perfused rat livers. *PSEBM* 1989;191:147–152.
210. Noel J, Fukami K, Hill AM, Capiod T. Oscillations of cytosolic free calcium concentration in the presence of intracellular antibodies to phosphatidylinositol 4,5-biphosphate in voltage-clamped guinea-pig hepatocytes. *Biochem J* 1992;288:357–360.
211. Capiod T, Combettes L, Noel J, Claret M. Evidence for bile acid-evoked oscillations of $Ca^{2(+)}$-dependent K^+ permeability unrelated to a D-myo-inositol 1,4,5-triphosphate effect in isolated guinea pig liver cells. *J Biol Chem* 1991;266:268–273.
212. Farrell GC, Duddy SK, Kass GE, Llopis J, Gahm A, Orrenius S. Release of Ca^{2+} from the endoplasmic reticulum is not the mechanism for bile acid-induced cholestasis and hepatotoxicity in the intact rat liver. *J Clin Invest* 1990;85:1255–1259.
213. Moore EW. The role of calcium in the pathogenesis of gallstones: Ca^{++} electrode studies of model bile salt solutions and other biologic systems with an hypothesis on structural requirements for Ca^{++} binding to proteins and bile acids. *Hepatology* 1984;4:S228–S243.

214. King JE, Schoenfield LJ. Cholestasis induced by sodium taurolithocholate in isolated hamster liver. *J Clin Invest* 1971;50:2305–2312.
215. Bouchard G, Yousef IM, Tuchweber B. Decreased biliary glutathione content is responsible for the decline in bile salt-independent flow induced by ethinyl estradiol in rats. *Toxicol Lett* 1994;74:221–233.
216. Ballatori N, Truong AT. Glutathione as a primary osmotic driving force in hepatic bile formation. *Am J Physiol* 1992;263:G617–G624.
217. Kuipers F, Radominska A, Zimniak P, Little JM, Havinga R, Vonk RJ, Lester R. Defective biliary secretion of bile acid 3-O-glucuronides in rats with hereditary conjugated hyperbilirubinemia. *J Lipid Res* 1989;30:1835–1845.
218. Ballatori N, Truong AT. Cholestasis, altered junctional permeability, and inverse changes in sinusoidal and biliary glutathione release by vasopressine and epinephrine. *Molec Pharmacol* 1990;38:64–71.
219. Raiford DS, Sciuto AM, Mitchell MC. Effects of vasopressor hormones and modulators of protein kinase C on glutathione efflux from perfused rat liver. *Am J Physiol* 1991;261:G578–G584.
220. Graf J. Canalicular bile salt-independent bile formation: concepts and clues from electrolytes transport in rat liver. *Am J Physiol* 1983;244:G233–G246.
221. Alpini G, Lenzi R, Zhai WR, Slott PA, Liu MH, Sarkozi L, Tavaloni N. Bile secretory function of intrahepatic biliary epithelium in the rat. *Am J Physiol* 1989;257:G124–G133.
222. Anwer MS. Mechanism of bile acid induced $HCO_3^-(-)$ rich hypercholeresis: an analysis based on quantitative acid-base chemistry. *J Hepatol* 1992;14:118–126.
223. Dumont M, Erlinger S, Uchman S. Hypercholeresis induced by ursodeoxycholic acid and 7-ketolithocholic acid in the rat: possible role of bicarbonate transport. *Gastroenterology* 1980;79:82–89.
224. Lorenzini I, Sakisaka S, Meier PJ, Boyer JL. Demonstration of a transcellular vesicle pathway for biliary excretion of inulin in the rat. *Gastroenterology* 1986;91:1278–1288.
225. Yousef IM, Tuchweber B, Weber A, Roy CC. Contribution of fluid phase endocytosis to bile flow in cholestasis and choleresis in rats. *PSEBM* 1988;189:147–151.
226. Scholmerich J, Baumgartner U, Miyai K, Gerok W. Hepatic passage of bile acids increases oxygen uptake by perfused rat liver. *Res Exp Med* 1990;190:69–75.
227. Lee MJ, Whitehouse MW. Inhibition of electron transport and coupled phosphorylation in liver mitochondria by cholanic (bile) acids and their conjugates. *Biochim Biophys Acta* 1965;100:317–328.
228. DeLange RJ, Glazer AN. Bile acids: antioxidants or enhancers of peroxidation depending on lipid concentration. *Arch Biochem Biophys* 1990;276:19–25.
229. Sokol RJ, Deverneaux M, Khandwala R, O'Brien K. Evidence for the involvement of oxygen free radicals in bile acid toxicity to isolated rat hepatocytes. *Hepatology* 1993;17:869–881.
230. Takikawa H, Ookhtens M, Stolz A, Kaplowitz N. Cyclical oxidation-reduction of the C3 position on bile acids catalyzed by 3 alpha-hydroxysteroid dehydrogenase. II. Studies in the prograde and retrograde single-pass, perfused rat liver and inhibition by indomethacin. *J Clin Invest* 1987;80:861–866.
231. Takikawa H, Stolz A, Kaplowitz N. Cyclical oxidation-reduction of the C3 position on bile acids catalysed by hepatic 3 alpha-hydroxysteroid dehydrogenase. I. Studies with the purified enzyme, isolated rat hepatocytes, and inhibition by indomethacin. *J Clin Invest* 1987;80:852–860.
232. Hallbrucker C, Ritter M, Lang F, Gerok W, Haussinger D. Hydroperoxide metabolism in rat liver: K^+ channel activation, cell volume changes and eicosanoid formation. *Eur J Biochem* 1993;211:449–458.
233. Dahm LJ, Hewett JA, Roth RA. Bile and bile salts potentiate superoxide anion release from activated rat peritoneal neutrophils. *Toxicol Appl Pharmacol* 1988;95:82–92.
234. Quist RG, Ton-Hu HT, Lillienau J, Hofmann AF, Barrett KE. Activation of mast cells by bile acids. *Gastroenterology* 1991;101:446–456.
235. Botla R, Spivey JR, Gores GJ. Ursodeoxycholate (UDCA) inhibits the mitochondrial membrane permeability transition induced by glycochenodeoxycholate: a mechanism of UDCA cytoprotection. *J Pharmacol Exp Ther* 1995;272:930–938.
236. Krahenbuhl S, Talos C, Fischer S, Reichen J. Toxicity of bile acids on the electron transport chain of isolated rat liver mitochondria. *Hepatology* 1994;19:471–479.
237. Rosser BG, Gores GJ. Liver cell necrosis: cellular mechanism and clinical implications. *Gastroenterology* 1995;108:252–275.
238. Ballardini G, Bianchi FB, Mirakian R, Fallani M, Pisi E, Bottazzo GF. HLA-A, B, C, HLA-D/DR and HLA-D/DQ expression on unfixed liver biopsy sections from patients with chronic liver disease. *Clin Exp Immunol* 1987;70:35–46.

239. Calmus Y, Arvieux C, Gane P, Boucher E, Nordlinger B, Rouger P, Poupon R. Cholestasis induces major histocompatibility complex class I expression in hepatocytes. *Gastroenterology* 1992;102:1371–1377.
240. Calmus Y, Gane P, Rouger P, Poupon R. Hepatic expression of class I and class II major histocompatibility complex molecules in primary biliary cirrhosis: effect of ursodeoxycholic acid. *Hepatology* 1990;11:12–15.
241. Innes GK, Nagafuchi Y, Fuller BJ, Hobbs KE. Increased expression of major histocompatibility antigens in the liver as a result of cholestasis. *Transplantation* 1988;45:749–752.
242. Hillaire S, Boucher E, Calmus Y, Gane P, Ballet F, Franco D, Moukthar M, Poupon R. Effects of bile acids and cholestasis on major histocompatibility complex class I in human and rats hepatocytes. *Gastroenterology* 1994;107:781–788.
243. Hirano F, Tanaka H, Makino I. Chenodeoxycholic acid-dependent induction of major histocompatibility complex class I mRNA expression in a human hepatoma cell line. *Biochem Biophys Res Comm* 1993;195:1408–1414.

Toxicology of the Liver, 2nd ed.,
Edited by Gabriel L. Plaa and William R. Hewitt
Copyright © 1998 Taylor & Francis

12

Cholestasis Produced by Combinations of Manganese and Bilirubin

Gabriel L. Plaa and Alexandra B. Duguay

Université de Montréal, Montréal, Québec, Canada H3C 3J7

Lena M. King

Parke Davis Research Institute, Mississauga, Ontario, Canada L5K 1B4

William R. Hewitt

SmithKline Beecham Pharmaceuticals, Collegeville, PA 19426-0989

The mechanisms involved in drug-induced cholestasis are poorly understood. One of the major reasons for this deficiency lies in the fact that the drug-induced cholestatic syndrome seen in humans is very difficult to reproduce in animals. It is possible, however, to produce cholestatic effects in animals with selected bile acids, some steroids, and certain chemicals that have no therapeutic utility (1, 2). The time course, duration, and biochemical features of the different models vary, but all produce decreased bile flow and accumulation of biliary secretory products in blood in the absence of any mechanical obstruction of the biliary tree (3–8). These models have served as laboratory tools to unravel hepatobiliary mechanisms possibly involved in intrahepatic cholestatic responses. Steroid- and bile acid–induced cholestasis are described elsewhere in this volume. The interesting cholestatic model described in this chapter is the intravenous combination of manganese and bilirubin in the rat. The model even may have some applicability to humans in view of recent reports of manganese as a contributing factor to cholestasis in patients receiving long-term parenteral nutrition (9, 10).

HEPATIC EFFECTS OF MANGANESE

In 1968, Witzleben et al. (11) described the morphologic changes occurring in the liver of rats 20 hr after an acute intravenous administration of manganese sulfate. This substance produced ultrastructural alterations in the hepatocyte that resembled those observed in cholestasis. In particular, the bile canaliculi became dilated with loss and swelling of the microvilli. In addition, increased prominence and dilatation of the Golgi apparatus were observed. The biliary excretion of bilirubin was very markedly reduced in rats 5 hr after the administration of manganese. Although the hepatocytes showed ultrastructural changes after manganese administration alone, no alterations in ductules were observed at this time. After 6 hr, multiple small foci of hepatocellular necrosis were observed; by 12 hr all animals exhibited hepatocellular necrosis involving either single cells or, commonly, patchy areas with no marked zonal distribution. There was no clear correlation between the severity of the necrosis observed and the extent of the cholestatic morphologic changes observed.

INTERACTION WITH BILIRUBIN

The effect of bilirubin in the cholestatic response to manganese was shown later. A brief reversible decrease in bile flow caused by manganese was markedly enhanced in a dose-related manner following an infusion of bilirubin (12–15). In addition, the bile collected from animals given both agents was turbid. The turbidity was not present in bile collected from rats given only manganese, but it could be produced in vitro by adding manganese sulfate to bile collected from normal rats infused with bilirubin. Klaassen (16) confirmed the finding that manganese followed by an intravenous dose of bilirubin resulted in a marked diminution in bile flow in the rat. He further observed, however, that the cholestatic effect no longer occurred if the bilirubin was administered before, rather than after, the manganese.

The early observations with manganese and bilirubin suggested that the observed cholestatic mechanism might be due to intracanalicular precipitation of a manganese/bilirubin aggregate. This hypothesis was supported by the finding of yellow acellular material in the bile ducts, although canalicular plugs were not evident. With electron microscopy, the infusion of bilirubin after injection of manganese resulted in more severe ultrastructural alterations than those observed with manganese given alone. The abnormalities included increased canalicular dilatation, the presence of prominent cytoplasmic vacuoles and swollen areas of pericanalicular cytoplasm. In addition, fibrillar electron-dense material was observed within the canaliculi, vacuoles, pericanalicular ectoplasm, and bile ducts; these findings were not observed in animals treated only with manganese. The ultrastructural alterations were consistent with an obstructive process. If the infusion of bilirubin followed the injection of manganese by 24 hr, the effects on bile flow and hepatic ultrastructure were very mild and not different from those of rats given manganese alone.

The infusion of only bilirubin itself does not result in the cholestatic picture described above. Bilirubin alone infused at rates high enough to saturate the hepatic excretory capacity can produce a diminution of bile flow in the rhesus monkey (17) but not in the isolated perfused rat liver (18). The addition of bilirubin to manganese-loaded animals, however, results in very profound cholestatic effects, the extent of which depends both on the dose of bilirubin and the interval after manganese loading. Witzleben reported (14) that bile flow had partially recovered by 24 hr and appeared to be normal by 48 hr. The cytoplasm of the bile duct epithelial cells also showed prominent alterations, with inclusions of amorphous or fibrillar material. By 48 hr, the canaliculi remained dilated with loss of microvilli, although the presence of intraluminal material was greatly reduced; fibrillar material was still evident at this time, although less so than at 24 hr; the bile duct cells contained less osmophilic material than that observed at 24 hr, but the epithelium itself was even more abnormal. To explain the bilirubin enhancement, the possibility was raised that manganese and bilirubin might act synergistically on the hepatocyte directly to affect bile formation, although alterations in bile salt composition had not been demonstrated in animals treated with manganese.

Sulfobromophthalein (BSP) was shown to protect against the cholestatic response in animals simultaneously infused with bilirubin and BSP (19). Bile flow rates obtained 4 hr after the initial injection of manganese in animals treated with bilirubin and BSP were indistinguishable from those observed in the control rats. BSP infusion, however, exerted no effect on biliary bilirubin concentrations 30–60 min after the infusion of bilirubin, indicating that the concentration of bilirubin in bile was not a determinative factor in the cholestatic response following manganese and bilirubin. A direct relationship between biliary manganese content and the severity of the cholestasis also proved elusive (20). In situations where BSP protected against cholestasis, manganese biliary excretion was actually increased rather than decreased. While bilirubin infusion itself was found to increase the manganese concentration in bile, the total amount of manganese excreted was not altered. These data suggested that manganese concentration itself in the bile was not a determinative factor. Regardless of the mechanisms involved, the discovery that manganese and bilirubin can interact to cause a physiologic and a morphologic cholestasis has produced an interesting experimental model.

CHARACTERISTICS OF Mn-BR CHOLESTASIS

The Mn-BR effect was further developed as a reversible model of experimental cholestasis by Plaa and his associates. De Lamirande and Plaa (21) demonstrated that even nonnecrotic dosages of manganese, which were not cholestatic when given alone, produced a reduction in bile flow in the rat provided bilirubin was injected after manganese within a specific time period. The cholestatic regimens of low, nonnecrotic doses of manganese and bilirubin also cause morphologic changes synchronous with the induction of cholestasis, in that the bile canaliculi progressively lose their microvilli while vacuolization occurs in the pericanalicular area and subsequently in the cytoplasm. BSP affords protection not only to the induced cholestasis but also to the morphologic changes (22). The severity of the cholestatic effect (ranging from a 10% to a 100% decrease in bile flow, 1 hr after bilirubin injection) was shown to be related to the bilirubin dosage independent of the manganese load (23).

Temporal Aspects

The time interval between manganese and bilirubin injections is critical for the induction of cholestasis (21, 23). If one waits too long after manganese to administer the bilirubin, decreased bile flow is not observed. The length of the time interval during which cholestasis can still be elicited with the manganese–bilirubin injection combination depends upon the dosage of manganese administered. This interesting dose–time relationship is depicted in Fig. 1. In this experiment performed in rats, the manganese dosage was varied, but the amount of bilirubin injected kept constant. For each separate manganese dosage, the time interval between the injections of manganese and the bilirubin injections was increased from 0.25 to 4 hr, and the resultant decrease in bile flow was measured 1 hr following bilirubin administration. Bilirubin had to be injected within 15 min after the smallest dosage of manganese (4.5 mg/kg) to get the largest decrease in bile flow, while 3 hr could elapse between the injections with a dosage of 9.0 mg/kg to yield the same result (23). With four different dosages of manganese, the "critical time interval" that could be used without abolishing the cholestatic effect was estimated from the descending portion of the bile flow curve (Fig. 1) for each manganese dosage. A 50% decrease in bile flow was used as the reference parameter; the "critical time interval" was defined as the time between injections during which one could still elicit a 50% decrease in bile flow. A positive linear regression was observed: as the dosage of manganese increased, the critical time interval also increased ($y = -2.4 + 0.21x$, where y is the time interval, expressed in hours, and x is the dosage, expressed in mg/kg).

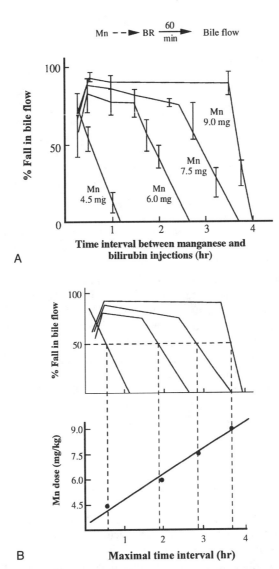

FIG. 1. Dose-effect relationships for manganese-bilirubin (Mn-BR) combinations on bile flow. At time 0, manganese (4.5–9 mg/kg intravenously) was injected, followed by bilirubin injection (25 mg/kg intravenously); bile flow was measured 60 min after bilirubin injection. (A) Effect of manganese dosage on bile flow when the time interval between manganese and bilirubin injections is varied. The ordinate is the maximum decrease in bile flow, expressed as a percentage of bile flow during the control period before manganese injection. The abscissa is the time interval between manganese and bilirubin injections. The influence of manganese dosage on the time interval pattern is depicted by the four separate curves. (B) Critical time intervals to attain a 50% decrease in bile flow after Mn-BR injections when manganese dosage is varied. The ordinate is the dosage (4.5–9 mg/kg intravenously) of manganese injected before bilirubin. The abscissa is the time interval between manganese and bilirubin injections, during which a 50% decrease in bile flow can still be observed 60 min after bilirubin injection. (Data taken from [23].)

BSP Protection

BSP inhibits the Mn-BR cholestatic effect if injected 10 min before bilirubin (21). Biliary excretion studies (23) demonstrated that the protection occurs only when biliary BSP excretion is incomplete at the time the bilirubin is injected. Furthermore, the degree of protection seems related to the amount of unexcreted BSP remaining. BSP is conjugated with glutathione prior to its biliary excretion. Only unconjugated BSP, however, and not BSP-glutathione, affords protection against the effect of Mn-BR (21). A linear relationship was demonstrated between the minimal protective dosage of BSP and the cholestatic dosage of bilirubin. A critical molar ratio of 0.74 between BSP and bilirubin dosages, independent of manganese load, was established experimentally, thus further supporting the concept that BSP exerts its protective action on the bilirubin moiety.

On the basis of these observations, it was proposed that an intermediate step is involved between manganese and the subsequent interaction with bilirubin to eventually lead to cholestasis (23). Manganese might act on the hepatic handling of bilirubin. A direct action on the biotransformation of bilirubin, however, seems unlikely even though it cannot be completely ruled out. The metabolic pattern of bilirubin in bile after administration of cholestatic regimens of the Mn-BR model was shown to be altered, but hydrostatic obstruction of bile flow also resulted in similar changes in metabolic patterns, indicating that altered bilirubin excretory pattern was a consequence, rather that the cause of, cholestasis (24). Also, it was shown that the bilirubin component involved in Mn-BR cholestasis could likely be the unconjugated form of bilirubin (25, 26), since bilirubin ditaurate (a synthetic stable form of conjugated bilirubin) does not provoke cholestasis in the Sprague-Dawley rat (26). Unfortunately, experimental data of hepatocellular events before bilirubin excretion and the influence of manganese on these events are not available.

THE HEPATOCYTE AS A SITE OF ACTION

The first mechanism suggested to explain the cholestasis produced by Mn-BR combinations was the presence of a physical obstruction in the canaliculus with hepatocellular morphologic changes secondary to a primary physical obstruction (1). The bile of rats treated with manganese or an Mn-BR combination is cloudy (1, 12, 13, 16). Several lines of experimental data, however, are inconsistent with a mechanical obstruction theory: Ultrastructural evaluation of liver does not show canalicular precipitates; manganese alone, albeit at high doses, causes cholestasis; and the biliary excretion patterns of bilirubin, BSP, and manganese do not appear to correlate with a physical obstruction (1, 19–21). Subsequent investigations strongly support the hypothesis that the cholestasis is initiated by hepatocellular changes.

The canalicular membrane as a target site for Mn-BR cholestasis has been investigated. The morphologic changes observed are predominant in the biliary pole, and this region has been implicated as a target in other cholestatic models. As well, it is possible that Mn^{2+} could affect membrane fluidity, since another divalent cation, Ca^{2+}, can influence membrane fluidity (27–29).

Biliary Tree Permeability

Biliary tree permeability has been shown to be markedly altered by cholestatic combinations of manganese and bilirubin. Ayotte and Plaa (30) applied the segmented retrograde intrabiliary injection (SRII) technique, devised by Fujimoto's group (31–33), to measure biliary permeability in rats following Mn-BR injections. Inulin and mannitol were used as marker substances to assess biliary tree permeability. When given by SRII, inulin, a large-molecular-weight compound, probably passes from the canalicular lumen to the blood via the tight junctions, whereas mannitol, a small-molecular-weight compound, is thought to pass through both the canalicular pathway and the tight junctions (32). Globally, in Mn-BR–treated animals, a decrease in recovery of inulin and mannitol in recovered bile after SRII indicated that both tight junctions and canalicular membranes were modified by the Mn-BR treatment. Based on the characteristics of both markers, and on the selective protection afforded by BSP against the Mn-BR–induced decrease in mannitol recovery, the conclusion was that an alteration of the canalicular membrane permeability could be critical in the sequence of events leading to bile flow impairment. In addition, a slight increase in intrabiliary pressure noted with the Mn-BR treatment suggested that the Mn-BR–induced decrease in marker permeability might also be accompanied by a decreased permeability of water at the canalicular membrane level. These initial observations were confirmed by Dahlström-King et al. (34), who further showed that the alterations in biliary tree permeability were dose-dependent on bilirubin. The various dose-dependent relationships for both bilirubin enhancement and BSP protection of Mn-BR cholestasis correlated very well with the effects of these agents on mannitol and inulin recoverability in the bile after retrograde intrabiliary injection. When the data presented by Ayotte and Plaa (30) are considered with those of Dahlström-King, coutare and Plaa (34), an excellent association is observed between maneuvers that lead to Mn-BR–induced cholestasis and those that alter biliary tree permeability as measured by SRII. Canalicular membrane permeability is probably more critical to Mn-BR cholestasis than changes in junctional complexes.

Bile acid secretion in the Mn-BR model has been assessed (35). From 15 to 90 min after bilirubin administration (the cholestatic phase), biliary bile acid concentration increased ~45%, while bile acid excretion rates were not appreciably modified during the same periods. When bile flows were plotted as a function of the corresponding bile acid excretion rates 90 min after bilirubin administration, a logarithmic (ln) model was found to best fit the data obtained. Mn-BR treatment resulted in a significantly less steep slope when compared to the one obtained in noncholestatic animals (35). This could theoretically be explained by regurgitation of bile through a paracellular pathway; alteration of the osmotic force generated by the active secretion of bile acids, perhaps through increased micelle size; reduction of the bile acid–dependent fraction, or diminution of fluid entry in the canaliculus in response to the osmotic force. The regurgitation hypothesis appears unlikely, since it is incompatible with the increase in biliary bile acid concentration observed during Mn-BR cholestasis. Since after Mn-BR treatment biliary phospholipid concentration was diminished, while bile acid concentration was elevated (35), micelle size should be accordingly smaller than in noncholestatic conditions; therefore, the altered osmotic force hypothesis also appears unlikely. Diminution of bile acid–dependent bile flow cannot be completely ruled out, but bile acid excretion rates were unaffected following Mn-BR treatment. Finally, several observations favor the "diminution of fluid entry" hypothesis. Changes in the permeability of the biliary tree were observed by the SRII technique (30, 34), and a diminution in bile canalicular permeability to water could account for the rise in intrabiliary pressure observed during these experiments (30). Furthermore, analysis of bile flow/bile acid excretion rate relationships (35) suggested that for the same amount of bile acid excreted, the quantity of fluid generated in the bile canaliculus was smaller in Mn-BR–treated animals. Can one speculate that Mn-Br treatment might reduce the osmotic water permeability coefficient of the canalicular membrane? The overall impression is that the bile canalicular membrane is physically altered following Mn-BR treatment, so that water flow through the membrane is hindered. Perhaps this results in cholestasis.

Membrane fluidity of bile canalicular and sinusoidal membrane fractions was assessed in rats treated with a Mn-BR combination to detect possible changes related to the onset of cholestasis. Microviscosity was measured by fluorescence polarization in vitro after incubation of membrane fractions with two molecular probes (36, 37). With a hydrophilic probe, decreased membrane fluidity was observed shortly after Mn-BR treatment in bile canalicular–enriched membrane fractions, whereas no alteration was detected with a more lipophilic probe describing the center of the lipid layer (Table 1). In contrast, with either probe, the fluidity of sinusoidal-enriched membrane fractions appeared to be unaffected by the cholestatic treatment. These results suggest

TABLE 1. *Microviscosity of bile canalicular- and sinusoidal-enriched membrane fractions following Mn-BR treatment*

Fraction	Control group		Mn-BR group	
	DPH	TMA-DPH	DPH	TMA-DPH
Canalicular membrane	0.190 ±0.006	0.233 ±0.007	0.193 ±0.003	0.244[1] ±0.003
Sinusoidal membrane	0.155 ±0.008	0.219 ±0.005	0.156 ±0.004	0.225 ±0.006

Rats received 4.5 mg Mn/kg intravenously, followed 15 min later with 25 mg bilirubin/kg intravenously; animals were killed 30 min after bilirubin treatment. Fluidity was measured by 1,6-diphenyl-1,3,5-hexatriene (DPH) and its 1,4-trimethyl-ammonium derivative (TMA-DPH) at 37°C using steady-state fluorescence polarization. Values are means ± SE for seven animals.
[1]Significantly different from control. (Data taken from [36, 37].)

that membrane alterations seem more likely to occur in the hydrophilic region of bile canalicular membranes and support the hypothesis that the canalicular membrane is the more likely site of action for the development of Mn-BR cholestasis.

Accumulation of Bilirubin and Manganese

Changes in the chemical composition of the bile canalicular membrane of rats treated with manganese and bilirubin have also been reported. The results of an early study (38) appear to indicate that an important shift in the recovery of protein from the plasma membrane to the bile canalicular membrane fraction occurred when cholestatic regimens of Mn-BR were administered. During these conditions bilirubin appeared to be incorporated into the bile canalicular–enriched membrane fraction, since the latter became yellow and the color was readily extracted by chloroform but not water. The incorporation of bilirubin into bile canalicular–enriched membrane fraction was later confirmed (39). In addition, a significant increase in both cholesterol and phospholipid content was observed in bile canalicular–enriched membranes after a cholestatic Mn-BR regimen, while the sinusoidal-enriched membrane fraction contents of cholesterol and phospholipids were not altered. However, bilirubin given alone increased the cholesterol content, while manganese alone increased the cholesterol and phospholipid content in the bile canalicular membrane without cholestasis. These observations suggest that the incorporation of bilirubin into the membrane is necessary to provoke cholestasis and that the increased content of cholesterol and phospholipids might facilitate the incorporation of bilirubin (39).

That the incorporation of manganese in canalicular membranes is likely a key event in Mn-BR–induced cholestasis, as well, has been demonstrated (40). After a large necrotic and cholestatic dose of manganese, the cation accumulates in both the canalicular and the plasma membrane fractions; a small nonnecrotic dose does not accumulate if administered alone. Nevertheless, the small nonnecrotic dose of manganese followed by bilirubin injection within the critical cholestatic time sequence leads to the subcellular accumulation of manganese at only one site, the canalicular membrane. Thus, bilirubin appears to facilitate manganese incorporation into the canalicular membrane selectively. The small dosage of manganese in conjunction with bilirubin produces manganese concentrations in canalicular membranes similar to those seen with the larger dosage of manganese alone. BSP administration partially reduces the manganese content (40). A critical amount of manganese present in canalicular membranes may be necessary before bile flow becomes affected, which may account for the characteristic time interval/bile flow response patterns observed (Fig. 1 A) with varying dosages of manganese combined with a fixed dosage of bilirubin (23).

A Mn-BR complex has been proposed as the cholestatic intermediate leading to diminished bile flow after the sequential administration of manganese and bilirubin in rats (40, 41). Bilirubin is known to form complexes with divalent cations, including manganese (13, 42). The concentrations of bilirubin found in the bile canalicular membrane 60 min after administration of manganese (4.5 mg/kg), followed 15 min later with bilirubin (25 mg/kg) were 407 ± 18 nmol/mg protein (39), while the manganese content was 1691 ± 91 nmol/mg protein (40), suggesting that the molar composition of a manganese/bilirubin complex might be as large as 4 : 1. Can a critical molar relationship be linked to the manganese–bilirubin bile flow relationship depicted in Fig. 1 B for varying dosages of manganese and bilirubin? This requires investigation. The putative Mn-BR complex might be transported to the canalicular locus of the hepatocyte membrane, where it could bind or incorporate, leading to alteration of membrane permeability. Alternatively, the putative complex might be formed directly at the canalicular membrane level, where it could precipitate and modify membrane permeability. BSP might exert its protective effect by either preventing the formation of the postulated complex or blocking its action on the canalicular membrane.

Taken together, these observations indicate that the accumulation of manganese and of bilirubin in the bile canalicular membrane of rats during Mn-BR cholestasis is evident. What is very unclear, however, is if the accumulation occurs as a complex or as separate manganese and bilirubin entities. The sequence of events leading to the accumulation is also not known, except that manganese administration, for some undetermined reason, must precede the injection of bilirubin (16, 21, 23). To further complicate the situation, cholesterol and perhaps phospholipids appear to be involved. Unfortunately, definitive critical experiments specifically designed to unravel the overall problem are sorely needed and have yet to be performed.

Accumulation of Cholesterol

Yousef and colleagues (43–46), studied bile acid–induced intrahepatic cholestasis in the rat and demonstrated that cholesterol was incorporated in bile canalicular membranes after lithocholic acid injections. Increased de novo cholesterol synthesis was believed to be the cause of this effect (43). The accumulation of cholesterol in vitro could be enhanced if cytosolic proteins were added to the incubation medium (45). One can abolish the cholesterol accumulation by pretreating animals with cycloheximide, an inhibitor of protein synthesis; interference with cytosolic binding of lithocholate, either by inhibition of binding proteins or by competition with lithocholate, might explain the protective effect (46).

Dahlström-King and Plaa (47) showed that unaltered protein synthesis is necessary for expression of maximal cholestasis in the Mn-BR model as well as in two bile acid models (lithocholic acid and taurolithocholic acid). The impact of cycloheximide on the reduction of bile flow after the Mn-BR combination was dependent on the severity of the response. The 40–60% reduction following the smaller dosage of bilirubin was virtually blocked by a small dose of cycloheximide given 18 hr earlier, whereas the 80% reduction following a larger dose of bilirubin was merely attenuated.

Due to the similarities between the bile acid and Mn-BR models, it appeared logical to investigate the role of cholesterol accumulation in Mn-BR intrahepatic cholestasis (36, 37, 48). Indeed, the cholesterol content of bile canalicular membranes is increased by twofold to threefold 45 min after Mn-BR treatment (Table 2). The increase was also observed in cytosol, but not in other subcellular fractions; a decrease was noted

TABLE 2. *Cholesterol content of bile canalicular membranes from control or Mn-BR cholestatic rats*

Cholesterol content (μmol/mg protein)	Control group	Mn-BR group
Total	1.244 ± 0.33	2.349 ± 0.30
Derived from de novo synthesis	0.389 ± 0.10	1.684 ± 0.21
Derived from hepatic pool	0.855 ± 0.23	0.665 ± 0.08

Rats received 4.5 mg Mn/kg intravenously, followed 15 min later with 25 mg bilirubin/kg intravenously; animals were killed 30 min after bilirubin treatment. Values are means $\pm$ SE for six animals. (Data taken from [37, 48].)

in microsomes. The source of the cholesterol accumulating in canalicular membranes was determined using ^{3}H-cholesterol to label hepatic pools and ^{14}C-mevalonic acid to label newly synthesized cholesterol. The results indicated that after Mn-BR treatment the contribution of newly synthesized cholesterol in bile canalicular membranes was greatly enhanced (Table 2). Furthermore, Mn-BR treatment favored the contribution of newly synthesized cholesterol rather than the contribution of intracellular preformed cholesterol pools in all subcellular fractions isolated 45 min after initiation of the cholestatic treatment. The newly synthesized cholesterol accumulating was calculated and shown to greatly exceed the estimated amount of newly synthesized cholesterol destined for biliary excretion by almost ten-fold, indicating that blockage of bile flow due to cholestasis cannot account for the actual amount of cholesterol accumulation observed in hepatic tissue. Thus, accumulation of newly synthesized cholesterol in bile canalicular membrane definitely appears to be an important feature of Mn-BR cholestasis. What is critical to establish, however, is the relationship of the cholesterol accumulation to the accumulation of manganese and bilirubin described previously, and, more important, the consequences of canalicular cholesterol accumulation on altered canalicular permeability after Mn-BR treatment.

POTENTIATION BY KETONES

A substantial body of data demonstrates that ketones and ketogenic substances can potentiate the hepatonecrogenic properties of chloroform, carbon tetrachloride, and a number of other halogenated hydrocarbons (2, 49, 50). Acetone was the first ketone described to possess this property (51); the phenomenon was later observed with methyl n-butyl ketone and 2,5-hexanedione (52). Among the ketogenic chemicals, isopropanol has been the subject of more detailed study (51, 53, 54). However, 1,3-butanediol, another ketogenic agent, was shown to potentiate the hepatonecrogenic properties of carbon tetrachloride, and it was established that the severity of the potentiation correlated remarkably well with the plasma and hepatic concentrations of β-hydroxybutyrate, the major metabolite of 1,3-butanediol (55, 56).

Potentiation of liver injury is not limited to necrogenic hepatotoxicants. With cholestatic agents, such interactions are observed as well. Rats maintained on 1,3-butanediol exhibit potentiated cholestatic responses to taurolithocholate or Mn-BR combinations; with α-naphthylisothiocyanate, the hyperbilirubinemia is enhanced but the decrease in bile flow remains unaffected (57). Methyl n-butyl ketone (MnBK) and methyl isobutyl ketone (MiBK) can aggravate taurolithocholate-induced cholestasis in rats (58).

1,3-Butanediol (BD) was among the first ketogenic agents tested against Mn-BR cholestasis (57). BD is relatively nontoxic in rats (oral LD50 > 10 g/kg) when given alone and is biotransformed into β-hydroxybutyrate and acetoacetate (56, 59). After 7 days of oral BD ingestion (about 10 g/kg/day), rats subjected to Mn-BR challenge demonstrated an enhanced responsiveness to the bile flow diminution of the combination, depending upon the severity of the Mn-BR treatment (57). Even the threshold dosage of manganese needed to elicit hepatobiliary dysfunction appeared to be smaller in BD-pretreated animals. Also, the decreased bile flow was more severe and lasted longer when nonmaximal dosages of bilirubin were administered after the initial treatment with manganese. Following a maximal dosage of bilirubin, however, which results in a maximal decrease in bile flow in non-pretreated animals, no potentiation was observed. Normally, BSP affords protection against Mn-BR cholestasis; this protective effect was diminished in BD-pretreated animals. To eliminate enhanced BSP biotransformation as an explanation of the reduced protective effect in BD-pretreated rats, experiments were performed with dibromosulfphthalein (DBSP), an analog of BSP that is not biotransformed but also protects against Mn-BR cholestasis. The protection conferred by DBSP was diminished in a dose-dependent manner by BD treatment. Two explanations for the enhancing effects of BD on Mn-BR cholestasis have been presented (57): The first supposes that bilirubin kinetics are altered and more bilirubin is available to form the putative Mn-BR intermediate; the second purports that cell susceptibility to manganese occurs or that the subsequent reaction of the intermediate with bilirubin is facilitated.

The oral administration of methyl isobutyl ketone (MiBK) to rats 18 hr before Mn-BR challenge results in a potentiated cholestatic response. The MiBK dose-dependent enhanced effect, however, was much more striking when the ketone was given daily for 3 days prior to challenge (60, 61). An interesting observation was that MiBK not only potentiated the decrease in bile flow observed after Mn-BR combination injections but also revealed bile-flow diminishing properties with a larger dosage of manganese administered alone without bilirubin. The two major metabolites of MiBK (4-methyl-2-pentanol [4MPOL] and 4-hydroxymethyl isobutyl ketone [4-OHMiBK]) also potentiate Mn-BR or manganese alone, but there are interesting differences between these metabolites (61). Daily pretreatment for 3 days showed that 4MPOL was a better potentiator than 4-OHMiBK in the Mn-BR model, while, with manganese given alone, 4-OHMiBK proved to be more effective. In terms of relative potency, 4MPOL appears quite similar to MiBK, while 4-OHMiBK seems less potent. When one considers that the biotransformation reaction of MiBK to the secondary alcohol 4MPOL is bidirectional, the latter compound could also be considered to be a ketogenic substance. Cycloheximide, an inhibitor of protein synthesis, reduces the bile flow diminution in Mn-BR–challenged animals pretreated with MiBK (unpublished observation) in a manner analogous to that observed with taurolithocholate-induced cholestasis after Mn-BR pretreatment (62); this suggests that protein synthesis may be involved in the MiBK potentiation phenomenon.

In laboratory studies on ketone-potentiated cholestasis, the ketones are usually administered orally by gavage, whereas occupational human exposure to MiBK or methyl n-butyl ketone (MnBK) usually occurs by inhalation. Consequently, the potentiating properties of these two ketones following inhalation (4 hr/day for 3 days before Mn-BR challenge) were investigated in rats (63–65). Both ketones can potentiate Mn-BR–induced cholestasis in a concentration-dependent fashion, but there are quantitative differences between these closely related structural isomers. In terms of exposure concentrations, MnBK was found to be a more potent potentiator than MiBK (65). The minimal effective concentrations (MEC) for MiBK and MnBK were estimated to be 400 and 150 ppm, respectively. MiBK tissue concentrations after inhalation were generally larger than those observed for MnBK (64). Perhaps differences in the potencies of the various metabolites might explain, in part, why MnBK appears to be a more potent potentiator than MiBK.

A possible effect of route of administration on MiBK potentiation of Mn-BR–induced cholestasis has been investigated, when oral bolus administration for 3 days was compared to 4-hr inhalation for 3 days (63). The minimal effective dose (MED) for potentiation after gavage was estimated to be 3 mmol/kg, and the MEC by inhalation was 400 ppm; 1.5 mmol/kg and 200 ppm were considered the no-effect dose (NED) and no-effect concentration (NEC), respectively. These MiBK pretreatment regimens yielded comparable plasma MiBK concentrations 1 hr after the last ketone treatment (Table 3). Nevertheless, a more severe diminution in bile flow was observed when MiBK was administered by inhalation (39% versus 72% decrease with 3 mmol/kg by mouth or 400 ppm, respectively; 50% versus 80% decrease with 6 mmol/kg by

TABLE 3. *Plasma concentrations of MiBK and its metabolites after oral administration or inhalation exposure*

Dose/concentration	MiBK	4-OHMiBK	4MPOL
1.5 mmol/kg	5.27 ± 0.98	1.10 ± 0.23	nd
200 ppm	5.02 ± 0.17	5.03 ± 0.89	nd
3 mmol/kg	8.45 ± 1.54	4.75 ± 0.81	nd
400 ppm	8.11 ± 0.30	6.14 ± 0.87	3.97 ± 0.11
6 mmol/kg	16.06 ± 6.40	13.27 ± 2.50	nd
600 ppm	14.30 ± 1.34	7.10 ± 0.37	4.78 ± 0.72

Rats were given MiBK orally (1.5, 3, or 6 mmol/kg) daily for 3 days or were exposed to MiBK (200, 400, or 600 ppm) by inhalation (4 hr/day daily for 3 days); dosages and concentrations represent 0.5, one, or two times the minimal effective dose (MED) or the minimal effective concentration (MEC) for potentiating Mn-BR-induced cholestasis. Animals were killed 1 hr after the last ketone treatment period. Values are means ± SE for six animals and expressed in μg/ml; nd signifies not detectable (<0.02 μg/ml). (Data taken from [63].)

mouth or 600 ppm, respectively). Perhaps the explanation for the apparent difference in severity is related to the fact that concentrations of 4MPOL, a major metabolite of MiBK, were greater when the ketone was administered by inhalation (Table 3).

The mechanisms responsible for the potentiation of Mn-BR cholestasis by ketones, in particular MiBK, are far from established. Ketone potentiation of necrogenic hepatotoxicants, such as carbon tetrachloride and chloroform, is thought to be largely due to enhanced bioactivation by cytochrome P450 (particularly CYP2E1) to yield reactive metabolites responsible for the liver injury (2, 50, 66). MiBK does induce cytochrome P450 isoforms and enhances the bioactivation of carbon tetrachloride at dosages that potentiate the acute hepatotoxic properties of carbon tetrachloride (67–69). Could a similar mechanism be involved in the potentiation of Mn-BR cholestasis? It appears that in rats over 90% of intravenously administered manganese is excreted into the bile, but not all of it is in a free cationic form (41,70, 71); in vitro, about 40% of manganese added directly to rat bile was found to be not ultrafiltrable, indicating binding to macromolecules (41). When the role of biotransformation products in chemical-induced cholestasis was reviewed in 1982 (72), however, there was no evidence suggesting that biotransformation of manganese or bilirubin occurs before these substances elicit hepatobiliary dysfunction; the situation has not changed in recent years. Furthermore, with taurolithocholate-induced cholestasis, which is also potentiated by MiBK, pretreatments with inducers of cytochrome P450 yielded mixed results when assessed for enhancing properties, while inhibitors of cytochrome P450 failed to protect against decreases in bile flow (73). Taken together, these observations support the premise that cytochrome P450 isoforms probably play only a minor role, if any, in the cholestatic response, but the matter remains unresolved.

Altered bile canalicular cholesterol content is thought to be a major event in Mn-BR–induced cholestasis (37, 48). Recently, it was shown (74) that rats exposed to MiBK by inhalation exhibit an even greater increase in cholesterol membrane accumulation when challenged with Mn-BR (Table 4). Other results indicate that after 600-ppm MiBK exposure the contribution of de novo cholesterol synthesis to the total cholesterol content of the various isolated hepatocellular fractions was more important

TABLE 4. *Cholesterol content of hepatocellular fractions from Mn-BR cholestatic rats pretreated with MiBK or air by inhalation*

Fraction	Air + Mn-BR group	MiBK + Mn-BR group
Canalicular membrane	2.349 ± 0.30	5.343 ± 0.90
Sinusoidal and lateral membranes	0.733 ± 0.05	1.024 ± 0.19
Cytosol	0.159 ± 0.04	1.057 ± 0.08

Rats were exposed to air or MiBK (600 ppm) by inhalation (4 hr/day, 3 days); 18 hr after the last exposure, they received 4.5 mg Mn/kg intravenously, followed 15 min later with 25 mg bilirubin/kg intravenously; animals were killed 30 min after bilirubin treatment. Values are means ± SE for six animals and expressed in μmol/mg protein. (Data taken from [37, 74].)

than the contribution of intracellular pools. Vesicle-mediated transport appears responsible for intracellular cholesterol exchange, whereas a carrier-mediated transport system seems implicated in the delivery of newly synthesized cholesterol to plasma membranes (75–78). MiBK and other ketones are known to induce cytochrome P450 isoforms (67, 69, 79–81); perhaps they induce other cytosolic proteins, as well. Consequently, MiBK might increase cytosolic proteins involved in cholesterol trafficking, thus increasing the contribution of newly synthesized cholesterol in bile canalicular membranes.

CONCLUSIONS

The Mn-BR model of experimental intrahepatic cholestasis in the rat is very interesting. Two substances, which when given alone exert no deleterious effect on bile flow or bile composition, result in a prompt dose-dependent diminution in bile flow when administered sequentially and in a precise order. The dose-effect relationships for each component of the combination differ from each other but yet are each critical for the overall cholestatic response. Unaltered protein synthesis appears necessary for expression of maximal cholestasis. The site of action appears to be localized at the bile canalicular membrane, where both chemical composition and physiologic function are altered. Finally, the overall hepatobiliary response can be modified by exposure to other chemicals before the Mn-BR challenge. Thus, the model serves as a useful laboratory tool for investigating normal bile formation, the pathogenesis of a form of intrahepatic cholestasis, and interactions between different classes of chemicals in the liver.

REFERENCES

1. Plaa GL, Priestly BG. Intrahepatic cholestasis induced by drugs and chemicals. *Pharmacol Rev* 1976;28:207–273.
2. Plaa GL. Toxic responses of the liver. In: Amdur MO, Doull J, Klaassen CD, eds. *Casarett and Doull's Toxicology*, 4th ed. New York: Pergamon Press, 1991:334–353.
3. Tuchweber B, Weber A, Roy CC, Yousef IM. Mechanisms of experimentally induced cholestasis. In: Popper H, Schaffner F, eds. *Progress in liver diseases*, vol. 8. New York: Grune & Stratton, 1986:161–178.
4. Reichen J, Simon FR. Cholestasis. In: Arias IM, Jakoby WB, Schachter D, Shafritz DA, eds. *The liver: biology and pathobiology*, 3rd ed. New York: Raven Press, 1994:1291–1326.
5. Vore M. Cholestasis. In: Siegers CP, Watkins JB III, eds. *Progress in pharmacology and clinical pharmacology: biliary excretion of drugs and other chemicals*. Stuttgart: Fischer, 1991:455–474.
6. Feuer G, DiFonzo CJ. Intrahepatic cholestasis: a review of biochemical-pathological mechanisms. *Drug Metab Drug Interact* 1992;10:1–161.
7. Fallon MB, Anserson JM, Boyer JL. Intrahepatic cholestasis. In: Schiff L, Schiff ER, eds. *Diseases of the liver*, vol. 1, 7th ed. Philadelphia: Lippincott, 1993:343–361.
8. Watkins JB III, Klaassen CD. Mechanisms of drug-induced cholestasis. In: Cameron RG, Feuer G, de la Iglesia FA, eds. *Handbook of experimental pharmacology: drug-induced hepatotoxicity*. Heidelberg: Springer Verlag, 1995:155–183.
9. Bayliss EA, Hambidge KM, Sokol RJ, Stewart B, Lilly JR. Hepatic concentrations of zinc, copper and manganese in infants with extrahepatic biliary atresia. *J Trace Elem Med Biol* 1995;9:40–43.

10. Fell JM, Reynolds AP, Meadows N, Khan K, Long SG, Quaghebeur G, Taylor WJ, Milla PJ. Manganese toxicity in children receiving long-term parenteral nutrition. *Lancet* 1996;347:1218–1221.
11. Witzleben CL, Pitlick P, Bermeyer J, Benoit R. Acute manganese overload: a new experimental model of intrahepatic cholestasis. *Am J Pathol* 1968;53:409–423.
12. Witzleben CL. Manganese-induced cholestasis: concurrent observations on bile flow rate and hepatic ultrastructure. *Am J Pathol* 1969;57:617–625.
13. Witzleben CL. Bilirubin as a cholestatic agent: physiologic and morphologic observations. *Am J Pathol* 1971;62:181–184.
14. Witzleben CL. Physiologic and morphologic natural history of a model of intrahepatic cholestasis. *Am J Pathol* 1972;66:577–588.
15. Boyce W, Witzleben CL. Bilirubin as a cholestatic agent. II. Effect of variable doses of bilirubin on the severity of Mn-BR cholestasis. *Am J Pathol* 1973;72:427–432.
16. Klaassen CD. Biliary excretion of manganese in rats, rabbits and dogs. *Toxicol Appl Pharmacol* 1974;29:458–468.
17. Gartner LM, Lane DL, Cornelius CE. Bilirubin transport by liver in adult Macaca mulatta. *Am J Physiol* 1971;220:528–535.
18. Bloomer JR, Zaccaria J. Effect of graded bilirubin loads on bilirubin transport by perfused rat liver. *Am J Physiol* 1976;230:736–742.
19. Witzleben CL, Boyce WH. Bilirubin as a cholestatic agent. III. Prevention of bilirubin-related cholestasis by sulfobromophthalein. *Arch Pathol* 1975a;99:492–495.
20. Witzleben CL, Boyce WH. Bilirubin as a cholestatic agent. IV. Effect of bilirubin and sulfobromophthalein (BSP) on biliary manganese excretion. *Arch Pathol* 1975b;99:496–498.
21. de Lamirande E, Plaa GL. Role of manganese, bilirubin and sulfobromophthalein in Mn-BR cholestasis in rats. *Proc Soc Exp Biol Med* 1978;158:283–287.
22. de Lamirande E, Tuchweber B, Plaa GL. Morphological aspects of Mn-BR induced cholestasis. *Liver* 1982;2:22–27.
23. de Lamirande E, Plaa GL. Dose and time relationships in Mn-BR cholestasis. *Toxicol Appl Pharmacol* 1979a;49:257–263.
24. de Lamirande E, Plaa GL. Bilirubin excretion pattern in Mn-BR cholestasis. *Arch Int Pharmacodyn* 1979b;239:24–35.
25. Witzleben CL, Boyer JL, Ng OC. Mn-BR cholestasis: further studies in pathogenesis. *Lab Invest* 1987;56:151–154.
26. Ayotte P, Plaa GL. Biliary excretion in Sprague-Dawley and Gunn rats during Mn-BR induced cholestasis. *Hepatology* 1988;8:1069–1078.
27. Galla HJ, Sackman E. Chemically induced lipid phase separation in model membranes containing charged lipids: a spin label study. *Biochim Biophys Acta* 1975;401:509–529.
28. Livingstone CJ, Schachter D. Calcium modulates the lipid dynamics of rat hepatocyte plasma membranes by direct and indirect mechanisms. *Biochemistry* 1980;19:4823–4827.
29. Storch J, Schachter D. Calcium alters the acyl chain composition and lipid fluidity of rat hepatocyte plasma membranes in vitro. *Biochim Biophys Acta* 1985;812:473–484.
30. Ayotte P, Plaa GL. Modification of biliary tree permeability in rats treated with a Mn-BR combination. *Toxicol Appl Pharmacol* 1986;84:295–303.
31. Olson JR, Fujimoto JM. Evaluation of hepatobiliary function in the rat by the segmented retrograde intrabiliary injection technique. *Biochem Pharmacol* 1980;29:205–211.
32. Imamura T, Fujimoto JM. Transit patterns of marker compounds given by segmented retrograde intrabiliary injection (SRII) in the isolated in situ perfused rat liver. *J Pharmacol Exp Ther* 1980;215:110–115.
33. Fujimoto JM. Some in vivo methods for studying sites of toxicant action in relation to bile formation. In: Plaa GL, Hewitt WR, eds. *Toxicology of the liver*. New York: Raven Press, 1982:121–145.
34. Dahlström-King L, Couture J, Plaa GL. Functional changes of the biliary tree associated with experimentally induced cholestasis: sulfobromophthalein on Mn-BR combination. *Toxicol Appl Pharmacol* 1990;108:559–567.
35. Ayotte P, Plaa GL. Biliary excretion in Sprague-Dawley and Gunn rats during Mn-BR-induced cholestasis. *Hepatology* 1988;8:1069–1078.
36. Duguay A, Couture J, Plaa GL. Alteration of bile canalicular membrane in Mn-BR induced intrahepatic cholestasis. *The Toxicologist* 1994;14:368.
37. Duguay A. Altération des lipides membranaires dans la potentialisation de la cholestase intrahépatique par un solvant cétonique, *Ph.D. Thesis*, Université de Montréal, 1997.

38. de Lamirande E, Tuchweber B, Plaa GL. Hepatocellular membrane alteration as a possible cause of Mn-BR-induced cholestasis. *Biochem Pharmacol* 1981;30:2305–2312.
39. Plaa GL, de Lamirande E, Lewittes M, Yousef IM. Liver cell plasma membrane lipids in Mn-BR-induced intrahepatic cholestasis. *Biochem Pharmacol* 1982;31:3698–3701.
40. Ayotte P, Plaa GL. Hepatic subcellular distribution of manganese in manganese and Mn-BR-induced cholestasis. *Biochem Pharmacol* 1985;34:3857–3865.
41. Klaassen CD. Biliary excretion of manganese in rats, rabbits and dogs. *Toxicol Appl Pharmacol* 1974;29:458–468.
42. Allen B, Bernhoft R, Blanckaert N, Svanvik J, Filly R, Gooding G, Way L. Sludge is calcium bilirubinate associated with bile stasis. *Am J Surg* 1981;141:51–56.
43. Kakis G, Yousef IM. Pathogenesis of cholic acid protection in lithocholate-induced intrahepatic cholestasis in rats. *Gastroenterology* 1978;75:595–607.
44. Kakis G, Yousef IM. Mechanism of cholic acid protection in lithocholate-induced intrahepatic cholestasis in rats. *Gastroenterology* 1980;78:1402–1411.
45. Yousef IM, Tuchweber B. Effect of lithocholic acid on cholesterol synthesis and transport in rat liver. *Biochim Biophys Acta* 1984;796:336–344.
46. Yousef IM, Tuchweber B, Weber A. Prevention of lithocholate-induced cholestasis by cycloheximide, an inhibitor of protein synthesis. *Life Sci* 1983;33:103–110.
47. Dahlström-King L, Plaa GL. Effect of inhibition of protein synthesis on cholestasis induced by taurolithocholate, lithocholate, and a Mn-BR combination in the rat. *Biochem Pharmacol* 1989;38:2543–2549.
48. Duguay AB, Yousef IM, Plaa GL. Newly synthesized cholesterol accumulation in bile canalicular membranes after Mn-BR-induced cholestasis. (submitted)
49. Hewitt WR, Miyajima H, Côté MG, Plaa GL. Modification of haloalkane-induced hepatotoxicity by exogenous ketones and metabolic ketosis. *Fed Proc* 1980;39:3118–3123.
50. Plaa GL. Experimental evaluation of haloalkanes and liver injury. *Fundam Appl Pharmacol* 1988;10:563–570.
51. Traiger GJ, Plaa GL. Relationship of alcohol metabolism to the potentiation of CCl4 hepatotoxicity induced by aliphatic alcohols. *J Pharmacol Exp Ther* 1972;183:481–488.
52. Hewitt WR, Miyajima H, Côté MG, Plaa GL. Acute alterations of chloroform-induced hepato- and nephrotoxicity by n-hexane, methyl n-butyl ketone, and 2,5-hexanedione. *Toxicol Appl Pharmacol* 1980;48:509–527.
53. Traiger GJ, Plaa GL. Differences in the potentiation of carbon tetrachloride in rats by ethanol and isopropanol pretreatments. *Toxicol Appl Pharmacol* 1971;20:105–112.
54. Traiger GJ, Plaa GL. Chlorinated hydrocarbon toxicity: potentiation by isopropyl alcohol and acetone. *Arch Environ Health* 1974;28:276–278.
55. Hewitt WR, Miyajima H, Côté MG. Hewitt LA, Cianflone DJ, Plaa GL. Dose-response relationships in 1,3-butanediol-induced potentiation of carbon tetrachloride toxicity. *Toxicol Appl Pharmacol* 1982;64:529–540.
56. Pilon D, Brodeur J, Plaa GL. 1,3-Butanediol-induced increases in ketone bodies and potentiation of CCl4 hepatotoxicity. *Toxicology* 1986;40:165–180.
57. de Lamirande E, Plaa GL. 1,3-Butanediol pretreatment on the cholestasis induced in rats by Mn-BR combinations, taurolithocholic acid, or α-naphthylisothiocyanate. *Toxicol Appl Pharmacol* 1981;59:467–475.
58. Plaa GL, Ayotte P. Taurolithocholate-induced intrahepatic cholestasis: potentiation by methyl isobutyl ketone and methyl n-butyl ketone in rats. *Toxicol Appl Pharmacol* 1985;80:228–234.
59. Mehlman MA, Tobin RB, Mackerer CR. 1,3-Butanediol catabolism in the rat. *Federation Proc* 1975;34:2182–2185.
60. Vézina M, Plaa GL. Potentiation by methyl isobutyl ketone of the cholestasis induced in rats by a Mn-BR combination or manganese alone. *Toxicol Appl Pharmacol* 1987;91:477–483.
61. Vézina M, Plaa GL. Methyl isobutyl ketone metabolites and potentiation of the cholestasis induced in rats by a Mn-BR combination or manganese alone. *Toxicol Appl Pharmacol* 1988;92:419–427.
62. Dahlström-King L, Plaa GL. Cycloheximide in methyl isobutyl ketone potentiation of taurolithocholic-acid-induced cholestasis. *The Toxicologist* 1987;7:58.
63. Duguay AB, Plaa GL. Plasma concentrations in methyl isobutyl ketone-potentiated experimental cholestasis after inhalation or oral administration. *Fundam Appl Toxicol* 1993;21:222–227.
64. Duguay AB, Plaa GL. Tissue concentrations of methyl isobutyl ketone, methyl n-butyl ketone and their metabolites after oral or inhalation exposure. *Toxicol Lett* 1995;75:51–58.

65. Duguay AB, Plaa GL. Ketone potentiation of intrahepatic cholestasis: effect of two aliphatic isomers. *J Toxicol Appl Environ Health* 1997;50:41–52.
66. Vézina M, Kobusch AB, du Souich P, Greselin E, Plaa GL. Potentiation of chloroform-induced hepatotoxicity by methyl isobutyl ketone and two metabolites. *Can J Physiol Pharmacol* 1990;68:1055–1061.
67. Kobusch AB, Bailey B, du Souich P. Enzyme induction by environmental agents: effect on drug kinetics. In: Plaa GL, du Souich P, Erill S, eds. *Interactions between drugs and chemicals in industrial societies*. Esteve Foundation Symposia, vol. 2, Amsterdam: Excerpta Medica, 1987:29–42.
68. Raymond P, Plaa GL. Ketone potentiation of haloalkane-induced hepato- and nephrotoxicity. I. Dose-response relationships. *J Toxicol Environ Health* 1995;45:465–480.
69. Raymond P, Plaa GL. Ketone potentiation of haloalkane-induced hepato- and nephrotoxicity. II. Implication of monooxygenases. *J Toxicol Environ Health* 1995;46:317–328.
70. Tichy M, Cikrt M. Manganese transfer into the bile in rats. *Arch Toxikol* 1972;29:51–58.
71. Tichy M, Cikrt M, Havrdova J. Manganese binding in rat bile. *Arch Toxikol* 1973;30:227–236.
72. Plaa GL, Hewitt WR. Biotransformation products and cholestasis. In: Popper H, Schaffner F, eds. *Progress in liver diseases*, vol. 7. New York: Grune & Stratton, 1982:179–194.
73. Dahlström-King L, Couture J, Plaa GL. Influence of agents affecting monooxygenase activity on taurolithocholic acid-induced cholestasis. *Toxicol Appl Pharmacol* 1992;63:243–252.
74. Duguay A, Plaa GL. Altered cholesterol synthesis as a mechanism involved in methyl isobutyl ketone-potentiated experimental cholestasis. *Toxicol Appl Pharmacol* (in press).
75. Van Meer G. Lipid traffic in animal cells. *Ann Rev Cell Biol* 1989;5:247–275.
76. Voelker DR. Lipid transport pathways in mammalian cells. *Experientia* 1990;46:569–579.
77. Reinhart MP. Intracellular sterol trafficking. *Experientia* 1990;46:599–610.
78. McIntyre JC, Sleight RG. Mechanisms of intracellular membrane lipid transport. *Curr Topics Memb* 1994;40:453–481.
79. Couri D, Hetland LB, Abdel-Rahman MS, Weiss H. The influence of inhaled ketone solvent vapors on hepatic microsomal biotransformation activities. *Toxicol Appl Pharmacol* 1977;41:285–289.
80. Kobusch A, Plaa GL, du Souich P. Effects of acetone and methyl n-butyl ketone on hepatic mixed-function oxidase. *Biochem Pharmacol* 1989;38:3461–3467.
81. Imaoka S, Funae Y. Induction of cytochrome P450 isoenzymes in rat liver by methyl n-alkyl ketones and n-alkylbenzenes: effects of hydrophobicity of inducers on inducibility of cytochrome P450. *Biochem Pharmacol* 1991;42:S143–S150.

Toxicology of the Liver, 2nd ed.,
Edited by Gabriel L. Plaa and William R. Hewitt
Copyright © 1998 Taylor & Francis

13

Evaluation of Chemical-Induced Bile Duct Proliferation

Claude Barriault

Université de Montréal, Montréal, Québec, Canada H3C 3J7

Alexis Desmoulière

CNRS-UPR 412, Institut de Biologie et Chimie des Protéines, Lyon, France

Andréa Monte Alto Costa

*CNRS-UPR 412, Institut de Biologie et Chimie des Protéines, Lyon, France
and Universidade do Estado do Rio de Janeiro, Rio de Janeiro, Brazil*

Ibrahim M. Yousef, and Beatriz Tuchweber

Université de Montréal, Montréal, Québec, Canada H3C 3J7

The liver is the largest visceral organ of the body. This organ has a double blood supply: the portal vein brings the venous blood from the intestine (which is rich in nutrients), and the hepatic artery contains blood rich in oxygen (1). This highly vascular organ performs several vital processes such as protein synthesis, detoxification of xenobiotics, phagocytosis of particulate material circulating in blood (Kupffer cells), and production and secretion of bile (hepatocytes and bile duct cells) (2).

These different functions are performed by the diverse cells that compose the organ. Hepatocytes form about 65% of liver cells but are responsible for 80% of the mass since they are larger than the other cells. Nonparenchymal cells (Kupffer, Ito, endothelial, and bile duct cells) form the rest of the organ (3).

Intrahepatic epithelial cells of the biliary tree represent 3–5% of the total hepatic cell population (4, 5) and about 0.14–0.43% of the organ volume (6). However, a common response of the liver to injury is bile duct proliferation, which may enhance the percentage of these cells in liver (7). Bile duct proliferation may be induced by toxic chemicals (8–10) or pathogens (11, 12) and can occur in conditions resulting from obstruction of the biliary tract both in animals and in humans (13–15).

This review will focus on chemical-induced bile duct proliferation in the liver and will discuss recent data on the possible origin of proliferated ducts.

BILIARY TREE

Bile Duct Anatomy and Function

Ductular cells and hepatocytes constitute the epithelial cell population of the liver. The ductular cells line the intrahepatic and extrahepatic ducts and are in direct contact with bile from the Hering canal to the Oddi sphincter.

Bile is formed and secreted by hepatocytes into the bile canaliculi; it flows into the cholangioles (or canals of Hering), which are short and fine epithelial channels. The cholangioles connect to bile ductules at the border of the portal tract and enter a branch of the intrahepatic bile duct. Cholangioles are formed by hepatocytes from the limiting plate and by low cuboidal biliary epithelial cells. Bile ductules are lined with simple and low cuboidal epithelial cells and are organized in the form of a rich anastomosing biliary plexus. The bile ductules join the bile ducts in the portal tracts, and, within each lobe of the liver, smaller bile ducts progressively merge to form hepatic ducts. In the rat, hepatic ducts unite to form the common bile duct. Bile ducts are essential for transporting bile to the duodenum and are also involved in bile formation (16, 17).

The ductular cells are a heterogenous cell population (18); within the biliary tree, the size of the cells varies between 6 and 15 μm, and they may be cylindrical or columnar in form. As has been described for hepatocytes (19), there may also be functional heterogeneity for the ductular cells, depending on their localization (18). Morphologically, they exibit numerous microvillosities on the apical aspect of the plasma membrane facing the canalicular lumen. Also, there is a basement membrane, and in the apical and basal poles of the cell there are clathrin-coated vesicles suggesting that receptor-mediated endocytosis occurs at both cellular poles (20). Junctional complexes are noted between ductular cells that maintain cell contact and limit the passage of molecules (e.g., proteins) derived from extracellular pathways (2).

By electron microscopy, ductular cells exibit a well-developed organelle system, with a significant number of small mitochondria and a Golgi apparatus in the apical pole of the cell in association with secretory vesicles, lysosomes, and multivesicular bodies (21).

As compared with hepatocytes, ductular cells exibit less mitochondria and endoplasmic reticulum membranes. On the other hand, the cytoplasmic microfilamentous network is well developed, and, as indicated before, cells exibit a basement membrane (18).

A peribiliary vascular plexus derived from the hepatic artery vascularizes the ductular cells. It has been proposed that substances secreted by the ductular cells into this vascular plexus could directly or indirectly reach the hepatocytes (16).

Knowledge of ductular cell function has significantly increased in recent years. For a long time, the only role attributed to these cells was a passive one, mainly that of bile transport from the site of formation in the hepatocyte to the duodenum, the site of action. However, it was evident that the role of ductular cells in bile transport was complex, by having an impact not only on the quantity but also on the quality of the bile they transported (5, 17). Today it is well established that ductular cells participate in bile formation, which is the result of the combined action of both hepatocytes and ductular cells (5, 21). The contribution of ductular cells to bile formation may range from 10% to 40%, depending on the animal species (5, 16, 22).

Ductular epithelial cells secrete significant amounts of water, sodium, chloride protein, and bicarbonate and can reabsorb these components as well as glucose, glutamate, and anions, thus modifying the bile composition and the secretory process (17). Recent data indicate that ductular cells could participate in lipid metabolism, as they synthesize cholesterol and appear to conjugate bile acid (23). This obviously raises a question as to whether they could also synthesize bile acids and metabolize liproproteins.

BILE DUCT PROLIFERATION

Generalities

Under normal circumstances, the adult liver presents little turnover, but, in response to injury, the principal epithelial cell population, the hepatocytes, may proliferate

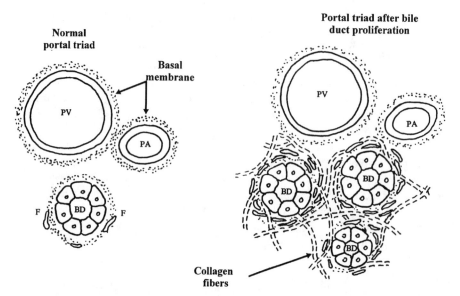

FIG. 1. Typical bile duct proliferation. The proliferation of bile duct epithelial cells leads to a significant increase in bile ductular structures associated with periportal fibrosis, which is likely related to proliferation and activation of periductular fibroblasts (F). BD, bile duct; PV, portal vein; PA, portal artery.

rapidly. Also, in several experimental and human conditions of hepatic tissue injury, a common feature observed is ductular epithelial cell proliferation, also known as ductular reaction (24) (Fig. 1). This cellular response consists mainly of proliferation of fine ductules, and some authors have drawn an analogy between this response and the proliferation of vascular capillaries observed during repair after tissue injury (8). It is important to point out that the ductular epithelial cells do not proliferate in random fashion but rather in organized ductule structures (7, 13).

When animals are exposed to chemical agents that induce hepatocellular necrosis, such as carbon tetrachloride or galactosamine, there is proliferation of hepatocytes and of nonparenchymal cells in the restitution phase (10). Other chemicals such as alpha-naphthylisothiocyanate (ANIT) and 4,4'-diaminodiphenylmethane (DDPM) can cause selective damage to bile duct cells and induce bile duct proliferation with little or no evidence of hepatocytic change (25, 26). After chemical-induced hepatic injury, the hepatic (hepatocytic or ductular) necrosis and the ductular reaction are accompanied by an inflammatory cell infiltrate and a portal fibrotic reaction. A recent study underlined the role of periductular fibroblasts in the portal fibrogenic process and the possibility that the very early ductular proliferative response may be related to the proliferation and activation of fibrogenic cells (15).

The response to injury may vary according to the origin of the new ductular structures. For mild to moderate liver injury, restitution is accomplished by the proliferation of mature liver cells that have retained the capacity to divide (27). This is a compartment that has been refered to as the amplification compartment (24). However, after

massive damage with substantial or complete loss of mature liver cells, liver regenerative mechanisms may involve a progenitor or stem cell compartment (28, 29).

Origin of Proliferating Bile Duct Cells

It has been well accepted that during ontogenesis, the intrahepatic bile ducts develop
from fetal hepatocytes or hepatoblasts. Early fetal hepatocytes are progenitors for
both adult hepatocytes and bile duct epithelial cells, suggesting that they are at least
bipotential precursors (30). Whether either or both of the cell lineages derived from
the hepatoblast retain the bipotential capacity of the precursor cells remains to be
elucidated. However, the gradual transformation of hepatocytes into bile duct–like
cells as seen in some liver diseases (e.g., chronic cholestasis) may reflect at least a
bipotential capacity of the hepatocyte (31).

   Despite much interest, there is controversy concerning the histogenesis of proliferated ductules found in various experimental and human liver diseases. In general the
proliferative response to injury may be divided into two categories (Fig. 2). In the first

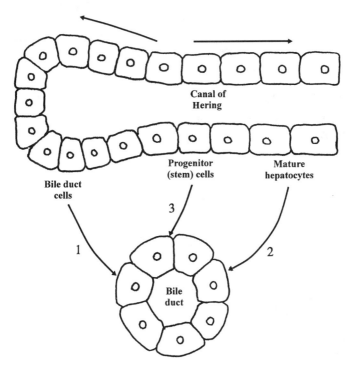

FIG. 2. Origin of bile duct cells. Proliferating ductular epithelial cells may arise from preexisting
duct cells (1), from hepatocytes gradually transforming to "ductular hepatocytes" (2), or from
progenitor (stem cells) (3) that also give rise to transitional cells capable of differentiating into
bile duct epithelial cells.

one, bile duct epithelial cells may arise by proliferation of the preexisting bile duct epithelium (typical proliferation) such as in bile duct ligature (13, 16) or ANIT-induced bile duct proliferation (16). Here, there may be tortuous changes and elongations of native bile duct and ductules. A second possibility implicates the transformation of progenitor cells where different cells types may appear (atypical proliferation). This includes the transformation of hepatocytes or a subpopulation of bipotential hepatocytes into bile duct cell type (28, 32–34). Present data suggest that the terminal ductular cells connecting the canals of Hering with the bile canaliculi or a distinct population of periductular cells consitute the progenitor or stem cell compartment (35). Among these cells are the so-called oval cells, which are small periportal cells with scant cytoplasm and ovoid nuclei. These oval cells fulfill the characteristics of bipotential stem cells giving rise to either hepatocytes or bile duct cells. From many studies of liver carcinogenesis, it was proposed that in some instances the oval cells may be a precursor for hepatic tumors (36).

Markers of Bile Duct Cells

The development of different markers to assess differentiation and to trace lineages of different hepatic cell populations has been a subject of intense research (29, 30). Hepatocytes express mainly cytokeratins (CK) 8 and CK 18, as well as albumin. Bile duct cell markers are CK 7, CK 8, CK 18, CK 19, and gamma-glutamyltransferase (GGT). The progenitor or stem cells express some of both hepatocyte and bile duct cell markers together with alpha-fetoprotein (AFP). The OV-6 mouse monoclonal antibody recognizing the common epitope of CK 19 and CK 14 is currently used to characterize normal hepatic bile duct and ductular cells as well as proliferating oval cells (37). In rats, an epitope (BPC$_5$) is expressed by progenitor cells, which correspond to epithelial cells present in the embryonic liver between days 10.5 and 16 (30).

Neveu et al. (38) showed that steady-state levels of connexin (Cx) 32, 26, and 43 mRNA transcripts each display unique patterns of temporal expression after a 70% partial hepatectomy: proliferating oval cells express diffuse Cx 43 immunoreactivity, but their differentiation into basophilic hepatocytes results in their expression of Cx 32 and Cx 26.

Recently, hepatic transcription factors (HNF 1 beta, HNF 3 gamma, and HNF4) have been used to characterize the early response of stemlike cells after chemical injury with 2-acetylaminofluorene (2-AAF) and after bile duct ligation; both are inducers of bile duct proliferation (39). It was noted that 2-AAF induced expression of HNF1 beta, HNF 3 gamma, AFP, and albumin in ductular cells within 24 hr after its administration. On the other hand, bile duct ligation had no effect on expression of these genes in ductal cells. This suggests that the oval cells compartment is implicated in the response after 2-AAF, while bile duct ligation could induce a mitogenic response in preexisting differentiated ductular cells. However, this needs to be corroborated.

The expression of glycoconjugates has been examined during intrahepatic bile duct development in rats using histochemical studies of lectin (40). During maturation, a change in staining was noted, with increases in the number and intensity of lectins binding to the biliary epithelium. Such a marker could be of use in studying the origin of the cells involved in the proliferative response in biliary disorders.

Specific cell surface components have been characterized and include HES_6 present in hepatocytes and BDS_7 on the surface of biliary epithelial cells (30, 41). In tumor cells such as in choliangiocarcinomal cells, it was shown that they exibit biliary epithelial cell phenotypes, while hepatocarcinoma cells generally lack HES_6, but can express BDS_7 (30). This may imply that hepatocarcinoma cells could derive from hepatic cells that are somehow blocked at an intermediate stage, defined by Marceau et al. (30) as the "differentiation window." At this stage, cells are allowed to express typical biliary epithelial cell features. The question remains, however, as to the origin of these cells, which may be from retrodifferentiating hepatocytes or differentiating (progenitor or stem) cells.

CHEMICAL-INDUCED PROLIFERATION OF DUCTULAR EPITHELIAL CELLS

Numerous agents have been reported to induce bile duct proliferation. However, depending on the agents used and the duration of injury, it seems that different cell lineages may be involved in the proliferative response. The aim of this chapter is to review the chemical agents that can cause extensive ductular epithelial cell proliferation. The model of damage induced by bile duct ligation in the rat, however, will be briefly described for comparative purposes, mainly to discuss the possible involvement of biliary obstruction in the development of the ductular reaction induced by some chemical agents.

The ductular proliferation seen with chemical agents appears to be quite different with agents that induce or do not induce hepatocarcinogenesis. In this review we will focus on the ductular proliferation induced by nonhepatocarcinogens and briefly discuss the complex and yet poorly understood response during carcinogenesis. The reader will find recent reviews on ductular epithelial cell proliferation during liver cancer development (42).

Alpha-Naphthylisothiocyanate (ANIT)

For many years, ANIT has been known to induce bile ductule epithelial cell proliferation (43, 44). By means of the [^{3}H]thymidine incorporation technique and immunohistochemical staining for various ductular cell markers it was shown that the progeny of proliferating cells were preexisting biliary epithelial cells that retained their characteristics (16). ANIT-induced ductular cells do not express AFP (a marker of stem cells) or albumin (a marker of stem cells as well as of hepatocytes). Furthermore, the proliferated structures can secrete water and electrolytes, indicating that the new cells are also functional (16). It is important to note the ANIT does not induce proliferation of oval cells and apparently does not lead to hepatocellular carcinoma.

Recently, Kossor et al. (26), using several doses of ANIT and various time periods of observation, reported a parallel between bile duct cell proliferation and obstruction of the bile ductules by cellular debris. Indeed, they showed that ductular epithelial cell proliferation occurred at doses/time points associated with cell damage and bile obstruction. Furthermore, the kinetics of ductular epithelial cell proliferation were comparable to that following bile duct ligation, suggesting that ANIT-induced epithelial cell proliferation may be the consequence of intrahepatic bile duct obstruction.

Bile Acids

Proliferation of bile ductules is a frequent finding described long ago in human hepatic disease, including obstructive jaundice. Thus, it is not surprising that many early studies examined biliary bile acids as agents that can induce ductular proliferation (45, 46). Of the normally occuring bile acids, lithocholic acid is the most hepatotoxic, inducing after acute parenteral treatment severe impairment of bile flow, or cholestasis (47). Its oral administration in high doses produces ductular epithelial cell proliferation in many animal species including rodents, reptiles, and primates (45, 46, 48–50). The ductular cell reaction is associated with an accumulation of inflammatory cells, but little or no hepatocytic necrosis. Prolonged lithocholate feeding can result in fibrosis and, eventually, cirrhosis, depending on the animal species (51). The mechanism of the ductular response after lithocholic acid is not known. A direct toxic effect of the bile acid on the ductular epithelium was suggested, as there was histologic evidence of damaged ductular cells (45). In cell cultures of bile ducts, lithocholate also exerted a toxic effect on ductular cells, but it did not influence their proliferative rate (52).

The potential hepatotoxic effects of long-term oral administration of chenodeoxycholic acid and ursodeoxycholic acid have attracted much attention in view of their use in humans in cholelithiasis and other hepatic diseases. Chronic studies in various animal species clearly showed that high doses of chenodeoxycholic acid and ursodeoxycholic acid can induce proliferation of bile ducts and inflammatory cell infiltration in portal areas, as well as fibrosis (51, 53–55). A moderate degree of focal hepatonecrosis was also observed. However, ursodeoxycholic acid produced less severe injury than the other bile acids (51). The mechanism of the liver toxicity is not known. Since these bile acids are converted to lithocholate by intestinal bacteria, it was assumed that liver changes may be attributed primarily to this monohydroxy bile acid (51, 53, 54). The hepatic damage may be limited in humans, as they can efficiently sulfate lithocholic acid and excrete it (54). But the type of conjugate of the sulfated bile acid is a critical factor, as glycine-conjugated forms remain toxic. Although high doses of ursodeoycholic acid may induce moderate bile duct epithelial proliferation (53), low doses reduce the bile ductular proliferation after bile duct ligation (56, 57). Enrichment of the biliary bile acid pool with the more hydrophylic bile acid could reduce the level of lithocholate and chenodeoxycholate.

Carbon Tetrachloride

It is well known that carbon tetrachloride is a hepatotoxicant that induces necrosis of centrolobular hepatocytes but virtually no bile ductular cell hyperplasia (58). However, when rats were subjected to bile duct ligation 4–6 weeks before administration of a single necrogenic dose of the toxicant, unusual "ductular hepatocytes" were observed in bile ductular hyperplasia areas, as was centrolobular necrosis typical of severe carbon tetrachloride hepatotoxicity. The size of these ductular structures was similar to those of surrounding proliferating ductules, and the structures were composed of biliary epithelial cells in association with one or more small "ductular hepatocytes" at different stages of maturation. It is of interest that hepatic cell cholangioles morphologically similar to those seen in the carbon tetrachloride/bile duct ligation model were described in the human liver after severe necrosis. These "ductular hepatocytes" did not express AFP or CK 19 but showed a marked positive reaction for H4, an antigen that seems to be exclusively expressed in hepatocytes of the normal as well as the bile duct–ligated rat. These observations led Sirica and Williams (58) to suggest that the "ductular hepatocyte" may originate from some cell within the hyperplastic bile ductules. The authors also proposed that the presence of "ductular hepatocytes" was the liver's means of adapting to massive liver injury by producing hepatocytes via biliary epithelium cell differentiation.

4,4′-Diaminodiphenylmethane (DDPM)

Fukushima et al. (59) were first to show that DDPM led to hyperplasia of bile ducts with little hepatocytic damage. Also, they observed a proliferation of oval cells but did not find hepatomas or cholangiocarcinomas.

Another study reported that DDPM did not induce oval cells or serum elevations of AFP, which has been correlated with early oval cell increase during liver carcinogenesis (25). The new ducts induced by DDPM did not express AFP and albumin and were surrounded by a layer of laminin, like normal duct structures.

Furan

The chemical agent furan, when given to animals in high doses, induces severe hepatonecrosis that is followed by a proliferative bile ductular response (60). Interestingly, as with the combined carbon tetrachloride–bile duct ligation treatment, "ductular hepatocytes" were also described, but in specific lobes of the liver (caudate and right lobes). If administration of furan (in low doses) is preceded by bile duct ligation there is an almost complete replacement of hepatocytes by well-differentiated bile ductular structures (61). The extent of bile duct proliferation was greater than that reported for bile duct ligation alone or treatment with chemical agents such as ANIT and DDPM. The mechanism underlying this response is unclear.

Galactosamine

Galactosamine, administered at a high dose (once or twice), is a hepatotoxicant that induces hepatitis associated with necrosis randomly distributed throughout the hepatic lobule. Twenty-four to 48 hr after treatment, proliferation of bile ducts has been observed in and around the portal tract areas (10, 63). These authors have also shown the occurrence of oval cells, and that the parenchyma contains a high proportion of small hepatocytes. It was proposed that these small hepatocytes originated from duct cells rather than from the replication of normal hepatocytes, as evidenced by labeling experiments. The oval cells expressed significant amounts of AFP mRNA and protein that were undetected in the normal hepatocyte population. The small hepatocytes were positive for AFP mRNA, which led to the suggestion that this cell subpopulation probably corresponds to transitional cells, with an intermediate state of differentiation between oval cells and hepatocytes.

Bile ductule proliferation may also occur following repetitive injections of galactosamine (9). Indeed, after 20–40 administrations of galactosamine (at a dose of 500 mg/kg, three times a week), expansion of portal tracts with prominent bile ductule proliferation was observed, like that observed after bile duct ligation in the rat. When galactosamine injections are continued (40–140 injections), formation of fibrous septa and, ultimately, cirrhosis develop.

Alcoholic and Some Other Liver Diseases

It has been reported that under these conditions, bile duct proliferation may occur (31, 32, 62). Biopsies of human liver in alcoholic liver diseases indicated that proliferated ductular cells were derived by transformation from hepatocellular cords (32). In this study, intermediate forms of hepatocytes were identified by light and electron microscopy as well as by markers of hepatocytes (glucose-6-phosphatase, glycogen).

By immunohistochemical technique, Van Eyken et al. (31, 62) have shown that in several human hepatic diseases such as primary biliary cirrhosis, primary sclerosing cholangitis, extrahepatic biliary obstruction, and alcoholic liver disease, some hepatocytes were weakly positive to CK 7 and 19, which are, in the normal liver, specific to biliary ductular cells. These results support the concept of "ductular metaplasia of hepatocytes." The same conclusion was reached in a study of hepatic nodular hyperplasia (64).

Recently, a high rate of proliferation of "ductular hepatocytes" was observed after submassive necrosis in humans (65). Although some of these cells expressed markers of hepatocytes or mature bile duct epithelium, most were a distinct population as evidenced by immunohistochemistry of various biomarkers. It was suggested that the "ductular hepatocyte" may represent a transient amplifying cell population derived from a progenitor cell in or in proximity to the canals of Hering. Interestingly, damaged hepatocytes expressed CK 19 and AE1, usually found in intermediate filaments of biliary ductular cells.

BILE DUCTULAR PROLIFERATION INDUCED
BY HEPATOCARCINOGENS

As discussed earlier, during the early stages of hepatocarcinogenesis induced by chemical agents, there is proliferation of ductular epithelial cells, which can persist when the carcinogenic stimulus is continued until the cancer occurs. Therefore, the relevance of the ductular reaction to hepatocarcinogenesis have been the subject of study for many years, and two main theories have been proposed to explain the carcinogenesis process. One theory is that the liver cancer appears from altered hepatocytes that undergo redifferentiation or retrodifferentiation and proliferate to form foci, hyperplastic nodules, and ultimately primary hepatocellular carcinoma (8). The other theory maintains that liver stem cells or oval cells are the progenitors, giving rise to primary hepatocellular carcinomas (66). The role of proliferating ductules is not clear, as there is no direct evidence that ductular cells can transform to intermediate hepatocytes, nodules, and cancer cells.

Proliferating ductular epithelial cells during liver cancer development have been described after exposure to numerous chemicals (42) including o-aminoazotoluene, azo dyes, 4-dimethylaminoazobenzene, 2-AAF, m-toluenediamine, dibenzcarbazole, tannic acid, ethionine, thioacetamide, aramite, aflatoxins, pyrrozilidine alkaloids and extracts of natural products.

NON-CHEMICAL-INDUCED BILE DUCT PROLIFERATION

Bile duct cell proliferation induced by ligature of the common bile duct has been studied by many investigators, and it is evident that proliferating bile ductular epithelial cells are the products of the existing biliary epithelium and retain its characteristics (13, 16). There is no evidence of participation of stem cells or ductular metaplasia of hepatocytes in this model of ductular proliferation.

FACTORS INVOLVED IN BILE DUCT EPITHELIAL
CELL PROLIFERATION

As discussed above, several conditions or agents may lead to proliferation of bile duct epithelial cells. Despite many studies, there is little knowledge of the factors that are involved in the proliferation of these cells.

Extensive studies have been carried out with hepatic regeneration models about mitogenic factors expressed in different liver cell subpopulations in relation to cell proliferation and differentiation. In the partial hepatectomy (PH) model, transforming growth factor-alpha (TGF-α), hepatocyte growth factor (HGF), epidermal growth factor (EGF), and acidic fibroblast growth factor (a-FGF) are expressed (67). In the 2-AAF/PH model, these factors are also expressed at high levels throughout the period of expansion and differentiation of the progenitor (oval) cells (68). The factors return to levels seen in normal livers at the end of the regeneration process (29).

TGF-α and a-FGF transcripts are found in both hepatic stellate cells and progenitor cells. HGF is produced by hepatic stellate cells, Kupffer cells, and endothelial cells, and it is the most potent liver mitogen. EGF is produced in extrahepatic tissues and may act in an endocrine fashion.

We can assume that these factors are implicated in bile duct proliferation observed after chemical injury, leading to the activation of progenitor or stem cells. In vitro, Joplin et al. (69) showed that human ductular epithelial cells proliferate in response to HGF. Thus, it may be that in conditions where this factor is enhanced, proliferation of ductular cells is increased.

Recently, Nagy et al. (70) examined the effects of infusion of EGF, HGF, and urokinase-type plasminogen activator (uPA) on the proliferation of ductal and periductal cells after their activation with 2-AAF. Interestingly, northern blot analysis had previously shown an association of uPA expression with oval cell proliferation. Infusion of EGF, HGF, uPA, or any combination for up to 7 days after previous treatment with 2-AAF resulted in increased numbers of [^{3}H]thymidine-labeled ductal and periductal cells expanding into the liver acinus. The administration of 2-AAF alone or in combination with infusion of HGF resulted in the proliferation of an almost equal number of ductal and hepatic stellate cells, while administration of 2-AAF with EGF or EGF and HGF resulted in 75–80% of the proliferating cells having a ductal phenotype. Futhermore, Nagy et al. (70) suggest that uPA enhances the proliferation of ductal cells by catalyzing the cleavage of monomeric pro-HGF to active dimeric HGF, and promotes the infiltration of ductal cells into the liver acinus by proteolytic degradation of matrix proteins.

In many situations after chemical injury, it has been shown that an equilibrium may exist between the number of cells entering mitosis and the number dying by apoptosis (programmed cell death). Certain growth factors appear to be capable of enhancing the survival of chemically activated cells. The expression of the c-myc protooncogene, which is a potent inducer of apoptosis, is down-regulated in the presence of growth factors (71). As suggested by Nagy et al. (70), the c-myc protein in combination with growth factors appears to be an important regulator determining, after chemical injury, the different aspects of oval cell activation and differentiation.

After CCl$_4$ or galactosamine administration to rats, blood levels of HGF increase rapidly. However, after CCl$_4$ administration, the lesion develops around the central vein while galactosamine induces primarily ductular proliferation; presumably, HGF does not act preferentially on specific target cells but induces the expansion of any chemically injured liver cell population.

After injury induced by bile duct ligation, TGF-α mRNA levels are not altered, even after the release of the obstruction (72). In contrast, HGF mRNA levels are elevated following ligation and show increased expression 1 day after decompression, peaking at 2 days of repair (72). These observations suggest that, in this model, HGF allows the proliferation of hepatocytes after decompression, in order to counterbalance the disappearance of ductular structures. Indeed, it has been shown that, after bile duct ligation, an important loss of hepatocellular mass per gram of liver occurs, induced by the portal area expansion (73).

After bile duct ligation, bile duct cell replication is significantly increased 24 hr after injury and diminishes to baseline by 1 week. Increased biliary pressure has been identified as an initiating factor in bile duct epithelial cell proliferation, but how this effect is mediated is not well known. Immunohistochemistry revealed low levels of TGF-β1 in the normal bile duct epithelium. In contrast, at 1 and 4 weeks after ligation, TGF-β1 is strongly expressed by the bile duct epithelium, suggesting that TGF-β1, together with its well known effect on extracellular matrix deposition, may play a role in the termination of the bile duct epithelial cell proliferative response (74). The expression of mannose 6-phosphate/insulin-like growth factor-II receptor, which facilitates the proteolytic activation of TGF-β1, is up-regulated in bile duct cells that are presumably involved in the activation of TGF-β1 (74). It is suggested that the role of TGF-β1 on the arrest of liver cell regeneration and atypical bile duct proliferation is linked to the pro-apoptotic action of TGF-β1 (75).

CONCLUSIONS AND PERSPECTIVES

Induction of bile duct cell proliferation in the liver may involve activation of both the normally quiescent hepatocytes and bile duct cells ("typical" proliferation of residual differentiated cells) or the multipotential ("atypical" proliferation) stem cell system.

The relationship between the involvement of different proliferating hepatic cells and the development of tumors remains to be clearly elucidated (hepatocarcinogenic versus non-hepatocarcinogenic chemical agents).

There is ample evidence to indicate that a stem cell system participates in the restitutive proliferative response after liver injury, if the response of more differentiated hepatic cells (hepatocytes and bile duct cells) is not sufficient to restore liver function.

It has been suggested that the ductular reaction could be a "pacemaker" in the development of progressive fibrosis leading to cirrhosis in diseases such as primary biliary cirrhosis and primary sclerosing cholangitis. We should point out that the ductular cells express TGF-β (76), one of whose functions is to stimulate periportal fibroblasts to produce extracellular matrix components. However, it has been shown that, in an ectopic graft of embryonic mouse liver (77) and in the mouse embryo (78), stem cells, for their differentiation in bile duct cells, should be in contact with connective tissue cells. We may suggest that portal fibrosis, which develops together with the bile ductular reaction, could stimulate the differentiation of stem cells or hepatocytes to bile duct cells. It remains to be determined whether under pathologic conditions, this sequence of events occurs, leading to the expansion of bile duct structures.

REFERENCES

1. McCoskey RS. Functional morphology of the liver with emphasis on microvasculature. In: Tavoloni N, Berk PD, eds. *Hepatic transport and bile secretion: physiology and pathophysiology.* New York: Raven Press, 1993:1–10.
2. Guyton AC, Hall JE. Secretory function of the alimentary tract. *Texbook of medical physiology.* Philadelphia: Saunders, 1996.

3. Ramadori G, Rieder H, Knittel T. Biology and pathobiology of sinusoidal liver cells. In: Tavoloni N, Berk PD, eds. *Hepatic transport and bile secretion: physiology and pathophysiology*. New York: Raven Press, 1993:83–102.
4. Grant AG, Billing BH. The isolation and characterization of bile ductule cell population from normal and bile-duct ligated rat livers. *Br J Exp Pathol* 1977;58:301–310.
5. Boyer JL. Bile duct epithelium: frontiers in transport physiology. *Am J Physiol* 1996;270:G1–G5.
6. Gall JA, Bhathal PS. A quantitative analysis of the liver folowing ligation of the common bile duct. *Liver* 1990;10:116–125.
7. Tavoloni N. The intrahepatic biliary epithelium: an area of growing interest in hepatology. *Semin Liver Dis* 1987;7:280–292.
8. Farber E. On the origin of liver cell cancer. In: Sirica AE, ed. *The role of cell types in hepatocarcinogenesis*. Boca Raton, FL: CRC Press, 1992:1–28.
9. Jonker AM, Dijkhuis FWJ, Hardonk MJ, Moerkerk P, Ten Kate J, Grond J. Immunohistochemical study of hepatic fibrosis induced in rats by multiple galactosamine injections. *Hepatology* 1994;19:775–781.
10. Tournier I, Legrès L, Schoevaert D, Feldmann G, Bernuau D. Cellular analysis of a-fetoprotein gene activation during carbon tetrachloride and D-galactosamine-induced acute liver injury in rats. *Lab Invest* 1988;59:657–665.
11. Masada CT, Shaw BW Jr, Zetterman RK, Kaufmann SS, Markin RS. Fulminant hepatic failure with massive necrosis as a results of hepatitis A infection. *J Clin Gastroenterol* 1993;17:158–162.
12. Lopez P, Tunon MJ, Gonzalez P, Diez N, Bravo AM, Gonzalez-Gallego J. Ductular proliferation and hepatic secretory function in experimental fascioliasis. *Exp Parasitol* 1993;77:36–42.
13. Slott PA, Liu MH, Tavoloni N. Origin, pattern and mechanism of bile duct proliferation following biliary obstruction in the rat. *Gastroenterology* 1990;99:466–477.
14. Morris JS, Gallo GA, Scheuer PJ, Path MRC, Sherlock S. Percutaneous liver biopsy in patients with large bile duct obstruction. *Gastroenterology* 1975;68:750–754.
15. Tuchweber B, Desmoulières A, Bochaton-Piallat ML, Rubbia-Brandt L, Gabbiani G. Proliferation and phenotypic modulation of portal fibroblasts in the early stages of cholestatic fibrosis in the rat. *Lab Invest* 1996;74:265–278.
16. Alpini G, Lenzi R, Zhai WR, Slott PA, Liu MH, Sarkozi L, Tavoloni N. Bile secretory function of intrahepatic biliary epithelium in the rat. *Am J Physiol* 1989;257:G124–G133.
17. Tarsetti F, Lenzen R, Salvi R, Schuler E, Dembitzer R, Tavoloni N. Biology and pathobiology of intrahepatic biliary epithelium. In: Tavoloni N, Berk PD, eds. *Hepatic transport and bile secretion: physiology and pathophysiology*. New York: Raven Press, 1993:619–635.
18. Desmet VJ. Organizational principles. In: Arias IM, Boyer JL, Fausto N, Jakoby WB, Schachter D, Shafritz DA, eds. *The liver: biology and pathobiology*. New York: Raven Press, 1994:3–14.
19. Gumucio JJ, Guibert EE. Zonal transport and functional compartmentation of the liver acinus. In: Tavoloni N, Berk PD, eds. *Hepatic transport and bile secretion: physiology and pathophysiology*. New York: Raven Press, 1993:71–82.
20. Ishii M, Vroman B, LaRusso NF. Isolation and morphologic characterization of bile duct epithelial cells from normal rat liver. *Gastroenterology* 1989;97:1236–1247.
21. Alpini G, Phillips JO, LaRusso NF. The biology of biliary epithelia. In: Arias IM, Boyer JL, Fausto N, Jakoby WB, Schachter D, Shafritz DA, eds. *The liver: biology and pathobiology*. New York: Raven Press, 1994:623–645.
22. Nathanson MH, Boyer JL. Mechanisms and regulation of bile secretion. *Hepatology* 1991;14:551–566.
23. Hylemon BP, Bohdan PM, Sirica AE, Heuman DM, Vlahcevic ZR. Cholesterol and bile acid metabolism in cultures of primary rat bile ductular epithelial cells. *Hepatology* 1989;11:982–988.
24. Burt AD, MacSween RNM. Bile duct proliferation: its true significance? *Histopathology* 1993;23:599–602.
25. Sell S. Comparison of oval cells induced in rat liver by feeding N-2-fluorenylacetamide in a choline-devoid diet and bile duct cells induced by feeding 4,4'-diaminodiphenylmethane. *Cancer Res* 1983;43:1761–1767.
26. Kossor DC, Golstein RS, Ngo W, DeNicola DB, Leonard TB, Dulick DM, Meunier PC. Biliary epithelial cell proliferation following α-naphtylisothiocyanate (ANIT) treatment: relationship to bile duct obstruction. *Fundam Appl Toxicol* 1995;26:51–62.
27. Bucher NLR, Strain AJ. Regulatory mechanisms in hepatic regeneration. In: Millward-Sadler M, Wright R, Arthur C, eds. *Wright's liver and biliary disease*. Philadelphia: WB Saunders, 1992:258–274.
28. Sirica AE, Elmore LW, Williams TW, Cole SL. Differentiation potential of hepatoplastic bile ductular

epithelial cells in rats models of hepatic injury and cholangiocarcinogenesis. In: Sirica AE, ed. *The role of cell types in hepatocarcinogenesis.* Boca Raton: CRC Press, 1992:183–208.

29. Thorgeirsson SS. Hepatic stem cells in liver regeneration. *FASEB J* 1996;10:1249–1256.

30. Marceau N, Blouin MJ, Noel M, Torok N, Loranger A. The role of bipotential progenitor cells in liver ontogenesis and neoplasia. In: Sirica AE, ed. *The role of cell types in hepatocarcinogenesis.* Boca Raton, FL: CRC Press, 1992:121–149.

31. Van Eyken P, Sciot R, Desmet VJ. A cytokeratin immunohistochemical study of cholestatic liver disease: evidence that hepatocytes can express 'bile duct-type' cytokeratins. *Histopathology* 1989;15:125–135.

32. Uchida T, Peters RL. The nature and origin of proliferated bile ductules in alcoholic liver disease. *Am J Clin Pathol* 1983;79:326–333.

33. Desmet JV. Intrahepatic bile ducts under the lens. *J Hepatol* 1985;1:545–549.

34. Sell S. Is there liver stem cell? *Cancer Res* 1990;50:3811–3815.

35. Thorgeirsson SS, Evarts RP. Growth and differentiation of stem cells in adult rat liver. In: Sirica AE, ed. *The role of cell types in hepatocarcinogenesis.* Boca Raton, FL: CRC Press, 1992:109–120.

36. Fausto N, Lemire JM, Shiojiri N. Ovals cells in liver carcinogenesis: cell lineage in hepatic development and identification of facultative stem cells in normal liver. In: Sirica AE, ed. *The role of cell types in hepatocarcinogenesis.* Boca Raton, FL: CRC Press, 1992:89–108.

37. Bisgaard HC, Parmelee DC, Dunsford HA, Sechi S, Thorgeirsson SS. Keratin 14 protein in cultures nonparenchymal rat hepatic epithelial cells: characterization of keratin 14 and keratin 19 as antigens for the commonly used mouse monoclonal antibody OV-6. *Mol Carcinog* 1993;7:60–66.

38. Neveu MJ, Hully JR, Babcock KL, Vaughan J, Hertzberg EL, Nicholson BJ, Paul DL, Pitot HC. Proliferation-associated differences in the spatial and temporal expression of gap junction genes in rat liver. *Hepatology* 1995;22:202–212.

39. Bisgaard HC, Nagy P, Santoni-Rugiu E, Thorgiersson SS. Proliferation, apoptosis, and induction of hepatic transcription factors are characteristics of the early response of biliary epithelial (oval) cells to chemical carcinogens. *Hepatology* 1996;23:62–70.

40. Sanzen T, Yoshida K, Sasaki M, Terada T, Nakanuma Y. Expression of glycoconjugates during intrahepatic bile duct development in the rat: an immunohistochemical and lectin-histochemical study. *Hepatology* 1995;22:944–951.

41. Blouin MJ, Lamy I, Loranger A, Noel M, Corlu A, Guguen-Guillouzo C, Marceau N. Specialization switch in differentiating embryonic rat liver progenitor cells in response to sodium butyrate. *Exp Cell Res* 1995;217:22–30.

42. Sirica AE, ed. *The role of cell types in hepatocarcinogenesis.* Boca Raton, FL: CRC Press, 1992.

43. Goldfarb S, Singer Ej, Popper H. Experimental cholangitis due to alpha-naphthyl-isothiocyanate (ANIT). *Am J Pathol* 1962;40:685–698.

44. Lopez M, Mazzanti L. Experimental investigations on alpha-naphthyl-isothiocyanate as a hyperplasic agent of the biliary ducts in the rat. *J Pathol Bacteriol* 1955;69:243–250.

45. Palmer RH, Hruban Z. Production of bile duct hyperplasia and gallstone by lithocholic acid. *J Clin Invest* 1966;45:1255–1266.

46. Hunt RD, Leveille GA, Sauberlich HE. Dietary bile acids and lipid metabolism. II. The ductular cell reaction induced by lithocholic acid. *Proc Soc Exp Biol Med* 1963;113:139–142.

47. Vu DD, Tuchweber B, Plaa GL, Yousef IM. Pathogenesis of lithocholate-induced intrahepatic cholestasis: role of glucoronidation and hydroxylation of lithocholate. *Biochim Biophys Acta* 1992;1126:53–59.

48. Hunt RD, Leveille GA, Sauberlich HE. Dietary bile acids and lipid metabolism. III. Effects of lithocholic acid in mammalian species. *Proc Soc Exp Biol Med* 1964;115:277–282.

49. Hunt RD. Proliferation of bile ductules (the ductular reaction) induced by lithocholic acid. *Fed Proc* 1965;24:431–439.

50. Stolk A. Induction of hepatic cirrhosis in Iguana iguana by 3-monohydroxycholanic acid treatment. *Experimentia* 1960;16:507–513.

51. Miyai K, Javitt NB, Gochman N, Jones HM, Baker D. Hepatotoxicity of bile acids in rabbits: ursodeoxycholic acid is less toxic than chenodeoxycholic acid. *Lab Invest* 1982;46:428–437.

52. Gall JAM, Bhathal PS. Isolation and culture of intrahepatic bile ducts and its application in assessing putative inducers of biliary epithelial cell hyperplasia. *Br J Exp Pathol* 1987;68:501–510.

53. Mamianetti A, Konopka HF, Lago N, Vescina C, Scarlato E, Carducci CN. Morphologic changes in livers of hamsters treated with high doses of ursodeoxycholic acid: correlation with bile acids in bile. *Pharmacol Res* 1994;29:187–195.

54. Okun R, Goldstein LI, Van Gelder GA, Goldenthal ET, Wazeter FX, Giel RG. National cooper-

ative gallstone study: nonprimate toxicology of chenodeoxycholic acid. *J Toxicol Environ Health* 1982;9:727–741.

55. Dyrszka H, Salen G, Zaki FG, Chen T, Mosbach EH. Hepatic toxicity in the rhesus monkey treated with chenodeoxycholic acid for 6 months: biochemical and ultrastructural studies. *Gastroenterology* 1976;70:93–104.

56. Frezza EE, Gerunda GE, Plebani M, Galligioni A, Neri D, Faccioli AM, Tiribelli C. Effect of ursodeoxycholic acid administration on bile duct proliferation and cholestasis in bile duct ligated rat. *Dig Dis Sci* 1993;38:1291–1296.

57. Poo JL, Feldmann G, Erlinger S, Braillon A, Gaudin C, Dumont M, Lebrec D. Ursodeoxycholic acid limits liver histologic alterations and portal hypertention induced by bile duct ligation in the rat. *Gastroenterology* 1992;102:1752–1759.

58. Sirica AE, Williams TW. Appearence of ductular hepatocytes in rat liver after bile duct ligation and subsequent zone 3 necrosis by carbon tetrachloride. *Am J Pathol* 1992;140:129–136.

59. Fukushima S, Shibata M, Hibino T, Yoshimura T, Hirose M, Ito N. Intrahepatic bile duct proliferation induced by 4,4′-diaminodiphenylmethane in rats. *Toxicol Appl Pharmacol* 1979;48:145–155.

60. Sirica AE, Gainey TW, Mumaw VR. Ductular hepatocytes: evidence for a bile ductular cell origin in furan-treated rats. *Am J Pathol* 1994;145:375–383.

61. Sirica AE, Cole SL, Williams T. A unique rat model of bile ductular hyperplasia in which liver is almost toatally replaced with well-differenciated bile ductules. *Am J Pathol* 1994;144:1257–1268.

62. Van Eyken P, Desmet VJ. A cytokeratin immunohistochemical study of alcoholic liver disease: evidence that hepatocytes can express bile duct-type cytokeratins. *Histopathology* 1988;13:605–617.

63. Lemire JM, Shiojiri N, Fausto N. Oval cell proliferation and the origin of small hepatocytes in liver injury induced by D-galactosamine. *Am J Pathol* 1991;139:535–552.

64. Van Eyken P, Sciot R, Callea F, Desmet VJ. A cytokeratin-immunohistochemical study of focal nodular hyperplasia of the liver: further evidence that ductular metaplasia of hepatocytes contributes to ductular "proliferation." *Liver* 1989;9:372–377.

65. Demetris AJ, Seaberg EC, Wennergerg A, Ionellie J, Michalopoulos G. Ductular reaction after submassive necrosis in humans: special emphasis on analysis of ductular hepatocytes. *Am J Pathol* 1996;149:439–448.

66. Sell S, Dunsford HA. Evidence for stem cell origin of hepatocellular carcinoma and cholangiocarcinoma. *Am J Pathol* 1989;134:1347–1363.

67. Michalopoulos GK. Liver regeneration: molecular mechanisms of growth control. *FASEB J* 1990;4:176–187.

68. Thorgeirsson SS, Evarts RP, Fujio K, Hu Z. Cellular biology of the rat hepatic stem cell compartment. In: Skouteris GG, ed. *Liver carcinogenesis*. Berlin: Springer Verlag, 1994:129–145.

69. Joplin R, Hishida T, Tsubouchi H, Daikuhara Y, Ayres R, Neuberger JM, Strain AJ. Human intrahepatic biliary epithelial cells proliferate in vitro in response to human hepatocyte growth factor. *J Clin Invest* 1992;90:1284–1289.

70. Nagy P, Bisgaard HC, Santoni-Rugiu E, Thorgeirsson SS. In vivo infusion of growth factors enhances the mitogenic response of rat hepatic ductal (oval) cells after administration of 2-acetylaminofluoren. *Hepatology* 1995;21:71–79.

71. Harrington EA, Bennett MR, Fanadi A, Evan GI. c-Myc induced apoptosis in fibroblasts is inhibited by specific cytokines. *EMBO J* 1994;13:3286–3295.

72. Aldana PR, Goerke ME, Carr SC, Tracy TF Jr. The expression of regenerative growth factors in chronic liver injury and repair. *J Surg Res* 1994;57:711–717.

73. Krahenbuhl S, Talos C, Lauterburg BH, Reichen J. Reduced antioxidative capacity in liver mitochondria from bile duct ligated rats. *Hepatology* 1995;22:607–612.

74. Saperstein LA, Jirtle RL, Farouk M, Thompson HJ, Chung KS, Meyers WC. Transforming-growth factor-beta 1 and mannose 6-phosphate/insulin-like growth factor-II receptor expression during intrahepatic bile duct hyperplasia and biliary fibrosis in the rat. *Hepatology* 1994;19:412–417.

75. Takiya S, Tagaya T, Takahashi K, Kawashima H, Kamiya M, Fukuzawa Y, Kobayashi S, Fukatsu A, Katoh K, Kakumu S. Role of transforming growth factor beta 1 on hepatic regeneration and apoptosis in liver diseases. *J Clin Pathol* 1995;48:1093–1097.

76. Milani S, Herbst H, Schuppan D, Stein H, Surrenti C. Transforming growth factors B1 B2 are differentially expressed in fibrotic liver disease. *Am J Pathol* 1991;139:1221–1229.

77. Shiojiri N. The origin of intrahepatic bile duct cells in the mouse. *J Embryol Exp Morphol* 1984;79:25–39.

78. Shiojiri N, Nagai Y. Preferential differentiation of the bile ducts along the portal vein in the development of mouse liver. *Anat Embryol* 1992;185:17–24.

Index